Little, Brown
Spiral Manuals

Alpert & Francis	Manual of Coronary Care
Alpert & Rippe	Manual of Cardiovascular Diagnosis and Therapy
Arndt	Manual of Dermatologic Therapeutics
Berk et al.	Handbook of Critical Care
Bochner et al.	Handbook of Clinical Pharmacology
Bordow et al.	Manual of Clinical Problems in Pulmonary Medicine: With Annotated Key References
Children's Hospital, Boston	Manual of Pediatric Therapeutics
Cloherty & Stark	Manual of Neonatal Care
Condon & Nyhus	Manual of Surgical Therapeutics
Friedman	Problem-Oriented Medical Diagnosis
Gantz & Gleckman	Manual of Clinical Problems in Infectious Disease: With Annotated Key References
Gardner & Provine	Manual of Acute Bacterial Infections
Hillis et al.	Manual of Clinical Problems in Cardiology: With Annotated Key References
Iversen & Clawson	Manual of Orthopaedic Therapeutics
Klippel & Anderson	Manual of Emergency and Outpatient Techniques
Niswander	Manual of Obstetrics: Diagnosis and Therapy
Papper	Manual of Medical Care of the Surgical Patient
Pavan-Langston	Manual of Ocular Diagnosis and Therapy
Roberts	Manual of Clinical Problems in Pediatrics: With Annotated Key References
Samuels	Manual of Neurologic Therapeutics
Shader	Manual of Psychiatric Therapeutics
Snow	Manual of Anesthesia
Spivak & Barnes	Manual of Clinical Problems in Internal Medicine: Annotated with Key References
Washington University	Manual of Medical Therapeutics

Manual of
Pediatric
Therapeutics

Manual of Pediatric Therapeutics

Second Edition

Department of Medicine
Children's Hospital Medical
Center, Boston

Edited by
John W. Graef, M.D.
Thomas E. Cone, Jr., M.D.

Little, Brown and Company
Boston

To
Charles A. Janeway
Physician, scholar, teacher,
humanitarian

Contents

Foreword

Who among physicians has not been stumped by an unusual complaint or has not been at a loss to know the appropriate medication for a given condition, or who would not welcome a quick consultation from someone more familiar with the problem at hand? It is the lot of all of us to seek authoritative advice from time to time.

Six years ago, Drs. Graef, Cone, and their many colleagues responded to that need with their highly successful *Manual of Pediatric Therapeutics*. The soft cover and spiral binding of the first edition was an implied statement that revisions would be forthcoming. In this new edition, the authors have updated or reorganized all chapters and have added chapters on adolescent gynecology and allergies.

This manual is designed to complement the more definitive textbooks and handbooks on pediatrics. Its origins were the notebooks of house staff, the "pearls" from the literature, and the accumulated wisdom of the faculty. Although no small volume can ever be the final word, the authors have done their best to summarize current practice as it takes place in the wards and clinics of the Children's Hospital Medical Center, Boston. They hope that their readers will find the second edition as useful as the first edition has been.

Mary Ellen Avery, M.D.
Physician-in-Chief

Preface

The gratifying response to the first edition of the *Manual of Pediatric Therapeutics* and the many helpful suggestions and comments from our readers have provided continuous encouragement throughout our preparation of the second edition. Nevertheless, the task of revision has been larger than we had anticipated, and the interval between the first and second editions longer than we had planned. We hope that this new edition, the result of many hours of rewriting and revision by our colleagues at the Children's Hospital Medical Center, will have been worth the wait.

The second edition is really a new book. Two new chapters have been added: Prepubertal and Adolescent Gynecology and Allergic Disorders. To make room for this new material, elements of the original chapter on special diagnostic problems have been incorporated elsewhere in the text (evaluation of *hematuria* in Chap. 9, *vomiting* in Chap. 11, *immunodeficiency* in Chap. 18, and *headache* in Chap. 21). The new, annotated *Manual of Clinical Problems in Pediatrics*, by Dr. Kenneth B. Roberts, we believe, fills the need for discussions of the evaluative aspects of clinical entities far more comprehensively than our space limitations permit.

Completely rewritten are chapters on renal, gastrointestinal, endocrine, and ear, nose, and throat disorders; and growth and development. New chapter sections include the sudden infant death syndrome (SIDS) and common psychiatric problems. In addition, all material that was retained from the first edition has been carefully reviewed, reedited, and updated.

Particular attention is called to the chapters titled Management of the Newborn, I and II, and Fluid and Electrolytes. These two areas, the "heart and soul" of contemporary pediatrics, have been completely rewritten to provide as much information as possible in the succinct format we utilize.

The material on the newborn is divided into two chapters. Management of the Newborn, I, discusses routine and emergency management of the full-term and the low-birth-weight infant. Management of the Newborn, II, discusses specific problems in the neonatal period, including respiratory, cardiac, hepatic, hematopoietic, infectious, and metabolic disorders. Obviously, there is considerable overlapping with other chapters, but with the exception of neonatal seizures (in Chap. 21), the specific discussions regarding the newborn can be found in these two chapters. (For a comprehensive guide to the management of newborns, the reader is referred to the *Manual of Neonatal Care*, by Drs. John P. Cloherty and Ann R. Stark.) The chapter on fluids and electrolytes is an up-to-date synthesis of current concepts in his field, and, unlike the majority of the chapters in the *Manual*, which can be read selectively, it is best read in its entirety.

The overall organization of the book has been changed as well. Although, as before, the first seven chapters are of general subject matter, the remainder has been organized into clusters of related disciplines. Thus, Fluid and Electrolytes (Chap. 8) is followed immediately by the chapters on renal, cardiac, and gastrointestinal disorders. Endocrine disorders, adolescent gynecology, and diabetes mellitus are clustered, followed by chapters dealing with infection and inflammation (Chaps. 15–19). The allergy chapter (No. 19) bridges those on inflammation

(Chap. 18) and pulmonary disorders (Chap. 20). The remaining chapters stand alone as close and important adjuncts to general pediatrics, and the emergency reference material on the inside front and back covers of the *Manual* should prove to be useful when needed.

Finally, a vignette and a caveat. One of the authors of this manual had occasion to consult its first edition for the treatment of thrush (oral candidiasis), one of the commonest of pediatric problems. Only at that moment did he discover (to his chagrin) that neither thrush nor oral nystatin was included and that he had to seek another source. Suffice it to say, thrush and idiopathic thrombocytopenic purpura (ITP), the other glaring omission from the first edition, are included in the second edition.

Like the first edition, however, the second cannot be, nor is it intended to be, a pediatric text. As before, evaluative material, though present, is kept to a minimum and intended *only* to guide the reader to utilization of the appropriate therapeutic plan. As a manual of therapeutics, the text is limited to discussion of those entities for which therapeutic guidelines can be agreed upon and whose benefits will clearly outweigh the risks of their misuse.

As before, the *Manual of Pediatric Therapeutics* is intended for use by pediatricians, family physicians, house officers, medical students, nurse practitioners, nurses, and nursing students. Availability of other reference material is assumed and recognition that other therapeutic approaches used at other teaching institutions may be as effective as those described here is implicit.

In the preparation of this second edition, we owe thanks to many persons. Invaluable advice and editorial assistance were received from Drs. Barbara Howard, Joseph Gootenberg, Ira Gewolb, Robert Tuttle, and Robertson Parkman.

Help with manuscript preparation was provided by Josephine Antczak, Cynthia Krusen, and Margaret Sherman. But our most devoted, patient, and diligent help came from our secretary, Annette Cardillo, and our production editor, Anne Najarian-Merian, whose patience and wise guidance were unflagging throughout.

Used with care, it is our hope that the second edition will prove to be as useful to readers as the first edition has been.

J.W.G.
T.E.C., Jr.

Manual of
Pediatric
Therapeutics

General Care of the Patient

I. CARING FOR CHILDREN Illness can be a frightening and unpleasant experience, particularly for children. Concern for the child's needs has helped to foster understanding of the impact of hospitalization on the child's growth and development. Hospital personnel are learning to consider how the child matures and learns, how he uses imagination and make-believe, the meaning of his toys and other possessions, and his capacity for adaptation to others. An older child may verbalize fear of an operation by angrily protesting the failure of a venipuncture. A 4-year-old may express the same feeling by mutilating a doll, and a 2-year-old, by biting other children or refusing to continue well-established toileting. Understanding age-dependent expressive abilities, often with the help of nurses and "play supervisors," can increase the physician's effectiveness in gaining the child's cooperation and in interpreting for the parents the new behaviors and their meaning in the context of hospitalization. By opening a discussion of the child's behavior, the physician not only addresses the disturbed behavior the parents have surely observed, but also allows the parents to express their own feelings about the illness. Making parents part of the team, that is, observing and interpreting the child's behavior, will help them to reacquire the important knowledge that they are needed and wanted collaborators in the medical management of the child both in the hospital and after the child returns home.

Children can feel and react even at times when they might appear uninterested or are absorbed by fear about their illness and the attendant hospital procedures. For this reason care must be taken to respect the modesty, integrity, and privacy of each child. And because children are likely to be afraid of situations they do not understand, they need to be told about their illness and its treatment in terms they can comprehend. Insincerity is a quality children quickly recognize, and deceiving a child is an abuse of trust that only serves ultimately to alienate him.

It should not be surprising if a child reacts angrily to painful procedures or is frustrated at his own lack of progress. An understanding physician views this anger as a normal reaction and should not feel threatened by it. It is the quiet and passive infant or child who may be a cause for concern. Older children, particularly, understand pain and even death and can be made unnecessarily anxious by bedside staff conversations that may be misinterpreted or misunderstood.

Both parents, but particularly a child's mother, are seen by the child uniquely, especially when the child is sick. The parents, in turn, know their child far better than those trying to help care for him. Listening to parents, carefully noting their observations, putting them at ease, and hearing out their worries even if they appear unrelated can help to provide them with the emotional resources needed to help their child. Impatience with or misunderstanding parents can impede their inclusion in the therapeutic process, particularly because parents will continue to care for the child after the illness—a point easily overlooked during the time of acute intervention.

To make their meaningful participation easier, parents need objective advice from the physician. While they should not be asked to make medical judgments, they have a legal and ethical right to be informed of the benefits and risks of therapy and to be included in the decision-making process.

Finally, a pediatrician's responsibility to a child does not end when the child has been cured of a physical illness. It is the unique role of those who care for children to help them fulfill their potential and take their rightful place as responsible adults. This may require the pediatrician to go far beyond traditional medical intervention into the area of schools, environment, and economic circumstances in the effort to assist the child.

II. THE HOSPITALIZED PATIENT

A. Medical orders   Written medical orders are the physician's instructions to the nursing staff concerning the care and treatment of the patient. They should be written clearly and accurately, with special consideration to dosage calculation and decimal points. Orders are the **legal responsibility** of the physician; each entry as well as each page (if there is more than one) should be correctly labeled with the time and date and properly signed. An incorrect entry should be canceled by drawing a single line through it, and *error* should be written nearby, so that there will be no confusion at a later time. Unusual orders should be discussed with the nurse at the time they are written and individualized for each patient. Properly written orders should cover diagnosis and treatment and provide for the patient's comfort and dignity. The following schemes may be utilized:

1. **Diagnosis**   List the diagnostic findings in order of significance. Indicate the condition of the patient, whether critical, fair, or satisfactory. When a patient's condition is listed as critical, the family should be informed **by the physician** to avoid misunderstanding.

2. **Disposition**   This includes the frequency of monitoring vital signs and weighing the patient, permitted activities, special observations, isolation procedures, and environmental conditions.

   a. Unnecessarily frequent determination of vital signs overburdens the nursing staff and may unnecessarily discomfit the patient.

   b. Bed rest for an ill child is often more constraining than limited activity, and the social environment will also affect the degree of activity. Hospitalized children, particularly those in isolation, should not be denied social interaction.

3. **Diet**   Choose the diet with the following considerations in mind: age, caloric needs, ability to chew, and special nutritional requirements necessitated by problems of absorption, intestinal irritation, residue, and transit time (see Chap. 11).

4. **Diagnostic tests**   Group in logical sequence (e.g., blood, radiographic). List all tests and the dates they are to be done. Diagnostic tests should be ordered after careful consideration of the costs, risks, and potential benefits, particularly regarding therapeutic implications.

5. **Drugs**   Include generic name, dose, route, frequency, and length of time to be administered. Review orders for narcotics *daily*. In general, separate drugs for specific therapy from drugs for symptomatic relief. Orders for respiratory or physical therapy must also be explicit as to duration, frequency, type, anatomic site of administration, and associated medication. Oxygen and aerosols require specific orders as well.

B. Common pediatric procedures

1. Venipuncture and intravenous infusion

a. Indications To withdraw venous blood or for continuous administration of solutions or drugs.

b. Site Hands, feet, scalp, or jugular or antecubital veins. The femoral veins should be avoided.

c. Technique

(1) Restrain the hands, feet, or arm with an armboard, or shave scalp aseptically.

(2) Place a tourniquet proximal to the puncture site. A rubber band with a small adhesive tag (for release) may be placed around the forehead to distend scalp veins in infants. Palpate the vein desired.

(3) Attach a short-beveled No. 21 or 23 scalp vein needle to a small syringe filled with sterile saline solution. If the puncture is to be used for blood collection, attach an empty syringe.

(4) Prepare the skin with 70% alcohol. (**This does not sterilize.** To prepare a sterile area for blood culture, iodine or thimerosal [Merthiolate] must be applied, then washed with alcohol.)

(5) Palpate the target vein with one hand and grasp the plastic "wings" of the needle with the other. Pierce the skin lightly to one side and 0.5 cm distal to the entry site. Infants' veins, especially on the scalp, are usually superficial, and a deep thrust may cause distal wall penetration and a hematoma. If venipuncture is for a blood sample only, *reverse* the direction of the thrust by the needle.

(6) Draw back on the syringe gently to avoid collapse of the vein.

(7) If blood returns, confirming venipuncture, *slowly* inject 1 ml of saline and observe the site for swelling. If swelling occurs, saline is infiltrating, and a new site must be selected and prepared.

(8) If saline enters the vein smoothly, tape the wings of the needle securely to the skin and attach the infusion set.

(9) Protect the infusion from accidental dislodging by taping an inverted paper cup or dish over the site with a "door" cut in one side to permit tubing to pass. Avoid using excess tape on the patient's skin. Do not cover the needle site closely, since covering may delay recognition of infiltration or phlebitis.

2. Arterial puncture

a. Indications Oxygen concentration determination; blood culture in endocarditis if venous blood cultures are negative; in cases of venous collapse or extreme difficulty in obtaining venous blood.

b. Sites Femoral, brachial, temporal, or radial artery.

c. Technique

(1) Prepare the skin with iodine solution, as described in **4.c.**

(2) No tourniquet is used.

(3) A 23- or 25-gauge straight or butterfly needle filled with heparin and a syringe rinsed with heparin are used.

(4) Locate the vessel by palpation.

(5) Infiltration with 1% xylocaine (Lidocaine) is optional, but may obscure the vessel.

(6) Puncture the skin and push the needle *through* the arterial site. Withdraw it slowly until blood is seen in the tubing.

(7) Blood will flow into a glass syringe without suction if the artery is punctured, or pulsations may be seen in tubing if a plastic syringe and scalp vein needle are used. Allow the blood to push all visible heparin solution out into the tubing before attaching the syringe (see **d**).

(8) After the needle is withdrawn, maintain compression at the puncture site for 3–5 min.

d. Cautions

(1) If you are drawing arterial blood gases, bear in mind that even small volumes of heparin (0.2 ml) may falsely lower pH, PCO_2, and HCO_3^- when small volumes of arterial blood (1 ml) are used. A 3-ml plastic syringe and butterfly scalp vein needle have a combined dead space of 0.41 ml.

(2) When drawing blood cultures, remove iodine from the skin to prevent vein irritation, and swab iodine from the tops of culture bottles before inserting needle to avoid sterilization of cultures.

3. Gastric gavage

a. Indications   When infants with normal GI function are slow to accept or cannot accept oral feeding.

b. Site   Preferably the nasal route.

c. Technique

(1) Wrap the child.

(2) Insert a lubricated, cooled, 10–14F feeding catheter into either nostril along the floor of the nares, aiming at the level of the ear lobes, and pass into the stomach. Estimate the length of tubing required by the distance from the nose to the ear plus the distance from the ear to the xiphoid process. Handle the tube with sterile gloves.

(3) Observe the patient's respiration. If the trachea is entered coughing will usually occur.

(4) Inject *2–3 ml* of air and listen over the stomach for an air rumble.

(5) Attach the funnel and pour the feeding *slowly*.

(6) Pinch the tube while withdrawing to avoid aspiration.

4. Lumbar puncture

a. Indications   Diagnostic evaluation of spinal fluid or as a route for therapy. Fundoscopic examination for evidence of increased intracranial pressure is a prerequisite.

b. Site   The 3rd or 4th lumbar interspace (at the level of the iliac crest in infants).

c. Technique

(1) Have an assistant hold the child in the lateral recumbent position on a flat table with one arm around the back of the child's neck and the other arm in the back of the knees. The child's head should be to the left of a right-handed physician. Children, especially neonates, may also be restrained sitting on the table. *The success of the pediatric lumbar puncture depends largely on the technique of holding.*

(2) Scrub the hands and wear surgical gloves and mask.

(3) Prepare the back with iodine solution and wash with alcohol; **residual iodine can cause dermatitis**. Move swabs in a widening spiral away from the site to avoid contamination. Do not cross an area already scrubbed with the same swab.

(4) Drape the area with sterile towels.

(5) In older children, infiltrate to the dura with a 1% xylocaine solution without epinephrine.

(6) A 20- or 21-gauge needle with a stylet is used in children. A 22- or 23-gauge needle (short) may be used in infants.

(7) Placing your finger or thumb on the 3rd or 4th lumbar vertebra, insert the needle below the vertebral spine in the midline, aiming for the umbilicus.

(8) A soft click is usually felt as the dura is entered.

(9) Remove the stylet to watch for fluid.

(10) If blood returns in the needle, replace the stylet and *leave the needle in place.*

(11) Repeat the procedure one interspace above, but no higher.

5. Thoracentesis   See also Chaps. 5 and 20.

a. Indications   Diagnostic evaluation of pulmonary diseases with pleural effusion; occasionally therapeutic in patients with empyema; to instill irritant chemicals in patients with recurrent pneumothorax who are not candidates for pleurectomy.

b. Site   In free pleural effusion, the 7th posterolateral intercostal space. If effusion is loculated, fluoroscopy or ultrasound should be utilized to locate the site of puncture.

c. Technique

(1) Always try to have the current chest x-ray in the treatment room, and recheck the physical findings (especially dullness to percussion) to assure that the puncture site is correct.

(2) Explain the procedure to patients who are old enough.

(3) Have an assistant hold the patient so that the most dependent site to be tapped is easily accessible to the instruments. The best position is usually sitting upright. The patient who is under traction or in decubitus for other reasons can be positioned on two chairs or on small tables, with the chest area exposed between the chairs. The patient who is in a sitting position and is old enough can rest the head and arms on a pillow placed on top of a bedside table raised to the proper height.

(4) Prepare the skin as in **4.c.**

(5) Palpate the ribs and count with the index and middle finger.

(6) In older children, infiltrate the parietal pleura with 2% xylocaine (Lidocaine).

(7) Place a hemostat or Kelly clamp across the needle approximately 1 cm from the tip, so that the needle will not inadvertently be thrust too far into the lung parenchyma.

(8) Insert the needle (20 gauge or preferably 18), connected to a three-way stopcock and sterile syringe over the upper edge of the lower rib (to avoid the intercostal vessels).

(9) In the majority of patients with fluid in abundance and some degree of pleural inflammation, there is a feeling of "going through leather." If a syringe is attached, a gentle pull of the plunger will aspirate fluid into the barrel.

(10) Use of the three-way stopcock will help to facilitate removal of aliquots of fluid and to prevent air leaks while changing syringes. If the fluid is clear, a new syringe is rapidly substituted for the syringe in use until enough material is withdrawn for diagnostic tests or until the area is "dry." This maneuver of rapidly utilizing clear fluid will avoid interference with the differential diagnosis encountered in cases of "bloody" tap, since it is at the end of the procedure that trauma to the lung tissue is most likely. Remember that many effusions will be rapidly replaced by fluid from the intravascular compartment. **As a rule, remove no more fluid than the volume of blood a child can tolerate losing.**

(11) With the child in maximal inspiration, remove the needle while maintaining negative pressure on the syringe. A plain bandage will suffice.

(12) Check the vital signs, and if they are satisfactory, take a control chest x-ray film to detect the presence or absence of pneumothorax and associated parenchymal disease, previously obscured by fluid.

(13) Complications

(a) Intercostal vessel bleeding usually is not significant unless biopsy needles are used. Its occurrence should be followed with observations of vital signs every 15 min for the next 2 hr and then hourly.

(b) Pneumothorax See Chaps. 5, Sec. **IC**, and 20, Sec. **VII**.

(c) Air embolism rarely occurs with thoracentesis, but could occur with the accidental aspiration of lung "juice."

C. Analgesia and sedation

1. Analgesia

a. General principles The following guidelines may be helpful (see also Table 1-1):

(1) If pain is present in multiple sites, only the *single* most severe source will be recognized by the patient.

(2) Although it is sometimes assumed that pain is not felt in children particularly in small infants, or is easily forgotten, local anesthesia should be provided for diagnostic procedures whenever feasible.

(3) True analgesics such as morphine may mask pain, while sedatives such as phenobarbital will not. For this reason, sedatives may be helpful in elucidating pain and tenderness, particularly in the acutely disturbed abdomen.

(4) Postoperative pain, although generally of shorter duration in children than in adults, may still be severe enough to require medication for several days.

(5) Neonates also feel pain, but are less able to express it. Do not forget to order analgesia for neonates when pain is expected to be present. When not otherwise contraindicated, pain relief can be achieved with smaller amounts of narcotics when combined with a sedative ("lytic cocktail," **3**, p. 12).

b. Specific therapeutics

(1) Nonnarcotic analgesics See Table 1-1.

(a) Acetylsalicylic acid (aspirin) is the most frequently used analgesic and has antipyretic properties as well (see Sec. **2.c**, p. 22, for the dose and route of administration).

i. Its analgesic properties are most suitable for the pain of headache, arthralgia, dysmenorrhea, or muscular ache. Doses in patients with acute rheumatic fever and juvenile rheumatoid arthritis are considerably higher (see Chap. 18, Sec. **I.A.3**) than for simpler analgesia.

ii. Enteric-coated preparations are available to reduce gastric irritation, but absorption of these preparations is variable.

able 1-1 Narcotic and Nonnarcotic Analgesics and Dosages for Pediatric Use

ame	Dose
onnarcotic:	
cetylsalicylic acid (aspirin)	65–100 mg/kg/24 hr in 4–6 doses
cetaminophen (Tempra, Tylenol)	Under 1 year 60 mg 1–3 years 60–120 mg 3–6 years 120 mg Over 6 years 240 mg
ropoxyphene (Darvon)	32–65 mg q3–4h prn
entazocine (Talwin)	30 mg q3–4h prn in adults. Not for children under 12
arcotic:	
odeine phosphate	3 mg/kg/24 hr in 6–8 divided doses. Antitussive: 1 mg/kg/24 hr
eperidine (Dermerol)	6 mg/kg/24 hr
ethadone	0.7 mg/kg/24 hr
orphine sulfate	0.1–0.2 mg/kg/dose
amphorated opium tincture (Paregoric)	0.25–0.5 ml/kg/dose

iii. **Toxic effects** include salicylism (see Chap. 3, Sec. **II.D**), G bleeding, iron deficiency anemia, abnormal clotting, altere thyroid function, decreased fasting blood sugar in diabete and increased cardiac load, which can aggravate incipien congestive heart failure and hemolysis in patients with glu cose 6-phosphate dehydrogenase (G-6-PD) deficiency.

(b) **Acetaminophen (Tempra, Tylenol)** Although this drug is mor valuable for antipyresis than for analgesia, its advantage i its availability in liquid form. It is also more expensive. Pea blood levels are achieved in 2 hr (see Sec. **III.B.2.c**). **Toxic effect** include methemoglobinemia, anemia, and liver damage, but i does not cause hemodialysis in G-6-PD deficiency. Overdose ca produce fulminant liver failure. **Phenacetin,** a sister drug, ha similar properties, although it is probably more toxic. It i often used with aspirin and caffeine (Empirin Compound), bu there is no evidence that this combination is more effectiv than aspirin alone.

(c) **Propoxyphene (Darvon)** is similar to codeine. Controlled tria place it as *less* effective than aspirin, with occasional patien finding it more effective. **Toxic reactions** include GI upset, ve tigo, and drowsiness, as well as pruritus and skin eruption Severe reactions include cyanosis, convulsions, coma, and re piratory depression. **It is not approved for use in children und 12.** Overdose is potentially lethal. If safer alternatives a available, propoxyphene should probably not be available at a in homes where small children reside.

(d) **Pentazocine (Talwin),** a morphine-related drug, produces wea morphine antagonism and morphinelike subjective effects. **It not approved for use in children under 12,** and because of i adverse effects on the CNS, **its use should be reserved for ho pitalized patients.** For an extensive discussion of this prepar tion, see *Med. Lett. Drugs Ther.* 18:45, 1976.

(2) **Narcotic analgesics** See Table 1-1.

(a) **Codeine,** a morphine derivative, is more effective than aspir but less so than morphine itself. It is also less addictive tha morphine and causes less disturbance of GI function, althoug seizures have been reported with its use. Its antitussive pro erties are well known, and it is frequently used for this pu pose; however, there is risk of its abuse for this indicatic Prolonged use of any narcotic is constipating. This may especially significant postoperatively.

(b) **Meperidine (Demerol)** is probably a more effective analge than codeine, partly because higher doses are tolerated. It highly addictive but less constipating and less depressing the respiratory center than is morphine. It is widely used as obstetric analgesic. *Because it does not constrict smooth mu cle*, meperidine can be used in the presence of asthma, though sedation in any case of respiratory distress is e tremely dangerous.

In combination with promethazine (Phenergan) and chl promazine (Thorazine), it can be used as a "lytic cocktail" produce rapid sedation with analgesia for painful diagnos procedures (see Table 1-1 and **3**, p. 12).

(c) Methadone is included because of its widespread use in anti-addiction programs and in cancer patients with ongoing severe pain. Its analgesic potency is roughly equivalent to that of morphine, and it is effective PO. Its respiratory depressant effect is considerable, but it causes less GI disturbance than does morphine. When an addict can substitute it for morphine or heroin, withdrawal may ultimately be eased, if more prolonged. Nevertheless, **methadone is addictive.** It merely produces less euphoria than morphine or heroin; thus, the psychological component of addiction is undermined by its use.

(d) Morphine is perhaps the most important and widely used narcotic analgesic and is effective in any age group. It has little sedative effect and produces concomitant euphoria, with the risk of addiction.

   i. Because PO and PR preparations, although effective, are somewhat unreliable in absorption and metabolism, parenteral use is generally advised, either SQ (20 min), IM (20 min), or IV (immediate but dangerous). Analgesia usually lasts 3–4 hr.

   ii. Morphine is excreted via the liver and **should be administered with caution to a newborn or a patient with liver disease.**

   iii. **Paregoric** or **camphorated opium tincture** makes use of the constipating properties of morphine to aid in relieving symptoms of diarrhea with spasm of the colon. **Camphorated opium tincture should never be confused with tincture of opium, which is 25 times more powerful.**

   iv. Because morphine is so addictive, its administration in the pediatric age group should be limited to patients with pulmonary stenosis and infundibular spasm, congestive heart failure, severe visceral pain of known origin, intractable pain, severe postoperative pain, and the pain of terminal disease. Although up to 14 days of administration is usually required to produce addiction, some adolescents may become addicted on only 1 or 2 doses.

   v. **Tolerance to morphine** includes tolerance to its CNS depressive properties, so that increasing the dose does not increase the likelihood of respiratory toxicity. The physician should remember that when a patient's dose is missed, an amount smaller than normal may suffice at the next dose. Death frequently occurs in addicts who administer *their usual high dose* after a few days off the drug, when tolerance is less.

   vi. **Toxic effects** include respiratory depression, increased intracranial pressure, arterial hypotension, nausea and vomiting, hyperglycemia, antidiuresis, urinary retention, addiction, and constipation.

   vii. A unique problem is the treatment of newborn infants of morphine-addicted mothers. Chlorpromazine, 0.7–1.0 mg/kg q6h IM, and paregoric, 2–4 gtt/kg q4h, have been used effectively to prevent withdrawal symptoms in these infants [see **3.b(2)**, p. 144].

Table 1-2 Preoperative Medication for Infants and Children[a]

Age	Average Weight (kg)	Pentobarbital[b] (Nembutal) (mg)	Morphine[c] (mg)	Atropin (mg)
Newborn	3.3			0.15
6 months	8.1	30 PR		0.2
1 year	10.6	45 PR	1.0	0.2
2 years	14.0	60 PR	1.5	0.3
3 years	15.0	60 PR	2.0	0.3
4 years	17.1	90 PR	3.0	0.3
5 years	19.4	90 PR	3.0	0.3
6 years	22.0	90 PR	4.0	0.4
7 years	24.7	90 PR	5.0	0.4
8 years	27.9	100 PO	6.0	0.4
9 years	31.4	100 PO	6.0	0.4
10 years	35.2	100 PO	7.0	0.4
11 years	39.6	100 PO	7.0	0.4
12 years	44.4	100 PO	7.0	0.4
13 years	49.1	100 PO	8.0	0.4
14 years	54.4	100 PO	8.0	0.4
15 years	58.8	100 PO	8.0	0.4
16 years	61.9	100 PO	8.0	0.4

[a] This guide is to be followed for average, well-developed patients. Increases c reductions in medication must be made for patients who do not fall into th guidelines, that is, hyperactive, obese, or poor-risk patients.
[b] The suggested guide for pentobarbital when followed by morphine is 4.0 mg/kg f rectal use (maximum, 120 mg) and 3.0 mg/kg for oral use (maximum, 100 mg Pentobarbital should be given at least 90 min before surgery.
[c] The suggested guide for morphine is 0.75 mg/year of age. Morphine should k given 35–45 min (IM or SQ) before surgery.

2. Sedation

a. **General principles** Among the most important characteristics childhood are curiosity and the drive to explore and learn. Sedatic can interfere with the child's capacity to interact with and learn fro the environment. It narrows the child's experience, which, lil childbirth for the mother, may be painful, but with help and suppor can also be rich and memorable.

(1) **Indications for sedation in children are few.** They include preane thesia (Table 1-2); painful diagnostic procedures such as bor marrow aspiration; agitation that contributes to morbidity, as respiratory diseases such as asthma or croup (in which sedatic should be used only with **extreme caution**); intubation or trached tomy for respiratory assistance; intractable pain; and occasional in the evaluation of severe visceral pain (e.g., acute appendiciti In this last case, sedation short of general anesthesia does n mask pain but permits its elucidation by reducing surroundir anxiety and factitious tenderness.

Table 1-3   Sedatives and Dosages for Pediatric Use

Name	Dose
Alcohol	10 ml brandy in 30 ml/H$_2$O in infants
Chloral hydrate	15–40 mg/kg/24 hr in 2–3 divided doses
Paraldehyde	0.15 ml/kg/dose
Antihistamine	Diphenhydramine 5 mg/kg/24 hr
	Promethazine 0.5 mg/kg/dose
	Hydroxyzine 2 mg/kg/24 hr
Chlorpromazine	2 mg/kg/24 hr
Barbiturates:	
Amobarbital (Amytal)	6 mg/kg/24 hr in 3 divided doses
Secobarbital (Seconal)	6 mg/kg/24 hr in 3 divided doses
Pentobarbital (Nembutal)	6 mg/kg/24 hr in 3 divided doses
Phenobarbital	6 mg/kg/24 hr in 3 divided doses
Demerol compound:	
25 mg meperidine	1 ml/15 kg IM, not to exceed 2 ml
6.25 mg chlorpromazine	
6.25 mg promethazine	
in 1 ml	

Any child who is paralyzed, either iatrogenically or by disease, may still be aware of his or her surroundings with all of the fear and pain as well as the loss of control entailed. Sedation in such a case is an important part of acute care.

In children, sedation is *not* the treatment of choice in insomnia or hyperactivity, and is used only as a last resort.

(2) The reaction of children to sedatives, particularly barbiturates, is unpredictable. At the toddler stage, sedatives may cause agitation. In addition, children have a higher incidence of idiosyncratic reactions to sedatives than do adults. For most purposes, the *weakest* effective sedative, such as hydroxyzine, is safe and least liable to cause unwanted side effects.

b. Specific therapeutics   See Table 1-3.

(1) Alcohol is an old-fashioned sedative, especially useful in infants; 10 ml brandy in 30 ml water PO or by gavage is usually effective.

(2) Chloral hydrate is probably the safest sedative and is inexpensive. It has a wide margin of safety, with the acceptable dose from 20–40 mg/kg/24 hr. Although the aftertaste is bitter, it is also available in PR form and seems to be well tolerated by children, particularly if offered in a small glass of juice. Peak activity usually occurs within 30–60 min of administration. **Caution should be used in patients with liver disease. Aspiration can produce fatal laryngospasm.**

(3) Paraldehyde (see p. 42, Sec. **III.E.4**) has the advantage of rapid action and is relatively safe. Used primarily for alcohol withdrawal in adults, it is particularly valuable in the management of seizures in children. **Caution should be exercised in patients with liver disease,** but it can be used in those with renal insufficiency. It is administered in corn oil PR; IV administration has been associated with polyethylene emboli from dissolved tubing.

(4) **Antihistamines** have a variety of clinical uses that have varying degrees of success. (For a more complete discussion of these agents, see *Med. Lett. Drugs Ther.* 19:1, 1977.)

(a) Antihistamines with the most effective sedative properties include promethazine (Phenergan), diphenhydramine (Benadryl), and hydroxyzine (Atarax). Cyclizine, meclizine, and promethazine are also clinically useful as antiemetics. Trimeprazine and diphenhydramine may reduce pruritus, possibly due to their sedative properties. Promethazine, chlorpromazine, and meperidine form a sedative compound (see **3** below), which produces rapid analgesia with sedation and is particularly useful for painful diagnostic procedures.

(b) **Serious side effects** are few, and the drugs are well tolerated PO.

(c) Because of the occasional stimulating effect of barbiturates in children under 2, antihistamines may be used to achieve a sedative effect, but in many children, no effect at all is seen.

(5) **Tranquilizers** With the exception of the phenothiazines, these drugs have little use in pediatrics (see *Can. Anaesth. Soc. J.* 5:177, 1958). Chlorpromazine is the most widely used phenothiazine and is the third component of the lytic cocktail. It has a relatively wide margin of safety and can be used effectively in agitated adolescents. It is one of the effective agents in the management of the infant of the heroin-addicted mother.

(6) **Barbiturates** are true hypnotic agents.

(a) Phenobarbital is used most widely in the control of seizure disorders and to antagonize stimulants such as caffeine or amphetamines (see **E.2**, p. 42 and **b**, p. 485).

(b) Secobarbital and pentobarbital are probably more useful sedative hypnotics because of their rapid action and are widely used as preoperative medication. They are not analgesics, so that pentobarbital in particular can be helpful in evaluating abdominal pain in the anxious small child.

(c) All three agents are available for use PO, PR, or parenterally.

(d) For PR administration of barbiturates, a suppository should be used; even then, effective absorption is variable. IM or IV injection is more reliable, but the individual reactions to a given dose preclude prediction of its effect.

(e) **Because of respiratory depression, extreme caution should be used in administering barbiturates IV,** although pentobarbital produces relatively little respiratory depression for the hypnotic dose used.

3. **Combined analgesia and sedation (lytic cocktail, Demerol compound)** To supply rapid analgesia and sedation, a compound preparation of meperidine, chlorpromazine, and promethazine has found wide acceptance at our institution. Ampules of 10 ml are made up in the proportions listed in Table 1-3.

D. **Transfusion therapy** Blood transfusion involves a significant risk. Absolute compatibility of blood is seldom met; the possibility of sensitization by subgroup factors is much more common than is appreciated by most physicians.

Donor blood is now routinely screened against the hepatitis-associated antigen by radioimmunoassay. However, this method is not sensitive enough to detect all infectious units of blood. Most cases of hepatitis that now occur following transfusion are non-A, non-B hepatitis (see Chap. 15).

1. Blood banking procedures

a. It is a universal practice for both donors and recipients to be separated into A, B, O and AB groups and Rh_0 (D) positive and Rh_0 negative types. The incidence of isoimmunization to the subgroups of the Rh factor and subsequent hemolytic reactions is not negligible. It is desirable that all Rh_0 (D)-negative bloods be tested for the Rh' (C), Rh" (E), and Rh^u (Du) factors.

b. The saline crossmatch detects complete antibodies and is a check on the donor's and patient's ABO grouping; however, neither this nor a serum crossmatch will detect a majority of the immunizations to the subtypes of Rh or other factors. The best assurance of at least in vitro compatibility includes the utilization of the indirect Coombs (antihuman globulin) technique, which detects incomplete antibodies.

2. Blood components

a. Fresh whole blood   Fresh whole blood is beneficial in massive transfusion. Platelet viability decreases after 6-hr storage as whole blood at 0–6°C; factor VIII is at a maximal level within the first 8 hr after collection; and factor V is present in adequate levels in blood stored less than 3 days.

b. Blood component therapy

(1) Packed (sedimented) red cells are the therapy of choice in anemic and chronically debilitated patients. The smaller volumes required to raise the hemoglobin level are less stressful than whole blood to the child with heart disease whose cardiac status is borderline and to the newborn. Some febrile reactions, especially in patients who have had repeated transfusions, may be due to the recipient's leukocyte antibodies. In such instances, leukocyte-poor red cells can be prepared by differential centrifugation or filtration, or, ideally, by the use of frozen deglycerolized red cells.

(a) If severe combined immunodeficiency or immunodeficiency secondary to cancer chemotherapy is present or suspected, only irradiated cells should be given because of potential graft versus host reactions.

(b) Patients who may require transplantation at some time during their illness should receive only frozen deglycerolized red cells to prevent immune sensitization.

(2) Platelets

(a) One unit of a platelet concentrate (the amount of platelets obtained from 500 ml of whole blood) for every 10 lb of the recipient's body weight should raise the platelet count $50,000/mm^3$ above the baseline level. Platelet concentrates can now be stored at room temperature for 48 hr with normal viability and hemostatic effect.

(b) In children who have idiopathic thrombocytopenic purpura or have had multiple platelet transfusions, platelet survival time is markedly shortened because of the formation of platelet antibodies.

(3) Factors VIII (antihemophilic factor) and IX   See Chap. 17, Sec. **VII.**

(4) Fibrinogen   A deficiency in production of fibrinogen occurs as a
rare congenital defect and in some patients with severe liver dis
ease. Acute hypofibrinogenemia can also result secondary to dis
seminated intravascular coagulation (DIC) or fibrinolysis. The
critical level of fibrinogen for normal blood coagulation is 100 mg
100 ml. At the present time, the therapy of choice is cryoprecipi
tated antihemophilic factor, which contains, on the average, 300
mg/U.

(5) Plasma expanders   One of the most urgent therapeutic emergen
cies is the treatment of shock associated with acute blood loss
severe burns, acute dehydration, or toxemia of infections (see
pp. 37, 38, and 40). The immediate need is to expand the circulating
blood volume until whole blood (in cases of hemorrhage) is avail
able. The agents of choice are

(a) A 5% solution of human albumin or other 5% fractionation
derivatives.

(b) A 25% albumin solution diluted to 5% concentration with nor
mal saline. **Note that undiluted concentrated 25% albumin is
contraindicated in a dehydrated patient.**

3. **General considerations**   A figure of 10 ml/lb packed red cells and 5 ml/lb
whole blood certainly represents a maximal pediatric transfusion in a
nonbleeding patient. Although many children can withstand this in
crease in blood volume, some will demonstrate signs of cardiac decom
pensation. Since severe anemia is often associated with borderline car
diac failure, elevated temperature, or infection, these children are least
tolerant of such a load. The following principles of transfusion therapy
are general guidelines that the physician must tailor to fit the specific
circumstance.

a. **Chronic anemia**   See also Chap. 17.

(1) Patients who may be helped by adequate medical therapy should
not receive a transfusion unless specific conditions coexist, such as
cardiac insufficiency, need for an operative procedure, or infection

(2) In general, a child in whom iron deficiency or other anemia has
gradually developed will rarely manifest symptoms unless the
hemoglobin concentration is 5.0 gm/100 ml or less.

(3) The more anemic the patient, the more likely that cardiac decom
pensation will be precipitated or aggravated by a rapid increase in
blood volume in transfusion. In such instances, a modified ex
change transfusion is necessary.

(a) Determining transfusion requirements   To determine the vol
ume of sedimented red blood cells required to reach the hemo
globin concentration desired, the following simple equation
may be used:

$$\text{Volume of cells} = \frac{\text{wt} \times V \times (\text{Hb}^b - \text{Hb}^a)}{\text{Hb}^s}$$

where wt = patient's weight in kilograms
   V = patient's blood volume (80 and 69 ml/kg are consid
      ered normal in infants and adults, respectively)
   Hb^a = hemoglobin level before transfusion
   Hb^b = desired hemoglobin level

Hb^s = hemoglobin concentration of sedimented red blood cells (22 to 24 gm/100 ml, depending on the degree of packing)

Thus, if it is desired to attain a hemoglobin level of 10 gm/100 ml in an infant weighing 12 kg with an initial hemoglobin of 5 gm/100 ml, one would substitute in the foregoing equation as follows:

Volume of cells

$$= \frac{12 \text{ kg} \times 80 \text{ ml/kg} \times (10 \text{ gm/100 ml} - 5 \text{ gm/100 ml})}{23 \text{ gm/100 ml}}$$

Volume of cells = 218 ml

Since this child's initial hemoglobin was 5 gm/100 ml, one would accomplish this with two transfusions of 110 ml each. (Post-transfusion survival of blood stored less than one week is 92 percent; 7 to 14 days, 85 percent; and 15 to 21 days, 78 percent.)

(b) Recommendations The following recommendations are based on the practical application of this equation:

i. The adoption of 5 ml/lb of whole blood or 10 ml/kg of packed red cells as a maximal pediatric transfusion in the absence of acute blood loss.

ii. If the initial hemoglobin level is less than 5 gm/100 ml, the volume of transfusion should be 3 ml/lb.

iii. If cardiac decompensation is present, a modified exchange transfusion should be performed, using packed or sedimented red cells.

b. Massive transfusion The rapid infusion of blood in amounts approaching the patient's blood volume within a short period introduces several potential hazards.

(1) Biochemical changes depend on the anticoagulant solution and the duration of storage, as shown in Table 1-4.

(2) The transfusion of a large amount of stored blood can cause temporary thrombocytopenia and deficiencies of factors V and VIII.

(3) Rapid infusion of large quantities of **cold** blood can result in cardiac irregularities or arrest. Bringing the temperature of the blood to 30°–37°C from its normal of 1°–6°C is an acceptable alternative.

c. Special situations

(1) Emergency transfusions When there is not time for a complete crossmatch, the choices in order of preference are:

(a) Group and type-specific blood

(b) Group O, Rh-negative red cells suspended in AB-negative plasma or 5% albumin

(c) Group O, Rh-negative whole blood

(2) Exchange transfusion Duration of storage depends on the anticoagulant used.

(a) Heparin Blood should be no more than 24 hr old.

Table 1-4 Biochemical Changes in Anticoagulant Solutions

Storage (days)	ACD Solution			CPD Solution		
	pH	Potassium (mEq/L)	DPG	pH	Potassium (mEq/L)	DPG
0	7.0	9.5	Normal	7.2	4.2	Normal
7	6.8	19.6	35% of normal	7.0	9.5	Normal
14	6.75	27.2	10% of normal	6.89	20.1	40% of normal
21	6.72	34.5	Negligible	6.85	24.5	Negligibl

ACD = Acid, citrate, dextrose; CPD = Citrate, phosphate, dextrose; DPG = Diphosphoglycerate.

    (b) ACD Blood should be no more than 48 hr old.

    (c) CPD Blood should be no more than 5 days old. (ACD and CPD bloods can be converted to heparinized blood by initially adding 22.5 mg heparin to one unit of blood. After complete mixing, 2 ml of a 10% calcium gluconate solution should be added.)

  (3) Neonatal thrombocytopenia Platelets from random donors often do not survive because of a maternal isoantibody. In such instances, maternal platelets suspended and washed in AB plasma should be used.

d. Complications of transfusion

  (1) Hemolytic transfusion reactions occur when red cells are destroyed by antibodies in the plasma of the recipient or donor. Signs of a reaction may follow administration of as little as 25–50 ml of blood.

    (a) Signs and symptoms Chills, headache, chest or back pain, nausea, vomiting, a rapid rise in temperature, a fall in blood pressure, and concomitant hemoglobinemia and hemoglobinuria.

    (b) Treatment Stop treatment. Attempt to provoke a diuresis; 50–100 ml of 20% mannitol is given in 5 min, followed by an infusion containing 25 mEq sodium bicarbonate to produce a urine flow of 1–3 ml/min. The mannitol should be repeated with hydration adequate to maintain a urine output of 100 ml/hr. If urine flow is unsatisfactory, tubular necrosis may be presumed.

  (2) Febrile (nonhemolytic) reactions

    (a) Signs and symptoms may vary from mild chilliness and slight temperature rise to severe chills and high fever. There may also be muscular aches and pains, flushing, nausea, and vomiting. Often this cannot be distinguished from a hemolytic reaction, except that there is *no hemoglobinemia or hemoglobinuria*.

    (b) Treatment Stop the transfusion and administer antipyretics if necessary (see **2.c,** p. 22).

(3) Allergic reactions occur in approximately 2 percent of transfusions and are seldom severe.

 (a) Signs and symptoms are hives, itching, or a diffuse rash. Facial and periorbital edema with mild laryngospasm may sometimes occur.

 (b) Treatment Stop the transfusion. Give antihistamines, or steroids, or both.

III. COMMON MANAGEMENT PROBLEMS

A. Feeding For a complete discussion of infant feeding and formula constituents, see Chap. 4 and *Pediatrics* 63 (1):52, 1979.

1. General considerations Nutritional requirements (Table 1-5) vary according to general health, activity states, growth rate, intestinal absorption, and the presence of metabolic disturbances. Normal growth and development are the best measures of adequate nutritional intake.

 a. Breast milk is the preferred source of nutrition for either low-birth-weight or full-term infants and can be continued through 18–24 months of age. Failure, when it occurs, is most commonly due to maternal anxiety about quantity of intake, the unsatisfied infant, fears of cosmetic effects, cultural pressures, and lack of adequate instructions. For a detailed discussion of breast feeding, see p. 94.

 b. If commercial formulas are used (see Table 4-3), the frequent and often unjustified changing of formulas when feeding problems occur may serve only to increase anxiety in both mother and child.

 c. Supplementation with vitamins D and C, iron, and fluoride may be needed (see Chap. 4 for dosages and indications).

 d. Introduction of solids The infant fed by formula or with human milk usually does not need solid foods prior to 5 months of age. At that time, the order of introduction of particular foods makes little difference, but should include an iron-fortified dry cereal (see also Chap. 4).

 e. Parents of infants with family histories of **allergy** should be aware of the more troublesome foods in the first year of life (orange juice, nuts, fish, strawberries, chocolates, and egg whites). Delaying exposure to these foods has been shown to result in fever sensitivity reactions.

 f. Protein requirements are proportionately higher during childhood because of rapid growth rates (see Table 1-5). If protein sources are largely vegetables, foods must be more varied to ensure an adequate intake of amino acids and vitamins.

 g. Cooking, in general, increases the digestibility of protein foods, but prolonged heating reduces protein availability.

 h. Obese parents should be given long-term dietary instructions for their infants, since there is a tendency for obesity to be familial (see Chap. 12).

 i. A child's food intake is seldom constant and varies daily in quantity and quality. In general, parents can be reassured that a child will take in enough to grow. A special period of apparent, decreased intake seems to occur at 7–9 months along with the desire of babies to feed themselves, at 2–3 years along with the further need for inde-

Table 1-5 Recommended Daily Dietary Allowances, Revised 1974[a]

Fat-Soluble Vitamins

	Years (From up to)	Weight (kg)	Energy (kcal)	Protein (gm)	Vitamin A (RE)	Activity (IU)	Vitamin D (IU)	Vitamin E Activity (IU)
Infants	0.0–0.5	6	kg × 117	kg × 2.2	420	1400	400	4
	0.5–1.0	9	kg × 108	kg × 2.0	400	2000	400	5
Children	1–3	13	1300	23	400	2000	400	7
	4–6	20	1800	30	500	2500	400	9
	7–10	30	2400	36	700	3300	400	10
Males	11–14	44	2800	44	1000	5000	400	12
	15–18	61	3000	54	1000	5000	400	15
	19–22	67	3000	52	1000	5000	400	15
Females	11–14	44	2400	44	800	4000	400	10
	15–18	54	2100	48	800	4000	400	11
	19–22	58	2100	46	800	4000	400	12
Pregnant			+300	+30	1000	5000	400	15
Lactating			+500	+20	1200	6000	400	15

Water-Soluble Vitamins

	Years (From up to)	Weight (kg)	Ascorbic Acid (mg)	Folacin (µg)	Niacin (mg)	Riboflavin (mg)	Thiamine (mg)	Vitamin B₆ (mg)	Vitamin B₁₂ (µg)
Infants	0.0–0.5	6	35	50	5	0.4	0.3	0.3	0.3
	0.5–1.0	9	35	50	8	0.6	0.5	0.4	0.3
Children	1–3	13	40	100	9	0.8	0.7	0.6	1.0
	4–6	20	40	200	12	1.1	0.9	0.9	1.5

				20	1.8	1.5	1.8	3.0
15–18	61			20	1.8	1.5	1.8	3.0
19–22	67			20	1.8	1.5	2.0	3.0
Females								
11–14	44			16	1.3	1.2	1.6	3.0
15–18	54			14	1.4	1.1	2.0	3.0
19–22	58			14	1.4	1.1	2.0	3.0
Pregnant	60			+2	+0.3	+0.3	2.5	4.0
Lactating	60			+4	+0.5	+0.3	2.5	4.0

Minerals

	Years (From up to)	Weight (kg)	Calcium (mg)	Phosphorus (mg)	Iodine (μg)	Iron (mg)	Magnesium (mg)	Zinc (mg)
Infants	0.0–0.5	6	360	240	35	10	60	3
	0.5–1.0	9	540	400	45	15	70	5
Children	1–3	13	800	800	60	15	150	10
	4–6	20	800	800	80	10	200	10
	7–10	30	800	800	110	10	250	10
Males	11–14	44	1200	1200	130	18	350	15
	15–18	61	1200	1200	150	18	400	15
	19–22	67	800	800	140	10	350	15
Females	11–14	44	1200	1200	115	18	300	15
	15–18	54	1200	1200	115	18	300	15
	19–22	58	800	800	110	18	300	15
Pregnant			1200	1200	125	18+[b]	450	20
Lactating			1200	1200	150	18	450	25

[a] Modified from Committee on Dietary Allowances and Committee on Interpretation of the Recommended Dietary Allowances. Food and Nutrition Board, National Research Council, 8th rev. ed., 1974. Washington, D.C.: National Academy of Sciences.
[b] Requires supplemental iron.

pendence, and at 5–6 years. It is important for the pediatrician to all himself with the parents in staying calm about these periods despit the pressure from concerned relatives, since these behaviors ar normal developmental processes.

j. New foods may be refused initially because of their unfamiliarity.

k. Forced feedings are never useful at any age.

2. **Colic** Although colic refers to paroxysmal abdominal pain of intestin origin, the symptom in infancy is used loosely and includes moderate-t severe and otherwise unexplained bouts of crying. Infants in the first 3- months of life appear to be most susceptible. Once begun, the persisten of the intense, inconsolable crying can be distressing to parents.

   a. **Etiology** There is no single cause, but persistent crying shou stimulate efforts for an explanation. Hunger is one of the most fr quent causes of crying and must be differentiated from other possib causes such as failure to eructate swallowed air, otitis media, corne abrasions, and milk intolerance. Overfeeding may also cause intes nal discomfort.

   b. **Clinical pattern** The clinical pattern is rather characteristic. Usual the attacks begin suddenly with paroxysms of irritability an screaming. The cry is loud and may persist for several hours. The le are often flexed and the infant appears to be experiencing abdomin pain. Often the abdomen is distended and tense, and the face is co torted and congested. When the attacks terminate, the infant is fr quently exhausted. Sometimes there is some relief with the passa of flatus or feces.

   c. **Management** If through careful history and examination a speci cause of colic is found, preventive measures should be directed at th cause.

      (1) Underfeeding and overfeeding can be properly relieved. Air sw lowing, which may be responsible in part for discomfort, may aided with appropriate feeding and burping techniques.

      (2) Colic quickly becomes a family affair and the entire family shou participate in its management, not only to diffuse the responsib ity but also to help diminish the psychosocial stress brought abo by the tense screaming. Parents often feel guilty that they a doing something wrong, or they may feel frustrated and helple Physicians can play a supportive and directive role by foresee an end at about 4 months and thereby appropriately divert t focus of the parents to the positive and exciting aspects of th child's development.

      (3) The use of sedative and anticholinergic agents has not been eff tive, and the hazards of overdosage and toxicity are such that u of these drugs in small infants is not recommended.

3. **Constipation**

   a. **Diagnosis**

      (1) Constipation may be diagnosed by history with the finding of fe contents on abdominal or rectal examination. Abdominal p may suggest it.

      (2) Although constipation may accompany many syndromes (Chap. 11, Sec. I), it more often represents too little free water

the diet, inadequate intake of high-residue food, disruption of the child's daily habits, or a painful anal fissure that causes withholding of the stool.

(3) Passing a daily stool does not exclude constipation as a problem. Large, hard, or painful stools, sometimes large enough to clog the toilet, are significant signs even if they occur daily by history. Similarly, infrequent stools, even once every 1–7 days, can be normal in breast-fed infants.

b. Treatment A stepwise approach follows.

(1) To assist the child to pass a hard stool:

(a) Glycerine or bisacodyl (Dulcolax) suppository (one only).

(b) *Pediatric* Fleet's enema (may be repeated once).

(c) Mineral oil, 15 ml PO. Magnesium sulfate or sodium sulfate may help in passing a hard stool and softening a forming stool.

(d) Manual disimpaction, which is unpleasant for both child and physician, but may be necessary. There is no known simple or pleasant way to perform this time-honored physician's chore.

(e) Soapsuds or milk and molasses slurry enemas are helpful in resistant cases. Gastrografin or Mucomyst enemas can be useful in the impaction of cystic fibrosis, but have serious potential side effects, including electrolyte disturbances, intravascular depletion, and toxic absorption, and are expensive.

(2) To increase bulk and soften the stool:

(a) An increase in intake of free water.

(b) Natural dietary lubricants (e.g., prune juice, olive oil, tomatoes, and tomato juice).

(c) High-residue foods (e.g., green vegetables and fruits). The addition of bran and whole grain products is optimal for lifelong dietary changes.

(d) Pharmacologic stool softeners such as dioctyl sodium sulfosuccinate (Colace), 5 mg/kg/24 hr, malt soup extract (Maltsupex), or senna concentrate (Senokot). The dosage of stool softeners is as follows: age 1 month–1 year, ½ tsp bid; 1–5 years, 1 tsp bid; 5–15 years, 2 tsp bid. Large initial doses are essential; when the stools become soft, the dosage can be reduced. Regular daily dosage is continued for about 2–3 months and slowly reduced as bowel tone and regular bowel habits are reacquired. Relapses are common, and prolonged follow-up is advisable. Initially, Senokot, in particular, may produce cramping.

(e) To assist the child with anal fissures:

I. A glycerine or bisacodyl suppository may be necessary (one only).

II. Soften the stool as described.

III. Sitz baths tid for small children.

(f) If anatomic lesions have been ruled out:

I. Establish a pattern of bowel movement after meals (gastrocolic reflex) or at other times, but at the same time each

day by sitting the child on the toilet whether or not a bow
movement results.

   ii. Be sure that emotional stress and anxiety have been car
fully excluded as causes.

   iii. Relax.

  (g) If constipation persists and encopresis occurs, a psychiatr
evaluation is indicated, and long-term management by tl
pediatrician is required, see **H,** p. 174.

B. Fever control

1. **General considerations** Fever is a cardinal and often the first sign
illness in many children. Yet its pattern may be even more importa
than its presence. Therefore, any attempts to reduce a fever shou
never interfere with efforts to ascertain its cause. In addition, there
evidence that the presence of fever may be of biologic value in sor
cases. The following suggestions for the management of fever may pro
helpful.

  a. Clinical correlation The height of the fever does not necessarily cc
respond directly to the severity of its cause. Newborns with sep
may have subnormal temperatures.

  b. Dehydration Because dehydration can be associated with fever (s
B.1.a, p. 191), adequate amounts of fluid must be administer
either PO if tolerated or IV if necessary. If dehydration *is* present,
may contribute to the potential toxicity of aspirin, particularly
infants.

  c. Skin exposure Children can lose excess heat through the skin a
should be lightly clothed when febrile.

  d. Sponging A number of antipyretics are available, but all have und
sirable side effects and toxicities. Sponging, on the other hand, is sa
and effective *if done properly.*

2. **Specific measures**

  a. Hydration See Chap. 8.

  b. Sponging Only tepid water should be used. Alcohol or ice wat
while lowering skin temperature more rapidly, is **less** effective l
cause surface vasoconstriction prevents heat loss, is associated w
increased morbidity, particularly in small infants, and **should**
avoided. The skin may be rubbed briskly to increase skin capill
circulation and heat loss. Sponging may be done no longer than a h
hour every 2 hours.

  c. Antipyretics See Table 1-6.

    (1) Acetylsalicylic acid (aspirin) The most widely used medicat
available, aspirin still has side effects and toxicity that necessit
caution in its use. Cumulative levels occur, and the half-life of t
drug is long. Because of insolubility, it is available only as a tab
or suppository. Children's preparations are flavored tablets of
mg each and are now limited by law to bottles of 36 tablets. T
ordinary dosage for fever in children is 60 mg/year of age c
(doses in inflammatory disease are discussed in Chap. 18, Sec
Side effects and toxic reactions include GI upset, GI bleeding,
terference with platelet activity, and prolongation of prothrom
time. The rectal preparation can irritate the mucosa, and a tc

Table 1-6 Some Antipyretics Useful in Pediatrics[a]

Drug	Analgesic	Anti-inflammatory[b]	Suggested Antipyretic Oral Dose (mg/kg q6h)
Aspirin and other salicylates	+	+	10–20
p-Aminophenols	+	–	
Phenacetin			5–10
Acetaminophen			5–10
Acetanilid			...[c]
Salicylamide	±	–	10–20

The phenylpyrazoles, including aminopyrine, dipyrone, phenylbutazone, and oxyphenbutazone, are excluded from this list because their adverse potential precludes their use for simple antipyresis.
Specifically, antirheumatic.
Not recommended for general antipyretic use in children.
Modified from A. K. Done and D. D. Done, *Pediatr. Clin. North Am.* 19:171, 1972.

reaction is known to occur from this route due to variable absorption.

(2) **Acetaminophen,** a widely used liquid alternative to aspirin, has the advantage of somewhat greater accuracy of dosage and less gastric irritation. It lacks antirheumatic properties, but is equal to aspirin in effectiveness as an antipyretic. The dose is 5–10 mg/kg q4–6h.

(3) **Phenacetin,** because it is more toxic than aspirin or acetaminophen, has no advantage over either.

(4) **Salicylamide** is unrelated to aspirin, does not have antirheumatic properties, and is not as effective an antipyretic as aspirin or acetaminophen. It is well tolerated PO and produces few toxic reactions. Because it is a liquid, it is often used in infants, but is probably rarely useful and has little to recommend it.

(5) **Chlorpromazine** in small doses (0.1 mg/kg/24 hr) helps reduce fever by surface vasodilatation and inhibition of shivering (thermogenesis). Its use in this manner is generally reserved for hospitalized patients with core temperatures > 104°F.

V. IMMUNIZATIONS See Tables 1-7 and 1-8.

A. **Routine immunizations for infants and young children** The American Academy of Pediatrics and the Public Health Service Advisory Committee on Immunization Practices have recommended a schedule for routine, active immunization of normal infants and children (see Table 1-7). Routine immunization of normal infants can be started at age 2 months; this schedule is appropriate for premature and low-birth-weight infants, and for breast-fed and bottle-fed infants.

B. **Immunizations in special circumstances**

1. **Primary immunization of children not immunized in infancy** For children *under age 6* who have not previously received immunizations, the type of

Table 1-7   Schedule for Active Immunization of Normal Infants and Children

Age	Vaccine	
2 months	DTP[a]	TOPV[b]
4 months	DTP	TOPV
6 months	DTP	TOPV (optional)[c]
1 year		Tuberculin test
15 months	Measles, rubella, mumps[d]	
1½ years	DTP	TOPV
4–6 years	DTP	TOPV
14–16 years	Td[e] (repeat every 10 years)	

[a] DTP = diphtheria and tetanus toxoids combined with pertussis vaccine.
[b] TOPV = trivalent oral polio vaccine.
[c] A third dose of TOPV is optional and should be given in areas of high endemicity c poliomyelitis.
[d] May be given as measles-rubella or measles-mumps-rubella combined vaccines.
[e] Td = combined tetanus and diphtheria toxoids (≤ 2 Lf units potency) for thos more than 6 years of age.
Adapted from American Academy of Pediatrics, *Report of the Committee on Infec tious Disease*, 18th ed. (Red Book), 1977, p. 3.

immunization used is similar to that of infancy (see Table 1-8). If ther has been an interruption in the primary immunization course, or a dela between recommended doses, it is not necessary to start the series ove again regardless of the duration of the interruption.

For children *over age 6* and adults, the combined, and less antigenicall potent, tetanus-diphtheria toxoids (Td) with adjuvant are recommende (see Table 1-8). The triple depot antigen DTP *should not be used.*

2. **Immunization of children with neurologic disease**   The indication for va cination of children with neurologic disorders is controversial, and th risks and benefits should be discussed with the parents and/or patien prior to vaccination. The "Red Book" of the American Academy c Pediatrics presents these guidelines:

   a. If the neurologic disorder is static and unchanging, immunizatio with vaccines such as pertussis, measles, rubella, and mumps offer the benefit of protection against the known neurologic complication of these diseases and the benefit would appear to exceed the risk c immunization.

   b. If the neurologic disorder is still evolving, immunizations likely t cause fever or to be associated with adverse neurologic reaction should be avoided, since the vaccine may result in an adverse effe on the neurologic disorders or be blamed for events resulting from th natural evolution of the disease.

3. **Immunization of immunosuppressed children**   Immunization of childre receiving short-term immunosuppression should be deferred until th therapy has been discontinued. Immunization of children receivin *long-term* immunosuppression may include killed antigen such as DPT c influenza vaccine but *must not include* live vaccines such as measle mumps, rubella, and smallpox.

Table 1-8 Schedule for Active Immunization of Children Not Immunized in Early Infancy[a]

UNDER 6 YEARS OF AGE

First visit	DTP, TOPV, Tuberculin test
Interval after first visit	
1 month	Measles,[b] mumps, rubella
2 months	DTP, TOPV
4 months	DTP, TOPV[c]
10 to 16 months or preschool	DTP, TOPV
Age 14–16 years	Td (repeat every 10 years)

6 YEARS OF AGE AND OVER

First visit	Td, TOPV, Tuberculin test
Interval after first visit	
1 month	Measles, mumps, rubella
2 months	Td, TOPV
8 to 14 months	Td, TOPV
Age 14–16 years	Td (repeat every 10 years)

a Physicians may choose to alter the sequence of these schedules if specific infections are prevalent at the time. For example, measles vaccine might be given on the first visit if an epidemic is under way in the community.
b Measles vaccine is not routinely given before 15 months of age (see Table 1-14).
c Optional.
Adapted from American Academy of Pediatrics, *Report of the Committee on Infectious Disease*, 18th ed. (Red Book), 1977, p. 11.

Following cessation of immunosuppressive therapy, an additional dose of inactivated vaccine is recommended. Then, if the child does not have a primary immunosuppressive disorder, a live vaccine program may be resumed. It has *not* yet been recommended that children who have completed therapy for hematologic malignancy be given live vaccines.

4. **Immunization during pregnancy** The use of the live vaccines of measles, mumps, rubella, smallpox, polio, and yellow fever are contraindicated during pregnancy. The latter two may be given if unavoidable exposure is anticipated during foreign travel. The inactivated vaccines of influenza and rabies may be used when indicated and tetanus and diphtheria toxoids (adult Td) can be used as part of good antepartum care. The children or household contacts of pregnant women may receive any live or inactivated vaccine, including rubella.

5. **Recommendations for specific nonroutine immunizations**

   a. **Smallpox**[1] Vaccination is recommended only for laboratory workers who are likely to have contact with the variola virus and for travelers to countries that continue to require vaccination for entry. Routine vaccination of children or adults, including health workers, should be discontinued.

   b. **Influenza** Vaccination is recommended for those at high risk for severe influenza because of underlying chronic diseases such as cardiac, renal, or pulmonary disease; diabetes; sickle cell anemia; or malignancy. Vaccine should not be administered to persons who have had allergic reactions to previous influenza vaccinations or who have a

1 As of December 1978 no new cases of smallpox had occurred for one year.

history of hypersensitivity to eggs or egg products. At present, the subvirion (split virus) preparation is recommended for persons less than 12 years old.

c. Polio immunization in adults Anyone who has completed the primary TOPV series should be given an additional dose of TOPV when there is a substantial risk of exposure to poliomyelitis during travel. Adults who have never received a polio vaccination, and who are at risk of exposure to poliomyelitis while traveling or to vaccine virus following immunization of their children with TOPV, should receive inactivated polio vaccine (IPV). Three doses should be given at monthly intervals and a fourth dose 6–12 months after the third.

d. Meningococcal polysaccharide vaccines Three meningococcal polysaccharide vaccines (monovalent A, monovalent C, and bivalent A-C) are currently licensed for selective use in the United States. The selected indications for these vaccines include

(1) Travel to countries having epidemic meningococcal disease.

(2) Adjunct to antibiotic chemoprophylaxis for household contacts of meningococcal disease caused by serogroup A or C.

(3) Control of epidemic meningococcal disease caused by serogroup A or C.

The safety of meningococcal vaccines in pregnant women has not been established.

e. Pneumococcal vaccine A polysaccharide vaccine containing antigen to 14 types of pneumococci (American types 1, 2, 3, 4, 6, 8, 9, 12, 14, 19, 23, 25, 51, and 56), which account for 80 percent of all bacteremic pneumococcal disease, has been licensed in the United States. As with other polysaccharide vaccines, infants and toddlers have a poor antibody response and it is not recommended in those under age 2. Its use is suggested in persons with splenic dysfunction (e.g., sickle cell anemia or splenectomy patients) and in those with chronic illnesses having an increased risk of pneumococcal disease (e.g., diabetes or cardiopulmonary, hepatic, and renal disease).

C. Practical aspects of vaccine administration

1. Contraindications General contraindications for vaccination include

a. Acute febrile illness (*minor* infection without fever is *not* a contraindication).

b. Administration of blood components (immune serum globulin, plasma, whole blood) within prior 8 weeks.

c. Pregnancy Live virus vaccines are contraindicated except in certain situations (see **IV.B.4**), and certain newer vaccines have not been proved safe during pregnancy.

d. Immunosuppressive therapy including radiation therapy, corticosteroids, antimetabolites, alkylating agents, and cytotoxic agents: only **live** virus vaccines are contraindicated.

e. Immunodeficiency disorders, primary and acquired, including leukemia, lymphoma, and generalized malignancy: only **live** virus vaccines are contraindicated.

f. Simultaneous administration of a single, live vaccine except measles mumps-rubella, and measles-rubella, which are effective in combination.

g. Prior allergic reaction to the same or a related vaccine. Children who are allergic to eggs, chickens, or ducks should not receive vaccines grown in chicken or duck eggs (influenza, yellow fever, and duck embryo rabies vaccine). These children **may** receive vaccines grown in chicken and duck fibroblast tissue culture (measles, mumps, rubella).

2. Technique of administration   Subcutaneous injections with a 25-gauge needle, ⅝ in. long, are usually given in the extensor or lateral surface of the upper arm, but may be given elsewhere, including the abdomen (in rabies vaccination). Intramuscular injection is given with a 20–22-gauge needle, 1 to 1½ in. long in the upper outer quadrant of the buttocks, the midlateral areas of the thigh, or the deltoid muscle.

3. Side effects and adverse reactions   Side effects and adverse reactions of vaccines may be local or systemic. In general, these are mild, predictable, and self-limited and only rarely are severe. The parents and patient should understand the risks involved in immunization and appreciate the potential benefit to be derived. *Consult the package insert for a description of the specific side effects of each vaccine.*

V. DEATH OF A CHILD   See also *Pediatrics* 62:96, 1978. In the first week of life, more deaths occur than in any subsequent period of childhood. Between the first week of life and one year of age, the sudden infant death syndrome is the most common cause of death. (For a complete discussion of this syndrome see Chapter 2.) After one year of age, accidents exceed all other acquired causes.

The strongest of all grief reactions occurs when parents have lost a child. Much of parental grief is based on the concept of parent-infant bonding. The reciprocal interaction between a parent and a young infant results in early involvement and mutual investment of growing intensity. The death of a child brings a sudden and drastic end to that relationship. Parents react to the death of their child in a manner that reflects their family life, emotional structure, individual attachment, and the degree of specific circumstances associated with the loss. What health professionals do during this period is usually based upon their own feelings as well as upon assumptions that arise from customs, traditions, state and hospital health rules, and even research interests. Thoughtful and caring medical personnel can share and help to lighten the family's burden.

When a child has a fatal disease, the parents and immediate family face the loss of all their expectations for the child and an extended period of sadness. After learning of the diagnosis, parents usually cannot absorb the detailed information they are given about the disease and its clinical course. They require sufficient time and privacy to formulate their questions, and they need guidance to establish realistic expectations, especially if referral to a large medical center is to be made. Often, their questions are repetitious; sometimes they completely avoid certain topics.

Fathers may sometimes have less insight into the mechanisms of child rearing and child health risks than do mothers, and they may be less prepared to accept the fragility of life and the constraints on their own control over their children's environment or destiny. Fathers seem to limit their requests for help, or, even more often, such requests after the loss of their child are not recognized by health professionals. Given a chance to express their feelings, fathers can utilize the support constructively. If possible, the same physician should talk with both parents together and/or separately about the child's progress and remain aware of their individual needs.

Following a child's death, the physician's first responsibility is to inform the parents in a direct, sensitive manner; warmth and understanding provide a closeness with the family. Unless there are exceptional circumstances, a parent should *never* be informed of a child's death by telephone.

An important prerequisite in talking to parents about their child's death is knowledge of the circumstances in which it occurred. Not being given this information may serve to reinforce parents' doubts and guilts.

It may be helpful to provide sedation or a quiet place for the parents, who may prefer to be alone. The hospital staff can also help with funeral arrangements, inform other family members, or arrange transportation.

Similarly, viewing and touching the body may be important, to help the parents grasp the actuality of their child's death. They may need time alone to hold and talk to the deceased child as their last gestures of caring. In the case of a newborn, seeing the body is especially important to the parents. Though these parents have had little physical contact with their child, they had experienced pregnancy and had formulated plans and expectations that are suddenly ended. During the pregnancy, they may also have had the normal fears about deformed infants, and often, mothers may recall incidents during pregnancy that they feel could have influenced the eventual outcome. To quiet those fears, they may need to see that their baby was not grossly abnormal.

Not only the parents but surviving children may need help with their grief. Children under the age of 5 years view the death as a temporary and reversible situation. Children between 5 and 10 years of age may look at death in terms of responsibility—something or someone was responsible. By the time children are about 10 years old, they are able to understand that death is inevitable and irreversible. Surviving older children appear to be able to resolve the problem of loss, and do substantially better when they are included in the grief process. For this reason parents can be advised to be as open as possible with their explanations and their own reactions.

Clinicians may need to clarify that a sibling died of a special illness or one that affects only infants and not older children or parents. Children may also need to be reassured that their health is good and that the same event will not happen to them.

In the course of normal sibling rivalry, children might wish an infant brother or sister to die. Small children indulge in magical thinking, which can cause events to occur by wishing them. In this way they may implicate themselves and need assurance that they did nothing to cause the death.

Some children mourn losses for a long time. Their grief may be exhibited in school difficulties or sleep problems or special fears. These should be addressed individually, with the knowledge that sibling loss almost certainly plays a significant role in these behavior changes.

Follow-up visits with parents are important. If an autopsy has been performed, a visit to discuss the findings should follow its completion. Irrespective of an autopsy, visits should be made at 6 weeks and 6 months, to gauge the progress of grieving, anticipate unusual problems in adjusting to the child's death, and answer the many questions about the circumstances of the death and how to help siblings adjust to their feelings. Friends and relatives usually tire of discussing the death long before parents have worked through their own feelings.

When parents have lost a child, the decision to have another is complex. If they are able to complete the grief process, the psychological environment for the subsequent newborn will be healthier. Parents are too often advised to have a "replacement" child quickly. There is no replacement for a lost child, and it may be better advice to parents to allow more time following a loss before a subsequent pregnancy. The physician who was so intimately involved can not only be open to such discussions but can help to correct the inevitable distortions of events caused by grief.

Finally, physicians must be aware of and deal with their own feelings about the death of a patient. A feeling of failure is often present, particularly when complicated management did not suffice. There may be a desire to "make it up" to the family because of possible uncertainty surrounding the physician's participation. There is nothing wrong with feeling a sense of loss at the death of a patient or with the need to grieve, but it is the physician's hard task to put his own grief aside until the needs of the parents and family have been met.

2

Emergencies, Child Abuse, and Sudden Infant Death Syndrome

This chapter includes only the most commonly encountered problems in emergency management. Others may be found in chapters dealing with specific pathologic conditions.

I. CARDIAC ARREST The diagnosis of cardiac arrest must be rapid (absent pulse and respirations, cyanosis, dilated pupils).

A. Equipment

1. **Drugs** Sodium bicarbonate, epinephrine 1:1000, 50% glucose, 10% calcium gluconate, atropine.

2. Needles (19–23 gauge), syringes, scalpels.

3. Pediatric-size laryngoscope blades (various sizes), airways, endotracheal tubes (see **B.4**), and tracheotomy tube.

4. Pediatric-size masks and Ambu bags.

B. Ventilation

1. Clear the oral cavity of secretions. Insert an oral airway.

2. Begin bag-to-mouth or mouth-to-mouth ventilation at a rate of 30–50/min.

3. Insert an O_2 tube into the patient's mouth or attach to an Ambu bag.

4. If ventilation appears ineffective, double-check to assure proper bag and mask technique. The majority of patients can be ventilated sufficiently without intubation. Even if not ideal, less-than-perfect bag and mask ventilation is to be preferred over inept or—worse—unsuccessful attempts at intubation by unskilled or inexperienced emergency room personnel. Ideally, all emergency physicians should receive sufficient training to feel at ease with pediatric intubation.

5. If ventilation is unsuccessful, perform **intubation** with an endotracheal tube (see Table 2-1 and Chap. 23). If there is doubt, the correct size of endotracheal tube for a child can be estimated from the diameter of the child's fifth finger.

   a. **Atropine,** 0.1–0.6 mg IM, is useful in avoiding vagal slowing during intubation, but interferes with subsequent monitoring of pupil size.

   b. A **nasogastric tube** should be inserted as soon as possible after intubation is accomplished.

C. Circulation

1. While beginning ventilation, start external cardiac massage by sternal compression. Place the patient on a solid surface.

2. Do not attempt to ventilate at the same time as the sternum is compressed. If the next inspiration is begun as compression is maximal, the

Table 2-1 Endotracheal Tubes Used in Children of Various Ages

Age of Child	Tube Specifications	
	Number (French)	Size (mm)
Premature–3 months	12–14	2.5–3.0
3–18 months	14–18	3.5–4.0
18 months–5 years	18–22	4.0–5.0
5–12 years	22–28	5.0–6.5
12 years or more	28–34	6.5–8.0

incoming air will lift the chest as cardiac compression is released. This synchronizes the respiratory and cardiac resuscitation efforts. Alternate one breath and four sternal compressions; 60–80 compressions/min is adequate.

   3. Determine the effectiveness of circulation by palpating the femoral pulse. Core temperatures below 95°F are possible with exposure or even in a cold treatment room and may significantly hinder the establishment of normal sinus rhythm. Warming blankets or warming lamps help to reestablish normothermia.

   4. Do not attempt an IV infusion until help arrives.

   D. **ECG monitor** When help arrives, attach an ECG monitor and start an IV infusion (central line if possible) (see Sec. **II.B.1**).

   E. **Drug administration** See Table 2-2. In general, resuscitation drugs administered via secure peripheral venous access will arrive centrally within 30 sec with good chest massage technique. Many patients will respond well to this regimen, particularly if repeated doses of bicarbonate and epinephrine are used. If there is ineffective chest massage, no venous route, or no response to peripheral administration, the drugs can be given directly into

Table 2-2 Resuscitation Drugs

Drug	Dose	Preparation	Route
Atropine	*1 ampule*, once (range = 0.25–1.5 ml)	0.4 mg/ml/ampule	IV or IC
Bicarbonate	*1 ml/kg/5 min* until resuscitated	1 mEq $NaHCO_3$/ml 44 mEq/50 ml ampule	IV or IC
Calcium	*0.1 ml/kg* once	10% calcium gluconate ampule (100 mg calcium gluconate/ml, or 0.28 mEq Ca^{++}/ml)	IV or IC
Dextrose	*1 ml/kg* once	50% D/W	IV or IC
Epinephrine Infants (0–6 months)	*1 ml*	1:10,000 dilution or 1:10 dilution of 1:1000 solution	IV or IC
Children and adolescents	*1 ml*	1:1000 solution (1-ml ampule)	IV or IC

the right ventricular cavity, preferably by the subxyphoid method. The needle (with syringe attached) is inserted in the midline, directly below the xyphoid, with the needle aimed toward the inferior tip of the left scapula. Entry of the right ventricle should be confirmed by aspiration of blood *before* injection of drugs.

1. Administer $NaHCO_3$, 1–2 mEq/kg by IV push, to correct acidosis.

2. If asystole is present, administer epinephrine (0.5–2.0 ml of 1:10,000 in infants, or 0.1–1.0 ml of 1:1000 in older children) as a direct IV or intracardiac injection.

3. If QRS complexes are observed without adequate pulse, 10% calcium gluconate, 10 mg/kg (0.1 ml/kg), are administered IV or as an intracardiac injection. **Be sure the infusion is not intramyocardial.**

4. Hypoglycemia and abnormal potassium levels can be readily detected by the use of Dextrostix and by interpretation of T waves on the ECG.

F. Defibrillation   See also Chap. 10, Sec. **I.D.**

1. If ventricular fibrillation is present, defibrillate, placing one electrode over the apex and one over the sternal notch (Table 2-3).

2. If there is no response, two shocks of the same magnitude may be given in rapid succession.

3. Failure of defibrillation suggests metabolic imbalance (e.g., hypoxia, hypothermia, hypoglycemia). *BCDE* medications (see Table 2-2) should be repeated, followed in 90 sec by repeat defibrillation. If blood samples are obtainable and laboratory results are immediately available, metabolic studies can be helpful.

G. Blood pressure   Following resuscitation, dopamine, 50 mg (1.25 ml)/500 ml in 5% D/W at 1.0–2.5 ml/kg/hr, or isoproterenol (Isuprel), 1.0 mg/100 ml in 5% D/W IV at 5 ml/hr, may be useful adjuncts in maintaining cardiac output. The drip should be titrated to the patient's response (see **II.C.2.a**, p. 38).

H. The cause of the cardiac arrest should be diagnosed and treated as soon as possible.

II. SHOCK   The various causes of shock in children are detailed in Table 2-4.

A. The aim of therapy is to restore circulation to peripheral vascular beds, thereby breaking the cycle in which metabolic dysfunction results in extravasation and pooling of blood and further loss of circulatory volume.

B. Evaluation   Infants in shock are usually hypotonic and have a weak or absent cry. Older children may be disoriented or stuporous. The skin may be mottled, gray or pale in color, and cool. Capillary filling in the fingers and toes is poor. Respirations may be shallow. The pulse is rapid and weak and

Table 2-3   Defibrillation Values

Type of Patient	Weight (kg)	Watt-Sec
Infant	12	25–50
Small child	12–25	100
Large child	25	100–200

Table 2-4 Causes of Shock in Children

	Common Preexisting Conditions	
Etiology	Newborn	Older Child
Hemorrhage	Via placenta or cord Intracerebral Fetomaternal, twin-twin	Trauma to abdominal organs, liver, spleen Thrombocytopenia DIC
Fluid loss	Gastroenteritis	Gastroenteritis Severe burn Diabetes mellitus and insipidus
Gram-negative sepsis	Congenital pneumonia Amnionitis Infected umbilical catheter	Pyelonephritis Meningococcemia Immunologic deficiency
Cardiogenic and vascular obstruction	Hypoplastic left ventricle Coarctation of aorta Endocardial fibroelastosis	Coxsackie myocarditis Rheumatic heart disease Pulmonary embolus Thrombotic thrombocytopenic purpura
Neurogenic disturbance	Cord injury following breech delivery	Spinal cord transection Epidural hematoma Other causes of acutely increased intracranial pressure
Anaphylaxis	(Rare)	Allergy to food or drugs
Adrenal disorder	Adrenogenital syndrome Adrenal necrosis following breech delivery	Adrenogenital syndrome Pituitary insufficiency
Respiratory disorder	Diaphragmatic hernia Severe hyaline membrane disease Neonatal pneumonia Pulmonary atresia	Pneumothorax Severe pneumonia
Upper airway obstruction	Choanal atresia, stenosis, goiter, oropharyngeal tumors	Epiglottitis, croup, foreign-body aspiration

sometimes cannot be obtained by palpation of the radial or femoral arteries. Blood pressure is diminished or unobtainable. Urine output is decreased or absent. Hemorrhage from venipuncture sites or from the GI tract may be present if shock has been complicated by disseminated intravascular coagulation (DIC) (see Chap. 17, Sec. **V.B**).

1. **Pulse** Continuous ECG monitoring is indicated for the patient in shock as a check on heart rate and rhythm. Silver chloride electrodes are convenient in the newborn because of their small size.

2. **Blood pressure**

   a. **In the newborn** Accurate arterial blood pressure measurements should be obtained even in the smallest of premature infants. Auscul tation and palpation methods are usually ineffective in newborns. However, the flush method provides a good measure of mean arterial blood pressure, especially in the absence of methods for the direct measurement of arterial pulse pressure via an arterial cannula.

(1) Flush blood pressures in the newborn are obtained with a 5.0-cm cuff applied to the wrist or ankle. The corresponding hand or foot is then compressed by wrapping with a soft rubber drain or bandage 3.5 by 50 cm, beginning at the tips of the digits and working proximally to the edge of the cuff. The cuff is inflated to 300 mm Hg, the wrap is released, and pressure is decreased at the rate of approximately 5 mm Hg/sec while the extremity is maintained at the level of the heart.

(2) During the first week of life, mean flush blood pressure at the wrist is 41 ± 8 (±2 standard deviations) mm Hg, and flush pressure between 1 and 12 months is 72 ± 10.5 mm Hg. *Changes in the trend of successive pressure recordings are more significant than are individual recordings.*

(3) A 3½F, 5F, or occasionally 8F Argyle catheter may be passed via the umbilical artery into the thoracic aorta proximal to the diaphragm for blood gas determinations and arterial blood pressure measurements via a pressure transducer (see **II.D.2**, p. 109).

b. In older children   Blood pressures in the older child are obtained with a cuff of a width two-thirds the length of the upper arm. Mean systolic blood pressure is 65 mm Hg at 1 day of age, 90 mm Hg at 1 year, 100 mm Hg at 6 years, and 113 mm Hg at 12 years.

3. Central venous pressure (CVP)

a. In the newborn   See **3**, p. 110.

(1) An umbilical vein catheter is positioned in the superior vena cava at a level above the diaphragm. **Never insert a catheter unless the free end is attached to a closed syringe,** since a low CVP combined with negative intrathoracic pressure may drain air from the catheter into the vena cava, resulting in air embolism.

(2) CVPs are measured from the midaxillary line to the top of the column of liquid while the child is in the supine position. The fluid column should vary with respiration and pulse. Pressures of 4–7 cm of H_2O are usually within the normal range in premature and full-term newborns.

b. In infants and older children

(1) Catheterization of the external jugular vein may be used in infants, while in older children the preferable site is in the antecubital fossa via the median basilic vein into the superior vena cava.

(2) Silastic is the material of choice for catheters inserted from a peripheral vein because it is pliable, radiopaque, and inert.

(3) A CVP of 0–6 cm H_2O is low in children and should be corrected with plasma expanders (see p. 37). A pressure of 6–15 cm H_2O is within the normal range; a pressure **greater than 15 cm H_2O is dangerously high.**

4. Urine output is measured hourly in newborns and infants. While unnecessary catheterization of the bladder is usually avoided in children, shock is one clinical situation in which the advantages of accurate hourly measurements of urine output usually outweigh the disadvan tages of catheterization. The closed urinary drainage system is rela tively effective in preventing bladder infection. Urine output should not be permitted to fall below a minimum of 0.5 ml/kg/hr.

5. Airway and oxygen

a. In the newborn Even if there is no gross pulmonary or cardiac dis ease, children in shock should be given the benefit of an increased inspiratory O_2 concentration.

(1) Added O_2 should be warm and moist.

(2) Isolettes maintain high O_2 concentrations poorly; a hood should be used. Hoods similar to the Olympic Oxyhood are satisfactory, pro viding inlets for IV tubing, nebulized oxygen, monitoring probes and a thermometer. Hoods are available in three sizes, for infant ranging in weight from 2½–18 lb. The tops may be removed for suctioning.

(3) Inspired O_2 concentration is monitored by serial arterial blood gas determinations and kept below 100 mm Hg.

b. In older children Infants and older children frequently do not toler ate nasal O_2, and O_2 via face mask is usually indicated. An oral airway is especially helpful, and orotracheal intubation may sometimes be necessary.

6. Temperature The mortality of sick newborns is significantly increased if the temperature is allowed to fall below 95°F (see p. 103). Skin tempera ture should be relatively constant. Isolette temperature should be main tained by a servomechanism activated by the infant's skin temperature A continuous record of Isolette temperatures should be maintained Hypothermia is a significant problem for any child undergoing resuscita tion.

7. Blood gas measurement and correction of acidosis See also Chap. 8.

a. A severely asphyxiated infant may have a base deficit of 25 mEq/L in the cord blood. Ventilation can lower this to 16 mEq/L, and the re maining metabolic component of the acidosis can be corrected by in fusing bicarbonate. If blood gas determinations are not available 5–10 mEq $NaHCO_3$ solution can be given IV to the full-term newborn over 2–5 min.

b. Before infusion, bicarbonate must be diluted 50% with 5% D/W to reduce its hypertonicity. (Rapid infusions of hypertonic bicarbonate solution have resulted in seizures, and hepatic necrosis may occur if the solu tion is given directly into the liver through a malplaced umbilical catheter.)

8. Evaluation for **infection, electrolyte imbalance, and renal function** should be done as the patient is stabilized.

C. Treatment The key to successful treatment of shock is rapid correction of circulatory insufficiency and its causes. A physician should be in atten dance until the critical stages are passed, and *attention to detail is of the utmost importance, especially when treating the premature or full-term new born infant.* Maintenance of temperature can make the difference between survival **and** death in a newborn. Even excessive handling can contribute to the stress experienced by the newborn, and manipulations and proce dures should be kept to a minimum in any child.

1. **Volume expansion**   Rapid expansion of the intravascular volume is critical in patients with shock in whom the CVP is low (less than 6 cm H_2O in older children; less than 4 cm H_2O in the newborn) and in whom there is evidence of poor peripheral circulation. Intravascular volume should be expanded *before* pressor agents are given.

   a. **Fluids for volume expansion**   See also Chaps. 1 and 8.

      (1) **Albumin**   Five percent albumin (salt-poor albumin, human) in isotonic saline is probably the best volume expander in shock. It does not carry the risk of hepatitis, does not have to be crossmatched, and does not cause allergic reactions so often as does blood or plasma; 25% albumin can be obtained in units of 20, 50, and 100 ml and can be stored at room temperature; 5% albumin solutions are obtained in 250-ml aliquots.

      (2) **Plasmanate,** which may be used as an alternative to 5% albumin, is a 5% solution of plasma protein fractions containing 88% normal human albumin, 7% alpha globulin, and 5% beta globulin. Electrolyte concentrations of Plasmanate are as follows: sodium, 110 mEq/L; potassium, 0.25 mEq/L; and chloride, 50 mEq/L. *Blood group agglutinins and coagulation factors are absent from Plasmanate.* Plasmanate has the same effective volume expansion as 5% albumin.

      (3) **Blood**   If albumin or plasmanate is not available, whole blood crossmatched against the patient's blood may be used, although the risk of hepatitis is therefore increased (see Chap. 1, Sec. **II.D**). Freshly drawn heparinized blood is best because of its low acid and potassium content. **Avoid infusing unmatched type O negative blood** during the early stages of shock because this leads to errors in crossmatching at a later time. In severe exsanguination, however, the use of unmatched type O negative blood may be unavoidable. If fresh blood is not available, acid-citrate-dextrose (ACD) blood not more than 6 days old should be given.

      (4) **Isotonic solution**   Saline is not the treatment of choice for shock because the absence of colloid fails to prevent loss of saline from the intravascular space. However, in progressive shock, there is probably loss of extracellular, extravascular fluid in addition to intravascular fluid; thus, some saline may be given in addition to the colloid necessary to expand intravascular volume, improve urine flow, and provide for ongoing fluid losses. When albumin, plasma, or blood is unavailable, saline is given as a stopgap measure to restore circulation.

      (5) **Fresh frozen plasma**   Plasma is also less desirable as a volume expander because of the risk of hepatitis, especially in pooled plasma preparations. Fresh frozen plasma can be used in shock when clotting factors are needed, such as in hemophilia.

   b. **Rate of administration**   In general, plasma expanders should be given as rapidly as possible until a blood pressure can be obtained and the CVP increases.

      (1) **In the newborn**   An initial volume of 5% albumin in isotonic saline may be given at a dose of 10 ml/kg over ½ hr. If the blood pressure is still low and the CVP is still less than 4.0 cm H_2O, the dose may be repeated.

(2) In infants and older children Give 10–15 ml/kg 5% albumin in isotonic saline over ½ hr. Repeat if there is no pulse, blood pressure, and CVP response. Higher rates of infusion through more than one venous line are indicated in cases of severe hemorrhage.

2. **Drugs** See Table 2-5.

  a. **Isoproterenol hydrochloride** The value of pressor agents in shock is unproved. Only after adequate attempts to restore circulation by volume expansion fail may pressor agents be used.

   (1) Isoproterenol is titrated as a drip until the heart rate begins to increase and the blood pressure just begins to fall.

   (2) Do not give isoproterenol and epinephrine concurrently because of the risk of arrhythmias.

   (3) Continuously monitor ECG during isoproterenol infusions.

  b. **Levarterenol and metaraminol** These agents **should probably not be used except in cases of impending cardiac arrest.** No attempt should be made to bring blood pressure to normal values with these agents, because excessive doses cause severe renal arteriolar constriction and reduce urine output.

  c. High doses of **corticosteroids** have been used in patients with severe hypovolemic shock as well as gram-negative sepsis, but their use is still experimental.

  d. **Mannitol** If CVP is adequate, blood pressure has been restored, and urine output is still less than 8 ml/24 hr, a single IV dose of mannitol may be given in an attempt to establish adequate urine flow. Mannitol is supplied as a 25% solution containing 250 mg/ml. **Mannitol should not be given when the serum is hyperosmolar,** as in children with hypertonic dehydration or diabetes mellitus with extreme dehydration and hyperglycemia.

3. **Treatment of specific shock syndromes**

  a. **Cardiogenic shock** See also Chap. 10, Sec. **II.**

   (1) Oxygen, diuretics, digoxin, morphine, upright positioning, and aminophylline are important.

   (2) CVP measurements are essential. If the CVP is low, give IV fluids; if it is high, phlebotomy may be indicated.

   (3) Monitor the ECG carefully and measure urine volume hourly.

   (4) Use an isoproterenol infusion for impending cardiovascular collapse, but **watch carefully for tachycardia and arrhythmias.**

  b. **Neurogenic shock** Severe injury to the spinal cord may result in loss of vasomotor tone, pooling of venous and arterial blood, and hypotension.

   (1) Monitor the CVP and give plasma expanders until the CVP returns to normal.

   (2) In the rare instances when volume expansion has not restored circulation in neurogenic shock, give vasopressin or an alpha adrenergic stimulator such as methoxamine (Vasoxyl) or phenylephrine (Neo-Synephrine).

Drug	Mechanism of Action	Dose

Isoproterenol hydrochloride (Isuprel)	Beta-adrenergic
	Increases
	  Inotropic heart action
	  Chronotropic heart action
	Decreases
	  Arteriolar resistance
	  Venous capacitance
	  Airway and pulmonary vascular resistance
		Use a solution of 1.0 μg/ml; give by IV drip at a rate of 0.05–4.0 μg/min

Dopamine (Intropin)	Dopaminergic Increases cardiac output, peripheral blood flow, renal perfusion	IV drip; begin at 2–5 μg/kg/min; increase to maximum of 20 μg/kg/min*

Methoxamine (Vasoxyl)	Alpha-adrenergic pressor amine
	Increases
	  Peripheral resistance
	Decreases
	  Renal blood flow
		0.25 mg/kg as a single IM dose, up to maximum dose of 15 mg IM
		Effective over 60–90-min period

Phenylephrine hydrochloride (Neo-Synephrine)	Increases Smooth muscle arteriolar tone	0.10 mg/kg as a single IM dose; maximum dose 7.0 mg IM
Vasopressin (Pitressin)		0.125–0.50 ml (20 U/ml) given as a single IM dose

Hydrocortisone (Solu-Cortef)	Increases
	  Cardiac output
	  Enzyme synthesis (use in shock is controversial)
		25 mg/kg IV initially, followed by 12 mg/kg/24 hr in divided doses

Dexamethasone (Decadron)	Decreases
	  Peripheral resistance
	  Lactate production
		2 mg/kg IV initially, followed by 1 mg/kg/24 hr in divided doses

Mannitol	Osmotic diuretic	1 gm/kg/IV

* Alpha-adrenergic effects become increasingly apparent between 8–20 μg/kg/min, with vasoconstriction and interruption of blood flow to the extremities being significant hazards.

c. Bacteremic shock

(1) Obtain cultures of blood, spinal fluid, urine, and other infected sites available for culture.

(2) Begin antibiotics as soon as possible. (For treatment of meningitis and bacteremic sepsis, see Chap. 15, Sec. **IV.M.**)

(3) Measure the CVP and expand the intravascular volume if the CVP is low.

(4) Give high doses of corticosteroids IV.

(5) If the CVP is normal and poor perfusion persists, start an isoproterenol drip (see **2.a**).

(6) Monitor for DIC at the beginning of treatment and at frequent intervals. If laboratory evidence suggests DIC, and restoration of blood pressure does not result in a normal coagulation profile consider exchange transfusion (Chap. 17).

d. Anaphylactic shock

(1) Delay absorption of antigen from the injection site by placing a tourniquet proximal to the site so as to impede lymphatic and venous drainage, but not arterial flow.

(2) Give 1:1000 aqueous epinephrine SQ at the injection site to retard absorption of antigen (0.01 ml/kg initially, followed by the same dose at 20-min intervals for a total of 3 doses).

(3) If laryngeal edema seriously impairs respirations at the time of the initial evaluation, the first dose of epinephrine may be given IV as a dilution in 5–10 ml normal saline.

(4) Measure the CVP and restore circulation rapidly with albumin if the CVP is low (see **3**, p. 35).

(5) For bronchospasm, give aminophylline, 4 mg/kg IV, over ½ hr. For persistent bronchospasm, give aminophylline, up to 20 mg/kg/24 h in divided doses q6h.

(6) For a severe or prolonged anaphylactic reaction, give, in addition 10 mg/kg hydrocortisone stat IV, followed by hydrocortisone, 1 mg/kg 24 hr in divided doses IV q4–6h. Dexamethasone (Decadron) may be used as an alternative to hydrocortisone.

(7) Antihistamines may be of some help. Give diphenhydramine (Benadryl) in 4 divided daily doses PO, IV, or IM. Do not exceed 150 mg total per day.

III. **SEIZURES** cause much parental anxiety and always carry the threat of hypoxic CNS damage. Thus, evaluation and therapy must be a coordinated reasoned effort by emergency room personnel (see Chap. 21).

A. Evaluation

1. History

a. Known seizure disorder

b. Medications child is taking

c. Illnesses that may be associated with seizures, e.g., hypertension

d. Acute illness prior to the seizure

2. Description of the seizure

   a. Localized or generalized

   b. Duration

   c. Incontinence

   d. Cyanosis

B. Diagnostic studies at initial presentation should include the following: electrolytes, BUN, blood sugar, calcium, pH, TCO_2, toxicology screen, blood lead level, urinalysis, and lumbar puncture.

C. General evaluative and supportive measures for any patient who has a seizure

   1. Determine the adequacy of the airway; i.e., is vomitus or saliva obstructing the airway? Are the clothes too tight about the neck?

   2. Suctioning may often be necessary, and to expedite it, the child's head should be lower than the trunk.

   3. Oxygen administration is advisable whether or not cyanosis is present.

   4. If the tongue is obstructing respirations, an oral airway may be tried empirically while respirations are monitored simultaneously. Use of a tongue blade is of questionable value.

   5. Make certain the child will not fall off the bed or strike hard objects during the seizure.

   6. Perform a brief but thorough physical examination with special reference to the neurologic system. Look for a Medic Alert tag or identification card on the patient's person, and inquire about a history of seizures.

   7. Monitor vital signs carefully.

   8. Draw blood for appropriate chemistries and save a clot tube for anticonvulsant levels. Make a Dextrostix determination and rule out or confirm hypoglycemia with administration of 50% D/W IV, 2 ml/kg stat.

   9. An IV infusion of 5% D in 0.25% saline is started.

   10. After adequate ventilation is maintained and cardiac status is stable, drug treatment should be started to arrest the seizures. Effective therapy depends on the following information:

      a. Is there a history of epilepsy and status epilepticus?

      b. Is this the initial episode, *or*

      c. Does it accompany a known metabolic epileptogenic disorder?

   11. If the patient is known to have epilepsy and is taking anticonvulsants, one may assume that he has not received them regularly, or the dose has been inadequate or ineffective, or there is a precipitating cause, often infection.

D. General treatment of status epilepticus

1. Diazepam

   a. Although still investigational in children under 12, IV diazepam (Valium) is the drug of choice in doses of 2 mg q3–5 min up to 10 mg. It is supplied as 5 mg/ml and given undiluted close to the infusion site; the IV line is flushed. In many children there will be a prompt and lasting effect from this regimen.

b. **Hypotension and respiratory arrest are known complications of this therapy, and pressor agents and assisted ventilation must be available.** If the episode is terminated, then recurs 5–15 min later, another course of up to 10 mg may be given IV. *IM administration of diazepam has no place in the management of status epilepticus.* Once the seizures are terminated, treatment with phenytoin sodium (Dilantin) should begin.

2. **Phenytoin sodium,** 8–10 mg/kg, is given slowly IV in saline (not to exceed 25 mg/min); in addition, 3 mg/kg is given IM. If successful, this is followed by daily maintenance of 5–8 mg/kg in 3 divided doses IM or PO.

   The major cause of death in status epilepticus is cardiac or respiratory failure closely following the IV use of a hypnotic agent. *An accurate flow sheet must be kept, with vital signs recorded q5–10 min and all medications listed.*

E. Specific therapy: febrile seizures

1. Begin fever control with tepid water sponging and rectal aspirin, 60 mg/year of age up to 600 mg.

2. Give 2–3 mg/kg phenobarbital IM. If this is not effective in 10 min, give an additional 2–3 mg/kg IM. A maximum dose of 120 mg is advised. If the patient has been taking phenobarbital prior to the seizure, adjust the stat dose so it will not exceed 5 mg/kg/day. The use of IV phenobarbital is not warranted.

3. As previously discussed, diazepam is also effective as an initial drug in seizures. However, since it is investigational in children and is a cardiorespiratory depressant, its use in febrile seizures, which are, by definition, self-limited, should be approached with caution. **It should not be used in conjunction with phenobarbital.** The dose is as listed in **D.1.a.**

4. **Paraldehyde** may be used initially or in conjunction with diazepam or phenobarbital. It is given by high rectal tube in a dose of 0.3 ml/kg, up to 6.0 ml. It is mixed with an equal volume of mineral oil injected in the tube, and 10 ml of normal saline is used to flush the mixture through the tube. The buttocks are then taped together.

5. Phenytoin sodium is not recommended for simple febrile seizures.

F. Specific therapy: hypoglycemia   See also Chaps. 5 and 14.

1. Provide the general supportive measures outlined previously.

2. Give 1 ml/kg IV of 50% D/W stat.

3. Then begin a drip of 15% D/W initially at a rate of 100 ml/kg/24 hr.

G. Specific therapy: hypertension

1. Provide the general supportive measures outlined previously.

2. Direct primary therapy to the hypertension (see Chap. 9, Sec. III).

3. Paraldehyde, or phenytoin sodium, or both may be used acutely via the routes and in the dosages outlined in **D.2** and **E.4.**

4. Phenobarbital may also be used, with the precautions already mentioned.

H. Specific therapy: meningitis or encephalitis

1. Provide the general supportive measures outlined previously.

2. In patients with meningitis, antibiotic therapy is paramount (see Chap. 15, Sec. **IV.M**).

3. Fluids administered by the IV route should be given with caution and with a careful watch for signs of cerebral edema, in appropriate ADH or centrally mediated cardiovascular responses. The management of cerebral edema is outlined in Table 2-6.

4. Paraldehyde, or phenytoin sodium, or both may be used acutely by the routes and in the dosages previously outlined. Phenobarbital may also be used, but **be alert for respiratory depression.**

I. **Specific therapy: hypocalcemia**

1. Provide the general supportive measures previously outlined.

2. Give 1.5 ml/kg IV of a 10% solution of calcium gluconate over a 20-min period. During this therapy, ECG monitoring is important.

3. After the 20-min infusion, start maintenance therapy with 10% calcium gluconate in a dosage of 15.0 ml/kg daily IV. The specific therapy for electrolyte imbalance is discussed in Chap. 8.

J. If these measures fail to control a seizure in a 1-hr period, general anesthesia must be considered. However, if ventilation and oxygenation are adequate, the risk associated with a prolonged seizure is reduced, and further efforts to end the seizure can be instituted in an orderly manner.

IV. THE UNCONSCIOUS PATIENT: A GENERAL PLAN OF MANAGEMENT

A. **Preliminary evaluation**

1. Evaluate vital signs and level of consciousness. If shock is present institute emergency measures (see Sec. **II.C**).

2. Briefly examine the patient for fractures or penetrating wounds (especially of the back).

3. Smell the patient's breath for signs of ketosis, alcohol, hydrocarbons, or other substances.

4. Check for Medic Alert tag, examine the contents of pockets, wallet, and so on.

B. **Initial measures**

1. Institute treatment for vital functions that are compromised.

2. Draw blood for CBC, type and crossmatching of whole blood, electrolytes, BUN, glucose, SGOT, LDH, bilirubin, arterial blood gases where indicated, prothrombin time, and toxicology screen. Save two tubes of clotted blood for further studies.

3. Start an IV infusion and administer 50% glucose at 1 ml/kg.

C. **History**

1. Be certain head trauma is ruled out by a *reliable* history. Obtain data on the chronology and progression of symptoms.

2. If the patient is unattended, assign a co-worker to contact the family by telephone.

D. **Physical examination**

1. Perform a detailed examination to include the respiratory pattern and pupillary, oculocephalic, and oculovestibular reflexes.

2. Note muscle tone and tendon reflexes.

   3. Look for needle marks in older children as evidence of self-administered drugs.

E. Have a co-worker start a flow sheet of vital signs and treatment.

F. Obtain a urine sample by catheter if necessary for routine urinalysis and ferric chloride determination to rule out salicylate and phenothiazine ingestion.

G. Reevaluate the patient and perform any other studies likely to yield a diagnosis.

V. CEREBRAL EDEMA (acute brain swellings)   Signs of transtentorial herniation, prolonged status epilepticus, rapidly increasing intracranial pressure, acute lead encephalopathy, and severe cerebral anoxia are present. Temporizing therapeutic measures should be undertaken until a mass lesion is ruled out. When a patient with a known posterior fossa lesion shows signs of rapidly increasing intracranial pressure, definitive surgical decompression or placement of a central ventricular drainage catheter is the preferred mode of therapy (see Table 2-6). Osmotic agents and fluid restriction are titered against

Table 2-6   Management of Cerebral Edema[a]

Stage of Treatment	Treatment	Dosage and Method
Initial, immediate treatment	Mannitol	20% (20 gm/100 ml IV) *or* 50-ml ampules containing 12.5 gm
Following initial treatment[b]	Mannitol with glycerol via nasogastric tube for chronic osmotic diuresis	1 gm/kg/q6h PO or PG
Acute and chronic[c]	Fluid restriction	0.5–0.67 maintenance fluids
	Hypothermia	Reduce core temperature to 89.6°F by cooling blankets. Use small doses chlorpromazine (0.1–0.2 mg/kg/dose) cautiously (hypotension) to avoid shivering.
	Hyperventilation	Mechanical ventilation used to lower $PaCO_2$ to about 20 mm Hg
Simultaneous acute administration	Dexamethasone (Decadron)	Day 1: 3 mg q6h IV
Continued treatment	Dexamethasone	Each subsequent day: 2 mg q6h IV or IM

[a] Careful attention must be directed to fluid and electrolyte balance in cerebral edema patients, and an indwelling catheter should be placed. Maintenance fluids should be provided.
[b] Fluids must be maintained to avoid iatrogenic dehydration due to osmotic diureses.
[c] Avoid noxious stimuli, e.g., distended bladder, excessive manipulation, examination.

serum osmolality, with an osmolality of about 295–300 mOsm as a goal. A surprisingly accurate estimation of the serum osmolality is possible using this formula:

$$mOsm = \left[\frac{mEq\ sodium}{Liter,\ serum}\right] + \frac{blood\ urea\ nitrogen\ (mg/100\ ml)}{2.8}$$
$$+ \frac{serum\ glucose\ (mg/100\ ml)}{18}$$

VI. CENTRAL NERVOUS SYSTEM RESUSCITATION AND PRESERVATION

A. "Standard" measures

1. **Fluid restriction**   Fluids are restricted to avoid hypertension due to volume overload.

2. **Restriction of noxious stimuli**   Endogenous release of adrenergic hormones with pain, bladder distention, and anxiety exacerbate raised intracranial pressure (ICP).

3. **Hypothermia**   If core temperature is lowered to 89.6°F using cooling blankets, CNS requirements for oxygen and glucose are reduced. Despite decreased central blood flow, the method appears to provide a net benefit to the patient following an anoxic insult, particularly if instituted within the first 8–12 hr after it occurs. Chlorpromazine in small doses (0.1–0.2 mg/kg/dose) helps to prevent shivering and central pooling.

4. **Hyperventilation**   Controlled ventilation is used to reduce the arterial CO_2 to 20 mm Hg, which by vasoconstriction reduces cerebral blood flow by as much as 50 percent. **A generous oxygen allowance is essential to avoid hypoxia in the face of the reduced flow.**

5. **Steroids**   Although of proved value only with focal ischemia or edema, steroids are widely used in postanoxic patients. No single dosage scheme has been established, but the following is one suggested schedule: Load with hydrocortisone, 1 mg/kg (infants) to 8 mg/kg (adolescents) and maintain with 0.25–0.50 mg/kg/24 hr in 4 divided doses IM or IV.

6. **Osmotic agents** are used to reduce ICP by diuresis and osmosis as well as by constricting the vascular compartment. Excessive use will trigger reflexes to raise blood pressure (see Sec. **V**).

B. Barbiturates
The use of high-dose barbiturates is still experimental. A few trials indicate beneficial effects on ICP, improved cerebral blood flow, containment of the toxic effects of cellular debris, and enhanced utilization of oxygen and glucose. No dosage regimen is recommended because data are lacking.

II. SEVERE ASTHMA ATTACK AND STATUS ASTHMATICUS
Status asthmaticus is a severe asthma attack that fails to respond to conservative therapy. In this condition, bronchospasm, mucosal edema, and excess mucous secretions combine to produce narrowing of airways, atelectasis, and impaired gas exchange.

An asthmatic attack is a frightening experience for both child and parents. Reassurance is extremely important during the acute stage. Agitation can be a manifestation of hypoxemia; even if it is not, the restless, anxious child can become exhausted from crying and purposeless resistance. Often, a parent at the bedside is the best sedative and can help the child to cooperate. (Obviously, an overly anxious parent may have the opposite effect.)

A. Evaluation

1. **History** includes age, duration of the attack, the course and severity of previous attacks, and a list, with doses, of all medications previously administered.

2. **Physical examination**

    a. **Ventilatory status** Assess the quality of breath sounds, the degree of dyspnea, and the extent of retractions.

    b. **Mental status** Look for somnolence, confusion, combativeness, or euphoria as signs of marked impairment of gas exchange.

    c. Determine vital signs frequently.

    d. Measure and follow pulsus paradoxicus, if present.

3. **Laboratory tests and ancillary studies** Infection is frequently the triggering event in status asthmaticus and is often hard to recognize clinically.

    a. **A complete blood count** should be obtained, if possible, before epinephrine is given; otherwise, the WBC count may be unreliable and difficult to interpret.

    b. BUN, sugar, and electrolytes.

    c. Urinalysis; repeated determinations of specific gravity.

    d. Nasopharyngeal studies include throat or sputum cultures (or both) and/or Gram stain.

    e. Chest roentgenograms can usually be delayed until initial therapy with adequate hydration has been provided; *radiologic evidence of pneumonia may not be demonstrable until adequate hydration has been given.* Oxygenation and appropriate supervision while the child is transported and the roentgenogram taken are extremely important.

    f. **Blood gases**

       (1) Venous pH and CO_2, obtained from free-flowing blood, without a tourniquet, will usually provide enough data to assess acid-base balance and ventilatory status at the outset of therapy.

       (2) Arterial blood gases should be measured and, in the severe attack in which the patient is unresponsive to therapy, the measurements should be repeated as necessary.

B. Therapy

1. **Oxygen Give humidified O_2 by nasal cannula or face mask to deliver 30–40% concentration in inspired air. A mist tent can be the most convenient way to deliver O_2 to the small, uncooperative child.** Patients with severe asthma attacks will uniformly present with *some* degree of hypoxemia secondary to perfusion of nonventilated, atelectatic segments of the lung (with right-to-left shunt as a result) and maldistribution of gas within the lung.

2. **Hydration and correction of acid-base abnormalities**

    a. Start an IV line with a scalp vein needle. In the absence of cardiac or renal impairment, it is safe to administer 20 ml/kg of 5% dextrose in 0.2 NS over 1–2 hr, to be followed by the same solution at 1½–2 times the maintenance rate. Fluids are essential to liquefy secretions and restore acid-base balance. Most severe episodes are accompanied by dehydration due to a combination of decreased intake, increased insensible water loss, and vomiting. Forcing fluids by mouth may be adequate in the mild or moderate attack, but will usually cause more vomiting in the patient with a severe attack.

b. Use sodium bicarbonate to maintain an arterial pH over 7.25; the initial dose may be calculated as 1–2 mEq/kg over 30 min or according to the following formula:

$$\text{mEq NaHCO}_3 = 0.3 \times \text{body weight (kg)} \times \text{base deficit (mEq/L)}$$

This dose can be repeated if necessary according to subsequent pH determinations.

c. The large majority of patients will present with a metabolic acidosis secondary to ketonemia of variable magnitude and accumulation of organic acid anions. If decreased alveolar ventilation supervenes, a rising $PaCO_2$ is a potential complication of $NaHCO_3$ use (see *Pediatrics* 42:238, 1968).

d. The use of tromethamine (THAM) is not recommended because of the hazard of respiratory depression.

3. Drugs

a. Bronchodilators   See also **B.2**, p. 476.

(1) Epinephrine

(a) Give 0.01 ml/kg SQ (maximum, 0.5 ml). If a beneficial effect is obtained, the injection can be repeated once or twice at 20-min intervals. When complete clearing of the attack is achieved, give 0.005 ml/kg of Sus-Phrine (epinephrine in a 1:200 dilution in thioglycollate suspension) 20 min after the last dose for longer-lasting action. If the patient is still in distress after 3 doses, or actually deteriorates after epinephrine administration, **do not give further doses. The excessive or inappropriate use of epinephrine can induce serious cardiac arrhythmias and cause increased restlessness and anxiety.**

(b) Hypoxemia and acidosis, tenacious mucous plugs blocking the airways, and pneumothorax are among the causes of lack of bronchomotor responses to epinephrine. Correction of acidosis may restore the response to epinephrine.

(2) Isoproterenol

(a) Use 0.5 ml of a 1:200 preparation and add 2 ml of saline (1:1000 dilution). Deliver via aerosol using a Bird respirator, Mark 8, for intermittent positive pressure breathing (IPPB) connected to a source of 100% O_2 (see Chap. 20, Sec. II). Give IPPB for 5–10 min with frequent pauses and repeat q2–4h as required. It can be alternated with nebulized saline aerosol to loosen secretions further and reduce airway resistance.

(b) Isoproterenol is a potent stimulator of beta receptors. It is frequently effective in the epinephrine-resistant patient. The age and cooperation of the child are important for its adequate administration.

(c) The use of IPPB with isoproterenol requires careful monitoring for the onset of serious cardiac arrhythmias.

(3) Isoetharine (Bronkosol)

(a) Administer as in **(2).(a)**, but use 0.5 ml of respiratory saline. IPPB administration is not more helpful than aerosol administration and may trigger bronchoconstricting reflexes.

(b) Preferentially stimulates beta-2 receptors and thus has less arrhythmia potential than isoproterenol. It should not be administered within 15 min of administration of other adrenergic drugs (epinephrine).

(4) Aminophylline

(a) Give 5–7 mg/kg in 30–50 ml of IV fluids to run over 20 min. The dose can be repeated q6–8h, but the total daily dose should not exceed 20 mg/kg. If serum aminophylline levels can be determined, this should be done in patients who require high doses of the drug, since there is substantial variation in absorption and excretion from patient to patient.

(b) When the bronchomotor response to epinephrine is inadequate, parenteral aminophylline may be effective in reducing the high airway resistance. Before administration, ascertain carefully the total amount of xanthine derivatives received in the previous 12 hr. If previous administration has been excessive (more than 8 mg/kg/12 hr) or in the presence of such symptoms as excitation, tremor, frequent vomiting, hematemesis, and convulsions, further use of aminophylline should be carefully considered or postponed for 6 hr after the last administered dose. **Rapid IV infusion of aminophylline can lead to cardiac arrhythmias, hypotension, and death.**

b. Expectorants (See Chap. 20, Sec. **II.D.**) IV **sodium iodide**, 25 mg/kg day, may be useful in loosening secretions and promoting cough. Administration may be distributed evenly over 24 hr, or it can be given in 1 dose over 4 hr.

c. Corticosteroids

(1) If after the preceding measures the patient shows no improvement or actually deteriorates, give hydrocortisone IV, 5–10 mg/kg q6h, by IV push or drip.

(2) Corticosteroids should be started early in the attack if the child is on long-term corticosteroid therapy or has a previous history of severe attacks leading to acute respiratory failure, or a complicated hospital course, or both.

d. Antibiotics Consider their use in the presence of

(1) Significant fever

(2) Elevated WBC (15,000 cu mm) and left shift obtained prior to epinephrine administration

(3) A sputum stain showing purulent secretions *or*

(4) Radiologic evidence of pneumonia (often difficult to differentiate from atelectasis)

e. Sedatives Chloral hydrate, 15–40 mg/kg, may be given PO or PR q6–8h as required. Opiates and barbiturates should be avoided because of the danger of respiratory depression and arrest. Other tranquilizers may pose a similar risk.

4. Physical therapy See also Chap. 20, Sec. I.C.

   a. Encourage the patient to cough at regular intervals to help in the removal of secretions. Percussion of the chest will improve the efficiency of coughing, especially after bronchodilators have produced their effect.

   b. Give breathing instructions to teach the patient how to perform abdominal inspirations, followed with deeper inspirations, and finally how to expire the breath through pursed lips. These instructions are often beneficial if the child is old enough to follow them.

   c. Sitting in an upright position will facilitate diaphragmatic excursions.

   d. When bronchospasm has ceased, therapy consisting of postural drainage, percussion, and vibration is recommended.

III. RESPIRATORY FAILURE IN STATUS ASTHMATICUS Despite appropriate therapy, respiratory failure can develop in a few children and lead to cardiorespiratory arrest and death. The management of the patient in respiratory failure requires a team approach, specialized equipment, and intensive care facilities, which must be arranged for in advance by the child's physician so that this therapy can be instituted electively before coma and arrest occur.

A. Diagnosis

   1. The clinical criteria for diagnosis of respiratory failure (*Pediatrics* 42: 238, 1968) are

     a. Decreased or absent inspiratory breath sounds.

     b. Severe inspiratory retractions and use of accessory muscles.

     c. Depressed level of consciousness and response to pain.

     d. Generalized muscle weakness.

     e. Cyanosis in 40% O_2.

     f. Agitation secondary to hypoxia.

   2. When three or more of these criteria are present, the partial pressure of CO_2 in arterial blood ($PaCO_2$) is usually ≥ 65 mm Hg. Some children who meet these criteria still respond well to vigorous medical therapy over one to several hours. When a rising $PaCO_2$ and absence of inspiratory breath sounds appear in a child who is becoming fatigued, the need for more aggressive intervention has to be considered.

   3. When interpreting arterial blood gases in asthmatic patients, note the progression seen, as highlighted in Table 2-7. Note that in stage III, only

ble 2-7 Arterial Blood Gases in Asthma

age	Degree of Obstruction	PaO_2	$PaCO_2$	pH	Acid-Base Status
I	+	Normal	↓	Alkaline	Respiratory alkalosis
I	++	↓	↓	Alkaline	Respiratory alkalosis
I	+++	↓↓	Normal	Normal	Normal
	++++	↓↓↓	↑	Acidosis	Respiratory acidosis

odified from J. S. Bacles, *Med. Clin. North Am.* 54:493, 1970.

hypoxia indicates the severity. It is critical to know the concentration of oxygen being inspired at the time the test is made.

B. Monitoring

1. A **central venous line** should be started.

2. Establish an **"arterial line"** by percutaneous insertion of a plastic cannula into the radial artery (or through direct visualization of the artery by cutdown). Then connect the cannula to a T connector (Abbott Laboratories No. 4612) and then to a constant infusion pump with continuous flushing of a dilute heparin solution of 1 U/ml of normal saline at 3 ml/hr. This has to be handled using a strict aseptic technique. The arterial cannula is used in direct transducing of systemic pressure. Repeated specimens of arterial blood can be drawn as necessary for evaluation of ventilatory and acid-base status.

3. **Record heart rate, blood pressure, and temperature** q30 min–1h. Connect a cardiac monitor to the patient.

4. **Intake and output**   Place a three-way lumen Foley catheter and provide catheter sterile care. Measure hourly urine output.

5. **Respirator variables**   Rate, volumes, positive end-expiratory pressure (PEEP), dead space.

6. **Inspired O2 concentration** (with an air O_2 analyzer).

7. **Chest x-ray films** as indicated clinically and by the arterial blood gases.

8. Tracheobronchial sterile **aspirates** should be smeared for Wright and Gram stains and sent for culture.

9. An intensive care **flow sheet** should be used for proper recording and monitoring of all variables involved.

C. Therapy   At present, there are two ways of aiding the child in status asthmaticus and respiratory failure:

1. **Intravenous isoproterenol**   The use of this drug has been reported as a successful alternative to artificial ventilation, with lesser risks than with the latter. **This form of therapy** *should not be attempted* **unless proper monitoring is used and methods of dealing with the potential complications are available.**

2. **Mechanical ventilation**   The primary aim of mechanical ventilation is to correct acidosis and hypoxemia, provide an easier way of draining tracheobronchial secretions, and gain time for medications to take effect.

   a. Induction on controlled ventilation

      (1) Use 100% O_2 by bag and mask with manually assisted ventilation.

      (2) Aspirate upper airway secretions (10–15 sec).

      (3) Aspirate the stomach with a large-size catheter (14F in an infant, 16–18F in an older child).

      (4) **Myoneural blockade**   After obtaining qualified help from personnel skilled in intubation procedures, provide myoneural blockade. The following drugs can be used IV:

         (a) Tubocurarine at 0.6 mg/kg

         (b) Succinylcholine by slow infusion of 10–50 mg (it has a very short duration of action)

         (c) Gallamine in a dose not to exceed 1.0 mg/kg

(5) Intubate the child under direct laryngoscopy. It is best to use a Smith Porter Ivory Tube (available with a prestretched cuff in sizes over 6 mm in diameter). A clear polyvinylchloride endotracheal tube can be used satisfactorily in its place. Under emergency conditions or with lack of skill, an orotracheal tube can be placed initially. It is best if a skilled person places the nasotracheal tube. **Leaving an orotracheal tube in place is dangerous,** since mouth and tongue motion can dislodge the tube into the esophagus, provoking vomiting. The associated aspiration and hypoxia can lead to rapid demise. The nasotracheal tube is "splinted" in place by the nasopharynx and is much better tolerated.

(6) Ventilate with 100% O_2.

(7) Aspirate tracheobronchial secretions.

(8) Listen to both sides of the chest for breath sounds, and change tube position if indicated.

(9) Prepare the skin with tincture of benzoin and fix tube with waterproof adhesive tape.

(10) Use a chest x-ray film to check the tube position and for diagnosis of pneumothorax.

b. Maintenance of controlled ventilation See also Chap. 20, Sec. **III.**

(1) A volume preset ventilator (Emerson, Engstrom, Bennett MA 1) should be used, since a tidal volume will be delivered to the patient irrespective of airway resistance or compliance.

(2) Set inspiratory and expiratory rates. Provide a prolonged expiratory time. Tidal volume is usually calculated as 7–10 ml/kg. Initial respiratory rate should be set between 15–40/min, according to the age of the child. One must often rely on visual and auscultatory evidence of ventilation during the initial adjustments and readjust the tidal volume and respiratory rate according to serial arterial gases and pH determinations. Multiple variables such as the patient's temperature and arterial pH and the characteristics of each ventilator make the management of the patient a complicated task, involving all the principles of intensive care.

(3) In a patient with diffuse alveolar collapse, PEEP may permit reduction of inspired O_2 concentration (FIO_2) to lower levels by substantially improving arterial oxygenation. A PEEP of 3–10 cm H_2O can be used.

(4) **Humidification** of the inspired air at the proper temperature is essential. If any air leak is present around the tube, the ambient air should also be well humidified to prevent development of thick, tenacious secretions that may suddenly block the tube. If a cuffed endotracheal tube is used, do not inflate the cuff above pressures of 20 mm Hg, to avoid pressure necrosis of the tracheal wall.

(5) When arterial blood gases have stabilized, start instillations of sterile saline (2–5 ml) in the tracheal airway at hourly intervals, followed by changes in chest position, percussion, vibration, and then sterile aspiration. The patient should not remain off the respirator for more than 15–20 sec.

(6) Institute manual hyperventilation (5–10 breaths) q30 min to pre vent atelectasis, and use an "artificial coughing" technique t help the drainage of secretions.

(7) Provide **continuous myoneural blockade** with

    (a) Tubocurarine, 1 mg/kg q30 min or as required, *or*

    (b) Gallamine, 1 mg/kg q30 min or when needed.

    (c) Morphine, 0.2 mg/kg (2–10 mg IV). Monitor for hypotension.

(8) If further **sedation** is considered necessary, give

    (a) Diazepam, 0.1–0.2 mg/kg IV prn, *or*

    (b) Pentobarbital, 1 mg/kg IV.

(9) Hydration is continued at 2–2½ times the maintenance rat **Watch the CVP carefully.** Patients on mechanical ventilation ma have increased ADH secretion and impaired fluid output.

(10) Continue the use of **aminophylline, sodium iodide,** and **cortico steroids** as discussed in **V.B,** p. 48. Isoproterenol via IPPB ca also be used after stabilization and initial improvement in ve tilatory and general status.

(11) **Acid-base balance** Effective artificial ventilation will usuall reduce the $PaCO_2$ and increase the pH to satisfactory levels. Th may not happen if there is a strong metabolic component to th acidosis. Sodium bicarbonate in the dosages discussed in Se **VII.B.2.b–d** should then be used. If the response is inadequate if hypernatremia is present, THAM can be used (1–2 mEq/kg IV infusion). With mechanical support of ventilation, the haza of respiratory depression is avoided.

c. Discontinuance of mechanical ventilation

(1) The child who becomes able to maintain stable arterial blood gas at 30–40% O_2 in inspired air, is usually ready to be switched from controlled to an assist mode, in which the patient can trigger t ventilator. Discontinue the muscle relaxant, allow spontaneo respirations to recur, and then set the ventilator to "Assist."

(2) If, after 1–4 hr of assisted ventilation, the $PaCO_2$ remains under mm Hg and the PaO_2 remains over 100 mm Hg at 50% or less FI(a program for discontinuing ventilation in stages can usually initiated. Progressively larger intervals without mechanical ve tilation, starting with 5–10 min and with arterial blood gases termined at the end, are carried out. During those periods t patient is breathing 40–60% humidified O_2 through a Briggs ada tor.

(3) Once the patient can tolerate spontaneous ventilation for sever hours, consider removing the tracheal airway. The endotrache tube is removed after careful suctioning.

(4) Then place the patient in a high-humidity, oxygen-enriched mosphere.

(5) Provide adequate physical therapy during the recovery phase.

(6) Start oral fluids and gradually increase as the patient's conditi allows.

(7) If aminophylline, sodium iodide, corticosteroids, and antibiotics are being used, change from parenteral to oral administration.

(8) Discontinue IV fluids after oral intake is satisfactory.

(9) Remove the arterial line after the patient is extubated and arterial gases are stable.

IX. COLD INJURY[1] may be divided into generalized injury (exposure, or accidental hypothermia) and local injury (frostbite, immersion foot).

A. In **accidental hypothermia (exposure)** the body temperature is less than 95°F. The onset is insidious, with abnormal behavior, apathy, clumsiness, weakness, and cessation of shivering. Progression to profound depression, with no audible heart sounds, no respiratory effort, and dilated pupils, may occur.

1. General measures   In the moribund patient, start artificial ventilation and cardiac massage. A central venous cutdown should be placed. **All patients should be placed on an ECG monitor** because of the high risk of arrhythmias during rewarming. BUN, electrolytes, and pH should be determined and monitored during the course of therapy.

2. Rewarming should be started as soon as possible. Several methods are possible:

   a. External rewarming

   (1) Passive (slow method)   Place the patient in a warm room and cover him with blankets.

   (2) Active (rapid method)   Apply external heat to the body surface, either with a hyperthermic blanket or a warm water bath, at a temperature of 98.6°F.

   b. Core rewarming

   (1) Extracorporeal rewarming is by pump oxygenator or artificial kidney. This is rapid and avoids the problem of rewarming shock. Although it is theoretically the best method when it can be done immediately, it has the major disadvantage of the delay involved in assembling the necessary medical-surgical team.

   (2) Warm peritoneal dialysis has been used, but this is a slow method of rewarming.

3. Complications

   a. Rewarming shock is caused by peripheral vasodilation associated with external rewarming. It is treated as hypovolemic shock (see Sec. **II.C**).

   b. Arrhythmias are a frequently encountered hazard (Chap. 10, Sec. I). Bradycardia, different types of heart block, "U waves," and ventricular arrhythmias may occur. Treat with external cardiac massage. If ventricular fibrillation occurs, *defibrillation cannot be effective until the patient's temperature is at least 82.4°F.*

   c. Acidosis and electrolyte imbalance should be treated appropriately (see Chap. 8, Sec. **II**).

The discussion in this section does not apply to the newborn.

  d. Convulsions may occur and should be treated appropriately (see Sec. III.C-J, pp. 41–43. Give 50% D/W, 1 ml/kg IV, stat because of the danger of hypoglycemia.

  e. Frostbite may be present (see **B**).

B. Frostbite and immersion foot frostbite result from exposure to extremely cold temperatures, usually for a prolonged time. Immersion foot occurs in the presence of moisture and at higher temperatures than frostbite. The pathologic changes of immersion foot are similar to but less severe than those of frostbite.

  1. Rewarming The method of choice for frostbite is rapid rewarming in hot water (104–111°F) for about 20 min. **Higher temperatures cause more injury** and must be avoided. Meperidine, 0.5–1.0 mg/kg IM (maximum, 100 mg), may be administered for pain.

  2. Avoid rubbing the skin, since it will increase tissue damage. The patient should also avoid smoking, because it causes peripheral vasoconstriction.

  3. Tetanus toxoid or antitoxin should be given (see Chap. 15, Sec. **IV.D**).

  4. Local care The open method with a protective cradle is recommended. Strict asepsis (gown and mask) is advised. Gentle debridement should be done. Bullae should not be ruptured.

  5. Antibiotics should be used if evidence of infection arises (see Chap. 15).

  6. Physical therapy is recommended during convalescence.

  7. Amputation should be delayed until optimal healing has occurred, which may be as long as 2 or 3 months.

  8. Malnutrition is often present, and a high-protein diet may be beneficial.

X. HEAT STROKE[2] Heat stroke is a failure of the usual heat-dissipating mechanisms. The three cardinal signs are hyperpyrexia, CNS disturbance, and hot and dry skin.

  A. Hyperpyrexia Remove the patient's clothing and place the patient in ice water, with vigorous massaging of the extremities to promote vasodilation. Check rectal temperature q10 min, and discontinue the bath when the temperature falls to 100°F. Promethazine, 0.5 mg/kg IM, may be used to facilitate temperature loss, but hypotension may occur.

  B. The general status of the patient should be carefully monitored. If shock develops, a central venous line should be placed, and the shock should be treated (see Sec. **II.C**). BUN and electrolytes should be determined and monitored and fluid losses replaced (see Chap. 8).

  C. Urine output should be monitored closely. Acute tubular necrosis may accompany heat stroke.

  D. Convulsions may occur and should be treated (see Sec. **III.D–J**).

  E. The ECG should be monitored and arrhythmias treated.

  F. Liver function studies should be made, since liver damage may occur, leading to liver failure (see Chap. 11).

  G. Watch for bleeding, which may arise because of increased capillary fragility and decreased prothrombin levels. DIC may develop and should be treated (see Chap. 17, Sec. **V.B**).

[2] The discussion in this section does not apply to newborns (see Chap. 5).

XI. BURNS Extra fluid loss through the skin due to the denuded areas in burns is minimized by the use of wet dressings. Urinary output is diminished because of an increased release of ADH, and low renal perfusion secondary to low plasma volume. Because of sequestered plasma at the burn sites, the severely burned patient has an "internal loss" of fluid.

A. Evaluation The severity of the burn will depend on its depth and the percentage of the surface area involved.

    1. First-degree burn Vasodilation occurs. There is very little edema.

    2. Second-degree burn Capillary damage is present. Fluid may accumulate beneath the skin (blisters, bullae). Some protein loss occurs in blistered areas.

    3. Third-degree burn The entire skin is destroyed, and capillaries are thrombosed; edema is maximal at 48 hr after the burn, but may last for weeks.

    4. The estimate of surface area burned is made by the "rule of nines" in the patient who is more than 12 years old. For the younger child, the rule must be modified and a greater area attributed to the head and face.

B. Therapy

    1. Day 1 Because of hypovolemia, an isotonic solution should be used to expand the extracellular fluid volume. Although isotonic saline could be used, the chloride load may cause hyperchloremic acidosis, and thus Ringer's lactate is preferred. A colloid solution (e.g., plasma or whole blood) may be substituted, but Ringer's lactate is more readily available.

        a. Replacement volume

        2 ml Ringer's lactate × % burn surface × weight (kg)

        b. Maintenance Give 1500–2000 ml/M²/24 hr.

        c. Precautions

            (1) If the burn area involves more than 50% of the body surface, the calculation for replacement assumes only 50%.

            (2) The first 24 hr of fluid is given in two portions: the first 8 hr **after the burn occurred** constitutes the **first** segment, and the remainder is given over the next 16 hr.

        d. Examination of the urine is crucial; volume and concentration should be monitored hourly; urine Na^+ and K^+ are also useful. In most cases, diminished urine volume is due to low renal perfusion, but with major burns **acute renal failure** is possible and will manifest itself as a low urine osmolality and a high urinary Na^+ content (Chap. 9, Sec. **IV**).

    2. Day 2 The patient should receive full maintenance fluid and two-thirds of the replacement volume calculated in the first 24 hr. The rate of infusion can be even over the day if the patient has a steady urine output and normal CVP.

    3. Day 3 Only maintenance fluid should be given, and careful monitoring of vital signs is mandatory. There usually is a diuretic phase as well as absorption of pooled fluid into the circulation: Observe for signs of pulmonary edema and for possible hyponatremia.

XII. DROWNING

A. Physiologic effects Most submersions are fatal after 2–3 min; by the third minute of submersion, respiratory arrest occurs and muscle tone disappears. During the fourth minute there is cardiac arrest. Interruption of submersion before the third minute usually will result in spontaneous resuscitation. Animal models clearly demonstrate the differences between freshwater and saltwater submersion, but the differences are not so readily applicable to humans. Note that with significant hypothermia due to cold water accidents, excellent CNS recoveries have been reported even after prolonged submersion.

1. In the animal model, **freshwater drowning** will result in hemodilution massive hemolysis (leading to hyperkalemia, hemorrhage pneumonitis and hemoglobinuria), and ventricular fibrillation.

2. In **saltwater drowning,** animal studies demonstrate hemoconcentration hypernatremia, and pulmonary edema due to the local osmotic effect of the high Na^+ aspirate in the lung.

3. When humans are submersed in either salt or fresh water, the change observed in the animal model, with the exception of pulmonary complications, are *not* so apparent. The electrolyte and hematocrit imbalance are *not* easily predictable, and close monitoring of *both* is necessary Seldom is the water free of debris and bacteria, so that antibiotics and corticosteroids must be added to the therapy. In an effort to minimize O consumption, hypothermia may also be indicated.

4. The main cause of death is the pulmonary damage and edema. Thus, it is important not to overload the patient with fluids, and CVP and urinary output should be monitored, along with vital signs.

B. Therapy

1. Initial therapy

a. **Respiratory support** Clear the airway and administer **O_2** by mask or if not available, by mouth-to-mouth breathing.

b. **Cardiac support** Give closed chest massage if necessary. An occasional case of auricular or ventricular fibrillation has been reported.

2. Subsequent therapy

a. Corticosteroids (see Chap. 20).

b. Antibiotics (see Chap. 15).

c. **IV fluids** In both saltwater and freshwater drowning, some hemoconcentration occurs. In the former there is a tendency toward hypernatremia; in the latter there may be hyperkalemia (from hemolysis).

3. Maintenance therapy Because of the danger of pulmonary edema, initial maintenance is kept at insensible losses ($\sim$ 800 ml/M^2/day) until it is clear that edema is *not* a problem or until there is a good urine output (ml/kg/hr).

4. Treatment for shock 10–20 ml/kg of plasma over 1 hr (use low Na plasma for saltwater submersion and low K^+ for freshwater submersion If plasma is unavailable, dextran in saline is used for freshwater drowning and dextran with 5% D/W for saltwater drowning. Packed cell may also be used in freshwater drowning to combat shock.

XIII. CHILD ABUSE AND NEGLECT

A. Objectives and problems

1. Recognition or suspicion of child abuse should be met by a long-range therapeutic plan, with attention to the establishment of supportive relationships. The goal of the initial process of management is protection of the child while the parents are helped through an acute family crisis.

2. Problems include parental personalities in which denial and projection serve as the principal modes of ego defense; the family's anxious confusion in facing an array of clinical specialty services and social agencies, often working in an uncoordinated manner to protect the child; and the exigencies of poverty, including mistrust of community institutions, racism, unemployment, and drugs. The clinical team may be frustrated by missed appointments, angry parental confrontations, time-consuming contacts with outside agencies, and conflicts among the responsible personnel stemming from the emotions brought forth by prolonged contact with disturbed families.

B. Diagnosis

1. Clinical findings   Suspect child abuse or neglect whenever a child presents with any one or a combination of the following clinical findings:

   a. Fractures that a simple fall would be unlikely to produce.

   (1) Different stages of healing in multiple fractures.

   (2) Metaphyseal fractures.

   (3) Epiphyseal separations.

   (4) Subperiosteal calcifications.

   b. Subdural hematomas.

   c. Multiple ecchymoses that may resemble purpura.

   d. Intestinal injuries, ruptured viscera.

   e. Burns of any kind, especially in infants.

   f. Poor hygiene.

   g. Inadequate gain in weight or height.

   h. Marked passivity and watchfulness, fearful expression.

   i. Bizarre accidents, multiple ingestions.

   j. Malnutrition.

   k. Developmental retardation.

2. Some frequent behavior patterns of abusive or negligent parents   They may

   a. Use severe punishments.

   b. Give a past history of abuse in their own upbringing.

   c. Display suspicion and antagonism toward others.

   d. Lead isolated lives.

   e. Make pleas for help in indirect ways, such as

   (1) Bringing the child to the clinician or emergency room for no specific reason or for repeated minor medical complaints.

(2) Insisting that the child be admitted to the hospital for a minor illness and expressing anxiety if he is not.

f. Leaning on their children for support, comfort, and reassurance.

g. Sampling a variety of health care facilities without establishing a relationship with any particular one.

h. Displaying poor impulse control or an openly hostile attitude toward the child.

i. Being unable to carry out consistent discipline, yet threatening or punishing the child if he does not live up to an expectation or whim.

j. Understanding little about normal child development and seeming unable to integrate the information offered about it.

C. Axioms of management

1. Once child abuse or neglect is diagnosed, the child is at great risk of reinjury or continued neglect.

2. Protection of the child must be a principal goal of initial intervention, but this protection must go hand in hand with a program to help the family through its crisis.

3. Traditional social casework cannot in itself protect an abused or neglected child in the dangerous environment. Medical follow-up is also necessary, and day-to-day contact with a child care center may help significantly to encourage the child's healthy development.

4. If the child is reinjured and medical attention is sought anew, the parents are likely to seek care in a facility other than that where the diagnosis was originally made or suspected.

5. Public social service agencies in both urban and rural areas do not have sufficient well-trained personnel, and the quality of administration and supervision in these agencies often is not high. These factors militate against their operating effectively in isolation from other social agencies. Simply reporting a case to the public agency mandated to receive child abuse case reports may not be sufficient to protect an abused or neglected child or to help the family.

6. Early attempts by the hospital staff to identify the agent of an injury or to determine if neglect was "intentional" may be ill advised. There is rarely a need to establish *precisely* who it was who injured or neglected a child and why. Clinical experience has shown that it is more important to establish confidence and trust in the hospital personnel. This may be jeopardized by overly aggressive attempts to ferret out the specific circumstances of the injury. On the other hand, lack of evidence for parental "guilt" is not a criterion for discharge of the patient.

7. If there is evidence that the child is at major risk, hospitalization to allow time for assessment of the home setting is appropriate. Children under the age of 3 are frequent victims; infants under 1 year of age with severe malnutrition or failure to thrive, fractures, burns, or bruises of any kind are especially at risk of reinjury or neglect. Prompt and effective intervention is vital to assure their survival.

D. Assessment of the child and family

1. An adequate general medical history and physical examination are necessary at the time the child is brought to the clinician. Photographs and a skeletal survey are made when indicated by the child's condition and the clinician's impression.

2. If a social worker is available, he or she is called promptly at the time of the family's visit. The physician should introduce the social worker as someone interested and able to help them through this difficult period. After the interview the physician and social worker should confer.

3. **Interviewing the parents**

   a. In the initial interviews and in subsequent contacts, **no direct or indirect attempt to draw out a confession from the parent is made.** Denial is a prominent ego defense in virtually all abusive parents. Their often bizarre stories of how their child was injured should not be taken as intentional falsifications. These odd accounts frequently indicate a parent's profound distress in acknowledging infliction of an injury or failure to protect a child. In the face of such a threatening reality, they repress it and may offer a blatant fabrication, which one must accept for the moment.

   b. One should not accuse the parent or he or she may use more primitive defenses than denial; i.e., a desperate resistance to talking about the problem at all, angry outbursts directed at the interviewer or hospital, and threats to take the child home immediately. This in turn may threaten information gathering and continuing helpful professional relationships and may endanger the child.

   c. A good interview technique allows parent and child to maintain the integrity of ego and family. It is appropriate to emphasize the child's need for hospital care and protection from harm. At this time, the clinician should demonstrate concern and the ability to help the *parents'* distress as well.

4. In explaining the legal obligation to report the case, the clinician's compassion and honesty will go far to allay the family's anxiety.

5. The opportunity to observe parent-child interaction and the child's physical and psychological milestones, which might lead to insight into the familial causes of a child's injury or neglect, may not be available to a clinician in an ambulatory setting.

XIV. DRUG ABUSE (See also *Med. Lett. Drugs Ther.* 9(3):1, 1977.)

A. Children and adolescents are seen by a physician or nurse for a variety of drug-related problems.

1. The state of consciousness may be altered as a result of drug overdose or unexpected effect.

2. The child may be experiencing acute anxiety or a panic reaction.

3. Secondary medical problems such as hepatitis or pneumonia may be present.

4. Parents may request examination for real or imagined drug effects.

B. **Initial approach** Young people using drugs usually enter an emergency room as a last resort. The clinician then has an unusual opportunity not only to give immediate help but also to initiate long-term care.

1. Approach the patient in a nonthreatening manner.

2. Make him or her comfortable in a chair or stretcher.

    3. Remove all unnecessary personnel from the room.

    4. Avoid restraints.

    5. Demonstrate that your knowledge, concern, and experience can be of help.

    6. Keep parenteral injections and blood drawing to a minimum.

C. Drug identification

    1. See Table 2-8.

    2. If necessary, send blood, urine, and gastric contents for toxicologic analysis.

    3. Correlate symptoms with the known effects of commonly abused drugs (see Table 3-1).

D. Therapy in specific ingestions See also Chap. 3, Sec. **II.**

    1. Barbiturates

      a. Maintain an adequate oral airway with frequent suctioning. If necessary, intubate via endotracheal or nasotracheal tube.

      b. Give humidified O_2 as needed via catheter at 4–6 L/min or via oronasal mask at 2–4 L/min.

      c. Maintain blood pressure (see Sec. **II.C**).

      d. Introduce a central venous catheter if necessary.

      e. If the patient is alert, induce emesis with 15 ml syrup of ipecac. If the patient is obtunded, endotracheal intubation may be required, using

Table 2-8 Glossary of Slang Terms for Various Drugs

Marihuana	Opiates	Cocaine	Amphetamines	Barbiturates	LSD
Pot	Dollies	Bernice	Bennies	Barbs	Acid
Hash	H	Coke	Blue Devils	Candy	A
Tea	Harry	Corine	Blue Velvet	Downers	D
Weed	Horse	Dust	Bombido	Goofballs	Blue Cheer
Flower	Joy-powder	Flake	Cartwheels	Nimby	Cube
Grass	Miss Emma	Gold Dust	Crossroads	Peanuts	Green Flats
Hay	Scag	Star Dust	Co-pilots	Pinks	Pink Swirls
Hemp	Gum	Cecil	Dexies	Rainbows	
Mary Jane	Morph	Girl	Footballs	Red Devils	
Griefo	Dope		Hearts	Seggy	
Reeker	Junk		Oranges	Tooies	
Rope	Thing		Peaches	Yellowjackets	
Herb	Smack		Roses	Blue Bullets	
			Truck Drivers		
			Wakeups		
			Whites		
			Browns		
			Speed		
			Uppers		

a cuffed endotracheal tube to prevent aspiration. Follow intubation with gastric lavage. Before removing the gastric tube, instill activated charcoal, 1 gm/kg/dose.

f. Avoid analeptic drugs.

g. Keep the patient's head down by elevating the feet to prevent aspiration.

h. Treat hypothermia, if present, with blankets.

i. Hemodialysis or peritoneal dialysis may be necessary.

2. Ethyl alcohol   See also Chap. 24.

a. Remove unabsorbed alcohol by gastric lavage or emesis.

b. If intoxication is severe (blood alcohol 0.3–0.5%), treat for aspiration hazard, airway obstruction, hypotension, and hypothermia, as in severe barbiturate intoxications.

c. Determine blood glucose. If hypoglycemic, give 50% dextrose, 1.0 ml/kg/dose, diluted ½–⅓ in an IV solution.

d. Check the ECG for evidence of cardiomyopathy.

e. Keep the urine slightly alkaline with $NaHCO_3$, 1–2 mEq/kg/dose IV, or 2 gm/250 ml water PO q2h.

f. Avoid administration of excess fluids.

g. Avoid depressant drugs.

h. Hemodialysis is indicated if the blood level is above 0.5%.

3. Amphetamines

a. Emesis with ipecac is generally preferred to gastric lavage in the alert patient.

b. For patients with mild intoxication or acute panic reactions, give emotional support.

c. Support respirations and blood pressure.

d. Acidify the urine with ammonium chloride, 2–6 gm daily PO.

e. Control convulsions with

(1) Paraldehyde, 0.3 ml/kg PR, diluted in an equal volume of mineral oil.

(2) Phenytoin sodium, 2–5 mg/kg/dose, slowly IV (50 mg/min). Repeat ½ dose after 30 min if seizures continue. Do not exceed 400 mg/day.

(3) Barbiturates should be used cautiously because of the already depressed state that may be present in amphetamine overdose.

f. Treat hypertension with phentolamine (Regitine), 5 mg slowly IV, or phentolamine hydrochloride, 5 mg/kg daily PO in 4 divided doses.

4. LSD (lysergic acid diethylamide)

a. Induce emesis.

b. Give emotional support. This may involve listening to the patient converse for hours, a procedure known as "talking down."

c. For young adults, use diazepam, 5–10 mg PO or slowly IV, for acute anxiety reactions. **Do not leave the patient alone.**

  d. Chlorpromazine may be helpful but is contraindicated if adulterants are present, such as strychnine, belladonna, phencyclidine, or dimethoxy-methylamphetamine ("STP").

  e. Long-term follow-up is important, since "flashbacks" and acute psychotic breaks have been known to occur after apparent recovery from the acute effects of LSD ingestion.

5. Glue sniffing

  a. Give emotional support in the emergency and at the time of follow-up visits.

  b. Obtain blood for liver and kidney function tests.

6. Narcotics

  a. If taken orally, induce emesis or lavage.

  b. Maintain respirations, airway, and blood pressure as in patients with barbiturate overdose (see **1**).

  c. Antagonize narcotic effects with naloxone hydrochloride (Narcan) 0.01 mg/kg/dose for children and 0.4 mg/dose for adults. If there is no response, repeat the dose after 3 min. If there is still no response narcotic overdose may not have occurred. If the patient responds to the antagonist, then relapses, give additional doses as necessary to relieve symptoms.

7. Glutethimide (Doriden) Treatment is substantially the same as for barbiturate intoxication (see **1**).

8. Phencyclidine (Angel Dust) See Chap. 3, Sec. **V**, for discussion.

E. Medical and psychiatric follow-up Young people abusing drugs are in need of ongoing emotional and medical support, which can be given by a physician alone or in collaboration with a school guidance counselor, clergyman, or social worker.

  1. The physician should know that young patients often fail to keep appointments, yet demand that the counselor be available.

  2. Common behavior characteristics of children who abuse drugs are

    a. An unrealistic sense of trust and demand for love

    b. Denial of the reality of time

    c. Flight from their own emotions and feelings

    d. Tendency toward severe depression

    e. Isolation of physical sexuality from psychological mutuality

    f. Behavioral passivity

  3. The family history often indicates an early lack of parental emotional nurturance and an early and continual failure of one parent to protect the child from the irrational demands of the other.

  4. Treatment attempts to bring the child back to normal activity slowly. The counselor may share his or her own family thoughts and experience with the child. Some children may require residential care or hospitalization at times of crisis.

F. Talking to parents It is useful to ask young patients how they plan to inform their parents that they have been on drugs. In the best of circumstances the patient will have enough rapport with the parents to discuss the problem with them, especially if given encouragement. Fortunately, child, parents, and physician are sometimes able to discuss together the problems common to both child and parent. Suffice it to say that difficulties arise when a counselor violates the trust placed in him by a fearful child who prefers to hide his or her activities from the parents.

XV. SUDDEN INFANT DEATH SYNDROME   Sudden infant death syndrome (SIDS) is the leading cause of death in infants between 1 week and 1 year of age. In the United States the incidence is **2–3 deaths**/1000 live births. The mortality is similar in rural and urban areas. Although typical cases have been reported in infants under 1 week and over 1 year of age, the peak incidence is between **2–4 months.**

A. Clinical findings   Most cases of SIDS occur during times of **sleep.** Typically, a well-cared-for infant is placed in a crib at night and is found dead in the morning. In a study of over 400 infants, 74 percent died quietly during the early morning hours. In none of these infants was there an agonal outcry, and the dying event went unobserved in all. In this study, one-third of the deaths occurred while *another person was sleeping in the same room.* The quiet nature of the death has been further substantiated by reports of deaths that occurred in car seats while the infant was sleeping and a parent was driving. There have been some infants, however, who have been found in a corner of the crib or grasping blankets, which may indicate a silent, terminal motor turmoil. This circumstance, when it does occur, has not been helpful in determining the pathogenesis.

B. Epidemiology   Epidemiologic studies have provided some data on SIDS that are suggestive.

1. There is a higher incidence of SIDS in the **winter months.** This observation is *independent of temperature* and holds true even for cities where there is little seasonal temperature variation.

2. Although SIDS has a slightly higher incidence in the lower socio-economic groups, victims come from all social classes.

3. The incidence is higher in **males** than in females and in **low-birth-weight infants.** Approximately 20 percent of the infants in two studies had a birth weight below 2500 gm.

4. SIDS occurs in both breast-fed and bottle-fed infants, and victims who have been fed only breast milk have been recorded. The incidence is slightly higher in siblings, but there is no predictable genetic pattern.

5. The least susceptible populations are **orientals** (0.51/1000 live births), followed by **whites** (1.32), then **Mexican-Americans** (1.74), and **blacks** (2.92). Most vulnerable are **American Indians** (5.93).

6. **Twins** are more susceptible than nontwins (3.87/1000 live births), and triplets are probably at greatest risk (8.33).

7. In some American cities, a decrease in the incidence of SIDS has recently been seen.

C. Mechanism

1. Almost all hypotheses proposed to explain the ultimate mechanism of death in SIDS have been disproved. Refuted theories include spinal hemorrhage, aspiration, hypogammaglobulinemia, and allergy to cow's milk. There has been insufficient evidence for rickets, renal dysfunction, tracheal collapse, enlarged thymus, bacterial sepsis, and overwhelming

viremia. Studies on diving reflexes, cardiac arrhythmias, and vagal reflexes have been inconclusive. Hypotheses must sufficiently account for
the (a) age and racial distribution, (b) predisposal to occur during sleep
hours, (c) incidence in the winter months, (d) lack of premonitory signs,
and (e) failure to find a cause of death on autopsy examination. Also, the
rapidity and apparent serenity of the death must be explained.

2. New findings have shifted attention from the immediate events of death
toward a search for chronic abnormalities. If high-risk profiles can be
developed, some deaths may be preventable.

   a. Currently, most investigative interest is focused on **apnea**. In several
studies of children with documented apnea who died suddenly, autop-
sies revealed no demonstrable cause of death. Since these initial
studies, respiratory physiologists have published additional data
about apnea and its possible relationship to SIDS.

   b. Histologic evidence of the effects of **chronic hypoxia** has been demonstrated in some infants who have died of SIDS. It has been theorized
that **chronic underventilation** of the lungs occurs during sleep, and
many of the infants have chronic hypoxemia prior to death. Hyper-
trophied pulmonary arteries have been found among infants who
have died of SIDS. The investigators considered this evidence of
chronic hypoxemia and are now investigating other possible
hypoxemic markers, such as extramedullary hematopoiesis, abnormal retention of periadrenal brown fat, abnormal proliferation of as-
troglial fibers in the brainstem, and postnatal growth slowdown.

   c. Neonatal abnormalities have been cited that may suggest evidence of
prenatal problems. These abnormalities include

      (1) Feeding patterns

      (2) Temperature regulation

      (3) Motor tone

      (4) Underactivity

      (5) Abnormal cry

      (6) Breathless and exhausted episodes during feeding

   d. In another kind of research, increased levels of **phosphoenolpyruvate
carboxykinase** have been demonstrated in some SIDS victims. The
researchers have raised the unresolved issue of the role of defective
gluconeogenesis in sudden death.

   e. **Postmortem evidence of mild infection,** usually upper respiratory infection, is found in 30–50 percent of SIDS victims, but **multiple viruses**
have been recovered, and, at present, researchers are reviewing the
relationships between immunity and respiratory viruses. Infants
when infected, appear to have an increased incidence of apneic episodes.

D. Reaction to sudden infant death

  1. Parents   The loss of a well-cared-for, healthy child, who in the first year
of life is the focus of family enthusiasm, evokes, especially for mothers,
the most painful type of grief reaction. Parents turn inward and blame
themselves for the death of their child. Typically, they recreate in their
own minds the few hours before the death of their child, to search for
evidence that they could have, in some way, prevented the terminal
event.

Although the immediate effect on parents is overpowering, the initial shock gives way to guilt, which often persists in spite of rational explanations. In the usual grief process, an early stage is internal bargaining. When sudden death is due to a known cause, the concrete character of the event can be incorporated into the normal rationalization of mourning. When, however, death is due to an unknown mechanism, as in SIDS, feelings of self-condemnation and inadequacy of mothering are reinforced. Fathers, who may consider themselves defenders and guardians of the family, also suffer harsh feelings of failure and are often unable to help. This type of death denies parents the prior mourning process that in other terminal illnesses may begin at the time of diagnosis. For young parents, this loss may be their first experience with death of a family member. They may often suffer further remorse because of innuendos in the remarks of poorly informed relatives and friends that the parents are at fault.

2. **Surviving children** are often the most neglected family members in cases of SIDS. Parents sometimes forget that children have both feelings and fantasies about death. Children may be excluded from the mourning by being separated from immediate family members, which effectively prohibits them from discussing the death.

Children under the age of 5 years view death as a temporary and reversible situation, akin to sleep or short absences. Children 5–10 years of age may look at death in terms of responsibility—something or someone was responsible. By the time most children are 10 years old, they are able to understand that death is inevitable, irreversible, and final. Surviving older children appear to be able to resolve the problem of loss, and they do substantially better when they are included in the grief process. For this reason, parents are advised to be as honest as possible with their explanations and their own emotional reactions.

In the course of normal sibling rivalry, children might wish an infant brother or sister to die. Small children indulge in magical thinking, which entails the belief that one can cause events by wishing for them to occur. Or a child may have lightly touched the infant on the night of the death or taken away a blanket or bottle and, because of an immature understanding of death, may implicate himself or herself in the cause. For this reason, siblings need to be assured that the death was unrelated to their feelings or actions.

E. **The role of the physician** The physician has the difficult responsibility of explaining SIDS to grieving parents and thus should have some understanding of how the death of a child affects parents. Without this understanding, there is a risk of reinforcing the parents' preconceived notions and adding to their guilt feelings.

It should be emphasized that the parents were in no way responsible for the death, that SIDS is unrelated to suffocation, feedings, and sleeping position. In reviewing the few hours before the death, parents often search for minor omissions for which to blame themselves. These should be discussed patiently and gently refuted. Parents may also blame relatives or baby sitters tending the child at the time of death. This also should be discussed openly. Parents need guidance in future family planning with surviving siblings.

In such circumstances, explaining a death requires compassion and, particularly, sensitivity, since *any insinuation of parental neglect* is distorted and misinterpreted. By such an approach, the physician provides some comfort to parents who have lost their child suddenly and unexpectedly.

3

Poisoning

Children under 5 years of age account for 80 percent of recorded cases of poison ingestion. Most children ingesting poison are seen before symptoms develop. Often, the clinician generally can determine the nature of the ingested substance from the history. When the nature of the substance ingested is unknown, the list of common signs and symptoms shown in Table 3-1 may be useful.

I. EMERGENCY MANAGEMENT

A. Identification of the poison Usually, the ingested material can be identified by a careful history. The drugs available in the home as well as the place where the ingestion took place often help in identifying the poison.

1. The initial history should include what and how much was taken (a swallow for a 3-year-old child is approximately 4–5 ml), when the ingestion occurred, and the present condition of the child.

2. If a substance is *not* a caustic or a hydrocarbon, and if the child is *not* comatose or having a seizure, removal by **emesis** may be instituted.

3. The physician should accept the largest estimated amount ingested in determining therapy.

4. Physical examination will often reveal supporting evidence for a particular ingestion. All vomitus and urine, as well as all containers and bottles, should be saved to assist in later identification.

5. The specific substance causing a poisoning should be confirmed by qualitative—and, when possible, quantitative—analysis performed on blood or urine.

B. Removal of the poison Removal prior to absorption and onset of symptoms is the primary aim. Enhancement of excretion and various methods of dialysis may be useful with more serious ingestions.

1. **Mechanical methods** The use of blunt objects and lavage are less effective in inducing emesis than are chemical emetics.

   a. The disadvantages of the use of lavage include emotional and physical trauma, ineffectiveness in removing tablets and, to a lesser extent, liquids, and the delay involved in bringing the patient to the hospital.

   b. For the comatose patient, a cuffed lavage tube or prior intubation with a cuffed endotracheal tube followed by passage of a lavage tube may be indicated.

   c. **Gastric lavage procedure**

      (1) Equipment: Catheter, 8–12F; 4-oz Asepto syringe; lavage with ½ NS.

      (2) Place the patient on the left side, with the head hanging over the table during lavage.

Table 3-1 Common Signs and Symptoms of Toxic Ingestions

Signs and Symptoms	Drugs Involved
Disturbance of cardiac function:	
Arrhythmias	Digitalis, quinidine
Tachycardia	Amphetamines, caffeine, ephedrine, cocaine
Bradycardia	Barbiturates, chloral hydrate, digitalis, quinine, opiates
Hypotension	Chloral hydrate, nitrites, quinine, chlorpromazine
Nervous system symptoms:	
Depression and coma	Barbiturates, alcohols, tranquilizers, antihistamines, chloral hydrate, paraldehyde, chloroform, ether, cyanide, CO, atropine, CO_2, nicotine, phenols, scopolamine, hydrogen sulfide, insulin, bromides, benzene, zylene, morphine and its derivatives, lead
Convulsions	Strychnine, parathion and other organic phosphate esters, amphetamines, ammonium salts, camphors, picrotoxin, cyanides, chlorinated hydrocarbons, lead, barium, cocaine, belladonna group, ergot, nicotine, salicylates, CO
Delirium	Belladonna group, alcohol, cocaine, marihuana, amphetamines, antihistamines, camphor, benzene, barbiturates, aniline
Gastrointestinal symptoms:	
Nausea, vomiting, and diarrhea	Heavy metal salts, alcohol, acids and alkalis, halogens, yellow phosphorus, phenols, muscarine, digitalis, aspirin, fluoride, parathion and other organic phosphate esters, many poisonous plants
Eye signs:	
Dilated pupils	Belladonna and derivatives (atropine), alcohol, chloroform, cocaine, meperidine, nicotine, amphetamine, ephedrine, epinephrine, tripelennamine, ether, isoproterenol, psychedelic drugs such as LSD, antihistamines
Constricted pupils	Morphine and derivatives, parathion and other organic phosphate derivatives, parasympathomimetic drugs, barbiturates, chloral hydrate, caffeine, nicotine
Blurred vision	Atropine, physostigmine, cocaine, dinitrophenol, nicotine, methyl and ethyl alcohol, indomethacin, carbon tetrachloride
Colored vision	Digitalis, quinine, CO, marihuana
Scotomas	Quinine, salicylates
Skin:	
Cyanosis (methemoglobinemia)	Nitrobenzene, aniline dyes, acetanilid, carbon dioxide, chloral hydrate, amyl nitrite, nitrites, methane, morphine

Table 3-1 *(Continued)*

Signs and Symptoms	Drugs Involved
Skin (Continued):	
Staining and coloring	Iodine, black; bromide, deep brown; nitric acid and picric acid, yellow; silver nitrite, bluish gray; CO, cyanide, pink; atabrine, yellow; methemoglobinemia, brown; atropine, flushed face
Jaundice	Aniline dyes, nitrobenzene, primaquine, benzene, arsenic, chromates, mushrooms, quinacrine, nitro compounds, phosphorus, carbon tetrachloride, phenothiazines, thiazides, diuretics
Discoloration of the gums	Lead, mercury, bismuth (usually chronic poisoning), arsenic
Tinnitus	Salicylates, quinines, streptomycin, camphor, ergot, methyl alcohol, tobacco
Alopecia	Thallium, x-rays, radium, arsenic, ergot, hypervitaminosis A
Salivation:	
Decreased salivation	Belladonna group, atropine, morphine, diphenhydramine hydrochloride, ephedrine
Increased salivation	Lead, mercury, thallium, other heavy metals, mushrooms
Sweating:	
Increased sweating	Parathion and other organic phosphate esters, alcohol (acute), insulin, nitrates, muscarine, pilocarpine, mercuric chloride, arsenic, aspirin, fluoride, nicotine, ammonia
Hyperpyrexia	Atropine, quinine, zinc fumes, boric acid, dinitrophenol, phenolphthalein, salicylates
Hyperventilation	Salicylates, nicotine, aromatics, CO_2, cyanide, atropine, camphor, cocaine
Abnormal odor on breath:	
Odor of alcohol	Phenols, chloral hydrate, alcohol
Odor of acetone	Lacquer, alcohol
Odor of coal gas	CO
Odor of wintergreen	Methyl salicylate
Odor of garlic	Phosphorus and arsenic
Odor of bitter almonds	Cyanide
Odor of shoe polish	Nitrobenzene
Pearlike odor	Chloral hydrate
Other odors	Hydrocarbons, turpentine, camphor
Abnormal odor of tissues:	
Specific odor of chemical ingested	Phenol, creosote, chloroform, hydrogen sulfide, ethchlorvynol, ether, alcohol, paraldehyde

Table 3-1 *(Continued)*

Signs and Symptoms	Drugs Involved
Abnormal odor of tissues (Continued):	
Odor of garlic	Phosphorus, arsenic, parathion
Odor of shoe polish	Nitrobenzene
Odor of violets	Turpentine in urine
Odor of pears	Chloral hydrate
Odor of bitter almonds	Cyanide
Abnormal color of gastric aspirate:	
Pink or purple	Potassium permanganate
Green	Nickel salts
Blue	Iodine, if starch is present
Abnormal color of urine:	
Dark green	Phenol, resorcinol
Brown or black	Antipyrine trinol (after long use)
Yellow	Picric acid
Bright yellow, changing to scarlet on adding caustic alkali	Santonin

    (3) Cool the tube with ice; use jelly to facilitate insertion.

    (4) Measure the distance to the stomach, and ensure entrance into the stomach by checking for bubbles under water or injecting air with auscultation over the stomach.

    (5) Aspirate the gastric contents prior to lavage.

    (6) Perform lavage 10–12 times or until the return is clear.

    (7) If indicated, leave a specific antidote or activated charcoal in the stomach on completion.

    (8) Pinch the tube on removal to prevent aspiration.

  2. Chemical methods Ipecac syrup and apomorphine are the most effective chemical methods of removal.

    a. Ipecac syrup is now the method of choice because it induces emesis in 15–20 min in 85 percent of patients with 1 dose and in 96 percent of patients in 30–40 min with 2 doses. It removes approximately 40 to 50 percent of an ingested product when administered within 1 hr of ingestion. It is available without prescription and has a long shelf life which allows for storage at home for emergency use. It is safe when taken in the recommended dosage (30 ml over 1 year of age and 10 ml under 1).

      (1) Its use is **contraindicated** in patients who have ingested caustic agents or hydrocarbons or in those who are comatose or having seizures.

      (2) For the patient 1 year and older, within or outside a hospital setting, 15 ml (1 tbsp) of ipecac syrup is given, followed by 200 ml clear fluid. If vomiting does not occur within 20 min, the same dose may be repeated once, followed by lavage, if necessary.

(3) For children age 6 months–1 year, 10 ml is given once only, followed by clear fluids and activity. If this is ineffective, lavage is indicated.

(4) For the adolescent, 30 ml of ipecac syrup is given along with clear fluids. If vomiting does not occur in 20 min, the dose may be repeated once, followed by lavage, if necessary.

b. Apomorphine causes emesis in 100 percent of patients within 2–5 min of its use. As in lavage, the patient must come to the hospital or to physician's office for its administration. The recommended dosage is 0.07 mg/kg/dose SQ. A respiratory depressant, its effect may be reversed with naloxone (Narcan), 0.01 mg/kg/dose. *Apomorphine is particularly effective when impending obtundation requires rapid induction of emesis.*

3. Enhanced excretion Methods of enhancing excretion should be used only in serious poisoning, since they involve some risk. Most cases are handled conservatively, allowing the patient to excrete or metabolize the ingested drug. Only a small percentage will require the following, more radical forms of therapy.

a. Fluid diuresis enhances excretion by increasing the rate of glomerular filtration, so that the resorptive sites in the distal tubules have a shorter exposure to the ingested drug. Fluid diuresis will enhance excretion of drugs normally handled by the kidneys. A sustained diuresis of 2–3 times normal is recommended.

b. Ionized diuresis is based on the principle that excretion is favored when a drug is maintained in its ionized state. Excretion of acidic compounds such as salicylates and long-acting barbiturates is enhanced by sustained alkalinization of the urine. The more acidic the ingested drug, the more effective is alkalinization in enhancing excretion.

(1) For salicylates sodium bicarbonate ($NaHCO_3$), 2–3 mEq/kg, is given q4h. Urinary pH is monitored, and additional $NaHCO_3$ is used if a pH above 7.5 is not maintained. Serum and urinary electrolytes, calcium, and magnesium should be monitored as well.

(2) Acidification of the urine with ammonium chloride 75 mg/kg q6h in poisoning with basic compounds (e.g., amphetamines and phencyclidine) will also enhance excretion.

c. Osmotic diuresis Osmotic diuresis (see Chap. 8, Sec. **I.B**) is based on the principle of an osmotic load preventing resorption of an ingested drug in the proximal tubules, Henle's loop, and distal tubules.

(1) A diuresis of 2–3 times the normal excretion is recommended.

(2) Contraindications to the procedure are cardiac disease, oliguria or anuria, hypotension, and pulmonary edema.

(3) Close monitoring of serum and urinary electrolytes, body weight, and central venous pressure (CVP) is indicated.

(4) Mannitol, 0.5 gm/kg/dose IV of a 25% solution q4–6h, may be used.

d. Diuretics Ethacrynic acid, 1 mg/kg/dose IM or IV at 2–3-hr intervals (or when urinary output decreases), has been used to enhance excretion. An output of 2–3 times normal in a child is sought. Furosemide

(Lasix), 3 mg/kg/dose IM or IV, has also been used. Urinary and blood electrolytes should be closely monitored (see Chap. 9).

4. **Dialysis** Exchange transfusions, peritoneal dialysis, and hemodialysis are not part of the usual emergency management of poisoning. Their use is reserved for the most severe cases, with the decision based on the degree of CNS involvement, the patient's ability to maintain respiration, blood pressure, and an adequate urinary output, and, finally, the inherent toxicity of the ingested drug (Table 3-2). **Coma may not be an indication for dialysis if blood pressure and respiration can be maintained and the patient is not anuric.**

   a. **Exchange transfusion** is generally effective in small children in poisoning with drugs that are tightly protein bound and have low volumes of distribution.

   b. **Peritoneal dialysis** is useful in children in instances of electrolyte and acid-base disturbance and with drugs that have high dialysis clearance across the peritoneum.

   c. **Hemodialysis** and **lipid dialysis** are less commonly used in children (The reader should consult *Trans. Am. Soc. Artif. Intern. Organs* 23:762, 1977, for a review of the dialyzability of drugs as well as of toxins.)

C. **Catharsis, dilution, and neutralization**

1. **Catharsis** Cathartics may hasten transit through the GI tract, thus decreasing absorption of poisons not removed by emesis. Enemas are effective for removing overdoses given PR.

2. **Dilution** is a relatively ineffective method, its greatest benefit being its calming influence. In the case of barbiturates, it may increase absorption by hastening transit of the ingested poison into the lower parts of the G. tract, from which subsequent removal will be difficult.

3. **Neutralization** of ingested bases with acids and ingested acids with bases **is no longer advised.** It is generally instituted too late to be effective, and the resultant exothermic reaction may cause secondary tissue damage.

D. **Supportive therapy** While allowing normal renal and hepatic processes to rid the body of the ingested drug, the principles of supportive therapy must be observed. These principles include the following:

1. **Respiratory** Assuring adequate respiratory exchange by clearing secretions, utilizing an oral airway, supplying sufficient O_2 and humidity, and turning the patient often to prevent pneumonia. Rarely, intubation and mechanical respiration will be required.

Table 3-2 Currently Known Dialyzable Poisons

Barbiturates*	**Glutethimide*–1, 2**
Barbital–1, 2	**Depressants, Sedatives,**
Phenobarbital–1, 2	**and Tranquilizers**
Amobarbital–1, 2	Diphenhydramine–1, 3
Pentobarbital–1, 2	Diphenylhydantoin–1, 2
Butabarbital–1, 2	Primidone–2
Secobarbital–1, 2	Meprobamate–1, 2
Cyclobarbital–1, 2	Ethchlorvynol*–1, 2, 3

Table 3-2 *(Continued)*

Ethynylcyclohexyl carbamate–1
Methyprylon–1, 2
Methaqualone–1, 2
Heroin–1
Gallamine triethiodide–1
Paraldehyde–1, 2
Chloral hydrate–1
Chlordiazepoxide–1

Antidepressants
Amphetamine–1, 2
Methamphetamine–1, 2
Tricyclic secondary amines–1
Tricyclic tertiary amines–1
Monoamine oxidase inhibitors–1
Tranylcypromine–1
Pargyline–1
Phenelzine–1
Isocarboxazid–1
Imipramine–1

Alcohols
Ethanol*–1, 2
Methanol*–1, 2, 3
Isopropanol–1
Ethylene glycol–1, 2

Analgesics
Acetylsalicylic acid*–1, 2, 3
Methylsalicylate*–1, 2, 3
Acetophenetidin–1
Dextropropoxyphene–1, 2
Paracetamol–1, 3

Antibiotics
Isoniazid–1, 2
Carbenicillin–1, 2
Streptomycin–1
Kanamycin–1, 2
Neomycin–1, 2
Vancomycin–1
Penicillin–1
Ampicillin–1
Sulfonamides–1
Cephaloridine–1
Chloramphenicol–1
Tetracycline–1
Nitrofurantoin–1
Polymyxin–1

Cycloserine–2
Quinine–1, 2
Metals
Arsenic–1, 2
Calcium–1, 2
Iron–1, 4
Lead–1
Lithium–1
Magnesium–1
Mercury–1, 4
Potassium–1, 2
Sodium–1, 2
Strontium–1
Halides
Bromide–1
Chloride–1
Iodide–1
Fluoride–1
Endogenous Toxins
Ammonia–1, 2, 3
Uric acid*–1
Bilirubin–1, 2, 3
Lactic acid–1, 2
Cystine–1
Endotoxin–1
Water intoxication–1, 2
Miscellaneous
Thiocyanate*–1
Aniline–1, 2, 3
Sodium chlorate–1, 2, 3
Potassium chlorate–1, 2, 3
Eucalyptus oil–1, 2
Boric acid–2
Potassium dichromate–1, 4
Chromic anhydride–1
Digoxin–1, 2
Sodium citrate–1
Dinitro-o-cresol–1
Amanita phalloides–1
Carbon tetrachloride–1
Ergotamine–2
Cyclophosphamide–1
5-Fluorouracil–1
Methotrexate–1
Camphor–1
Trichlorethylene–1, 2
CO–1

1 = hemodialysis, 2 = peritoneal dialysis, 3 = exchange transfusion, 4 = chelation and dialysis.
* Kinetics of dialysis thoroughly studied, or clinical experience extensive, or both.
Adapted from G. E. Schreiner, *Trans. Am. Soc. Artif. Intern. Organs* 23:762, 1977. By permission.

2. **Cardiac** Correction of shock (see Chap. 2, Sec. **II.C**).

3. **Fluid homeostasis** Replacement of previous and ongoing losses, as well as correction of electrolyte derangements (see Chap. 8, Sec. **III**).

4. **Hematologic** Correction of hemolytic anemias with packed cell transfusions or whole blood transfusions for external losses of blood (see Chap. 1 Sec. **II.D**).

5. **Central nervous system** CNS involvement may require control of seizures with barbiturates, paraldehyde, phenytoin sodium, or diazepam supportive measures for prolonged coma, adequate suctioning, and preventive measures against self-injury (see Chap. 2, Sec. **III**, and Chap. 21 Sec. **B**).

6. **Renal failure** will require fluid and electrolyte management. Dialysis ma be needed (see Chap. 9).

7. **Antibiotic therapy** for bacterial superinfection. Prophylactic antibiotic are discouraged (see Chap. 15, Sec. **I.A**).

8. **General supportive measures** include the monitoring of vital signs avoidance of CNS stimulants, and the use of analgesics as indicated.

E. Antidotes

1. **Local antidotes**

   a. The universal antidote (a mixture of charcoal, magnesium hydroxide and tannic acid) is ineffective and in fact is hepatotoxic. **It should no be used.**

   b. **Activated charcoal,** an odorless, tasteless, black powder, is the residue from the distillation of wood pulp. It forms a stable complex with the ingested toxin, thus preventing absorption.

      (1) **It should not be given before ipecac syrup,** since it will bind the syrup and make it ineffective. Its effectiveness depends on it small particle size and large surface area. It should be used fo drugs against which it is known to be effective (Table 3-3); it is no effective against cyanide, ethyl and methyl alcohol, alkali, or acid.

      (2) The dose is 1 gm/kg PO in 8 oz of water. It may be given followin induced emesis or via a nasogastric tube after lavage. The dose in the adolescent patient is 30 gm mixed in 8 oz of water.

2. **Specific antidotes** The number of ingestions for which there is a specifi antidote are few. The following list includes the drugs or substances fo which an antidote is available.

   a. **Dimercaprol** (British antilewisite [BAL]), for arsenic, bismuth chromium, cobalt, copper, iron, lead, magnesium, radium, selenium and uranium. The dose is 3–4 mg/kg/dose IM at intervals of 4–8 hr fo 5 days and then 3 mg/kg/dose q12h (see Sec. **III**).

   b. **Ethylenediaminetetraacetate** (EDTA), for lead, iron, mercury, copper, nickel, zinc, cobalt, beryllium, and manganese. The dose is 50–7 mg/kg/day IM or IV in 2–3 divided doses for 5–7 days. Add procaine fo IM use.

   c. **Penicillamine,** for lead, copper, and mercury. The dose is 25–50 mg/kg day PO in 4 divided doses for 5 days. The maximum dose per day is gm (see Sec. **III**).

Table 3-3 Drugs Absorbed by Activated Charcoal

Amphetamines	Phenytoin sodium	Penicillin
Antipyrene	Glutethimide	Phenol
Aspirin	Iodine	Phenolphthalein
Atropine	Ipecac	Propoxyphene
Barbiturates	Methylene blue	Primaquine
Camphor	Morphine	Quinine
Cantharides	Muscarine	Salicylates
Chlorpheniramine	Nicotine	Sulfonamides
Cocaine	Opium	Stramonium
Colchicine	Oxalates	Strychnine
Digitalis	Parathion	

Adapted from D. G. Corby and W. J. Deckers, *Pediatrics* 54:324, 1974. By permission.

d. Amyl or sodium nitrite and thiosulfate, for cyanide. The doses are amyl sodium nitrite, 0.33 ml/kg of a 3% solution IV at a rate of 2.5–5.0 ml/min, followed in 15 min by sodium thiosulfate, 1.65 ml/kg of a 25% solution IV at a rate of 2.5–5.0 ml/min.

e. Naloxone hydrochloride (Narcan), for narcotics. Give 0.03 mg/kg/dose IV. Continue therapy until a narcotic effect is no longer present.

f. Vitamin K_1, for warfarin and bishydroxycoumarin. The dose is 2–5 mg/kg IM or IV.

g. Deferoxamine, for iron. The dose is 1–2 gm or 50 mg/kg IM q4–6h. For severe intoxication, give IV at a rate *not to exceed* 15 mg/kg/hr. Do not exceed 6 gm in 24 hr. (See also Sec. **II.C.3.d.**)

h. Ethanol, for methanol and ethylene glycol. The dose of a 50% solution is 0.75–1.5 ml/kg IV, followed by 0.5 ml/kg q4h to maintain the blood ethanol level between 100–150/100 ml.

i. Atropine sulfate or pralidoxime iodide (2-PAM iodide), for insecticides (cholinesterase inhibitors). Doses are atropine, 1–4 mg or 0.05 mg/kg IV, with repeat doses of 2 mg at intervals of 2–5 min until full atropinization is achieved and then as necessary to maintain atropinization; 2-PAM iodide, 250 μg given slowly IV and repeated in 12 hr as needed.

j. Methylene blue, for methemoglobinemia induced by nitrites, aniline dyes, chlorates, phenacetin, nitrobenzene, sulfonamides, and quinones. The dose of methylene blue is 1–2 mg/kg IV as a 1% solution and is repeated in 4 hr if needed.

k. Chlorpromazine, for amphetamines. The dose is 1 mg/kg IM or IV q6h. Titrate subsequent doses to the clinical response.

l. Diphenhydramine (Benadryl), for phenothiazine extrapyramidal reactions. The dose is 1–2 mg/kg IV q6h for 4 doses.

m. Oxygen for carbon monoxide (100% O_2 for 30 min).

n. *N*-acetylcysteine, for acetaminophen. Give 140 mg/kg as a loading dose PO and then 20 mg/kg/dose for 18 doses (see Sec. **II.E**).

F. Prevention No course of therapy, no matter how trivial the ingestion, is complete without a discussion about why the poisoning occurred and a

Table 3-4   Common Ingestions of Low Toxicity

No Treatment Required	Removal Necessary if Large Amounts Ingested
Ballpoint inks	Aftershave lotion
Bar soap	Body conditioners
Bathtub floating toys	Colognes
Battery (dry cell)	Deodorants
Bubble bath soap	Fabric softeners
Candles	Hair dyes
Chalk	Hair sprays
Clay (modeling)	Hair tonic
Crayons with A.P., C.P., or C.S. 130–46 designation	Indelible markers
Dehumidifying packets	Matches (more than 20 wooden matches or 2 books of paper matches)
Detergents (anionic)	Nodoz
Eye makeup	Oral contraceptives
Fishbowl additives	Perfumes
Golf balls	Suntan preparations
Hand lotion and cream	Toilet water
Ink (blue, black, red)	
Lipstick	
Newspaper	
Pencils (lead and coloring)	
Putty and Silly Putty	
Sachets	
Shampoo	
Shaving cream and shaving lotions	
Shoe polish (occasionally, aniline dyes are present)	
Striking surface materials of matchboxes	
Sweetening agents (saccharin, cyclamate)	
Teething rings	
Thermometers	
Toothpaste	

review of ways to ensure that the incident will not be repeated. Recognition that the agent, an unpredictable child, and an emotionally unstable milieu may all play a part in a poisoning is essential in such discussions.

II. SPECIFIC INGESTIONS   Table 3-4 lists certain common substances of low toxicity that either require no treatment when ingested or require only emesis when ingested in large quantities. The specific ingestions listed in this section are chosen because their management remains complex and difficult.

  A. Caustics

   1. Etiology   The severity of the caustic burn is related to the concentration and duration of contact rather than to the amount ingested. Following ingestion, a burn ensues during the first week, granulation tissue during the second week, and fibrosis during the third week. Typical acids in gested are toilet-bowl cleaners, metal-cleaning fluids, and some bleaching products. Typical alkalis ingested are powerful detergents, toilet-bowl cleaners, and dishwasher and laundry granules.

2. Evaluation and diagnosis

    a. Immediate severe pain is experienced in the mouth and retrosternal area. The absence of oral burns is reassuring but is not sure evidence against esophageal involvement. Other symptoms include vomiting, signs of vascular collapse, and coma.

    b. Esophageal perforation with mediastinitis and gastric perforation with peritonitis may occur. Aspiration may lead to pulmonary necrosis or glottic edema. Bacterial superinfection may occur during the first and second weeks and esophageal stricture formation in later weeks. If a skilled surgeon is available, esophagoscopy may be performed within the first 2 days to determine the presence and extent of injury.

3. Treatment

    a. Emesis and lavage are contraindicated.

    b. The caustic should be washed off the esophagus with water or milk. Neutralization with acids or alkalis is not indicated.

    c. Opiates may be used for pain.

    d. Blood, albumin, and saline are used for shock (see Chap. 2, Sec. **II.C**).

    e. Liquids and soft foods may be given when the patient can swallow.

    f. If evidence points to an esophageal burn (clinical evidence or a burn demonstrated by esophagoscopy), corticosteroids should be begun within 48 hr (prednisone 2 mg/kg/day) and continued for 3–4 weeks. A barium swallow is indicated following corticosteroid therapy to confirm the presence or absence of stricture formation; if present, subsequent dilations will be necessary.

B. Hydrocarbons

1. Etiology and evaluation

    a. Gasoline, kerosene, lighter fluid, paint thinners, and industrial rubber solvents produce both CNS and pulmonary involvement. Furniture polishes and waxes (mineral seal oils) produce mainly pulmonary damage.

    b. The type of pathologic changes in the lung will depend on the type of hydrocarbon ingested. The mineral seal oils produce low-grade chronic pulmonary inflammation, while kerosene and naphtha derivatives (Table 3-5) produce a more fulminant course.

    c. CNS involvement generally is produced by hydrocarbons as a result of absorption from the lungs. Pulmonary involvement is caused by aspiration during ingestion or subsequent vomiting.

    d. The liver, kidney, spleen, myocardium, and bone marrow may also be involved.

2. Diagnosis

    a. Ingestion of a hydrocarbon causes mucous membrane irritation. Vomiting, bloody diarrhea, and perianal excoriation occur.

    b. Pulmonary involvement is evidenced by coughing, gagging, dyspnea, cyanosis, and rales.

Table 3-5 Petroleum Products: Estimation of Aspiration Hazard and Systemic Toxicity

Product	Source(s)	Systemic Toxicity	Aspiration Hazard*
Petroleum, ether, or benzene	Industrial or rubber solvents	4+	—
Gasoline	Fuel	3+	2+
Naphtha	Solvent, lighter fluid, dry cleaner, thinner	3+	3+
Kerosene	Fuel, charcoal lighter fluid, thinner, pesticide solvent	2+	2+
Mineral seal oil	Furniture polish	3+	4+
Fuel or diesel oil	Fuel, heating oil	1+	1+
Mineral oil		—	—
Lubricating oil	Motor oil, cutting oil, transmission fluid	—	—

* Formulations with increased viscosity have decreased aspiration hazard.

    c. Central nervous system manifestations include restlessness, confusion, drowsiness, and coma. Pneumothorax and pleural effusions may complicate the pulmonary picture.

  3. Treatment

    a. Removal should be deferred in the case of hydrocarbons, the danger from aspiration being greater than the risk from GI absorption. Removal is indicated if a very large amount (10–12 ml/kg) has been ingested, or if a more toxic compound is ingested along with the petroleum distillate hydrocarbon.

    b. Present evidence now suggests that in the *alert* patient, **emesis** with ipecac syrup is a safer method of removal than lavage. In the *obtunded* patient, protection of the lungs with a cuffed endotracheal tube and subsequent **lavage** constitute the therapy of choice.

    c. The use of activated charcoal and olive oil may lead to spontaneous vomiting and should thus be avoided.

    d. For pulmonary involvement, O_2, humidity, bronchodilators for bronchospasticity, and antibiotics are recommended.

    e. Present evidence does not support the use of corticosteroids for mild to moderate caustic burns.

    f. Infiltrates may take 1–2 weeks to resolve fully; waxes and polishes may take even longer.

    g. Management of CNS, liver, and renal involvement is supportive.

    h. Due to myocardial irritability, sympathomimetic drugs should be avoided.

C. Iron

  1. Etiology Because iron tablets and vitamins with iron are ubiquitous in homes, iron ingestion is common.

2. Evaluation and diagnosis

    a. Symptoms generally occur 30 min–2 hr following ingestion and are often severe. Early symptoms include vomiting, bloody diarrhea, drowsiness, and, less commonly, shock and coma.

    b. A period of improvement (6–24 hr after ingestion) is followed by a **recurrence** of symptoms, which include fever, metabolic acidosis, hepatic impairment, restlessness, convulsions, shock, and coma.

    c. **Stricture of the GI tract** is an infrequent and late complication, occurring 3–4 weeks after ingestion.

    d. Initial laboratory studies should include a CBC, serum electrolytes, serum iron, and an x-ray film of the GI tract to detect the presence of radiopaque iron tablets.

3. Treatment

    a. Early emesis with ipecac syrup is indicated if 1 gm or more of ferrous sulfate has been taken.

    b. IV fluids, sodium bicarbonate, and volume expanders will be needed to correct acidosis and fluid loss.

    c. Sodium bicarbonate by mouth may relieve abdominal discomfort, prevent intestinal erosion, and decrease absorption of iron.

    d. Deferoxamine treatment

        (1) Indications

            (a) Coma and shock.

            (b) A serum iron level exceeding the iron-binding capacity.

            (c) Symptoms other than minimal vomiting and diarrhea.

            (d) Positive provocative chelation (burgundy-colored urine on challenge with 50 mg/kg of deferoxamine).

        (2) Administration The parenteral route is preferable to either the PO or IV route. The IM dose is 1–2 gm q3–12h, depending on the amount ingested, the clinical state of the patient, and the serum iron level. The urine will turn burgundy red when the serum iron level is 500 μg/100 ml or greater. In cases of hypotension, the IV route should be used; give 1 gm by slow infusion at a rate not to exceed 15 mg/kg/hr. Generally, the serum iron level falls within 12–18 hr, and clinical improvement is seen in 6–12 hr. Cessation of therapy will generally be possible from 12–36 hr after beginning therapy.

        (3) Dialysis Ferrous sulfate is not dialyzable except when bound to deferoxamine. Dialysis is indicated in the presence of oliguria or anuria.

D. Salicylates are the most frequent cause of poisoning in children.

    1. Etiology Accidental ingestion or excess salicylate used at therapeutic doses.

    2. Evaluation

        a. Salicylates produce an initial respiratory alkalosis due to hyperventilation secondary to central stimulation. The body compensates by excreting base via the kidneys. A state of metabolic acidosis, especially in young children, is quickly superimposed. Dehydration and worsening acidosis occur due to hyperventilation, renal solute loss, and increased metabolic rate, and vomiting. Presenting symptoms in the younger child generally include metabolic acidosis and respiratory alkalosis. The adolescent presents with respiratory alkalosis alone.

b. The first symptoms seen in both alkalosis and acidosis are deep, rapid respiration, thirst, vomiting, and profuse sweating. In severe intoxication, confusion, delirium, coma, convulsions, circulatory collapse and oliguria may ensue.

c. Salicylates increase body metabolism, prolong prothrombin times, cause platelet dysfunction, and may induce either hyperglycemia or hypoglycemia. They are first excreted in the urine within ½ hr after ingestion, and peak serum levels occur 2 hr after ingestion. Of an ingested load of aspirin, 75 percent is excreted through the kidneys and 25 percent is handled by oxidation.

d. Initial laboratory studies include a CBC, electrolytes, blood gases, serum ketones, blood glucose, prothrombin time, serum salicylate level, and urine acetone, pH, protein, and ferric chloride.

3. Diagnosis Ingestion of 150 mg/kg will cause symptoms. A salicylate level of 50 mg/100 ml causes mild symptoms; 50–80 mg/100 ml produce symptoms of moderate severity; and 80–100 mg/100 ml produces severe symptoms. The nomogram in Figure 3-1 will be of assistance in determining the expected severity of clinical illness following a single dose ingestion of aspirin. A level of 50 mg/100 ml or any symptoms (except mild hyperventilation) generally indicate that hospitalization is necessary.

4. Treatment

a. Induction of emesis with ipecac syrup is required when a toxic dose (greater than 150 mg/kg) has been ingested.

b. IV fluids to replace fluid losses (see Chap. 8, Sec. III) and adequate glucose to correct hypoglycemia.

c. Lowering of temperature elevation with tepid sponging.

d. Vitamin K to combat bleeding due to hypoprothrombinemia.

e. Alkalinization of the urine (2–3 mEq/kg of $NaHCO_3$ q4–6h) and monitoring of the urinary pH (keeping it above 7.5) will result in enhanced excretion of salicylates with serum half-lives being lowered from 24–36 to 6–8 hr. Generous amounts of potassium (3–5 mEq/kg day) are necessary to replace potassium loss and *allow alkalinization of the urine.*

f. Potentially fatal serum levels (100–150 mg/100 ml), oliguria or anuria and cardiac disease are all indications for dialysis. A poor response to $NaHCO_3$, coma, and seizures are *relative* indications for dialysis.

E. Acetaminophen

1. Etiology At present, acetaminophen is used more than aspirin as an analgesic and antipyretic. It is consequently widely available in homes and is thus one of the drugs most frequently ingested by children and adolescents.

2. Evaluation

a. The major target organ of acetaminophen overdose is the liver.

b. Signs and symptoms within the first 12–24 hr of ingestion include nausea, vomiting, and diaphoresis. Evidence of hepatotoxicity ap

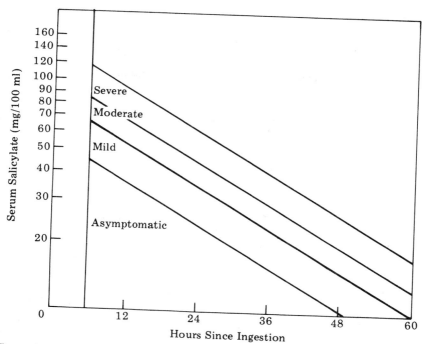

Figure 3-1 Nomogram relating serum salicylate levels to expected clinical severity of intoxications following a single dose of salicylates. (From A. K. Done, *Pediatrics* 26:800, 1960. Copyright by the American Academy of Pediatrics, 1960.)

pears 24–36 hr after ingestion and includes hepatic enlargement with tenderness and jaundice, hyperbilirubinemia, hyperammonemia, and prolongation of the prothrombin time. Liver biopsy shows focal hepatocyte cytolysis and centrizonal necrosis. Serum transaminase activity peaks by 3–4 days following ingestion and returns to normal within a week in those who recover.

c. Metabolites of acetaminophen, rather than the parent compound, are hepatotoxic. In overdose, normal metabolic pathways are saturated, and reactive intermediates are consequently formed that bind to liver macromolecules, causing liver necrosis.

d. The consequences of acetaminophen ingestion cannot be anticipated from the initial nonspecific signs. Although the history is often unreliable, a single ingested dose of 3 gm in a 2- or 3-year-old (approximately 150 mg/kg) and a dose greater than 8 gm in the adolescent may result in hepatic damage.

e. *An acetaminophen blood level drawn 4 hr following ingestion is the best predictor of subsequent hepatotoxicity.* When interpreted on the Rumack-Mathews nomogram (Fig. 3-2), a plasma concentration greater than 200 mg/ml at 4 hr or 50 mg/ml at 12 hr after ingestion is associated with liver damage. A half-life that exceeds 3 hr is also predictive of subsequent liver damage.

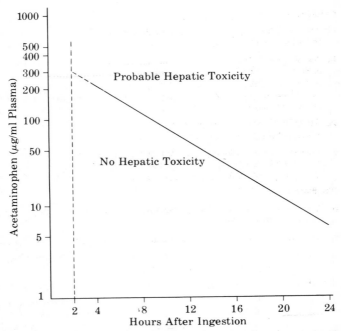

Figure 3-2 Semilogarithmic plot of plasma acetaminophen concentration versus time based on data from adult patients. Patients with concentrations above the line at the corresponding times after ingestion may develop hepatotoxicity. Patients with concentrations below the line have a low probability of developing hepatotoxicity. (From B. H. Rumack and H. Mathews, *Pediatrics* 55:871, 1975. Copyright by the American Academy of Pediatrics, 1975.)

    f. Acetaminophen overdose must be distinguished from the Reye syndrome, amino acid disorders, and alpha₁-antitrypsin deficiency in the child and from drug abuse (alcohol, heroin, volatile hydrocarbons) and Wilson's disease in the adolescent.

3. Treatment

    a. Removal of the ingested dose with ipecac syrup or gastric lavage when the patient is seen within 4 hr of ingestion.

    b. Activated charcoal will bind acetaminophen. **Its use should be deferred if *N*-acetylcysteine (Mucomyst) is to be used,** since it will bind the antidote, thereby reducing its effectiveness.

    c. Avoid enzyme inducers such as phenobarbital and alcohol.

    d. Avoid forcing fluids or ionized diuresis.

    e. When acetaminophen has been taken in high doses, or when acetaminophen levels are in the range likely to cause hepatotoxicity, *N*-acetylcysteine may be administered under an investigational protocol coordinated by the Rocky Mountain Poison Center. The Center should be contacted (1-800-332-3073) for the specifics of the protocol.

F. Phencyclidine

    1. Etiology   Phencyclidine (PCP) is a widely available abused drug.

2. Evaluation

a. In overdose, adverse effects begin within 1–2 hr of exposure. The duration of effect ranges from hours to weeks.

b. Signs and symptoms referable to the CNS include disorientation, confusion, restlessness, excitation, hallucinations, seizures, and coma. Speech is slow and slurred and memory impaired. The pupils are often miotic, with horizontal and vertical nystagmus. Ataxia, increased muscle tone, and brisk deep tendon reflexes are common.

c. Complications include respiratory depression, aspiration pneumonia, arrhythmias, hypertension, and rhabdomyolysis.

d. Phencyclidine is rapidly absorbed by the oral and respiratory routes. It is widely distributed throughout the body, is excreted primarily by the liver, and undergoes enterohepatic recirculation.

3. Treatment

a. Removal by ipecac syrup if the patient is alert or gastric lavage if the patient is obtunded.

b. Activated charcoal and magnesium sulfate or citrate for GI catharsis.

c. Tight restraints and excess stimulation should be avoided (do not attempt to "talk the patient down").

d. Diazepam is preferred as an anticonvulsant and for acute anxiety.

e. Removal of the drug from the body may be enhanced by continuous nasogastric drainage and acidification of the urine (pH < 5) with ammonium chloride (2.75 mEq/kg q6h) via a nasogastric tube and ascorbic acid (2 gm q6h) IV. Furosemide (see Table 10-1) may also be used to increase PCP excretion through the urine. This therapy should be used until CNS signs have disappeared.

III. LEAD POISONING

A. Etiology   Lead poisoning results from the ingestion of plaster or other objects saturated or coated with lead-based paint (lead content > 0.06 percent); from inhalation of lead vapor or fumes; from ingestion of foods stored in lead-lined containers, or of ceramics coated with lead glazes and fired below 1800°F; and from absorption from lead-saturated soil.

Airborne lead probably contributes to increased lead absorption by ingestion of fallout on soil or dust rather than inhalation. Children of lead workers and children living in pre-World War II dilapidated housing, near major highways, bridges, or freeways, and downwind from lead smelters are at particular risk.

There is no racial predilection, but malnutrition enhances lead toxicity in vitro.

Although figures vary by target population and geographic area, virtually no industralized area or large city is spared. Indeed, in many rural areas, particularly in the northeastern United States, the incidence is higher than in some urban locations (e.g., in the Southwest). Recognizing that the incidence is variable, public health workers have screened target populations in urban centers, revealing elevated lead levels in 10–30 percent of children 1–6 years of age. Firm data from screening for free erythrocyte protoporphyrin (FEP; see text) are not yet available but appear comparable. Of particular interest, even the incidence of elevated lead levels in areas considered unlikely, e.g., some suburbs, middle-class neighborhoods, is 1.5–3 percent.

B. Evaluation

1. **History** Data should be obtained on the size of the family and the location, age, and condition of the home or other frequented areas. Whethe
or not there is a history of pica should be determined, but pica is not
sine qua non in lead poisoning. Questions should be asked about th
child's appetite, bowel habits, and general behavior, as well as abou
signs of irritability and lethargy.

2. **Complete physical examination** should include a complete neurologic e:
amination, as well as a developmental assessment and psychometric e
amination, if possible.

3. **Laboratory studies**

   a. Blood lead levels may be determined by a micromethod, either atom
   absorption spectrophotometry or anodic stripping voltammetry. I
   experienced hands, the laboratory error should be ≤ 5 percen
   Whenever possible, venous samples should be obtained to avoid tl
   problem of skin contamination by lead-laden soil. If a finger-stio
   sample is used, the finger should be carefully washed and rinsed
   minimize such contamination.

   b. Free erythrocyte protoporphyrin (FEP) or zinc protoporphyrin (ZP)
   is widely accepted as reflecting lead toxicity. Since the interpretatio
   of values is complicated by the effect of iron deficiency on FEP or ZI
   levels, **absolute criteria for lead poisoning are difficult to establish.**
   general, values above 100 μg/100 ml probably reflect lead effect a:
   values above 250 μg/100 ml are almost certainly due to lead with
   without concomitant iron deficiency. Rare exceptions occur, includi:
   erythrocytic protoporphyria.

   Because 1–3 weeks of lead exposure is required to elevate protopo
   phyrin levels, it is theoretically possible for lead levels to be elevat∢
   in the presence of normal FEP or ZPP. This is sometimes seen
   adults with acute, chance industrial or other lead exposure, but it
   uncommon in children, in whom lead exposure tends to be chronic a:
   insidious.

   For a complete discussion, see the Center for Disease Contro
   pamphlet *Preventing Lead Poisoning in Young Children.*

   c. **Other blood tests** Blood tests in any child with elevated blood lea
   FEP, or both should include a CBC, with attention to basophi
   stippling of the erythrocyte, iron and iron-binding capacity, BU
   and serum creatinine. Delta-amino levulinic acid and delta-ami
   levulinic acid dehydratase are also sensitive to elevated lead leve
   but are not widely available, and such determinations have few cli
   cal advantages over FEP or ZPP. In the absence of clinical anem
   elevated levels of FEP or ZPP can be due to either lead, iron de
   ciency, or both, although with sufficiently long exposure, some degr
   of anemia usually is found. Similarly, because FEP or ZPP refl∢
   events at the cellular level, serum iron and iron-binding capacity c
   be normal when FEP and ZPP are not.

   Urinary coproporphyrin is less well correlated with increased le
   burden than FEP or ZPP, but the assay can be performed by t
   clinician and may be helpful when other tests cannot be done.

   d. X-ray films of the skull to detect widening of sutures (encephal∢
   athy) are helpful, as are x-ray films of the knees to detect wideni
   and increased density of the zones of provisional calcification in ⊥
   distal femur, proximal tibia, and proximal fibula (chronic ingesti

and anteroposterior views of the abdomen for radiopacities (acute ingestion). Knee films in children 18–30 months of age should be in-·terpreted cautiously, since a wide range of normal changes during rapid growth can mimic "lead lines." However, when widening and increased density of the zone of provisional calcification include the proximal fibulas as well as the proximal tibia and distal femur, the likelihood is increased that chronic exposure to a heavy metal, most probably lead, is responsible.

e. Hair and teeth can be assayed for lead, which, if elevated, reflects chronic ingestion.

f. Lead mobilization test (provocative chelation) In children with only moderate elevations of blood lead, in whom the results are conflicting or who have already undergone chelation therapy, the lead mobilization test can clarify the size of the *mobilizable* pool of lead. Since this pool has been correlated with indicators of toxicity, a positive lead mobilization test should be considered an indication for therapy except in asymptomatic adults.

Up to 50 mg/kg/24 hr of calcium disodium EDTA is administered by IM or IV drip. The dose may be divided or given in toto in a single dose. Urine is collected quantitatively for up to 24 hr. The test is positive if the 24-hr collection yields more than 1 μg lead/mg EDTA injected.

Alternatively, a shorter collection (6–8 hr) of urine may be used, with a concomitant reduction in the yield of lead. In this case the dose of EDTA is given in toto at the beginning of collection. Because the large bulk of lead is excreted within 6–12 hr following the EDTA dose, an excretion of > 0.5 μg lead/mg EDTA injected is considered positive. This modification permits the test to be performed on an outpatient basis.

Note that determinations of the urinary concentration of lead are *not* helpful. It is the *absolute* excretion of lead/time interval/chelation dose that is measured, requiring quantitative urine collections and good hydration during the test, which is no mean feat in the toddler who is not yet toilet trained.

Indications for the lead mobilization test are given in Table 3-6.

g. Lumbar puncture is contraindicated unless it is certain that cerebrospinal fluid pressure is not increased. Lumbar puncture adds little to the evaluation, and the findings do not affect therapy.

h. In encephalopathy, the electroencephalogram shows diffuse changes or may be normal.

i. Nerve conduction times may be abnormal in chronic lead poisoning, reflecting segmental demyelination. This is seen particularly when lead poisoning is present in children with sickle cell disease.

Table 3-6 Indications for Lead Mobilization Test

---

1. Venous blood lead $\geqq$ 30–60 μg/100 ml and FEP $\geqq$ 100 μg/100 ml
2. Venous blood lead $\geqq$ 30–60 μg/100 ml and FEP $\geqq$ 50–100 μg/100 ml with positive findings on x-rays of abdomen *or* knees
3. To assess need for further chelation in patient under therapy, in whom lead level and FEP may be misleading

Table 3-7 Clinical and Laboratory Evidence of Lead Intoxication and Asymptomatic Lead Burden

Lead Intoxication	Asymptomatic Increased Lead Burden
Clinical	*Clinical*
Anorexia, constipation, irritability, clumsiness, lethargy, behavior changes, hyperactivity (sequela), abdominal pain, vomiting, fever, hepatosplenomegaly, ataxia, convulsions, coma with increased CSF pressure	History of pica Environmental lead source Positive family history Sequelae: fine motor dysfunction, language delay, hyperactivity
Laboratory	*Laboratory*
FEP (ZPP) $\geqq$ 250 μg/100 ml Microcytic, hypochromic anemia Basophilic erythrocyte stippling	Blood lead > 30 μg/100 ml FEP $\geqq$ 100 μg/100 ml[a] Hair lead > 100 μg/100 ml in proximal segment
Increased urinary coproporphyrin	24-hr urinary lead excretion > 80–100 μg
Increased metaphyseal densities on x-ray	Lead mobilization test > 1 μg/mg EDTA injected/24 hr[b]
Aminoaciduria, glucosuria	Radiopacity in GI tract on x-ray
Prolonged nerve conduction time	Elevated tooth lead

[a] FEP $\geqq$ 50 μg/100 ml is elevated. However, at moderate elevations, iron deficiency alone may be responsible.
[b] See text.

    j. Routine urinalysis may show pyuria, casts, glucosuria, or aminoaciduria. These findings are usually seen in chronic, severe plumbism in association with circulating blood lead levels above 100 gm/100 ml. A Fanconi-type tubular acidosis characterized by aminoaciduria, glucosuria, and hypophosphatemia may be found in such patients.

C. Diagnosis See Table 3-7.

D. Therapy **At all costs, the source of lead must be removed despite the existence of other problems.**

    1. Commonly used chelating agents are EDTA, BAL, and D-penicillamine. (For a complete discussion of the use of chelating agents, see *J. Pediatr.* 73:1, 1968, and *Pediatrics* 53:441, 1974.)

        a. EDTA

            (1) Mechanism of action EDTA binds lead preferentially to calcium; when the calcium disodium salt (Versenate) is used, 1 mole of calcium is released for each mole of metal bound, thereby avoiding hypocalcemia. Lead is removed from the soft tissues and CNS, but *not* from red blood cells. Whether or not EDTA removes lead directly from bone is not clear. However, bone pools of lead are reduced after multiple chelations with EDTA. It is of importance that EDTA enhances removal of other metals, notably zinc and iron [see **(5)**]. Urinary lead excretion is increased twentyfold to fiftyfold.

(2) Route of administration EDTA may be given IV or IM. When given IV, a slow drip provides the best results. When this is impractical, the dose should be divided by four or six and each dose administered slowly over 1–3 hr. In IM administration, EDTA should be given with procaine in deep injection. The usual procaine concentration is 0.5 percent, but higher concentrations (up to 2 percent) do not alter the effectiveness or distribution of the EDTA.

Although oral preparations of EDTA are available, absorption is variable. Worse, these have been shown to enhance absorption of lead from the gut, and so **oral EDTA is contraindicated in childhood plumbism.**

(3) Pharmacokinetics Calcium disodium EDTA remains stable for months when refrigerated. It is ubiquitously distributed through the body, both when given IV and IM, and is rapidly excreted in the kidney. The half-life is about 35 min for either preparation.

(4) Dose Under most circumstances, a total daily dose of 50 mg/kg will provide sufficient lead diuresis. This dose is administered up to 5 days sequentially and then discontinued for at least 48 hr to permit clearance of the lead-EDTA complexes and permit some reequilibration of lead stores. Under these conditions, as many 5-day courses of EDTA as indicated can be administered. As a rule, the longer the hiatus between courses of EDTA, the lower the risk of toxicity. In severe lead poisoning (blood lead 80 μg/100 ml or symptoms are present), the dose can be increased to 75 mg/kg, although the risk of renal toxicity is thereby also increased.

(5) Toxicity The kidney is the principal site of toxicity, with renal effects seen at doses as low as 65 mg/kg/24 hr. Lead-EDTA complexes are more toxic than EDTA itself, and thus the risk of toxicity is increased in patients with very high lead burdens. During chelation, urinalyses and careful monitoring of BUN, creatinine, and calcium should be done. Although hypocalcemia is avoided by the use of the calcium salt of EDTA, *hyper*calcemia, usually mild, can be seen with prolonged therapy. Other toxic effects include removal of zinc, iron, and other metals (although only zinc and iron appear to present clinical problems). When chelation therapy is completed, replacement of iron and, if indicated, zinc should be undertaken.

b. BAL actually removes more lead from the body than does EDTA because it enhances fecal as well as urinary excretion. In addition, it diffuses well into erythrocytes. It can be administered in the presence of renal impairment because it is predominantly excreted in bile.

(1) Mechanism of action Two molecules of BAL combine with one of heavy metal to form a stable complex. To a degree, BAL protects sulfhydryl enzymes from deactivation and, if given early in the course of intoxication, can reactivate already affected enzymes.

(2) Route of administration BAL is only available for IM administration in oil.

(3) Pharmacokinetics BAL is detoxified in the liver, and urinary excretion of sulfur is increased for several hours after its administration. Peak levels occur in 30 min, with complete detoxification in 4 hr.

(4) Dose   The usual dosage is 12 mg/kg/day and up to 24 mg/kg/day in severe cases, in 3–6 divided doses. Since it is mainly used to lower the blood lead rapidly, it need not be given for a full 5 days with EDTA (see Sec. **E.2.d**). 48–72 hr may suffice, **provided EDTA is continued.**

(5) Toxicity   Toxic reactions may occur in as many as 50 percent of patients. A febrile reaction peculiar to children occurs in 30 percent, which may lead to the erroneous conclusion that infection is present. The presence of a transient granulocytopenia may further confuse the observer. In both adults and children, other reactions include transient hypertension, nausea, headache, burning sensation of the oropharynx, conjunctivitis, rhinorrhea and excessive salivation, paresthesias, burning sensation in the penis sweating, abdominal pain, and occasional sterile abscesses. Such reactions are most likely with the inappropriate use of BAL, that is, when heavy metal concentration is relatively low.

c. D-Penicillamine, the only available oral chelating agent, is probably somewhat less efficient than EDTA and BAL in removing lead from the body; it does not remove lead from erythrocytes. The D-isomer has relatively low toxicity and can be given over a long period. Side effects can be minimized by beginning with a lower dose and gradually increasing to the full dose [see (4)].

(1) Mechanism of action   D-Penicillamine enhances urinary excretion of lead, although not as effectively per mole as EDTA. Excreted lead is not necessarily in the form of chelated complexes, and the specific mechanism is not well understood.

(2) Pharmacokinetics   D-Penicillamine is well absorbed PO and rapidly excreted in urine. It is stable in vivo, even more so when acetylated.

(3) Route of administration   The D-isomer is administered PO. It is currently available as both 125-mg and 250-mg tablets. These capsules may be opened and dissolved in liquid, if necessary.

(4) Dose   The usual oral dose is 20–40 mg/kg. Side effects can be minimized by initiating therapy with small doses; e.g., 25 percent of the expected dose and increasing after one week to 50 percent and again after one week to the full dose, as well as by monitoring for toxicity.

(5) Toxicity and side effects   The D-isomer of penicillamine is relatively nontoxic. As many as 20 percent of patients receiving the drug will experience some form of toxicity, usually reactions resembling those of penicillin sensitivity, including fevers, rashes leukopenia, thrombocytopenia, and eosinophilia. Anorexia nausea, and vomiting are infrequent. Of most concern, however are isolated reports of nephrotoxicity, possibly from hypersensitivity reactions. Toxicity may be reduced by concurrent administration of pyridoxine, although no careful studies of this effect are available. **D-Penicillamine should not be administered to patients with known penicillin allergy.**

2. Monitoring chelation therapy   Urinary lead excretion may be used to monitor the effectiveness of chelation therapy, since the blood lead can be misleading in the presence of these agents.

    a. During chelation therapy, serum calcium, BUN, and lead in the blood and urine, as well as urinalyses, are monitored for evidence of hypocalcemia or renal toxicity due to EDTA. If such evidence is present, EDTA can be reduced or discontinued, and renal function usually returns to normal.

    b. Occasionally, symptoms may worsen during therapy. This phenomenon is not understood, but removal of lead should continue, with attention to CNS changes suggestive of cerebral edema (see **E.3**).

    c. EDTA is administered for up to 5 days at a time. In general, urinary lead excretion tends to fall off after the fourth day regardless of the lead burden, while the risk of EDTA nephrotoxicity increases after the fifth day. For this reason, EDTA chelation is interrupted after 5 days, and a "rest period" of at least 48–72 hr is initiated. If the lead burden, indicated by initial blood lead and urine lead excretion, is very high, chelation is again begun after 48–72 hr, and a new 24-hr urine lead is obtained for comparison. In this manner, as many chelations as are indicated by the lead burden can be undertaken without significant risk until such time as the initial 24-hr urine lead excretion fails to yield $1 \geqq \mu g$ lead/mg EDTA. Therapy is then discontinued and long-term follow-up begun. Subsequent chelation may well be necessary, but a longer hiatus between chelations can now ensue.

    d. Because of the "rebound" phenomenon during reequilibration of body lead stores, blood lead and FEP levels immediately following chelation tend to be misleading and are best obtained 2–3 weeks following therapy.

    e. The ultimate goal of therapy is to reduce body lead burden to safe levels (i.e., blood lead $< 30 \ \mu g/100 \ ml$) and FEP to normal (i.e., $< 50 \ \mu g/100 \ ml$). Because chelation therapy tends to be less efficient as the body burden is lowered, the clinician must exercise judgment to decide when enough therapy has been administered. Such factors as the child's age, degree of exposure, likelihood of continued exposure, discomfort, and side effects of parenteral chelation must be weighed. In general, the most complete therapy should be applied to children under 3 years of age.

E. Management of plumbism The criteria for chelation therapy proposed in Table 3-8 are intended as guidelines. Each child is different. Important variables include age, duration of exposure, risk factors such as iron deficiency, sickle cell disease, and metabolic acidosis, and developmental levels.

    1. Asymptomatic increased absorption

        a. *If* the child is asymptomatic, and *if* the lead source is found and removed, and *if* there is no biochemical evidence of intoxication, *no* treatment is necessary. The child may be followed by monthly blood lead determinations (if FEP $\leqq 100 \ \mu g/100 \ ml$) and, if indicated (see Table 3-5), by a lead mobilization test.

Table 3-8 Indications for Chelation Therapy

1. Venous blood lead $\geqq 60 \ \mu g/100 \ ml$ on two successive occasions, *or*
2. Venous blood lead $\geqq 30$–$60 \ \mu g/100 \ ml$ and FEP $\geqq 250 \ \mu g/100 \ ml$ *or*
3. Positive lead mobilization test

Factors contributing to indications:
  Age, degree of exposure, underlying developmental level, iron deficiency

b. *If* there is anemia, or *if* the blood lead is increasing, or *if* the child is at risk of further ingestion, a single dose of 50 mg/kg EDTA can be given each morning for 5 days, discontinued for 48 hr, and begun again as long as the elevated lead burden persists. Hospitalization is not necessary for this purpose, and BUN, urinalysis, and blood leads can be obtained on days 1, 3, and 5.

c. *If* prolonged therapy is required, D-penicillamine, 20–40 mg/kg PO, may be administered instead of EDTA (therapy can be continuous, without 48-hr intervals).

2. Acute lead intoxication, mild to moderate

a. Hospitalize the child.

b. Give maintenance fluids.

c. Administer EDTA IV if possible or IM if necessary (50 mg/kg daily in 3 divided doses). If the IM route is chosen, the dose can be bid or even a single injection.

d. If the lead burden appears high on the basis of urinary excretion, add BAL IM in 3 divided doses of 12–24 mg/kg/24 hr for 48–72 hr.

e. Monitor BUN, blood, 24-hr urine lead, and the urinalyses.

f. After chelation is completed, administer iron (see Chap. 15, Sec. **I.A.3**).

3. Acute lead intoxication (severe, with encephalopathy)

a. **This is a medical emergency.**

b. Give maintenance fluids.

c. Begin EDTA IV, 75 mg/kg/day in 3 divided doses by slow drip.

d. Begin BAL IM, 24 mg/kg/day in 3–6 divided doses.

e. Treat cerebral edema with mannitol and dexamethasone (Decadron) (see Chap. 2, Sec. **V**).

f. *Continue chelation therapy at all costs, since cerebral edema will not respond to therapy until the lead burden is reduced.*

g. Treat seizures with anticonvulsants (see Table 14-1).

h. After 5 days, discontinue therapy for 48 hr and restart.

i. Monitor BUN, calcium, EEG, urinalysis findings, and blood and 24-hr urine lead.

j. Continue with a close monthly follow-up as long as the child is at risk.

4. Sequelae
Evidence is accumulating that both symptomatic and asymptomatic lead poisoning produce sequelae. Gross screening tests are generally not sensitive enough to distinguish subtle deficits and are frequently performed in children too young to provide reproducible results.

All children with histories of increased lead burden, whether symptomatic or asymptomatic, should undergo thorough neuropsychological evaluation prior to entering school, ideally at ages 5–6. At a minimum this should include evaluation of visual-motor skills, expressive and receptive language skills, visual and auditory perceptual skills, and fine and gross motor skills. I.Q. testing may be misleading because it fails to reflect specific functional deficits. With these results in hand, the clinician can alert the school to a child's difficulties and recommend remedial or special education where deficits exist. Conversely, when none is found the family and school authorities can be appropriately reassured. Behavior problems related to lead poisoning, such as hyperactivity, may respond to pharmacologic therapy.

F. Prevention   **Lead poisoning is a preventable disease.** Strong laws are in effect in some states requiring removal of lead paint from the market and strong penalties for nonremoval from houses in cases of plumbism. Intensive screening of children to identify those at risk, widespread inspection of housing, and stringent enforcement of sanitary and housing codes can reduce morbidity in this disease.

4

Management of the Newborn, I

I. GENERAL PRINCIPLES OF NEWBORN EVALUATION AND CARE

A. Delivery room

1. Fetal and maternal history

a. Maternal factors

(1) **Prior obstetric history,** e. g., abortions, premature births, congenital anomalies, and infants dying shortly after birth.

(2) **Maternal diseases** Chronic disorders such as renal disease and diabetes may predispose to malnourished infants, require premature birth, or cause delayed maturation.

(3) **Maternal infections** Syphilis, gonorrhea, tuberculosis, or TORCH (*t*oxoplasmosis, *r*ubella, *c*ytomegalovirus, *h*erpesvirus).

(4) **Medications,** e. g., teratogenicity, fetal depression, narcotic addiction, fetal alcohol syndrome, and cigarette smoking.

(5) **Perinatal maternal factors,** including toxemia, abruptio placentae, placenta previa, prolonged labor, multiple births, and prolonged rupture of membranes.

b. Fetal factors

(1) **Gestational age** relates to timing of elective delivery, therapy for jaundice, temperature, feeding, and postnatal growth rate.

(2) **Pulmonary maturation** The amniotic fluid lecithin-sphingomyelin ratio (L/S) is an indicator of pulmonary maturation.

(3) **Oxytocin challenge test** Fetal distress following an oxytocin-induced uterine contraction gives a relative index of fetal risk.

(4) **Fetal monitoring** during labor will predict asphyxia.

2. Delivery room care of high-risk infants

a. Preparation

(1) Be aware of the maternal and fetal history.

(2) **Equipment**

(a) Radiant warmer bed, blankets.

(b) Flow-through anesthesia bag capable of delivering 100% oxygen.

(c) Infant face masks of various sizes.

(d) Stethoscope.

(e) Laryngoscope with No. 0 and No. 1 blades, batteries, and bulbs.

(f) Cole orotracheal tubes with 2.5, 3.0, and 3.5-mm internal diameters, two of each.

(g) Drugs $NaHCO_3$, 0.5 mg/ml; epinephrine, 1:10,000; dextrose, 25 or 50%; calcium gluconate 10%; atropine; naloxone (Narcan) 0.2 mg/ml; saline; and albumin.

(h) Umbilical catheterization tray with No. 3.5F and 5F catheters.

(i) A heated, warmed incubator with a portable oxygen supply.

b. Delivery

(1) Place the infant on a warming table.

(2) Suction the nares and mouth with a suction bulb. Gastric aspiration and deep suctioning in the first 5 min of life may produce bradycardia and should not be done routinely.

(3) If thick meconium is present, suction the oropharynx and trachea before the onset of breathing.

(4) Dry the infant.

(5) Evaluate by the Apgar Score (Table 4-1).

(a) Apgar 3–4 If the heart rate is below 100, clear the airway and ventilate with bag and mask with pressures of 20–25 cm H_2O at 30 breaths/min.

(b) Apgar 0–2 For treatment of infants whose Apgar scores are 0–2, see Fig. 4-1.

(6) All infants should have a brief general examination for anomalies.

(7) If the mother is awake and the infant appears well, permit her to hold the infant as soon as she wishes.

B. Nursery care

1. Feeding and nutrition Requirements for full-term neonates are between 110–130 kcal/kg/day. The protein requirement is 2–3 gm/kg/day. Fat intake makes up 55–65 kcal/kg/day, and the balance is carbohydrate.

Table 4-1 Apgar Score*

Sign	0	1	2
Heart rate	Absent	Slow, less than 100	100 or over
Respiratory effort	Absent	Weak cry, hypoventilation	Crying lustily
Muscle tone	Flaccid	Some flexion, extremities	Well-flexed
Reflex irritability	No response	Some motion	Cry
Color	Blue, pale	Blue hands and feet	Entirely pink

* Score infant at 1 and 5 min of age.

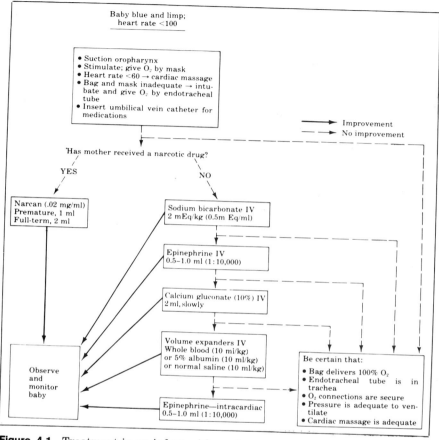

Figure 4-1 Treatment in an infant with an Apgar score of 0–2. (Adapted from J. Kattwinckel, Continuing Education Program, University of Virginia.)

a. Breast-feeding

(1) Breast milk is of proved nutritional and emotional value for the feeding of the full-term infant, and should be encouraged for all full-term infants and most premature infants.

(2) Whether or not breast milk is nutritionally adequate for the premature infant is disputed. The protein in breast milk is 60% whey (β-lactoglobulin and lactalbumin) and 40% casein and relatively digestible by the premature. However, the low total protein content of breast milk may be inadequate to support optimal growth in premature infants. Prematures not growing adequately on breast milk may therefore require protein supplementation (up to 2 gm/day) (see Table 4-5). Some prematures may also have a transient lactase deficiency that requires lactose-free formula.

(3) Human milk contains a number of antimicrobial components not found in infant formulas: Immunoglobulins, leukocytes, lactoferrin, the third component of complement in colostrum, and lysozymes. In areas where sanitation is poor, the use of nonhuman milk formulas has been clearly associated with increased infant mortality from infection.

(4) Fostering successful breast-feeding

(a) Both the obstetrician and the pediatrician should discuss nursing prenatally with the mother.

(b) Experienced nursing mothers should be available to discuss the satisfactions and techniques of breast-feeding with expectant mothers.

(c) Obstetric ward and neonatal unit practices should be altered to foster successful nursing. Some of these changes include

i. Decreasing the amount of sedation or anesthesia given to mothers.

ii. Allowing the mother to nurse the infant immediately after delivery, if possible.

iii. Encouraging "rooming in" to avoid separation of mother and infant.

iv. Having infants fed on demand rather than on a rigid schedule.

v. Seeing that the personnel caring for new mothers are actively supportive of breast-feeding.

(5) There are few contraindications to breast-feeding. These are chronic debilitating disease or active tuberculosis in the mother.

(6) **Drug use** Although the literature on the excretion of drugs in breast milk is not extensive, there are a few areas of general agreement on drugs to be avoided by mothers who are breast-feeding. These include chloramphenicol, nitrofurantoin, sulfonamides (in infants with glucose 6-phosphate dehydrogenase deficiency [G-6-PD]), and possibly tetracycline, phenindione, antimetabolites, antithyroid drugs, methadone, morphine, propoxyphene (Darvon), excess alcohol, lithium, and any isotopically labeled pharmaceutical (e.g., ^{131}I, ^{99m}Tc, and ^{67}Ga). The safety of many drugs for use *during* nursing is not known. (See *Med. Lett. Drug Ther.* 21(5) : 1979, and discussion on drug use during lactation in J. Cloherty and A. Stark (eds.), *Manual of Neonatal Care*, Boston, Little, Brown, 1980.)

b. **Formula feeding** (See also Chap. 1, Sec. **III.A.**) A number of commercially available formulas are adequate (Tables 4-2 to 4-4). Those based on cow's milk (e.g., Similac, Enfamil) are the usual formulas for full-term infants.

(1) Similac PM 60/40 or similar formulas are best for premature infants in the first weeks of life because of the whey-casein and calcium-phosphorus ratios.

(2) Soy-based formulas and formulas whose caloric density is greater than 20 cal/oz are for special situations.

(3) Protein, medium-chain triglycerides (MCTs), and glucose-polymer

caloric supplements (Table 4-5) should be used only for babies who require caloric supplementation. These supplements may increase the likelihood of late metabolic acidosis and prevent absorption of Ca^{++} and other minerals. They are also expensive.

c. Supplements (vitamins, iron, and calcium)

(1) Breast-feeding

(a) Breast-fed infants need supplementation with 400 IU/day of vitamin D. Although vitamins A and C are not necessary, they will not be harmful in the doses provided in commercially available vitamin preparations (vitamin A, 1500 IU; vitamin D, 400 IU; vitamin C, 50 mg).

(b) The use of iron supplements in breast-fed infants is controversial (see *Pediatrics* 63:52, 1979). Some have suggested a dose of 2 mg/kg/day of elemental iron.

(c) If infants are fully breast-fed they should receive fluoride supplementation as in **(2).(b)** even if the mother drinks fluoridated water.

(2) Formulas

(a) Formulas usually contain adequate vitamins (1 quart formula/day), though iron supplementation after 4–8 weeks of age may be necessary (2 mg/kg/day elemental iron).

(b) Fluoride should be supplemented if babies are not receiving fluoridated water (0.25 mg/day up to age 2, 0.50 mg/day age 2–3 years, 1.0 mg/day 3–16 years).

(c) Small prematures should be given vitamin E (25–50 IU/day) for prevention of hemolysis.

(d) Vitamin K, 0.5 mg IM weekly, should be given to infants not being fed orally or on antibiotics.

(e) Supplemental calcium (150 mg/kg/day elemental Ca^{++} is the recommended total daily consumption) may be necessary, since formulas contain approximately 1 mg Ca^{++}/cal.

d. Special nutritional needs of the low-birth-weight infant

(1) Fluid intake of the low-birth-weight infant should increase from 75 ml/kg/day on day 1 to approximately 150 ml/kg/day after day 5. Daily caloric requirements are 50–100 kcal/kg by 3 days of age and 110–150 kcal/kg during later growth.

Low-birth-weight infants usually tolerate feeding q2–3h better than larger feedings q4h.

(a) If the infant is under 1250–1500 gm, start an IV with 10% D/W at about 100 ml/kg/day. Continue IV until PO feedings are 100 ml/kg/day.

(b) Follow Dextrostix at ½, 1, and 2 hr of age, then q4h prn. The Somogyi effect can occur if the IV infiltrates.

(2) First feeding, 5% D/W; second and third feedings, half-strength formula without iron, or breast milk; subsequent feedings, full-strength formula or breast milk.

(3) Close monitoring of urine and specific gravity, skin turgor, body weight, serum and urine osmolarity, and electrolyte concentrations is necessary.

Table 4-2 Nutrient Sources in Infant Formulas

Formula	Sources		
	Carbohydrate	Protein	Fat
Breast milk	Lactose	Lactalbumin, casein	High in olein, lower in volatile fatty acids
Regular			
Enfamil (MJ)	Lactose	Nonfat milk	Soy and coconut oils; E:PUFA, 0.8:1
Similac (Ross)	Lactose	Nonfat milk	Coconut, soy, and corn oils
Humanized			
Similac PM 60/40	Lactose	Nonfat milk, partially de-mineralized whey	Corn and coconut oils
SMA (Wyeth)	Lactose	Nonfat milk, demineralized whey	Oleo (destearinated beef fat); coconut, safflower, and soy oils
Designed for specialized needs			
CHO-Intolerance CHO-Free (Syntex)			
Hypoallergenic ISOMIL (Ross)	Corn syrup, sucrose, modified corn starch	Soy protein isolate	Soy oil
	Sucrose, tapioca starch	Soy protein isolate	Soy, coconut, and corn oils
Nutramigen (MJ)		Hydrolyzed casein	Corn oil

Malabsorption			
Portagen (MJ)	Lactose, dextrose, maltose, sucrose	Casein	MCT, corn oil
Pregestimil (MJ)	Dextrose, tapioca (no lactose)	Hydrolyzed casein, L-cystine, L-tyrosine, L-tryptophan	MCT, corn oil
Inborn errors of metabolism			
Lofenalac (MJ)	Corn syrup, solids, modified tapioca starch	Casein hydrolysate (most phenylalanine removed). Fortified with tyrosine, tryptophan, histidine, methionine	Corn oil
Adjusted caloric density			
Similac 13 (Ross)	Lactose	Nonfat milk	Coconut, soy, and corn oils
Similac 24	Lactose	Nonfat milk	Coconut, soy, and corn oils
Premature (MJ)	Lactose, sucrose	Nonfat milk	MCT, corn and coconut oils

Table 4-3 Nutrient Content of Infant Formulas

Formula	cal/oz	Per 100 ml				mg/100 ml	
		Protein	CHO	Fat	Calcium	Phosphorus	Iron
Breast milk	22	1.2	6.8	3.8	34	14	0.05
Regular							
Enfamil (MJ)	20	1.5	7.0	3.7	55	46	0.15 (with iron 1.2)
Similac (Ross)	20	1.5	7.1	3.6	60	44	Trace (with iron 1.2)
Humanized							
Similac PM 60/40 (Ross)	20	1.6	7.6	3.5	40	20	0.26
SMA (Wyeth)	20	1.5	7.2	3.6	40	32	1.2
Designed for specialized needs							
CHO-Intolerance	20						
CHO-Free (Syntex)	with CHO added	1.8	6.4 with CHO added	3.5	94	60	0.83
Hypoallergenic							
ISOMIL (Ross)	20	2.0	6.8	3.6	73	52	1.2
Nutramigen (MJ)	20	2.2	8.8	2.6	63	47	1.27
ProSobee (MJ)	20	2.5	6.8	3.4	79	53	1.27
Malabsorption							
Portagen (MJ)	20	2.4	7.8	3.2	63	47	1.27
Pregestimil (MJ)	20	2.2	8.8	2.8	63	47	1.27
Inborn errors of metabolism							
Lofenalac (MJ)	20	2.33	8.8	2.7	63	47	1.27
Adjusted caloric density							
Similac 13 (Ross)	13	1.2	4.5	2.3	45	35	Trace
Similac 24	24	2.2	8.3	4.3	83	64	1.50 (with iron)
Premature (MJ)	24	2.2	9.2				
Water and electrolyte maintenance							
Lytren (MJ)	9		7.6				
Pedialyte (Ross)	6		5.0				
5% Glucose	6		5.0				
10% Glucose	12		10.0				

Table 4-4 Approximate Electrolyte Content in Infant Formulas

Formula	mEq/L			mOsm/L	Estimated Renal Solute Load (mOsm/L)
	Na⁺	K⁺	Cl⁻		
Breast Milk	7	13	11	133	75
Regular					
Enfamil (MJ)	1	19	15	262	120
Similac (Ross)	10.9	19.2	16.6	262	109
Humanized					
Similac PM 60/40 (Ross)	6.9	14.9	12.9	275	105
SMA (Wyeth)	6.5	14.4	10.4	272	105
Designed for specialized needs					
CHO-Intolerance				131	
CHO-Free (Syntex)	15.8	22.6	9.4	355 without glucose	120
Hypoallergenic					
ISOMIL (Ross)	12.6	18.2	14.9	208	126
Nutramigen (MJ)	13.9	17.4	13.2	416	132
ProSobee (MJ)	18.3	19.0	11.9	233	149
Malabsorption					
Portagen (MJ)	13.9	24.0	16.3	211	150
Pregestimil (MJ)	13.9	17.4	13.2	539	140
Inborn errors of metabolism					
Lofenalac (MJ)	13.9	17	13.2	407	135
Adjusted caloric density					
Similac 13 (Ross)	10.0	15.0	11.3	155	84
Similac 24	13.5	26.2	21.4	310	149

(4) Supplements as needed for oral supplementation to increase caloric concentrations of formula should never be over 25 cal/oz (see Table 4-5).

(a) Carbohydrates Glucose polymer (Polycose), 4 cal/gm

(b) Fat MCT oil (medium-chain triglycerides), 8.3 cal/gm, 9 cal/gm

(c) After 1 week

i. 25–50 IU vitamin E (Aquasol E) qd PO.

ii. 1 ml multivitamins qd PO (including vitamin D, 400 IU; vitamin A, 1500 IU; vitamin C, 25–50 mg).

iii. 0.25–1.0 mg folate qd PO.

iv. Vitamin K₁, 0.5 mg weekly, if the patient is on long-term antibiotics or total parenteral nutrition.

v. Calcium gluconate 10% (9 mg Ca⁺⁺/ml) added to the formula for a calcium dose of 150 mg/kg (this should be done gradually over 1 week).

Table 4-5 Commonly Used Supplements to Increase Calorie Content of Formula

Product	Cal/gm	Cal	CHO (gm)	Protein (gm)	Fat (gm)	Na (mg)	Food Sources
Casec (MJ)	4	17		4		7.1	Calcium caseinate (88%, milk fat)
Glucose	4	35	8.75				
Karo Syrup	4	60	15			22	Corn syrup/tbsp: 4 gm glucose, 1 gm sucrose, 2 gm maltose, 2 gm trisaccharides, 5.5 gm polysaccharides
Lipomul-Oral (Upjohn)	9	90			10		Corn oil
MCT oil (MJ)	9	115			13.8		Coconut oil, MCTs easily absorbed; need no bile salts or lipase for absorption
EMF	4	60		15			Predigested collagen
Polycose (Ross)	4	30	7.5			10	Hydrolyzed cornstarch, glucose polymer

102

(5) Keep gastric intake *below* 200 ml/kg/day to avoid aspiration. Infants who need to suck in excess of their appetite can be appeased with pacifiers.

(6) On discharge, discontinue vitamin E and begin iron (2 mg elemental iron/kg/day).

(7) Infants who are unable to tolerate oral gavage feedings need parenteral nutrition (see Chap. 11).

    (a) Fluid needs are as described in Table 8-8, but they may vary, depending on the need to restrict fluid (e.g., as in hyaline membrane disease) or the need to give extra fluid (e.g., small prematures with large insensible water losses, who may have fluid requirements up to 200 ml/kg/day).

    (b) On day 2, 3 mEq/kg/day of sodium and 2 mEq/kg/day of potassium are required.

    (c) Caloric requirements are initially provided as **dextrose** 8–10% (4 kcal/gm) as tolerated and as **protein** (4 kcal/gm) as protein hydrolysates or free amino acids in gradually increasing dosage from 1 gm/kg/day on day 2 to 2.5 gm/kg/day on days 4–7.

    (d) **Fat** (9 kcal/gm) is given as 10% soybean emulsion. *Intralipid* may be used to provide additional calories without excessive fluid intake if the infant is receiving inadequate calories *after* the first week of life (see Chap. 11) or when bilirubin is under 8 mg/100 ml (5 mg/100 ml for small prematures).

2. Temperature control Heat loss may be minimized by placing an infant in a neutral thermal environment (NTE). The NTE is the thermal condition at which heat production is minimal yet core temperature is within normal range (see Table 4-6).

    a. Healthy infant The skin should be dried and the infant wrapped. Examination in the delivery room should be performed under a radiant warmer with a skin probe, keeping the skin temperature at 36.5°C.

    b. Sick infant The skin should be dried and the infant wrapped and transported in a heated incubator. A radiant warmer with a ser-

Table 4-6 Neutral Thermal Environmental Temperatures

Birth Weight (kg)	(lb)	Incubator Air Temperature (°C)	First 24 Hours (°F)
	2	35.0	95.0
		34.9	94.9
	3	34.2	93.6
.5		34.0	93.2
	4	33.7	92.7
		33.5	92.3
	5	33.3	92.0
.5		33.2	91.8
	6	33.1	91.6
		33.0	91.4

vocontrol is used for procedures. Very sick neonates, access to whom is important, may be kept in an open radiant warmer with servocontrol of skin temperature; a small, clear-plastic heat shield will prevent loss by convection and radiation and may be used when observation is less important.

C. Physical examination of the newborn   At no other time than at birth is more information obtained from the general overall visual and auditory appraisal of a naked infant and less information obtained from an exhaustive system-by-system examination. Three categories are of utmost importance: **cardiorespiratory status,** the **presence of congenital anomalies,** and the **effects of gestation, labor, delivery, anesthetics, and signs of infection or other disease.**

1. **Initial examination**   A fretful infant should be quieted with a nipple. The usual order of examination is as follows:

   a. **Respiratory**   Evaluation of respiratory status includes color, presence of acrocyanosis, and respiratory rate (normal 40–60 and often periodic), including the presence of apnea. Rales and questionable breath sounds are usually insignificant if the infant is otherwise well. On the other hand, retractions, nasal flaring, and respiratory grunting are significant in the absence of crying. Percussion has little value.

   b. **Cardiac**   Evaluation of the heart includes the position of maximal impulse, palpation of femoral and brachial pulses, and auscultation of the heart for rate, rhythm, and presence of murmurs. Because of rapid alterations in systemic and pulmonary pressures, murmurs do not always reflect the pressure of significant heart disease.

   c. **Abdomen**   Observation for asymmetry, including the musculature, masses, and fullness is critical. Palpation with gentle pressure from lower to upper quadrants is most useful. Bowel sounds may or may not be present initially. The normal liver may be as much as 2.5 cm below the right costal margin. Palpate for both kidneys.

   d. **Genitalia and rectum**   Observe for symmetry, presence of both testicles, and normal placement and patency of the urethral orifice and anus.

   e. **Extremities, spine, and joints**   Observe for anomalies of the digits, structural abnormalities, hip dislocation, and positional anomalies.

   f. **Head, neck, and mouth**   Inspect for cuts, bruises, caput, cephalo-hematoma, mobility of suture lines, and skull molding. Measure the head circumference from occiput to midbrow. Observe for neck flexibility and asymmetry and cleft palate and lip.

   g. **Neurologic examination**   Observations for neurologic status can usually be made concurrently while handling the baby for the preceding examinations. Observe for tone, activity, symmetry of extremities and facial movements, alertness, consolability, and reflexes, including the Moro, suck, rooting, grasping, and plantar reflexes.

   h. **Eye examination**   (Periorbital edema from silver nitrate may interfere.) Usually the presence of cataracts and tumors can be evaluated by elicitation of the red reflex. Scleral hemorrhage and pupillary size can be assessed.

2. The **discharge examination** should include attention to cardiac status (congestive heart failure or new murmur), abdomen (masses), stools

urine, skin (jaundice, infection), cord (infection), feeding (amount), maternal competence, and follow-up.

D. Premature infants (under 37 weeks gestation)

1. **Delivery** If possible infants under 30 weeks gestation should be delivered in a hospital with an intensive care nursery. The need for infant transport adds to the mortality and morbidity of this group.

2. **Respiration** Hyaline membrane disease (HMD) can be prevented by the measurement of the L/S ratio in amniotic fluid and prenatal treatment of the mother with steroids when indicated. Perinatal hypoxia and apnea should be anticipated and treated.

3. **Cardiovascular** Fluid overloading should be avoided. Patent ductus arteriosus is common.

4. **Hematologic** Blood component therapy (packed cells, plasma, platelets) may be necessary for anemia, hypovolemia, or bleeding.

5. **Hyperbilirubinemia**, hypoglycemia, hypocalcemia, hyponatremia, temperature control problems, and special nutritional needs must be anticipated.

E. Small for gestational age (SGA) infants (birth weight below the 10th percentile for gestational age) Conditions associated with SGA infants are listed in Table 4-7.

1. **During pregnancy,** monitor fetal well-being by urinary measurements and ultrasonographic measurements of the fetus.

2. **At delivery,** anticipate fetal distress, meconium aspiration, hypoxia, and heat loss. In the **newborn** monitor for polycythemia, hypoglycemia, and hypocalcemia. Evaluate for fetal causes of poor growth, including anomalies and congenital infection. Examination of the placenta is frequently useful.

F. Large for gestational age (LGA) (birth weight over the 90th percentile for gestational age) Conditions associated with LGA infants are listed in Table 4-7.

These infants are at high risk of obstetric trauma, including dystocia, leading to fractures, brachial plexus injuries, or central nervous system injury. Polycythemia and hypoglycemia may be present.

Table 4-7 Disparities with Gestational Age

Large Infants for Gestational Age	Small Infants for Gestational Age	
Constitutionally large infants	Advanced maternal age	Chronic hypertension
	Multiparity	
Infants of diabetic mothers	Race	Sickle cell disease
Postmaturity	Infertility	Chronic disease
Transposition of the great vessels	Previous spontaneous abortions	Smoking
Erythroblastosis fetalis	Unwed state	Multiple fetuses
Beckwith syndrome	Drug abuse	Placental lesions
Parabiotic syndrome	Maternal heart or renal disease	Congenital anomaly
		Chromosomal anomaly
	Toxemia	Congenital infections

G. **Postmature infants** (gestation over 42 weeks) The etiology is usually un-known, but postmaturity is associated with anencephaly, trisomy 18, and Seckel's dwarfism.

1. **Management** during pregnancy includes careful estimation of fetal gestational age by dates, ultrasound, and monitoring of fetal well-being.

2. **Delivery** may be elective depending on lung maturity or fetal distress. Intrapartum asphyxia, meconium aspiration, neonatal hypoglycemia and polycythemia are seen in postmature infants.

II. INTENSIVE CARE OF THE NEWBORN See also Chaps. 2 and 20.

A. **Airway**

1. Remove foreign material such as meconium and vomitus by suction.

2. Establish patency of the airway using an oral airway (size 00 or 1) as necessary. The infant can usually be adequately ventilated by a bag and mask until preparations are made for intubation.

B. **Intubation**

1. **Equipment** In the delivery room or in an emergency, oral intubation is quickest and easiest with Cole tubes. Cole tube sizes are Nos. 14, 16, and 18 for a full-term infant and Nos. 10 and 12 for a premature infant.

   When the infant's condition is stabilized, Cole tubes are changed to a soft, cuffless nasotracheal tube (e.g., Portex) for chronic intubation. Portex tube sizes are as follows:

Infant Weight (gm)	Portex Tube Size (internal diameter in mm)
Under 1250 gm	2.5 mm
1250 to 2000 gm	3.0 mm
Over 2000 gm	3.5 mm

   Additional equipment includes a laryngoscope with size 0 and size blades, tincture of benzoin, adhesive tape, Magill forceps, sutures, and various-sized stylets. If possible, a clinician experienced in intubation of infants should be in attendance.

2. **Method**

   a. Suction the mouth and upper airway.

   b. If the intubation is elective, empty the stomach and attach a cardiac monitor to the baby.

   c. For nasotracheal intubation, measure for proper tube length **prior to intubation** (see Fig. 4-2).

   d. The baby should be ventilated with a bag and mask just prior to intubation.

   e. The infant's head should be in the neutral position, avoiding excessive extension of the neck. The laryngoscope is held between the thumb and first finger of the left hand, with the second and third fingers holding the chin and stabilizing the head. Pushing down on the larynx with the fifth finger of the left hand (or having an assistant do it) and keeping the infant's head straight may help to visualize the vocal cords (trachea). The laryngoscope is passed into the right side of the mouth and then to the midline, swinging the tongue out of the way.

   f. The endotracheal tube is held with the right hand and inserted be-

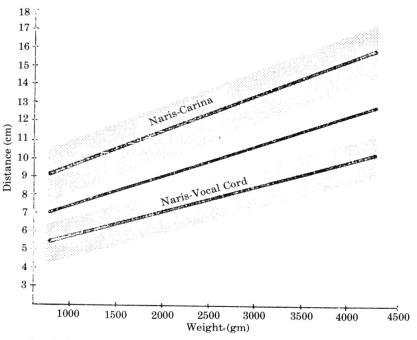

Figure 4-2. Relation of naris-carina and naris-glottis distance to body weight. From T. Aceto, Jr., *Pediatrics* 42:825, 1968. Copyright by the American Academy of Pediatrics, 1968.)

tween the vocal cords to about 2 cm below the glottis. During naso-tracheal intubation, Magill forceps can be useful to guide the tube between the cords. If the fifth finger is pressing on the trachea, the tube can be felt as it slips into place.

g. Check the tube position by auscultation to ensure equal aeration of both lungs. If air entry is poor over the left chest, pull back the tube until aeration is improved.

h. During the procedure, one person should continually observe the infant and monitor heart rate. The infant should not be allowed to become hypoxic or have bradycardia during intubation. If bradycardia occurs, stop the procedure and ventilate the infant with a bag and mask. Attaching an anesthesia bag on one side to 100% oxygen and on the other to the intubation tube adapter will deliver 100% oxygen to the pharynx during the intubation procedure. (An in-line pop-off valve should be present so that pressures do not exceed 25 cm H_2O.)

i. Intubation in the delivery room is usually temporary, and the tube can be held in place by hand. If prolonged ventilation is required, the tube should be secured by paper tape, and an x-ray obtained to check its position.

C. Ventilation   See also Chaps. 2 and 20.

   1. Principles

   a. Delivery room

   (1) Artificial ventilation is used to oxygenate the infant and, whe[n] necessary, to initiate spontaneous ventilation. Usually, the airwa[y] is cleared and ventilation is established with a mask and an anes[-]thesia bag capable of delivering an FIO_2 of 1.0.

   (2) A maximal pressure of 25 cm H_2O with a rate of 30 breaths/min [is] usually adequate. Pressure should be measured by an in-lin[e] manometer.

   (3) Pressure should be increased if the chest wall is not moving [in] spite of a tightly fitting face mask. A good response will be show[n] by a rise in heart rate, good skin color, and an increase in th[e] baby's activity. **If these signs are not observed, the baby should b[e] promptly intubated and ventilated.**

   b. Nursery

   (1) Continuous distending airway pressure   CDAP includes all arti[fi]cial methods that attempt to maintain aveolar distention (co[n]tinuous negative airway pressure, continuous positive airwa[y] pressure).
   CDAP is indicated

   (a) In HMD, when an FIO_2 greater than 0.4–0.6 is required to kee[p] arterial PO_2 (PaO_2) at 50–70 torr or when apnea does not r[e]spond to other therapy (see Sec. **II.D**).

   (b) In HMD, CDAP increases arterial PO_2, allowing the reducti[on] of FIO_2.

   (c) Contraindications to CDAP without positive-pressure ventil[a]tion are increasing $PaCO_2$, persistent acidosis, and diseases n[ot] associated with decreased pulmonary compliance.

   (2) Intermittent positive pressure ventilation   IPPV is indicated

   (a) In HMD, when the PaO_2 is less than 50 torr, FIO_2 is over 6[0] and CDAP is 10 cm H_2O.

   (b) When PCO_2 is over 70–80 from any cause.

   (c) In persistent respiratory acidosis.

   (d) When apnea does not respond to other therapy (see Sec. **II.[D**). The actual levels of arterial PO_2 and PCO_2 selected for inte[r]vention depend on the disease course. Respiratory support [is] adjusted so that PaO_2 = 50–70 torr, $PaCO_2$ = 35–50 torr, and p[H] = 7.30–7.40. These values are optimal and differ for certa[in] diseases.

   2. Methods   For detailed discussion of the methods used in providing co[n]tinuous distending airway pressure or intermittent positive pressu[re] ventilation (IPPV), and of the recommendations for ventilation and ca[re] of the infant on the respirator, consult Cloherty and Stark's *Manual [of] Neonatal Care.*

   3. Long-term complications of respirator therapy

   a. Bronchopulmonary dysplasia   Chronic lung disease in the form [of] BPD occurs in 5–30 percent of survivors of respirator therapy f[or]

HMD. These infants often require prolonged treatment with oxygen and respiratory therapy because of severe disease. Most recover slowly, although some may die of infection or cor pulmonale during the first year of life.

b. Retrolental fibroplasia Premature infants receiving oxygen therapy are at risk of retrolental fibroplasia. (To avoid visual impairment, close attention must be paid to O_2 concentration and blood gases must be frequently assessed.) All premature infants treated with oxygen should have an ophthalmologic examination **prior to discharge.** In very small prematures (weighing under 1000 gm) RLF may occur even if the PO_2 did not exceed 100.

c. Neurologic impairment is estimated to occur in 10–15 percent of the survivors of respirator therapy for HMD. Infants with less severe disease are presumably less affected.

d. Familial psychopathology Little is known about the long-term effects of HMD and its management on parent-infant interaction, although the incidence of child abuse is said to be higher in infants born prematurely, or ill, than in normal infants.

D. Procedures

1. Blood gases Samples may be obtained from a warmed heel in a heparinized Natelson tube by heel stick or by direct puncture of the radial, temporal, or posterior tibial arteries. **Brachial and femoral arterial punctures should be avoided.** If the infant's condition is unstable cannulation of the umbilical radial, posterior tibial, or temporal arteries may be necessary.

2. Umbilical artery catheter

   a. Umbilical artery catheters aid greatly in parenteral therapy, in monitoring blood gases, and in withdrawing blood samples. **However, indwelling arterial catheters carry great potential dangers, including life-threatening infection and thromboembolism.**

   b. Indications Umbilical artery catheters should not be used **unless** the infants under care are considered to have 30–50 percent risk of mortality from their primary disease (e.g., gross prematurity, birth weight 1000 gm, HMD, severe aspiration pneumonia, and severe shock).

   c. Methods

   (1) Complete sterility is required, including gloves, gown, and mask.

   (2) Cut the cord 1.0–1.5 cm from the skin. Tie the base with tape.

   (3) Identify arteries Gently insert the tip of iris forceps into the lumen of one artery. Allow the forceps to expand and dilate the artery while holding the cord stump between the thumb and forefinger.

   (4) Insert a saline-filled catheter (5F for infants over 1250 gm and 3.5F for infants under 1250 gm) into the artery for the appropriate distance (Fig. 4-3).

   (5) X-ray films should be taken after placement of all umbilical catheters. The tip should be either at or below the level of L3–L4 or just above the diaphragm (T6–T10).

   (6) When adequate placement is assured, the catheter should be se-

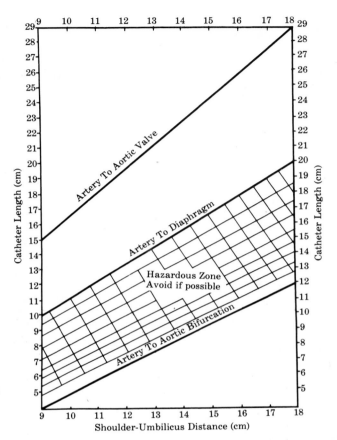

Figure 4-3 Shoulder-umbilicus distance measured above lateral end of clavicle to umbilicus versus length of umbilical artery catheter needed to reach designated level. (From P. M. Dunn, *Arch. Dis. Child.* 41:69, 1966. Reproduced by permission.)

               cured by a suture as well as by adhesive tape. The umbilical stump should be covered with an antimicrobial agent (e.g., Betadine ointment) and left open to air.

(7) The infusion solution should contain 1U of heparin/ml of infusate.

(8) Arterial catheters should be removed as soon as possible. Use of the transcutaneous PO_2 monitor and heel-stick blood gas determinations will permit this.

3. Umbilical vein catheters

    a. Indications   Umbilical vein catheters are used for emergency access to the circulation and for exchange transfusion. Because of the risk of thrombosis and infection they are not used for chronic care. Small prematures ($\approx$ 750 gm) may have to be managed *only* with umbilical vein catheters. In the latter case, it must be verified by x-ray that the

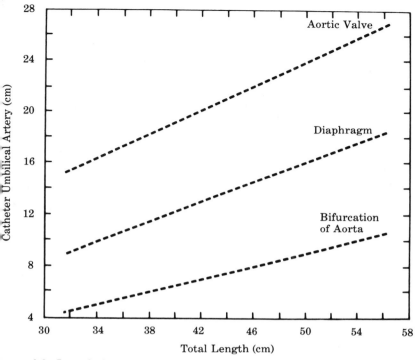

gure 4-4 Length from shoulder to umbilicus versus length of umbilical vein
atheter. (From P. M. Dunn, *Arch. Dis. Child.* 41:69, 1966. Reproduced by permis-
on.)

catheter is in the vena cava or right atrium before hypertonic infusions are begun.

b. Methods

(1) Prepare as for umbilical artery catheterization.

(2) Identify the vein, remove visible clots, and dilate with an iris forceps.

(3) Insert a saline-filled 5F (< 1250 gm) or 8F (> 1250 gm) catheter. A
multiholed catheter is used for exchange transfusions, a single-
holed catheter for long-term replacement (see Fig. 4-4 for position).

(4) When free blood flow is achieved (usually at a distance of 5–7 cm),
the catheter is adequately placed for exchange transfusion.

(5) Keep the catheter and surrounding area sterile during exchange
transfusion. In general, conditions as close to sterile as possible
should be maintained in long-term placement as well.

(6) Following exchange, place a purse-string silk suture around the
vein before removing the catheter. For subsequent exchanges the
cord should be soaked with warm saline until it is soft. The suture
will assist in identification of the vein and reinsertion of the catheter.

5

Management of the Newborn, II

I. RESPIRATORY DISEASES

A. Hyaline membrane disease (HMD)

1. Etiology HMD is caused by an **absence or deficiency of surfactant,** a phospholipid that normally lines alveoli. **Functional surfactant** appears at approximately the 34th week of gestation. HMD is therefore strongly associated with prematurity as well as with other factors that affect lung maturation.

2. Prenatal evaluation

   a. Measurement of the L/S ratio in amniotic fluid is a reliable index of fetal lung development in pregnancies that are not complicated by maternal diabetes or Rh sensitization. The incidence of HMD is under 2 percent if the L/S ratio is greater than or equal to 2:1. The L/S ratio must be greater than 3:1 to predict pulmonary maturity in infants of diabetic mothers.

   b. Use of maternal steroids If an infant of less than 33 weeks' gestation with evidence of pulmonary immaturity (L/S less than 2:1) must be delivered, alleviation of pulmonary immaturity may be accomplished by administration of glucocorticoids to the mother.
   A full course of dexamethasone, 4 mg IM q8h for 48 hr, or beta-methasone, 12 mg IM q24h for 48 hr, must be given to ensure a beneficial effect. If the infant remains undelivered for more than 7 days after the course of glucocorticoids and gestation is still less than 33 weeks, a repeat course must be given.

3. Postnatal evaluation

   a. A premature infant with grunting respirations, rapid respiratory rate, and hypoxia starting shortly after birth usually has HMD. However, other causes of respiratory distress must be considered.

   b. Laboratory studies

   (1) Gastric aspirate should be obtained during the first hour of life. The gastric aspirate is used for two tests:

   (a) Gram stain for neutrophils and bacteria (5 neutrophils/high-power field or the presence of bacteria in the first hour of life are associated with infection).

   (b) Gastric aspirate shake test to assess the amount of pulmonary surfactant in the newborn's lungs if the L/S ratio is not known.
   This test has an approximately 10 percent false-negative rate, but only 1 percent false-positive. It is performed as follows:

   i. Absolute alcohol, 0.5 ml, is added to 0.5 ml of gastric aspirate in 4-ml glass tube, 82.0 by 10.25 mm (No. 4852 Red

Stopper Tube, Becton, Dickinson & Co.) (as supplied new from the manufacturer). The test tube, capped by the thumb, is vigorously shaken for 15 sec and allowed to stand for 15 min.

ii. The test is then read as follows:

Negative   No bubbles
1+   Very small bubbles in meniscus extending one-third or less of distance around the test tube (a magnifying glass is usually required to determine that these small bubbles are indeed bubbles as opposed to particles).
2+   A single rim of bubbles extending one-third to all around the test tube (a magnifying glass is not necessary).
3+   A rim of bubbles all the way around the test tube.

iii. The test is interpreted as follows:

Negative   High risk of HMD
1+ or 2+   Intermediate risk of HMD
3+   Little chance of HMD

(2) Chest x-ray.

(3) Blood gases.

(4) An ECG and several blood pressure measurements should be taken.

(5) Cultures should be made of the skin (nose, throat, ear canal, umbilicus, and rectum), gastric aspirate, urine, and blood. Spinal fluid should be included if the infant's condition allows.

(6) Hematocrit, Ca^{++}, total protein, and bilirubin should be determined.

4. Treatment

a. Oxygen

(1) Dosage   Sufficient oxygen should be used to maintain PO_2 at about 60–70 mm Hg. Care must be taken to administer the *lowest* oxygen concentration required to maintain adequate arterial saturation. Oxygen should be fully but not excessively warmed and humidified and the humidity chamber changed daily to avoid bacterial growth. Oxygen should be administered via oxygen-air blenders that allow precise control over the concentration of administered oxygen. The oxygen concentrations being administered should be checked at least every hour. If an infant requires intermittent assisted ventilation with a Mapleson bag, the oxygen concentration administered via the bag should be similar to that usually required by the infant. When supplemental oxygen is used, PaO_2 should be checked no less than q6h. In older infants with chronic lung disease, arterial saturation need be checked no more frequently than daily.

(2) Toxicity   Arterial oxygen concentrations (PaO_2) over 100 torr are unnecessary and hazardous to the retina and pulmonary parenchyma.

(3) Delivery of oxygen   If the infant's oxygen requirement exceeds that which can be delivered by hood [see Chap. 4, Sec. **II.C.1.b.(1)**].

b. Normal fluid, electrolyte, and nutritional requirements should be pro

vided. Infants need a minimum of 100–120 cal/kg/day for adequate growth. Feeding by gavage may be attempted if the infant's condition is stable, even if the infant is on a respirator.

   c. The use of **antibiotics** is individualized. In general, infants with HMD should be started on appropriate antibiotics after full cultures are taken. If cultures are negative after 48 hr, antibiotics can be stopped.

B. Meconium aspiration   Meconium aspiration before or during birth can obstruct airways, interfere with gas exchange, increase pulmonary vascular resistance, and cause severe respiratory distress. There is a 10–20 percent incidence of pneumothorax or pneumomediastinum associated with meconium aspiration.

   1. Etiology   One-half of infants with meconium-stained amniotic fluid have meconium in the trachea on suction. Such infants frequently are postmature or have suffered intrapartum asphyxia.

     a. Prevention of passage of meconium in utero   Stress testing (oxytocin challenge test), nonstress testing with fetal monitoring, and scalp pH sampling should be done in all pregnancies with evidence of uteroplacental insufficiency. High-risk pregnancies include those with toxemia or hypertension, heavy smoking, chronic maternal disease, poor fetal growth, and postmaturity.

     b. Prevention of meconium aspiration

       (1) When thick particulate or "pea-soup" meconium is present, the obstetrician should attempt to clear the nose and oropharynx of the infant before the chest is born. This can be done with a bulb syringe followed by the passage of a de Lee catheter through the nose to the oropharynx.

       (2) When the birth is completed, the infant should then be passed to the anesthesiologist or pediatrician, who should suction the trachea with the largest orotracheal tube that will fit. The tube should be introduced **into the trachea** under direct laryngoscopy and sucked by mouth as it is being withdrawn. Usually two to four intubations are sufficient.

       (3) Oxygen by mask should be administered after the trachea has been cleared.

       (4) To the extent possible, the airway should be cleared and ventilation initiated *before* significant bradycardia occurs. Once the child has had a few breaths, meconium in the airway has moved from the trachea to the smaller bronchi, so exhaustive attempts to remove it at that point are unwise. Similarly, *no* positive pressure should be used until *after* the trachea is sucked out.

       (5) The trachea should also be suctioned in infants with thin meconium and Apgar scores of 6 or less.

   2. Evaluation and diagnosis

     a. The amount and thickness of the meconium is directly related to the severity of the disease.

     b. If tachypnea or respiratory distress increase, evaluation should include

       (1) A chest x-ray.

       (2) Arterial or heel-stick blood gas determination.

(3) Measurement of blood sugar, magnesium, and calcium levels.

c. If an infiltrate is seen on the chest x-ray, cultures of the blood, urine, skin, nasopharynx, and trachea are indicated because meconium enhances the growth of bacteria, and differentiating pneumonia from meconium aspiration is difficult.

d. Arterial desaturation due to right-to-left shunting is likely to be more of a problem than is carbon dioxide retention.

3. Therapy

a. Infants with significant aspiration often have severe difficulty. Following diagnosis

(1) Respiratory physiotherapy and oropharyngeal suction should be done q30min for the first 2 hr and qh for the next 8 hr. The trachea should be suctioned if a tube is in place.

(2) These infants may be acutely asphyxiated, with an associated metabolic acidosis, which should be corrected with bicarbonate (see Chap. 8).

b. If FIO_2 requirements are over 40 percent a trial of positive end-expiratory pressure (PEEP) in the range of 4–7 cm H_2O might be instituted. Results are variable.

c. The use of antibiotics is individualized, but, in general, if an infiltrate is seen on chest x-ray, antibiotics are used empirically after cultures have been obtained.

C. Air leak

1. Etiology Air leak in the newborn infant results from alveolar rupture or dissection of air into the pulmonary parenchyma outside the branching tree. Infants who have HMD or pneumonia, or who have required resuscitation or have sustained meconium aspiration, are at increased risk of pneumothorax.

2. Evaluation and diagnosis

a. Clinical signs of **pneumothorax** develop rapidly and include moderate to severe respiratory distress, cyanosis, a shift of the apex beat, change in breath sounds, a drop in blood pressure and perfusion.

b. **Pneumomediastinum** may be manifest by subcutaneous emphysema. A dramatic change in blood pressure or perfusion may indicate a shift of the mediastinum or dissection of air along the aorta.

c. **Pneumopericardium** will cause an immediate deterioration in blood pressure, heart rate, and arterial oxygen. This problem should be considered in the presence of pneumomediastinum and pneumothorax. It will lead to death unless diagnosed and treated quickly.

d. Anteroposterior and cross-table lateral x-rays will help differentiate these from other causes of respiratory distress.

e. For acute evaluation of an infant who deteriorates dramatically, the **fiberoptic transilluminator** may be used to diagnose pneumothorax.

3. Treatment

a. Pneumothorax

(1) Uncomplicated pneumothorax In infants with no underlying pulmonary disease or complicating therapy (respirator or PEEP and who are not in distress from pneumothorax or pneumomediastinum, there may be no continuing air leak. Under these conditions, conservative therapy may be adequate. This consists of observation in an incubator, frequent small feedings to minimize crying, and a follow-up x-ray. The extrapulmonary air will usually resolve in 24–48 hr.

The use of 100% oxygen, while effective in speeding the resolution of pneumothorax, **is not recommended** because of the danger of retrolental fibroplasia.

(2) Needle aspiration The occasional infant who has no underlying pulmonary problem or continuing air leak, but **who is in distress** from the pneumothorax may be treated by **needle aspiration.**

(a) Place the infant in a sitting position if possible.

(b) Attach a 25-gauge needle to a 50-ml syringe via a three-way stopcock. Place a hemostat about 1 cm from the needle tip to prevent deep penetration.

(c) The needle should enter through the second intercostal space in the anterior axillary line lateral to the pectoralis major muscle. Hit the rib with the needle and slide it over the top to minimize the chance of bleeding from the intercostal artery.

(d) If air continues to leak, a chest tube must be inserted. If the infant is breathing or crying after the visceral pleura opposes the parietal pleura, the needle tip may cause a bronchopleural fistula. This is not a common occurrence, but it is prudent to remove the needle as soon as possible.

(3) Chest tube placement Infants with a continuing air leak, underlying pulmonary disease causing continued distress, or on respirator therapy or PEEP require **chest tube placement** and suction for drainage of pneumothorax. This should be performed or supervised by experienced nursery personnel.

b. Pneumomediastinum Chest tubes are not placed in infants with pneumomediastinum alone.

c. Pneumopericardium

(1) Symptomatic pneumopericardium may be drained using a 20-gauge, 1½-inch needle attached via a three-way stopcock to a 10–20-ml syringe.

(a) Following surgical preparation, insert a needle at the subxyphoid region, aiming for the posterior left shoulder, and, with suction on the syringe, advance the needle until air appears.

(b) When air stops flowing, withdraw the needle.

(2) Often, a single aspiration results in clinical improvement. About 25–40 percent of patients will have a recurrent symptomatic pneumopericardium, which may be treated as just described.

(3) Infrequently, the pneumopericardium will act as if constant air drainage into pericardial space has occurred. Placement of a 16-gauge Intracath into the pericardial space seems appropriate in this situation.

D. Apnea An apneic spell is defined as cessation of effective respiration accompanied by bradycardia (heart rate under 100 beats/min) or cyanosis.

Bradycardia and cyanosis are usually present after 20 sec of apnea, although they may occur more rapidly in the small premature infant. After 30–45 sec, pallor and hypotonia are seen, and infants may be unresponsive to tactile stimulation. The majority of very small premature infants (under 30 weeks' gestational age) have occasional apneic spells. As many as 25 percent of all premature infants weighing under 1800 gm (about 34 weeks) will have at least one apneic episode. These spells generally begin at 1–2 days of age and may recur for 2–3 weeks postnatally, although most occur within the first 10 days of life.

1. **Etiology** Many clinical conditions have been associated with apneic spells; some may be causative. A partial list includes those related to

    a. Hypoxemia due to pneumonia; RDS (especially when weaning from CDAP); congenital heart disease, particularly PDA; anemia; or hypovolemia.

    b. Respiratory center depression due to hypoglycemia, hypocalcemia, electrolyte disorders, sepsis, drugs, intracranial hemorrhage, or seizures.

    c. Reflexes due to suction catheters; fluid in the upper airway during feeding or soon after delivery; lung inflation.

    d. **Temperature** Infants in Isolettes servocontrolled to maintain skin temperatures at 36.8°C have more frequent spells than those maintained at 36.0°C. Sudden increases in incubator temperature similarly increase the frequency of apneic spells.

    e. **Airway obstruction** due to passive neck flexion, pressure on the lower rim of a face mask, and submental pressure are all encountered during nursery procedures. Spontaneously occurring airway obstruction, which tends to occur when preterm infants assume a position of neck flexion, may contribute to the *prolongation* of apneic spells.

2. **Monitoring and evaluation**

    a. All infants of less than 34 weeks' gestational age should be placed on apnea monitors for at least 10 days. Since impedance apnea monitors may not distinguish respiratory efforts during airway obstruction from normal breaths, heart rate should also be monitored.

    b. When a monitor alarm sounds, the clinician should respond to the **infant,** not the monitor. Check for bradycardia, cyanosis, and airway obstruction.

    c. Following the first apneic spell, the infant should be evaluated for a possible underlying cause as discussed in **1,** and, if one is identified, specific treatment should be initiated. Particular attention should be paid to the possibility of a precipitating cause in infants of more than 33–34 weeks' gestational age.

3. **Treatment**

    a. Most apneic spells in premature infants respond to tactile stimulation. Infants who fail to respond should be ventilated during the spell with bag and mask, generally with an FIO_2 of under 0.40 or equal to the FIO_2 prior to the spell, to avoid marked elevations in arterial PO_2.

    b. For repeated prolonged spells, i.e., more than 2–3/hr or requiring frequent bagging, treatment should be initiated in the order of increasing invasiveness and risk.

       (1) Decreasing environmental temperature to the low end of the neu

tral thermal environment range may decrease the number of spells. Placing a heat shield around a small premature infant may prevent swings in temperature.

(2) Small increases in FIO_2 (0.25–0.26) may reduce the frequency of apneic spells. However, without a continuously reading oxygen electrode to monitor arterial oxygenation, the **risk of retrolental fibroplasia** makes this intervention relatively hazardous.

(3) A blood transfusion to elevate the hematocrit slightly (i.e., to about 45 percent) despite the absence of significant anemia may also reduce the frequency of spells and is relatively benign.

(4) Nasal CPAP at low pressures (3–4 cm H_2O) is effective in some cases.

(5) Theophylline in a dose of 2 mg/kg q4–6h often decreases the number of spells. A more recent recommended dosage in premature infants is an initial IV loading dose of 5.5 mg/kg given over 20 min, followed by 1.1 mg/kg q8h. Serum levels should be obtained during therapy, and the dosage should be adjusted to maintain theophylline concentration in the range of 7–13 gm/ml. The dosage should be reduced if tachycardia or GI toxicity become evident.

(6) Caffeine citrate may decrease the frequency of apneic spells. As with theophylline, the acute and long-term toxicity of caffeine in newborn infants is not well defined, although no significant heart rate changes are noted with caffeine. A suggested dosage schedule for caffeine citrate is a loading dose of 20 mg/kg PO or IV, followed by a maintenance dose of 5–10 mg/kg qd–bid for 3 days. The drug is then stopped for 24 hr and resumed if apnea recurs.

(7) If all these interventions fail, mechanical ventilation may be required, but this is seldom necessary.

II. CARDIAC DISEASE IN THE NEWBORN   Severe congenital cardiac disease occurs in approximately 1 out of 400 infants.

A. Congestive heart failure

1. Etiology   PDA in premature infants is the most common cause of congestive heart failure (CHF) in the newborn period. Other causes are hypoplastic left heart syndrome, complex congenital heart disease, myocarditis, arteriovenous fistula in the brain or liver, and idiopathic paroxysmal tachycardia.

2. Evaluation

a. Common signs of heart failure in the newborn are tachycardia, tachypnea, hepatomegaly, cardiomegaly, and diaphoresis.

b. Arterial blood gases, chest x-rays, electrocardiogram, echocardiography, radionuclide angiography, and cardiac catheterization are all useful in evaluation.

3. Diagnosis

a. Patent ductus arteriosus   Most premature infants with PDA do not require cardiac catheterization, since a PDA is usually evident by clinical examination, and its hemodynamic significance can be quantitated by noninvasive tests.

(1) For signs and symptoms see Table 5-1.

(2) The diagnosis of a PDA can be confirmed and the amount of the left-to-right shunt quantitated by echocardiography and a radionuclide angiogram (^{99m}Tc sodium pertechnetate).

b. The diagnosis of other causes of CHF are also given in Table 5-1.

4. Treatment

  a. **General medical treatment** is directed toward decreasing the work load on the heart.

   (1) Although digoxin has been the mainstay of treatment in all age groups for many years, recent work suggests that **digoxin may be of little benefit to the very immature preterm infant with CHF secondary to PDA** (see Chap. 10).

   (2) Other therapeutic measures include diuretics, fluid restrictions to under 120–150 ml/kg/day, use of a low-solute formula (e.g., Similac PM 60/40 or breast milk; see Chap. 1), maintenance of a neutral thermal environment (see Chap. 4, Sec. I.B.2), and decreasing the work of the feeding, e.g., gavage rather than nipple feedings.

   (3) Adequate oxygenation of the myocardium is sought by

     (a) Maintaining the hematocrit at over 40% (use packed red blood cells, 5 ml/kg, given over 2–4 hr and repeated as necessary).

     (b) Increasing FIO_2 as necessary to maintain the PaO_2 at 60–80 torr.

  b. **Cardiotonic drugs** are the cornerstone of CHF treatment.

   (1) For specific recommendations regarding **digitalis** and **diuretics,** see Chap. 10.

   (2) **Isoproterenol (Isuprel)** Isoproterenol can be used in severe CHF when other means fail to maintain adequate cardiac output (see Chaps. 2, 10, and 12).

   (3) **Dopamine** has been used in the newborn for the treatment of severe hypotension. It has also been used to reverse the hypotensive effects of tolazoline (Priscoline) when it is used in the treatment of persistent fetal circulation. For the dosage, see Appendix Table 5-1 at the end of this chapter.

B. Cyanosis Cyanosis can indicate life-threatening illness.

 1. Etiology

  a. The major cardiac causes of cyanosis in the newborn are transposition of the great arteries, critical pulmonary stenosis, or atresia, or both, tetralogy of Fallot, tricuspid atresia, anomalous pulmonary veins, and Ebstein's anomaly.

  b. Major pulmonary causes are HMD, meconium aspiration, pneumothorax, and persistent fetal circulation.

 2. Evaluation

  a. These infants must be evaluated rapidly by ECG, chest x-ray, right radial arterial blood gases in room air and 100% oxygen, and an echocardiogram. If available, a cardiologist should be promptly consulted.

  b. Early measurement of PaO_2 in 100% oxygen in a child with developing pulmonary disease can be helpful when cyanotic congenital heart disease is being considered later in the infant's course. Many infants with HMD may have a PaO_2 greater than 100 torr in 100% oxygen early in their disease, but not by day 2 or 3. A PaO_2 over 100 in an adequately ventilated infant virtually excludes significant cyanotic heart disease.

3. **Treatment** Treatment of cardiac causes of cyanosis in the newborn is a **medical emergency.** The infant must be given enough oxygen to keep the PaO_2 over 60 torr. Therapy for CHF as outlined in **A.4** must be given. Surgery is frequently required.

C. Rhythm disturbances See also Chap. 10.

1. **Bradycardia** Both sinus bradycardia and that due to congenital heart block are rare.

   a. **Etiology** Evaluate intracranial pressure, hypertension, potassium intoxication, hypothyroidism, and congenital heart disease. Congenital heart block may be secondary to maternal collagen vascular disease.

   b. **Treatment**

      (1) Treat the underlying cause if possible. If the low heart rate persists after treatment but there is no evidence of cardiovascular compromise, observation without treatment is a wise course. In general, infants with a heart rate between 50–70 beats/min may be asymptomatic and need no treatment if they remain well for over 72 hr with a normal QRS complex on the ECG.

      (2) In infants with a heart rate under 50, respiratory distress, cyanosis, and CHF are frequent. Treatment consists in the use of a chronotropic agent such as isoproterenol to raise the heart rate acutely (see **A.4**). If asymptomatic bradycardia persists when medication is withdrawn, insertion of a pacemaker may be necessary.

      (3) When fetal heart rate monitoring indicates a persistent fetal bradycardia, arrangements for a cardiologic consultation should be made prior to delivery.

2. **Paroxysmal atrial tachycardia** is relatively common.

   a. **Etiology** Congenital paroxysmal atrial tachycardia (PAT) may be associated with Wolff-Parkinson-White syndrome, structural congenital heart disease, or no evident cardiac abnormality.

   b. **Evaluation**

      (1) The heart rate is 200–300/min; P waves are rarely seen, and the QRS may be normal or abnormal.

      (2) If PAT is present prenatally, it carries a risk of CHF in utero, with a possibility of fetal hydrops, or stillbirth, or both. Treatment of the mother with digoxin should be instituted and early delivery planned in conjunction with determination of pulmonary maturity (L/S ratio).

   c. **Treatment** consists of attempts to convert the infant to a sinus rhythm. Infants in good condition at delivery can usually tolerate up to 24 hr of tachycardia without CHF.

      (1) Occasionally, infants respond to vagal stimulation (rectal examination) or pressure applied to the fontanelle.

Table 5-1 Presenting Signs and Findings in Congenital Heart Disease

Diagnosis	Age	Presenting Signs	Auscultation	X-Ray Findings	ECG
Transposition of the arteries					
Intact ventricular septum	First hours or days	Cyanosis	Unremarkable	Cardiac enlargement Pulmonary vasculature ↑	Right ventricular hypertrophy
Ventricular septal defect	First weeks	Congestive heart failure	Pansystolic murmur	Cardiac enlargement+ Pulmonary vasculature ↑↑	Combined ventricular hypertrophy
Ventricular septal defect and pulmonic stenosis	First days or weeks	Cyanosis	Pansystolic and stenotic murmurs	Cardiac enlargement Pulmonary vasculature →	Combined ventricular hypertrophy
Tetralogy of Fallot	First days or weeks	Cyanosis	Early stenotic murmur, single S_2 at lower left sternal border	Cardiac enlargement 0 Pulmonary vasculature ↓	Right ventricular hypertrophy
Pure pulmonary stenosis	First weeks or months, occasionally	Cyanosis	Late stenotic murmur, widely split S_2, faint P_2	Cardiac enlargement + Pulmonary vasculature ↓	Right ventricular hypertrophy marked

Hypoplastic left heart	First days	Cyanosis and congestive heart failure, with femoral pulses	Late stenotic murmur, single S_2	Cardiac enlargement++ Pulmonary vasculature $\uparrow\uparrow$	Right ventricular hypertrophy marked
Ventricular septal defect	First weeks	Congestive heart failure, loud P_2	Pansystolic murmur, narrowly split S_2	Cardiac enlargement+ Pulmonary vasculature $\uparrow$	Combined ventricular hypertrophy
Coarctation of the aorta	First weeks	Congestive heart failure with hypertension	Stenotic murmur across back	Cardiac enlargement+ Pulmonary vasculature (passive) $\uparrow$	Right ventricular hypertrophy
Patent ductus arteriosus with pulmonary artery hypertension	First weeks	Congestive heart failure Bounding pulses	Crescendic systolic murmur, ? early diastolic murmur, split S_2, loud P	Cardiac enlargement+ Pulmonary vasculature $\uparrow$	Combined ventricular hypertrophy

(2) Whether responsive to vagal stimulation or not, infants with PAT should be rapidly digitalized.

(3) If deterioration in the infant's clinical state occurs, cardioversion may be necessary. Begin at 10 watt-sec and increase by 10 watt-sec until successful reversion to sinus rhythm occurs. After normal sinus rhythm is established, digoxin therapy is usually maintained for 6–12 months.

III. HEMATOLOGIC PROBLEMS

A. Jaundice (including erythroblastosis)

1. Etiology

a. **Physiologic jaundice** is defined as unconjugated hyperbilirubinemia (total serum bilirubin < 2 mg/100 ml, direct fraction < 15 percent of the total) that appears on or after the third day of life and resolves prior to 10 days.

b. **Nonphysiologic jaundice** is jaundice due to an abnormality of bilirubin production, metabolism, or excretion.

(1) **Indirect hyperbilirubinemia**   Direct bilirubin is less than 15 percent of the total bilirubin.

(a) The major cause of indirect hyperbilirubinemia is **mother-infant blood group incompatibility**. There are three major categories, as follows:

i. AO or BO incompatibility. These incompatibilities range from being clinically unimportant to causing severe postnatal hyperbilirubinemia.

ii. Rhesus (Rh) incompatibility (Rh negative mother, Rh positive infant). A similar clinical spectrum is present, as in ABO disease. The most severely affected infants are born hydropic, with erythroblastosis fetalis.

iii. **Other minor blood group incompatibilities** (e.g., anti-Kell, anti-Duffy). A woman may be sensitized to any of these antigens by previous pregnancies, blood transfusions, or abortions.

(b) **Red blood cell membrane and enzyme defects** may cause indirect hyperbilirubinemia.

(c) A third cause of indirect hyperbilirubinemia is hemorrhage into an extravascular space (e.g., intracranial, pulmonary, retroperitoneal).

(d) Prolonged (10 days) indirect hyperbilirubinemia may be caused by hypothyroidism or be related to the ingestion of breast milk.

i. **Breast milk jaundice** is prolonged indirect hyperbilirubinemia possibly caused by inhibition of hepatic glucuronyl transferase by a pregnanetriol in breast milk. This is a rare cause of neonatal jaundice and usually *is not* an indication for discontinuing breast-feeding except for diagnostic purposes.

ii. A rare mother excretes large amounts of a substance that inhibits bilirubin conjugation, resulting in marked unconjugated hyperbilirubinemia in her newborn (Lucey-Driscoll syndrome).

   iii. Other causes are congenital familial nonhemolytic jaundice types 1 and 2 (Crigler-Najjar syndrome), novobiocin, and diabetes in the mother.

  (2) Direct hyperbilirubinemia (direct bilirubin > 15 percent of the total bilirubin)   Causes of direct hyperbilirubinemia are sepsis, intrauterine (TORCH) infections, neonatal hepatitis, intrahepatic biliary atresia syndrome, extrahepatic biliary atresia, biliary tract obstruction by an abdominal mass or anular pancreas, galactosemia, tyrosinemia, alpha$_1$-antitrypsin deficiency, posthemolytic disease of the newborn syndrome (inspissated bile syndrome), and prolonged total parenteral nutrition.

2. Evaluation and diagnosis

  a. The goal of evaluation is to decide at what serum bilirubin level treatment should be instituted to avoid **kernicterus** and **sublethal bilirubin encephalopathy**.

    (1) Kernicterus is a toxic effect of non-albumin-bound unconjugated bilirubin on the CNS. Susceptibility to kernicterus is increased by factors that decrease albumin binding (hypoalbuminemia, acidosis, hypoglycemia, organic anions) and factors that increase diffusion of free bilirubin into the brain (increasing concentration, and/or increased duration of exposure to elevated levels of bilirubin stress).

    (2) Sublethal bilirubin encephalopathy results in mild neurodevelopmental deficits.

  b. Infants who appear jaundiced have serum bilirubin levels greater than 6 mg/100 ml. A full-term infant whose bilirubin is over 5 mg/100 ml within the first 24 hr of life, over 10 mg/100 ml within the first 48 hr, or over 12 mg/100 ml after 72 hr requires investigation.

  c. For **initial evaluation** of indirect hyperbilirubinemia, the following tests will help place the infant in the correct diagnostic group and assess the risk of long-term problems:

    (1) Blood groups of mother and infant

    (2) Direct Coombs test on cord blood or the infant's blood and, if positive, identification of the antibody

    (3) Hematocrit (q4–8h) to evaluate the rate of rise of serum bilirubin

  d. Assessing bilirubin binding   If the serum bilirubin exceeds 18 mg/100 ml in full-term infants or ($\frac{2}{3}$) × (0.1) × (birth weight in grams) of an infant weighing under 2000 gm, a test must be done for the presence of non-albumin-bound bilirubin. These include the Sephadex column (Karnlute), which we use, and the salicylate binding test.

3. Therapy

The goal of therapy is to prevent the presence of unconjugated free (unbound) bilirubin in the serum of all infants.

  a. General   See Fig. 5-1.

    (1) Establish that the baby has adequate fluid intake. In breast-fed infants, supplement the diet with 10% D/W or formula if indicated. Give IV fluids if indicated.

    (2) Correct asphyxia, hypotension, hypoxia, and/or hypothermia.

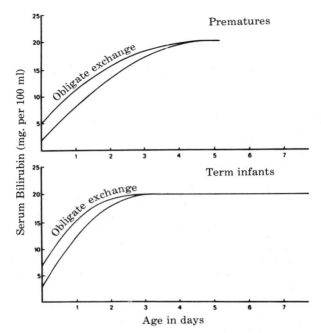

Figure 5-1 Serum bilirubin levels plotted against age in premature and full-term infants with erythroblastosis. Levels above the top line are predictive of an ultimate bilirubin level of over 20 unless the natural course is altered by treatment. Levels below the bottom line predict that the level will not eventually reach 20. Between the lines is an intermediate zone where the ultimate level could be below or above 20. (Adapted from J. Lucey et al., *Pediatrics* 41:1, 1968.)

b. Phototherapy

    (1) Principles

        (a) Indications Phototherapy should be instituted if there is a risk that unconjugated bilirubin will rise to levels that might saturate albumin-binding sites (resulting in free bilirubin) or that would possibly result in the need for an exchange transfusion. Prophylactic phototherapy may be indicated in special circumstances (i.e., in tiny infants in whom dangerous levels of bilirubin are likely to develop, in severely bruised prematures, in hemolytic disease while waiting for exchange transfusion). In hemolytic disease, phototherapy is used as an adjunct to exchange transfusion.

        (b) Toxicity No significant long-term toxicity has been described. However, phototherapy should be used with the same caution as with any other treatment (e.g., medications).

        (c) Effectiveness The amount of skin exposure and radiant energy impinging on the skin are of primary importance for effective phototherapy. Blue light (450–500 mm wavelength) is more effective in lowering bilirubin, but cool white light provides a better visualization of cyanosis in the infant.

(2) Technique of phototherapy

(a) Perform appropriate diagnostic studies before phototherapy is started (see **2**).

(b) Shield both eyes of the infant.

(c) Be certain all electric outlets are properly grounded.

(d) Use a Plexiglass cover or shield to prevent harm to the infant in case of lamp breakage and to screen out wavelengths below 300 μ, thus protecting the infant from ultraviolet light.

(e) Monitor temperature q2h. Use a control alarm if possible.

(f) Weigh the infant daily or, if the infant is small, twice daily and provide extra fluid as necessary.

(g) **Do not use skin color as a guide to hyperbilirubinemia in infants under phototherapy.** Instead, monitor bilirubin at least q12h.

(h) Change the lamps every 2000 hours of use (alternatively, change them all every 3 months). Monitoring the energy output in the range of 425–475 nm will give more precise information on energy output.

(3) Side effects include

(a) Increased insensible water loss, which requires a 20–30 percent increase in fluid intake.

(b) Transient rashes.

(c) Diarrhea.

(d) Bronze baby syndrome, a rare complication usually seen in infants with parenchymal hepatic disease who are treated with phototherapy. **Do not use phototherapy in infants with liver disease or obstructive jaundice.**

c. Exchange transfusion

(1) Indications Exchange transfusion should be instituted to correct severe anemia or if evaluation of bilirubin levels indicates any potential that free (unbound to albumin) unconjugated bilirubin could be present. If unbound bilirubin is already present, damage may result.

(2) Early exchange transfusion is often indicated in the presence of hydrops, a known sensitized infant, or an infant with a history of anemia. The critical indications for immediate (at birth) exchange transfusion are usually a cord hemoglobin less than 12 mg/100 ml and a cord indirect bilirubin greater than 3.5 mg/100 ml. Each case must be evaluated before any decision to exchange is arrived at. Figure 5-1 and Table 5-2 give useful guidelines.

When a severely hydropic infant is expected, cooperation among the pediatricians, obstetricians, and blood bank personnel is essential. In such an infant, immediate exchange transfusion may be lifesaving in correcting anemia and CHF and removing sensitized red blood cells.

(3) Late exchange transfusions in hemolytic disease are usually indicated when the bilirubin in full-term infants is 10 mg/100 ml at 24 hr and 15 mg/100 ml at 48 hr (see Fig. 5-1 and Table 5-2).

Table 5-2   Serum Levels of Indirect Bilirubin and Exchange Transfusion[a]

| Birth Weight (gm) | Serum Bilirubin Level for Exchange Transfusion (mg/100 ml) | |
	Normal Infants[b]	Abnormal Infants[c]
1000	10.0[d]	10.0[d]
1001–1250	13.0	10.0[d]
1251–1500	15.0	13.0
1501–2000	17.0	15.0
2001–2500	18.0	17.0
2500	20.0	18.0

[a] These are guidelines only.
[b] Normal infants are defined for this purpose as having none of the problems listed in footnote c.
[c] Abnormal infants have one or more of the following problems: (1) perinatal asphyxia, (2) persistent hypothermia, (3) acidemia, (4) persistent hypothermia, (5) hypoalbuminemia, (6) hemolysis, (7) sepsis, (8) hyperglycemia, (9) elevated free fatty acids or the presence of drugs that compete for bilirubin binding, (10) signs of clinical or central nervous system deterioration.
[d] There have been case reports of basal ganglion staining at levels considerably lower than 10 mg.
Source: Adapted from Committee on Phototherapy in the Newborn, *Final Report of the Committee on Phototherapy in the Newborn*, Washington, D.C., National Research Council, 1974; Committee on Fetus and Newborn, *Standards and Recommendations for Hospital Care of Newborn Infants* (6th ed.), Evanston, Ill.: American Academy of Pediatrics, 1977.

(4) Technique of exchange transfusion

(a) General   Sick infants need attention to asphyxia, hypoglycemia, acidosis, and temperature control before exchange transfusion. All infants should be exchanged under a **radiant heater**, servocontrolled to the infant, and a **cardiac monitor** should be in place.

An assistant experienced in resuscitation should be assigned to record volumes of blood, observe the infant, and check vital signs.

(b) Exchange transfusions are usually done through the umbilical vein. If the umbilical vein cannot be entered, the safest route is through a central venous pressure (CVP) line placed through the antecubital fossa. These lines can be left in for future exchanges.

It is not useful to check the position of umbilical venous catheters by x-ray because they often have to be moved around during the exchange. On the other hand, the position of central venous catheters *should be checked* by x-ray.

(5) Blood   Fresh (under 24 hr old) blood should be used. Irradiated blood should be used if the infant has received intrauterine transfusions.

(a) General   Heparinized blood is preferable, but if there is doubt about whether the exchange will occur, citrate-phosphate-dextrose (CPD) blood should be used so that the blood will not be wasted. Blood should be warmed to 37°C.

   i. Only blood compatible with the mother, with a low titer of anti-A and anti-B, should be used.

   ii. Subsequent transfusions should be done with blood compatible with that of the mother and infant.

   iii. Blood should be gently shaken frequently, since the RBCs will settle rapidly and the settling can lead to exchange with relatively anemic blood at the end of the exchange.

(b) Acid-citrate-dextrose (ACD) or CPD blood   Citrate binds Ca^{++} and Mg^{++}, leading to decreased ionized calcium. The clinical relevance of this is not known. Following cessation of exchange transfusion, the Ca^{++} levels rapidly return to normal values.

   i. It has been recommended that 0.5–2.0 ml 10% calcium gluconate be given following each 100 ml of exchange blood. However, this measure only temporarily increases the ionized Ca fraction. Most infants will not require additional calcium.

   ii. The dextrose may lead to hypertonicity and rebound hypoglycemia from hyperplastic islets.

   iii. Acid-base balance   The pH of donor blood is generally low. However, citrate is metabolized to alkali by the liver. If the baby is unable to metabolize citrate, the citrate can produce significant acidosis. Nevertheless, buffer should not be added because of the eventual conversion of citrate to HCO_3^-.

(c) Heparinized blood usually contains 25 mg of heparin/500 ml of blood.

   i. Coagulation   Heparin is usually metabolized within 4–6 hr; severe erythroblastosis may interfere with metabolism and may be further complicated by disseminated intravascular coagulation (DIC), thrombocytopenia, and decreased clotting factors. **Protamine** is administered following the exchange to neutralize the heparin estimated to be remaining in the baby (1 mg protamine per unit of heparin).

   ii. Since sugar in the heparinized blood may be low, a Dextrostix blood sugar should be checked on the blood and on the baby during the exchange. When citrated blood is used, the infant's blood sugar should be checked after the exchange; 10 ml of 5% dextrose can be given as an umbilical vein push after each 100 ml of blood if necessary. If the catheter tip rests above the liver, a more concentrated sugar solution may be used.

(6) Specific points

(a) Sick infants who are anemic (hematocrit under 35) are best given a partial exchange transfusion with packed red blood cells (25–80 ml/kg) to raise the hematocrit to 40%. After stabilization, more exchange transfusions can be given for hyperbilirubinemia. The blood for these exchanges should be set up

prior to delivery and packed with the plasma separated into a side bag, so that it can be remixed if a packed cell exchange is not necessary.

(b) Exchange in sick hydropic infants is best performed through umbilical arterial and venous catheters, so that blood may be removed and replaced simultaneously.

(c) An infant's blood volume is usually 80 ml/kg, and exchange transfusions are usually done using double the infant's blood volume (160 ml/kg), in aliquots of 10–20 ml, depending on the infant's tolerance for the procedure. (An aliquot should never exceed 10 percent of the infant's estimated blood volume.) A useful approach is to start with 10-ml aliquots, increasing to 20-ml aliquots in infants weighing over 2 kg if all goes well.

(d) The rate of exchange has little effect on the amount of bilirubin removed; however, small aliquots and a slower rate reduce the stress on cardiovascular adaptation. The recommended time for an exchange in a full-term infant is 1 hr.

(e) Albumin (salt-poor albumin, 1 gm/kg 1–2 hr, prior to exchange) increases the amount of bilirubin removed by the exchange. Albumin is contraindicated in CHF or severe anemia.

(f) A two-volume exchange removes 87 percent of the *infant's* red blood cells.

(g) When finishing an exchange transfusion, put a silk purse-string suture around the vein and leave a "tail," which, together with soaking, will make things easy for the one doing the next exchange.

(h) When the catheter is removed, snug up the cord tie for an hour or so. **Do not forget about it, or skin necrosis will occur.**

(i) When removing the venous catheter, pull it right out, or else blood will flow from the distal side hole, out the proximal side hole, and cause unnecessary anxiety to the operator.

(j) Although it is controversial, prophylactic antibiotics are recommended if a catheter was passed through an old, dirty cord; if there is great difficulty in passing the catheter; or if there are multiple exchanges.

(7) **Subsequent exchange** is indicated at bilirubin levels suggesting that unbound bilirubin is potentially present (see Fig. 5-1 and Table 5-2).

(8) **Complications of exchange transfusions**

(a) **Vascular**   Embolization with air or clots, and thrombosis.

(b) **Cardiac**   Arrhythmias, volume overload, and arrest.

(c) **Electrolytes**   Hyperkalemia, hypernatremia, hypocalcemia, and acidosis.

(d) **Clotting**   Overheparinization and thrombocytopenia.

(e) **Infections**   Bacteremia and serum hepatitis.

(f) **Miscellaneous**   Mechanical injury to donor cells, perforation of vessels, hypothermia, hypoglycemia, and possibly necrotizing enterocolitis.

B. Anemia (see also Chap. 17)   Since the neonatal period is unique, the anemias of this period will be considered separately.

  1. Blood loss can be fatal due to low total blood volume.

   a. Physical findings   Shock, extreme pallor, tachycardia, and tachypnea. Jaundice is absent.

   b. Etiology   Most commonly, fetal-maternal hemorrhage.

   c. Features

   (1) History of chills and back pain in the mother secondary to a transfusion reaction in fetal-maternal hemorrhage.

   (2) A Kleihauer-Betke preparation for hemoglobin F will detect fetal cells in maternal blood.

   d. Other causes   Twin-twin transfusion, placenta previa, placental abruption, umbilical cord rupture or hematoma, incision of anterior placenta or cord, traumatic amniocentesis, intracranial or pulmonary hemorrhage.

  2. Hemolysis

   a. Physical and laboratory findings   Jaundice, elevated or normal reticulocyte count, positive Coombs test (but not always).

   b. Etiology

   (1) Coombs-positive anemia

   (a) ABO incompatibility; no history of previous sensitization.

   (b) RH incompatibility; previous pregnancy or abortion.

   (c) Minor blood group incompatibility (Kell, "c," "E," etc.).

   (2) Coombs-negative anemia   Red cell membrane defects (e.g., spherocytosis), enzyme defect (e.g., G-6-PD deficiency), bacterial (or TORCH) infection, and metabolic disease (i.e., galactosemia). Vitamin E deficiency, usually affecting the premature infant weighing less than 1800 gm, is characterized by acanthocytes, a serum β-tocopherol level below 0.5 mg/100 ml, and a positive peroxide hemolysis test.

  3. Marrow failure

   a. Physical and laboratory findings   Signs and symptoms characteristic of the underlying disease; low reticulocyte count.

   b. Etiology

   (1) Infiltrative disease   Congenital leukemia, neuroblastoma, storage disease, and infection.

   (2) Red cell failure   Diamond-Blackfan syndrome, Fanconi's anemia, and other rare syndromes.

  4. Therapy

   a. Transfusion   See also Chap. 1, Sec. **II.D**, p. 12.

   (1) The maximal amount transfused should usually be 10 ml/kg of whole blood, monitoring the infant. Give more blood as needed (see Shock, p. 32).

   (2) Premature infants may be quite comfortable with hemoglobin in the range of 6.5–8.0 gm/100 ml. The level itself is *not* an indication for transfusion. However, if any other condition (e.g., sepsis, pneumonia, bronchopulmonary dysplasia) requires increased oxygen-carrying capacity, transfusions will be indicated.

b. Prevention or amelioration of anemia of prematurity

    (1) Vitamin E   Until the infant is 2–3 months of age, 25 IU of a water-soluble form is given daily.

    (2) Formulas similar to mother's milk in that they are low in linoleic acid are used to maintain a low content of red blood cell polyunsaturated fatty acids.

    (3) Iron is not used for the first 2 months, since therapeutic doses (8 mg/kg/day) enhance lipid peroxidation of red blood cell membranes.

    (4) After 8 weeks, iron supplements (2 mg/kg/day) as fortified formula or therapeutic iron are used to prevent late anemia of prematurity.

C. Polycythemia

  1. Etiology

    a. Placental overtransfusion.

    b. Placental insufficiency.

    c. Other causes, including maternal diabetes, congenital adrenal hyperplasia, Beckwith syndrome, neonatal thyrotoxicosis, Down syndrome, and trisomy D.

  2. Evaluation and diagnosis

    a. Most infants with polycythemia are asymptomatic.

    b. Suggestive symptoms include cyanosis (due to unsaturated hemoglobin), priapism, hypoglycemia, and jaundice (bilirubin load to the liver: 1 gm hemoglobin produces 34 gm bilirubin).

    c. Central hematocrits should be checked to diagnose or rule out polycythemia.

  3. Treatment

    a. Any **central hematocrit** above 60 is of concern.

    b. Any symptomatic child should have a partial exchange transfusion if the central hematocrit is **above 65.**

    c. Asymptomatic infants with a central hematocrit 60–70 can usually be managed by pushing fluids.

    d. Exchange transfusion is probably indicated with a central hematocrit more than 70 in the absence of symptoms (see **A.3.c**).

    Exchange is done with fresh frozen plasma if available or 5% albumin to bring hematocrit to 60 by the following calculation:

$$\text{Volume of exchange in ml} = \frac{\text{blood volume} \times (\text{observed Hct} - \text{desired Hct})}{\text{Observed Hct}}$$

D. Bleeding   See Chap. 17, Sec. **VII.A.1.**

IV. METABOLIC PROBLEMS

A. Infants of diabetic mothers (IDM)

1. **Pregnancy** Management during the diabetic pregnancy should include

   a. Close cooperation between the obstetrician, pediatrician, and internist.

   b. Frequent prenatal visits.

   c. Accurate dating of time of conception.

   d. Maintenance of maternal blood sugar and diet, or insulin, or both in a range that keeps glycosuria less than 20 gm/day. *Oral hypoglycemic agents should not be used because they cross the placenta and are associated with severe and prolonged neonatal hypoglycemia.*

   e. Fetal ultrasonography and/or measurement of alpha[1]-fetoprotein in maternal blood and amniotic fluid.

   f. Measurement of indications of fetal health (see Sec. I).

   g. Measurement of the L/S ratio.

   h. Elective delivery.

2. **Evaluation** Infants of diabetic mothers are subject to the following: hypoglycemia, hypocalcemia; hyperbilirubinemia; RDS; feeding problems; congenital anomalies; polycythemia and, rarely, renal vein thrombosis.

3. **Diagnosis**

   a. At delivery, a sample of amniotic fluid can be obtained for L/S ratio, shake test (Sec. **I.A.3**) for presence of surface active material, and Gram stain.

   b. Gastric aspirate should be obtained for the shake test and Gram stain.

   c. **Laboratory data** Determine the following:

      (1) **Blood sugar** at birth and at 1, 2, 3, 6, 12, 24, and 48 hr (Dextrostix reading).

      (2) **Calcium** at 6, 12, 24, and 48 hr.

      (3) **Hematocrit** at 1 hr and 24 hr.

      (4) **Bilirubin** as needed.

      (5) **Chest x-ray** and **blood gases** as indicated.

4. **Therapy** See Secs. **B.3** and **C.3**.

B. Hypoglycemia

in the neonate is defined as any blood sugar less than 40 mg/100 ml with hypoglycemic symptoms that disappear after IV glucose. Thus any blood sugar less than 40 mg/100 ml should be a cause for concern.

1. **Etiology** See Table 5-3.

2. **Evaluation and diagnosis**

   a. **Symptoms** include lethargy, apathy, and limpness, tremors, apnea, cyanosis, seizures, weak or high-pitched cry, and poor feeding.

   b. **Laboratory data** In the newborn, glucose oxidase methods that measure true glucose should be used rather than those that measure total reducing substances. Dextrostix with the Ames Eyetone Instrument can be useful.

Table 5-3 Etiology of Neonatal Hypoglycemia

Mechanism and Clinical Syndrome

Hyperinsulinism
  Infant of diabetic mother
  Leucine sensitivity
  Islet cell hyperplasia or hyperfunction
  Beckwith syndrome
  Maternal chlorpropamide therapy
  Erythroblastosis (rebound hypoglycemia after exchange with ACD blood with
    high blood sugar)
Decreased glucose stores
  Prematurity
  Intrauterine growth retardation
Other
  Sepsis
  Shock
  Asphyxia
  During exchange with heparinized blood that may have low blood sugar
  Glycogen storage disease
  Fructose intolerance
  Galactosemia
  Adrenal insufficiency

3. Treatment

  a. Anticipation and prevention is more important than treatment.

   (1) Well infants who are at high risk of hypoglycemia should have
   blood sugars measured at 3, 6, 12, 24 hr of age and be given early
   oral or gavage feedings with 10% glucose and water q2h until the
   sugar level is stable. At this point, they can be weaned to milk
   with continuing attention to their blood sugars for the first 2 days
   of life.

   (2) Any asphyxiated infant should be given parenteral glucose as part
   of the resuscitative effort.

  b. Symptomatic hypoglycemia is best treated by first drawing blood for
  appropriate studies and then giving the following:

   (1) Glucose, 0.5–1.0 gm/kg of body weight by IV push. This is done by
   giving 2.4 ml of 25% D/W per kilogram at a rate of 1 ml/min (e.g., a
   4-kg infant should receive 8–16 ml of 25% D/W over 8–16 min).

   (2) This should be followed by a continuous infusion of dextrose at a
   rate of 4–8 mg/glucose/kg/min. The glucose concentration of the
   fluid will depend on the daily fluid requirement. (On day 1, the fluid
   requirement is 65/ml/kg/day, or 0.045 ml/kg/min; 10% D/W provides
   4.5 mg glucose/kg/min, and 15% D/W provides 6.75 mg glucose/kg/
   min. Either may be used.) For most patients, 10% D/W at daily
   maintenance rates will provide adequate IV glucose.

   (3) The concentration of glucose and the rate of infusion are increased
   as necessary to maintain a normal blood sugar (e.g., some infants
   with hyperinsulinism will require 15% D/W).

   (4) Glucagon at a dose of 300 μg/kg IM can be administered to mobilize
   glucose in infants with adequate glycogen stores.

(5) Epinephrine, diazoxide, and growth hormone are to be used only with endocrinologic consultation in special cases of chronic intractable hypoglycemia.

C. Hypocalcemia

1. Etiology

a. First 3 days

(1) Maternal: Diabetes, toxemia, obstetric complications, severe dietary calcium deficiency, maternal hyperparathyroidism.

(2) Intrapartum: Asphyxia, prematurity, small-for-gestational age infants.

(3) Postnatal: Hypoxia, shock, sepsis, treatment with bicarbonate, exchange transfusions with citrated blood.

b. After 3 days   See Chap. 8.

2. Evaluation and diagnosis

a. Signs of hypocalcemia in the newborn are nonspecific, and the classic Chvostek sign and carpopedal spasm are helpful only if *present.*

b. Irritability, jitteriness, hypotonia, a high-pitched cry, and seizures are the most common presenting symptoms.

c. Calcium levels should be measured frequently in infants with the preceding conditions and substantiated if necessary with ECG measurement of the Q–OTC (Q–onset of T/R–R), or Q–T interval. They should be measured at 6, 12, 24, and 48 hr of age in infants of diabetic mothers; at 1, 3, 6, and 12 hr of age in intrapartum asphyxia; and at 12, 24, and 48 hr of age in small-for-dates infants.

3. Risks of treatment can be minimized by attention to details.

a. An IV push of calcium can cause a sudden elevation of serum calcium, leading to bradycardia or other cardiac arrhythmias.

b. Extravasation of calcium solutions into subcutaneous tissues can cause severe tissue necrosis. Therefore, calcium-containing solutions should not be infused into a peripheral vein by a pump except in unusual circumstances.

c. Calcium cannot be mixed with $NaHCO_3^-$, since this may produce $CaCO_3$ precipitation.

d. Calcium can cause necrosis of the liver if it is administered via an umbilical vein catheter that is in the portal system.

e. Calcium pushed into the aorta may be a factor in necrotizing enterocolitis. Therefore it should be given only by slow maintenance drip if an umbilical artery catheter is used.

4. Therapy

a. Preparations   It is preferable to use only one calcium salt (gluconate) for either IV or PO administration, e.g., calcium gluconate 10%, PO or IV (1 ml of 10% calcium gluconate = 100 mg of calcium gluconate = 9 mg of elemental calcium or 0.45 mEq/ml).

b. Doses

(1) For symptomatic hypocalcemia (Ca under 7 mg/100 ml without symptoms), give 5–10 ml/kg/day of 10% calcium gluconate. For maintenance calcium, give 45–90 mg/kg/day of elemental calcium PO or IV. Start with a low dose and increase the dose as needed.

(2) Acute symptomatic hypocalcemia

   (a) Give 2 ml/kg of 10% calcium gluconate IV stat.

   (b) The maximum dose is 5 ml for prematures and 10 ml for full term infants. This amount can be given slowly IV (1 ml/min) with careful observation of the heart rate and the vein if a peripheral vein is being used. This dose is conservative and can be repeated in 15 min if there is no clinical response.

c. Maintenance

   (1) Following the acute dose, maintenance calcium should be given parenterally or by mouth. A low-phosphate milk (e.g., breast milk or Similac PM 60/40) should be used when oral feeding is started. Calcium can be added directly to the formula if necessary.

   (2) Treatment of hypocalcemia is rarely necessary for more than 4–5 days unless other complications are present.
   During treatment, calcium levels should be monitored q12–24h and the dose gradually tapered as indicated. By 1 week of age most infants of diabetic mothers remain normocalcemic on a regular formula or breast milk and without supplements.

d. Hypomagnesemia

   (1) Hypocalcemia may be associated with **hypomagnesemia** and will not respond unless the hypomagnesemia is treated. Normal magnesium levels in newborns are 1.2–1.8 mEq/L, or 2.4–3.6 mg/100 ml.

   (2) Treatment consists in administration of 0.1–0.2 ml/kg of 50% $MgSO_4$ IV or IM, repeating if necessary q12h, as well as the addition of 3 mEq/L of magnesium to maintenance fluids.

e. Persistent hypocalcemia   If the infant remains hypocalcemic, despite adequate calcium supplementation and normal magnesium levels, a search for other causes of hypocalcemia must be started (see Chaps. 8, 9, and 12).

V. INFECTION   Infection accounts for 10–20 percent of infant deaths.

A. Congenital infections

  1. TORCH (toxoplasmosis, rubella, cytomegalic inclusion virus, herpes virus).

   a. Evaluation and diagnosis

   (1) Maternal history   Screening by serology should be considered when maternal factors suggest risk of congenital infection (see Sec. I).

   (2) Neonatal manifestations include

      (a) Prematurity, intrauterine growth retardation, failure to thrive.

      (b) Eye abnormalities, including glaucoma, cataracts, chorioretinitis, conjunctivitis, keratoconjunctivitis, and microophthalmia.

      (c) Skin abnormalities, including vesicles, purpura, maculopapular rash.

      (d) CNS abnormalities, including microcephaly, hydrocephalus, intracerebral calcifications (periventricular in cytomegalovirus disease and scattered in toxoplasmosis), meningoencephalitis, mental retardation, and deafness.

- **(e) Visceral abnormalities,** including hepatomegaly, splenomegaly, hepatitis, bony lesions on x-ray, and cardiac abnormalities, especially PDA with pulmonary stenosis.

- **(f) Hematologic abnormalities,** including prolonged jaundice, thrombocytopenia, or unexplained nucleated red blood cells in the peripheral smear.

- **(3) Laboratory examination**   See also Chap. 15.

  - **(a)** Draw sera for a TORCH screen (5–10 ml of blood) **(prior to transfusions)** or cord blood (serum) and pair with a sample from the mother, drawn at the same time. This should include a search for IGM-specific immunofluorescent antibodies. Convalescent serum from the mother and baby must be sent in 2–8 weeks, depending on the clinical situation. Sera may be required at 3–6 months.

  - **(b)** Viral cultures (herpesvirus from maternal or neonatal sores will grow in 3–4 days).

  - **(c)** Histologic study of the placenta.

  - **(d)** Tzanck prep of smear of vesicles from the infant or mother.

  - **(e)** Urine cytologic study after Millipore filtration for cytomegalic inclusion virus.

- **b. Treatment**   See also Chap 15.

  - **(1)** No specific treatment is available for rubella or cytomegalovirus infection. Therapy is symptomatic.

  - **(2)** Adenine arabinoside (ara-A) has shown some effectiveness in the treatment of neonatal herpesvirus infection (see Chap. 15, Sec. **V.B.3**). Topical IDU (see Chap. 24) eyedrops and large doses of gamma globulin (10–20 mg IM) have been used.

- **c. Prevention**

  - **(1)** Congenital **rubella** is prevented by adequate immunization of childbearing women (see Chap. 1).

  - **(2) Toxoplasmosis** (see Chap. 16) may possibly be prevented by avoidance of cats and raw meat during pregnancy.

2. Syphilis   See also Chap. 15, Sec. **IV.U.2.**

- **a. Etiology**   Transplacental transmission of *Treponema pallidum.*

- **b. Evaluation and diagnosis**

  - **(1) Perinatal** clinical signs include stillbirth, fetal hydrops, and prematurity.

  - **(2) Postnatal** manifestations include failure to thrive, persistent rhinitis, lymphadenopathy, rash, jaundice, anemia, hepatosplenomegaly, nephrosis, and meningitis.

- **c. Laboratory tests**

  - **(1) Mother**   Rapid plasma reagin (RPR) with titers and fluorescent-treponemal antibody absorption test (FTA-ABS) with titers.

(2) Infant

  (a) RPR with titer and FTA-ABS with titer.

  (b) If available IGM-FTA-ABS is most specific for fetal infection.

  (c) X-rays of long bones for evidence of metaphyseal demineralization or periosteal new bone formation.

  (d) Dark-field examination of any nasal discharge.

  (e) Cerebrospinal fluid examination.

d. Treatment   See also Chap. 15, Sec. **IV.U.**

  (1) Pregnant mother with primary, secondary, or latent or late latent syphilis

  (a) Benzathine penicillin G   The dose is 2.4 million U IM (1.2 million in each buttock initially). Repeat 7 days later. The total dose is 4.8 million U. Alternatively, give aqueous procaine penicillin G, 1.2 million U/day IM for 10 days.

  (b) In the presence of penicillin allergy, **cephaloridine**, 2 gm/day PO for 12 days, is given. **Erythromycin** PO in the same dose has been used, but it does not cross the placenta well. **Tetracycline** in the same dose is effective, but it may have teratogenic effects.

  (2) Infant

  (a) If the infant's serologic test results are negative and the infant has no disease, no treatment is necessary.

  (b) If the serologic test results are positive, treat the symptomatic infant. Treat the asymptomatic infant when

  i. The titer is 3–4 times higher than the mother's.

  ii. The FTA is 3–4+.

  iii. IGM is elevated (over 20 mg/100 ml).

  iv. The mother is inadequately treated or untreated.

  v. The mother is unreliable, and follow-up is doubtful.

  (c) If the baby has a positive RPR, or FTA, or both, and the history and clinical findings (including x-ray) make infection unlikely, it is safe to await the IGM report and repeat RPR and FTA titers. Any significant rise in titer or any clinical signs require treatment. If transferred antibodies, the baby should have a falling titer.

  (d) Give **procaine penicillin G** in aqueous suspension, 50,000 U/kg IM in 1 daily dose for 10–14 days or **aqueous penicillin G**, 50,000 U/kg/day, q12h IM for 10–14 days (see Table 15-14).

3. Gonorrhea

  a. Etiology   Intrapartum infection with *Neisseria gonorrhoeae.*

  b. Evaluation and diagnosis

  (1) Gonococcal ophthalmia is discussed in Chap. 24.

  (2) Other evidence of gonococcal infection includes rhinitis, anorectal infection, sinusitis, arthritis, sepsis, and meningitis.

  (3) In infants born to mothers with gonococcal infection, eye nasopharyngeal, ear, gastric, and anorectal Gram stains and cultures should be done.

    c. Treatment   Any Gram stain or culture from a neonatal source positive for *N. gonorrhoeae*, even without evidence of infection, should be treated (see Table 15-13).

B. Acquired infections (See also Chap. 15.)   Life-threatening neonatal infections (sepsis, meningitis) share some clinical features. The incidence of sepsis in the newborn is 2 in 1000.

   1. Sepsis and meningitis

     a. Etiology   Organisms associated with neonatal infections are listed in Table 5-4.

     b. Evaluation

       (1) Sepsis should be suspected in the following situations:

        (a) Any sudden change for worse.

        (b) Temperature control problems, metabolic acidosis, infant "not doing well."

        (c) Common symptoms include poor feeding, lethargy, apneic spells, spitting, or vomiting, or both, and diarrhea.

        (d) Signs include omphalitis, ileus, abdominal distention, cyanosis, petechiae, grunting respirations, and purpura.

        (e) Laboratory

          i. Culture and Gram stain of blood, cerebrospinal fluid (CSF), urine (bladder tap), stool, nose, and throat.

          ii. Gram stain of gastric aspirate.

          iii. Chest x-ray.

Table 5-4   Organisms Associated with Newborn Infection

Early Infection
Group A and B streptococci
Gram-negative organisms
Escherichia coli
Klebsiella-Aerobacter
Pseudomonas
Neisseria gonorrhoeae
Group A streptococci
Candida
Chlamydia
*Late Nursery Infection (> 5 days of age)**
Staphylococcus aureus
Gram-negative organisms
E. coli
Klebsiella-Aerobacter
Pseudomonas
Serratia

*The causative organisms vary with the flora of the nursery and its personnel.

iv. Total neutrophil and absolute band count.

v. Histopathology of the placenta and cord If no inflammation is seen, the risk of infection is low.

vi. Radionuclide scan if osteomyelitis is suspected.

(f) The **diagnosis** of sepsis is confirmed by a positive uncontaminated blood culture. **However, in a sick infant or when there is a high index of suspicion, therapy should not be withheld pending confirmation.**

(2) Meningitis

(a) Any infant suspected of sepsis should have a lumbar puncture. Normal values are given in Table 5-5.

(b) Neonatal meningitis is rapidly fatal, and few if any clinical signs may be present **up to and including** its terminal stages.

(c) A full fontanelle is a **late** sign of meningitis.

(d) Fever may or may not be present.

(e) Laboratory See **(1).(e)** above.

(f) The **diagnosis** is confirmed when more than 10 WBC/mm^3 are present (see Table 5-5) and by a positive CSF culture.

c. Treatment

(1) Sepsis

(a) Treatment should begin **before** culture results are available. Therapy can be modified or discontinued as indicated.

Table 5-5 Cerebrospinal Fluid Findings in High-Risk Neonates Without Meningitis

Laboratory Study	Term	Preterm
WBC count (cells/mm^3)		
No. of infants	87	30
Mean	8.2	9.0
Median	5	6
S.D.	7.1	8.2
Range	0–32	0–29
± 2 S.D.	0–22.4	0–25.
Percentage neutrophils	61.3%	57.2%
Protein (mg/100 ml)		
No. of infants	35	17
Mean	90	115
Range	20–170	65–150
Glucose (mg/100 ml)		
No. of infants	51	23
Mean	52	50
Range	34–119	24–63
CSF and blood glucose (%)		
No. of infants	51	23
Mean	81	74
Range	44–248	55–105

Source: Modified from L. D. Sariff et al., *J. Pediatr.* 88(3): 473, 1976.

(b) IV antibiotics should be initiated in high, frequent doses (see Appendix Table 5-1). Ampicillin, oxacillin, or penicillin G with kanamycin or gentamicin are recommended for initial therapy.

(c) Careful attention should be paid to temperature, hydration, caloric intake, and acid-base balance.

(d) When confirmatory cultures are ready, antibiotics should be "tailored" to the sensitivities of the organism or organisms recovered.

(e) IV therapy is continued for 10–14 days.

(2) Meningitis

(a) Broad-spectrum antibiotic coverage should be begun as soon as the diagnosis is confirmed and **before** culture results are obtained.

(b) If organisms are sensitive to penicillin, the appropriate penicillin should be initiated.

(c) The morbidity and mortality in **gram-negative** neonatal meningitis caused by penicillin-resistant organisms remain so high that early, aggressive therapy with aminoglycosides must be instituted.

(d) Chloramphenicol (see Chap. 15, Sec. **III.A.6**) in appropriate doses should be considered as an alternative or additional treatment to the use of aminoglycosides for gram-negative meningitis.

   i. Emergence of chloramphenicol resistance during the treatment of gram-negative infections has been reported.

   ii. Great care must be used if chloramphenicol is given in the presence of hemolytic anemia (due to the drug's toxic effect on bone marrow red cells) and of granulocytopenia. The drug should also be used cautiously in the presence of liver disease.

   iii. Measuring chloramphenicol levels in the blood and CSF is helpful in preventing dose-related chloramphenicol toxicity (bone marrow suppression and "gray baby syndrome"). The assay for chloramphenicol (as well as for all aminoglycosides) can be obtained from as little as 10 μL of serum. The ratio of CSF to serum chloramphenicol levels is 0.65 (range 0.48–0.99).

(e) Repeat cultures of blood and CSF should be obtained in the patient on therapy to ensure rapid sterilization of blood and CSF.

2. Group B streptococcal infection The group B streptococcus is now the major cause of sepsis and meningitis in most nurseries in the United States. The attack rate of group B sepsis is 2 in 1000 live births.

a. Etiology Group B streptococci are recovered from the vaginal cultures of 25 percent of American mothers at the time of delivery. Of these infants, 25 percent have positive skin or nasopharyngeal cultures, or both, and some will become ill.

b. Evaluation

(1) The early-onset type may present as mild respiratory distress or "transient tachypnea of the newborn," progressing rapidly to shock and death in an infant with few or no risk factors for infection. If the disease presents within a few hours of birth, mortality is high, irrespective of therapy.

(2) Late infections may present as meningitis at 2–4 weeks of age.

(3) Laboratory studies include CBC, chest x-ray, urinalysis "surface" cultures, lumbar puncture, and gastric aspirate.

c. The **diagnosis** is confirmed by positive blood and surface cultures.

(1) The chest x-ray may show pneumonia, "retained lung fluid," or a pattern not unlike hyaline membrane disease.

(2) The gastric aspirate may show gram-positive diplococci with neutrophils.

d. Treatment

(1) Infants suspected of having group B streptococcal pneumonia or sepsis should be treated with aqueous penicillin, 200,000–300,000 U/kg/day in 3–4 doses/day, or ampicillin, 200 mg/kg/day and gentamicin (see Appendix Table 5-1).

(2) If sepsis or meningitis is proved, treatment should be carried out for 14 days.

3. Pneumonia

a. Etiology

(1) Congenital pneumonia

(a) Transplacental agents include TORCH, enteroviruses, *Treponema pallidum*, *Listeria monocytogenes*, *Mycobacterium tuberculosis*, genital *Mycoplasma*, and pneumococci.

(b) Maternal **vaginal** causes are group B streptococci, *E. coli*, and other gram-negative enteric bacteria, staphylococci, pneumococci, anaerobic organisms, *Chlamydia*, *Mycoplasma*, and herpesvirus.

(2) Pneumonia acquired during birth may be due to maternal vaginal flora, but may not present until a few days after birth.

(3) Pneumonia acquired after birth may come from nursery personnel, other infants in the nursery, or nursery equipment. Staphylococci, gram-negative enteric bacteria, enteroviruses, *Chlamydia*, and herpesvirus are among the common agents.

b. Evaluation

(1) A **history** of maternal fever, premature delivery, prolonged rupture of membranes, excessive obstetric manipulation, or foul-smelling amniotic fluid should increase the suspicion of neonatal pneumonia.

(2) Physical examination Fever, lethargy, tachypnea, grunting, flaring of nasal alae, retractions, irregular breathing rales, and cyanosis may be present.

(3) Laboratory tests should include a CBC, a chest x-ray for evidence of pulmonary infiltrate or pleural fluid, and a gastric aspirate for Gram stain and culture (see Sec. **I.A.3**). The presence of neutrophils is correlated with pneumonia more than is the finding of bacteria. Cultures, and Gram stain of blood, urine, and spinal fluid and tracheal aspirate should be obtained.

(4) If pleural fluid is present, a pleural tap should be done. If necessary, direct lung aspiration (lung tap) is indicated.

c. Diagnosis The diagnosis of pneumonia is usually made by the presence of physical signs (see **B.2**) and a chest x-ray showing a pulmonary infiltrate.

d. Treatment

(1) General supportive measures include

    (a) Fluid, electrolyte, and acid-base balance.

    (b) Maintenance of hematocrit, blood volume, and blood pressure.

    (c) Nutrition.

    (d) Temperature control.

(2) Respiratory support includes

    (a) Respiratory physical therapy; oxygen as needed.

    (b) Intermittent positive pressure ventilation.

    (c) Drainage of pleural fluid if the fluid is compromising respiration.

(3) Antibiotics are used as in the treatment of sepsis, depending on the suspected cause.

4. Omphalitis The devitalized umbilical cord is an excellent culture medium for many bacteria. In areas where there is poor maternal immunity to tetanus and inadequate aseptic technique, neonatal tetanus due to omphalitis is a major cause of death.

a. Etiology The cord is colonized shortly after birth with the local flora. Infection with streptococci and staphylococci is common. **Phlebitis** may spread to the liver, causing liver abscess or thrombosis of the hepatic vein. **Arteritis** may interfere with postnatal obliteration of the umbilical vessels and cause bleeding.

b. Evaluation and diagnosis

(1) Infection can cause peritonitis and septic emboli to the lungs, pancreas, kidney, skin, and bone.

(2) If true omphalitis is present, the infant should have a full evaluation for sepsis, including blood, urine, and CSF cultures.

c. Treatment

(1) As in sepsis, IV antibiotics are administered before culture results are available. Because staphylococcus is a common agent, oxacillin and either gentamicin or kanamycin are preferred.

(2) Any catheter in the umbilicus should be removed.

(3) Leaving the cord open to the air to dry may decrease the number of flora.

C. Tuberculosis in the newborn In the United States, when maternal tuberculosis (TB) is present or suspected at the time of delivery, management of the newborn is a major clinical problem. For a brief discussion see Chap. 15, Sec. **IV.T.** For a complete discussion, see *Manual of Neonatal Care.*

VI. OTHER PROBLEMS

A. Necrotizing enterocolitis (NEC) is a severe, often fatal, disease seen in 1–10 percent of prematurely born infants.

  1. Etiology Factors suggested to cause mucosal damage are **ischemia**, feeding of hypertonic formula and some medications, bacterial invasion, and the absence of normal colostrum.

  2. Evaluation and diagnosis

    a. Signs and symptoms

      (1) Bloody diarrhea in a small premature, with abdominal distention and bloody or bile-stained gastric aspirates, suggests NEC.

      (2) Mucosal slough may be passed per rectum.

    b. Laboratory studies

      (1) A flat plate of the abdomen may show pneumatosis cystoides intestinalis. Free peritoneal gas or gas in the portal venous system may be present.

      (2) Cultures of the stool and blood should be obtained.

    c. Prevention of perforation

      (1) Impaired carbohydrate absorption may be an early sign of this disease. Monitoring stool for fecal reducing substance and decreasing feedings may **prevent** severe disease.

      (2) If early feeding must be initiated, breast milk is preferred.

  3. Treatment

    a. The infant should receive nothing by mouth.

    b. A nasogastric tube should be placed for drainage.

    c. Treat as sepsis (see p. 140).

    d. Serial x-rays should be obtained q6h as long as the infant is ill.

    e. Discontinue all umbilical lines.

    f. If symptoms improve, treatment should be continued for 7–10 days.

    g. If the baby worsens, surgical consultation and removal of any necrotic bowel may be necessary.

B. Drug withdrawal in the newborn

  1. Etiology Withdrawal symptoms may be seen in infants born to mothers taking narcotics, methadone, diazepam, phenobarbital, alcohol, ethchlorvynol, pentazocine, and chlordiazepoxide.

  2. Evaluation and diagnosis

    a. Maternal history Discreet, sensitive history taking is necessary to elicit a history of drug abuse.

    b. The **infant's symptoms** include disturbed patterns of sleeping and waking rhythms; nasal congestion, sneezing, and yawning; high-pitched cry; increased sucking, ravenous appetite; irritability, jitteriness; hypertonicity, hyperreflexia, and clonus; sweating and tachypnea; vomiting, diarrhea, and dehydration; fever; seizures; tremors.

    c. Infants of methadone-treated mothers may have severe, prolonged withdrawal. Some have "late" withdrawal that may be of the following two types:

(1) The first group shows symptoms shortly after birth, improves, then relapses at 2–4 weeks.

(2) The second group shows no symptoms at birth, but symptoms develop 2–3 weeks later. These infants may also have a history of a sudden, tremendous increase in appetite.

d. Blood and urine samples from the mother and infant for toxic screening within 24 hr after delivery may help, but drugs given to the mother during labor can sometimes confuse the results. Clinical suspicion and careful history usually lead to the diagnosis.

3. Treatment   The goal of treatment is an infant who is not irritable, is not vomiting, has no diarrhea, and can sleep between feedings, yet is not heavily sedated.

a. Swaddling, holding, and rocking may help infants who are not severely affected.

b. Drugs   Infants in whom the preceding therapy is inadequate will need medication.

(1) Phenobarbital, 5–8 mg/kg/day IM or PO in 4 divided doses, and tapered over 2 weeks, can be given. The side effects are sedation, poor sucking, and no control of diarrhea.

(2) Chlorpromazine, 1.5–3.0 mg/kg/24 hr in divided doses q6h, is given initially IM then PO. This dose is maintained for 2–4 days, then tapered as tolerated every 2–4 days. The length of treatment is from 1–6 weeks. Methadone-dependent infants tend to need a longer course of treatment.

(3) Paregoric, 0.05/ml/kg (2 drops/kg/dose), is given q4h. The dose is increased by 2 drops (0.05 ml) at the end of a 4-hr period if no improvement is seen. Some babies will need medication more often than q4h. Once the adequate dose is determined, it can be tapered by 10 percent daily. The length of treatment is 1–6 weeks. **Side effects** include sleepiness and constipation. **The effects of oral benzoic acid on bilirubin binding to albumin are not known. Camphor is a CNS stimulant.**

(4) Tincture of opium USP   For the above reasons, if a narcotic is to be used it may be best to use **tincture of opium USP,** a 10% solution (equal to 1.0% morphine). Dilute this 25-fold to a concentration equal to that of paregoric (0.4% opium or 0.04% morphine) and give in the same dose as paregoric.

(5) Diazepam   The dose is 1–2 mg IM q8h until symptoms are controlled. The dose is then halved, then changed to q12h, then halved again. The length of treatment ranges from 2–7 days, and it seems to be effective in a shorter time than are other medications. **Note that sodium benzoate included in parenteral diazepam interferes with bilirubin binding.**

(6) Methadone should not be routinely used until more data on toxicity are available. **Methadone is excreted in breast milk,** and thus methadone-treated mothers should not breast-feed. When administration has been necessary, the doses used have been 0.5–1.0 mg q4–8h.

c. The major problem for these children is proper disposition and follow-up. Most states require reporting of these infants as battered children, and social agencies should be involved in the decision for disposition (see Chap. 2, Sec. **XIII**, p. 57). Some risk factors to consider in sending infants home with their mothers are

(1) **Maternal age**   The risk increases as age decreases.

(2) **Length of drug use**   The risk increases as length of usage increases.

(3) Availability of a drug program.

(4) Drug use while on methadone.

C. Malformed infants

1. History

a. Talk to the parents and explain the need for a careful history and diagnostic evaluation. Discuss with them whether or not they should see the child.

b. Obtain a detailed family history, especially with regard to similar abnormalities in other family members, fetal death, or death in early childhood.

c. Confirm a pregnancy history of exposure to drugs, illness, and any environmental hazard.

2. Examination   Malformed infants who are either stillborn or die soon after birth are of special concern. Many of these infants have genetic disorders that will be identified only if a thorough diagnostic evaluation is performed.

a. Perform a careful physical examination (whether or not child is dead). Remember that the obvious deformity may not be the sole abnormality.

b. Photographs should be obtained, *especially* if the child dies.

c. X-rays should be obtained even if the child has died.

d. A postmortem examination should be done.

e. Chromosomal and blood studies should be done, but only if child is clinically well. If the child is moribund, determination is not feasible. A skin biopsy for fibroblasts should be done under sterile conditions (refrigerate and process immediately).

3. Do a literature search.

4. If the diagnosis is uncertain, obtain the best advice available. If possible, consult with a geneticist, who will also be helpful for long-term counseling.

5. Specific genetic counseling should deal with determining the diagnosis, etiology, prognosis, and possible treatment. The risk of recurrence and the feasibility of future prenatal diagnosis should be discussed.

Drug	Dose, Route, and Schedule	Comments
Antibiotics		
Ampicillin	100 mg/kg/day IM or IV q12h < 1 week old q8h > 1 week old	
Carbenicillin	*Initial dose* 100 mg/kg IV *Follow by* Newborns under 2000 gm body weight Under 7 days old: 225 mg/kg/day IV q8h Over 7 days old: 400 mg/kg/day IV q6h Newborns over 2000 gm body weight: Under 3 days old: 300 mg/kg/day IV q6h Over 3 days old: 400 mg/kg/day IV q6h	
Cephalexin	50–100 mg/kg/day IV q8h	
Chloramphenicol	*Premature newborns under 1 week old:* 25 mg/kg/day IV q8–12h *Full-term newborns under 1 week old:* 25–50 mg/kg/day IV q8–12h *All infants over 1 week old:* 50 mg/kg/day IV	IM chloramphenicol is erratically absorbed. *Toxic effects* are seen with serum levels over 50 μg/ml; serum levels should be kept under 25 μg/ml to avoid the "gray baby syndrome"
Gentamicin sulfate	*Premature or full-term newborns under 1 week old:* 5 mg/kg/day q12h IM or IV as a 1–2 hr infusion *Newborns over 1 week old:* 5.0–7.5 mg/kg/day q8h IM or IV as a 1–2 hr infusion	Optimal serum level is 4–10 μg/ml 1 hr after IV dose
Kanamycin sulfate	*Newborns under 7 days old* Under 2000 gm body weight: 7.5 mg/kg q12h IM or slow IV over at least 20 min Over 2000 gm body weight: 10 mg/kg q12h IM or slow IV over at least 20 min *Newborns over 7 days old* Under 2000 gm body weight: 10 mg/kg q12h Over 2000 gm body weight: 10 mg q8h	These doses exceed 15 mg/kg/day recommended by the manufacturer, but are effective and safe. Risks of ototoxicity and nephrotoxicity are increased when renal function is poor. Try to keep the total dose under 500 mg/kg, since ototoxicity is related to total dose. Therapeutic serum level is 15–20 mg

Appendix Table 5-1 (*Continued*)

Drug	Dose, Route, and Schedule	Comments
Oxacillin sodium	25–50 mg/kg dose IM or IV Under 2500 gm under 2 weeks old: bid–tid Under 2500 gm over 2 weeks old: tid–qid	Use higher dose more frequently in severe infection
Miscellaneous		
ACTH	3–5 U/kg/day in 4 divided doses IM	
Chlorpromazine (Thorazine)	2.0–2.5 mg/kg/day in 4 divided doses PO, IM, IV	
Meperidine (Demerol)	1.0–1.5 mg/kg/dose q4h PO or IM	
Dexamethasone	0.5–1.0 mg q6–8h IM, IV	For tracheal or CNS edema
Dopamine HCl (Intropin)	5–20 μg/kg/min IV starting with lower dose and working up to desired effect	
Glucagon	30–300 μg/kg. May repeat after 6–12 hr IM or IV	
Magnesium sulfate	0.2 mg/kg/dose 50% solution q4–8h IM (for tetanus neonatorum or other repeated convulsions)	Hypotension may occur
Protamine sulfate	12.5 mg/U of blood for exchange transfusion, slow IV 1.0 mg IV for each 1.0 mg heparin in previous 4 hr	

6

Growth and Development

The terms growth and development are not interchangeable. *Growth* refers to proportionate changes in size, *development* to increase in skill and complexity of function.

I. GROWTH

A. Characteristics of growth
Growth is such a conspicuous characteristic of the young of any species that one whose attention is occupied with infants and children may find it easy to take growth for granted.

Observations on growth should be part of every physical examination. Differences in segmental growth rates cause a change in the ratio of sitting height to total height. Sitting height represents about 70 percent of total height at birth, but falls rapidly to about 57 percent at 3 years.

B. Factors influencing growth

1. Endocrine system

a. Thyroid hormones are important prenatally and during the first year of life, when growth and development are rapid. Because thyroxine does not cross the placenta, it cannot prevent congenital hypothyroidism. However, it is transmitted in breast milk and while moderating the effects of neonatal hypothyroidism may delay diagnosis as well.

b. Pituitary The pituitary growth hormone is essential for normal growth after the second year of life. Hypopituitarism leads to concomitant failure of weight and height growth.

c. Androgens, which are produced by the adrenal cortex in both sexes, by the testes in the male, and, to a lesser extent, by the ovaries in the female, can cause the growth spurt at puberty. The androgens stimulate *growth* more than maturation.

2. Malnutrition
Any condition leading to an inadequate caloric intake will lead to growth retardation. This includes any disorder that limits the availability of food, hinders its transport, or interferes with its absorption. If malnutrition is sufficiently severe, there may be complete growth arrest. In general, weight is affected first, then length, and finally head growth. When the unfavorable condition is terminated, a sudden growth spurt usually occurs and may compensate entirely for the (duration of) growth arrest.

The calories required to restart growth may be as many as 200/kg/day. During refeeding, rapid head growth may simulate hydrocephalus, but without other neurologic signs.

3. Psychosocial deprivation
results in growth delay. Although not completely understood, this probably occurs through a combination of neuroendocrine alteration and caloric deprivation.

C. **Physical measurement**   Standards for height, weight, and head circumference according to age and sex are available in pediatric texts. In general, they have been based on middle-class Caucasian populations, but are useful as relative growth standards regardless of race.

   1. *Length* is the measurement of stature taken in the supine position; *height* is the measurement in the erect position.

   2. Hip width is obtained by obstetric calipers pressed firmly against the most lateral points of the iliac crests.

   3. Head circumference is obtained by applying a tape over the glabella and supraorbital ridges and the part of the occiput that gives the greatest posterior circumference. Routine measurements of head size should be part of the basic records on infants and young children. This is the age of very rapid growth of the brain, and departures from the normal or rapid changes in percentiles have both diagnostic and prognostic significance for such problems as microcephaly or hydrocephalus.

D. **Accelerated growth periods**   The normal growth of a child is not a uniformly continuous process but has three separate periods of acceleration. The velocity of human growth decreases from birth onward, but this decrease is interrupted once and perhaps twice. It is slowed markedly from 6–8 years, a period known as the juvenile, or midgrowth, spurt, about which we still have little information, and is entirely reversed from the ages of 13–15, the period known as the adolescent growth spurt and associated with the development of puberty.

E. **Variations in the rate of growth of different tissues**   The growth rate of different tissues and body organs varies considerably.

   1. Head   The head is disproportionately large at birth and has attained about 95 percent of its total growth when a child is 8–9 years old.

   2. Lymphatic tissue   The growth of this tissue is remarkable in that the total size of such organs as the thymus reaches its peak in the 5–10-year age group and then gradually regresses. The unique pattern of change exhibited by lymphoid tissue must be kept in mind when assessing tissues such as the tonsils and lymphoid tissue if judged by adult standards. It is likely that what is so often called "hypertrophy" of the tonsils during the preschool and early school years really represents a physiologic pattern of growth, since there is an initial spurt in fetal life and in infancy, followed by a long interval of relatively slow growth and then by a second growth spurt in adolescence.

F. **Patterns of growth**   Each child grows at his or her own rate, although all children go through the same stages of growth and development on their way from birth to maturity.

   1. Measurement

      a. A graphic method of plotting a child's body measurements on standard deviation charts will show how consistently the child is maintaining his or her percentile relationship to other children of the same age and sex.

      b. Repeated measurements of height and weight provide the simplest and still the best index of physical growth. The child should, of course, be assessed not only on height and weight but also on rate of growth, relative proportions, and state of maturity in relation to age.

      c. Radiologic examination is often used to determine whether the child's osseous development is delayed or advanced for his or her age. Dentition will also help to provide confirmatory evidence.

2. Changes in body proportions

a. There is a general cephalocaudal progression of growth at successive age periods. This accounts for the relatively large head and short lower extremities at birth and the progressive changes in these relationships.

b. From the second half of the first year to puberty, the extremities grow more rapidly than the trunk, and both more rapidly than the head. At puberty the rates of growth of trunk and extremities are about equal, but the trunk continues to grow after the extremities have ceased their growth in the postpubescent period.

3. Sex differences in growth
At birth and during early childhood, boys are slightly taller and heavier than girls. At about 6 years, girls may surpass boys in weight. Boys, maturing about 2 years later on the average than girls, do not catch up in weight until they are a little over age 14. Girls are taller than boys between about 10 and 14 years. Not all measurements follow this pattern. For example, at all ages boys exceed girls in chest circumference, and girls exceed boys in thigh circumference and skeletal maturity. The muscular development of boys exceeds that of girls at all ages. The stages of pubertal development are shown in Table 6-1.

4. Dentition
Individual variation in the date of eruption of the teeth is considerable, although teeth are usually cut in the following order and at the following time.

a. First set of teeth (primary dentition)

(1) Lower central incisors, 5–10 months

(2) Upper central and lateral incisors, 8–12 months

(3) Lower lateral incisors and lower and upper first molars, 12–14 months

(4) Lower and upper canines, 16–22 months

(5) Lower and upper second molars, 24–30 months

b. Second set of teeth (permanent dentition)

(1) First molars, 5 and 7 years

(2) Central incisors, 6½ and 8 years

(3) Lateral incisors, 7 and 9 years

(4) First bicuspids, 9 and 11 years

(5) Second bicuspids, 10 and 12 years

(6) Canines, 10 and 12 years

(7) Cuspids, 11 and 14 years

(8) Second molars, 11 and 13 years

(9) Third molars, 16 and 21 years (or later)

5. Skeletal maturation,
or bone age, is a means of classifying skeletal growth and should be regarded as a supplement to the general appraisal of the child.

a. Skeletal maturation is most variable at the onset of ossification.

b. The appearance of primary or secondary centers in the early ages, and the fusion of primary and secondary centers at puberty, deter-

Table 6-1 Tanner Stages of Pubertal Development

Tanner Stage	Breast Development	Pubic Hair	Male Genital Development
1	No palpable glandular tissue; areola not pigmented; no protrusion of breast from chest wall except for nipple	None	Genitals same size and shape as in early childhood
2	Glandular tissue coextensive with areola; nipple and breast project as single mound	Few wispy strands, usually on labia in girls	Scrotum and testes larger; scrotum redder
3	Further enlargement and elevation of breast and areola, with no separation of their contours	Darker, coarser hair extending over pubis	Penis larger and mostly longer; scrotum and testes have enlarged further
4	More glandular tissue and pigmentation; areola and nipple form secondary mound above breast	Dark, curly hair covering mons veneris but not on thighs	Penis larger, with enlarged glans; scrotum and testes larger and scrotum darker
5	Areola and nipple in smooth profile with breast	Mature, extends into thighs	Adult size and shape

Adapted from J. M. Tanner, *Growth and Adolescence* (2nd ed.), Oxford, England: Blackwell Scientific Publications, 1962.

Table 6-2   Average Daily Weight Gain by Birth Weight Groups

Birth Weight (gm)	No. Patients	Age in Months				
		0–2	2–4	4–6	6–8	0–8
1000	4	11.0	19.9	26.5	20.3	19.4
1000–1500	16	10.5	23.5	26.5	19.8	20.1
1500–2000	94	14.5	29.4	25.0	17.2	21.5
2000	49	14.8	30.0	24.7	17.0	21.6
Total	163	14.2	28.6	25.1	17.4	21.3

Adapted from K. Glaser et al., *Pediatrics* 5:130, 1950.

mine maturation. The times of onset and completion of various centers, for both sexes, may be found in the tables of maturation and growth in standard textbooks of pediatrics.

   c. In the older child, a single roentgenogram of the hand and wrist usually permits visualization of a sufficient variety of ossification centers for evaluation of bone age. In infants, a single knee film may also be needed.

   d. When short or tall stature is of concern or an endocrine abnormality is suspected, ultimate height can be estimated using tables in radiologic texts based on a comparison of chronological age, bone age, and present height.

6. Growth of the premature infant

   a. Weight curves are available for premature infants of varying gestational ages (see Fig. 5-3). The postnatal growth of premature infants resembles the growth pattern of fetuses of the same size rather than that of full-term infants of the same postnatal age.

   The most rapid daily weight gain occurs between 2 and 6 months of gestation and levels off to about 20 gm/day thereafter (Table 6-2). Rapid head growth occurs especially when initially ill prematures finally obtain adequate calories. Head growth faster than 1 cm/week should be watched with special care, since it could indicate hydrocephalus.

   b. After the first 2 years of life, the differences in height and weight levels between premature and full-term infants (except for the very smallest premature infants) are not significant.

7. Predicting height and weight with mnemonics

Remember that at 2 years of age the child is about half as tall as he or she will be at maturity. Remember also that at 3 years the child is 3 ft tall and at 4 years is 40 in. tall; or at 3½ years the average child weighs 35 lb and at 7 years weighs 7 times birth weight. Several predictive formulas (using mnemonics) have been added to those already in use (*A.M.A. J. Dis. Child.* 88:452, 1954). The values obtained from these formulas compare reasonably well with those in published growth charts.

   a. **Predicted weight (lb) from age** (3–12 months)

   Formula: weight = age (months) + 11

   b. **Predicted height (in.) from age** (2–14 years)

   Formula: height = $(2½ \times$ age$) + 30$

c. **Predicted weight (lb) as function of height** (2–12 years)

Formula: weight $= 48 + \left(\dfrac{\text{height}}{2} - 23\right) \times \left(\dfrac{\text{height}}{10}\right)$

d. The commonly accepted statement that the child at age 2 has achieved one-half his or her final height holds up well for boys. For girls, however, 10–12 cm (2.54–4.00 in.) is subtracted from the value obtained. When the length at 3 years is known, an approximation of final height can be obtained by multiplying by 1.87 for boys and 1.73 for girls.

e. The formula of Tanner et al. (*Arch. Dis. Child.* 31:372, 1956) demonstrated that height at 3 years correlates better with height at maturity than it does at any other age.

Adult height (cm) $= 1.27 \times H_3 + 54.9$ cm (males)
Adult height (cm) $= 1.29 \times H_3 + 42.3$ cm (females)

II. DEVELOPMENT

A. Norms of development Parents, grandparents, and teachers often focus concern on a child's development, specifically, his or her abilities in functioning. For parents, these issues are made more intense by feelings that the child's progress is a direct result of their parenting ability. Although the *sequence* of stages in development is nearly uniform in all children the *age* at which each stage is normally reached has a range rather than a certain time of occurrence.

B. Developmental lines It is useful to divide developmental stages into categories of functioning (Table 6-3).

1. **Motor** Physical movement is divided into **gross motor abilities** (posture, trunk, and lower limbs) and **fine motor abilities** (upper extremities).

2. The **social-adaptive** functions include interpersonal interactions and skills in dealing with the environment (e.g., dressing, feeding, toileting, and helping with household tasks).

3. **Language functioning** includes the first acquisition of words, followed by progressive command of verbal structures and definitions.

4. **Cognitive functioning** describes a child's understanding or mental construction of the world and his or her relation to it. Piaget has described periods of cognitive development (and the stages within each): the sensorimotor period, preoperational period, concrete operational period, and formal operational. (For a clear discussion of Piaget's theory, see H. Ginsberg and S. Opper, *Piaget's Theory of Intellectual Development*, Englewood Cliffs, N.J.: Prentice-Hall, 1969.)

C. Temperament is a person's *style of functioning* rather than his or her specific capabilities. Assessment of temperament includes characteristic activity level, rhythmicity, approval or withdrawal (to new experiences), adaptability, intensity of reaction and threshold of responsiveness, general quality of mood, distractability, attention span, and persistence. Clusters of extremes of these characteristics have been associated with an increased tendency toward behavioral or emotional problems independent of intelligence and social class (A. Thomas, S. Chess, and H. G. Birch, *Temperament and Behavior Problems in Children*, New York: New York University Press, 1968). Understanding of the role of temperament in a child's reactions may be central to fostering more acceptable behavior patterns.

Table 6-3 Developmental Lines

| Usual Age Range (months) | Motor | | Social-Adaptive | Language | Cognitive |
	Gross	Fine			
0–2	Head control	Hands to mouth; pre-reach movements while watching objects	Active elicitor; quiets or smiles differentially for caregivers	Varied cry patterns	Follows objects visually
2–5	Rolls over	Hands to midline, batting at objects	Begins to show preference for caregiver	Laughs and coos; reciprocal vocalization	Watches spectacles (e.g., mobiles), but only uses whole body activity to reinitiate spectacle
5–9	Sits alone	Unilateral reach	Peek-a-boo and pat-a-cake begin; resists toys being pulled from grasp; begins to be aware of strangers	Imitates speech sounds	Watches dropped object but does not look for hidden object; uses nonspecific means of exploring objects (e.g., mouthing, banging)
9–12	Crawls	Pincer grasp appearing (radialized)	May show upset with strangers	Repetitive consonants (babbling)	Recognizes object when only part is showing
	Stands, climbs	Shapes hands to object; begins to be skillful with tiny objects	Insists on trying things on own		
12–14	Walks	Fine pincer grasp complete	Insists on finger feeding; protests caregiver's leaving	Uses one word appropriately; uses three words; paragraph speech	Finds hidden objects; uses specific actions to explore and activate toys, e.g., pushes car
14–21	Runs, kicks ball	Skillful use of hands; allows for scribbles, piling blocks	Feeds self with spoon; negativism; assists in simple household tasks	Jargon; phrases; knows one body part	Uses key to wind up toy (i.e., sees and looks for indirect causes)

D. **Developmental assessment,** in general, relies on sequential observations over time. A history of past milestones must often substitute for such longitudinal study. However, such a history has the disadvantages of poor definition of skills and vague recall of ages at which these skills were noted.

   1. **Global delays** A child who is functioning with skills characteristic of younger children in all developmental lines is considered **globally delayed.** This may reflect conditions affecting the entire CNS, such as prematurity, prenatal or birth injury, severe or chronic illness, psychosocial deprivation, or a genetic defect. Multiply handicapped children are more difficult to assess for cognitive and language levels because their motor limitations interfere with the demonstration of other skills.

   2. **Isolated delays** If only one or two lines of development are delayed, more specific deficits must be suspected.

      a. **Gross motor delay** may signal structural disorders (e.g., dislocated hip, muscle diseases, myelodysplasia, mild or limited cerebral palsy).

      b. **Fine motor delay** may be a sign of impaired vision or cerebellar dysfunction.

      c. **Language delay** should always prompt audiologic evaluation and investigation of speech stimulation at home.

      d. **Social-adaptive delay** may be related to imbalance in interpersonal relationships within the family.

   3. **Advanced development** The greatest problem for children whose development is advanced, as for children who are large for their age, is the tendency of adults to expect their social and emotional functioning to be commensurate and therefore stress them with unrealistic expectations. Their advanced abilities in school may also isolate them socially from their peers. African and American black infants sometimes show precocious motor development and the former, advanced mental development as well. Developmental precocity has also been found in preindustrial societies in Latin America and Asia (J. Werner, *J. Crosscultural Psychol.* 3:111, 1972).

E. **Newborn assessment** Because the neonate is physically and socially dependent on the environment, discrete areas of independent function used to describe older infants are not applicable. Newborns have a developmental hierarchy of emerging abilities to organize their interaction with the environment. This organization has been divided into four levels of adaptation that can be used in assessment (see *J. Abnorm. Child Psychol.* 5:215, 1977). The series of behavioral parameters reflecting an infant's degree of homeostasis in each level of organization makes up the Brazelton Neonatal Behavioral Assessment Scale (T. B. Brazelton, *Neonatal Behavioral Assessment Scale,* Philadelphia: Lippincott, 1973). This scale goes beyond traditional neurologic assessments in describing the social interactions by which the neonate elicits and reinforces adult caregiving behaviors. It has been used primarily as a research instrument for investigation into the process of early behavioral development.

   The four levels of organization are also useful categories for pediatricians in structuring their assessments of the newborn. However, these levels also highlight the interactive abilities that are the most significant to the parents and also are the most sensitive discriminators between individuals in studies of infants at risk.

   1. **Physiologic organization** includes observations of the stability of the neo-

nate's cardiorespiratory, autonomic-alimentary system: respiratory and heart rates and rhythms, including yawning, hiccups, and apnea; skin color changes, including mottling; and GI function, including vomiting, burping, and defecation. All these functions are less well controlled in premature infants, for example, who may become dangerously unstable with stress.

2. **Motoric organization** includes observations of the quality (i.e., smoothness, range of motion, and coordination of different actions) of spontaneous limb and digit movements, as well as muscle tone and primitive reflexes.

   a. **Asymmetric reflexes** should always suggest a neurologic abnormality.

   b. **The primitive reflexes** generally disappear after 3 months of age, and their persistence may signal neurologic damage. They include

      (1) Plantar grasp   Plantar flexion of the toes on pressing against the ball of the foot.

      (2) Hand grasp   Gripping of the fingers on pressing the palms.

      (3) Automatic walking   Sequential advancement of the legs when the feet are placed on a surface with the body held upright.

      (4) Tonic neck reflex   Extension of the ipsilateral arm and leg and flexion of the contralateral when the head is turned to one side.

      (5) Rooting reflex   Deviation of the mouth and head, turning toward a stimulator of the lip or perioral area.

      (6) Sucking reflex   Coordinated sucking on introduction of a finger or nipple into the mouth.

      (7) Stepping reflex   Flexion of the leg and subsequent foot-placing when the dorsum of the foot is scraped on the edge of a surface.

      (8) Moro, or startle, response   Extension of arms and legs, followed by flexion as if to embrace, elicited by dropping the head backward but also occurring spontaneously or with sudden light or noise.

      (9) Incurvation reflex   Lateral flexion of the trunk on stroking the back near the spine.

3. **State organization** includes observations of variations in the state of consciousness, i.e., sleep and waking states (see *Clin. Child Dev.* No. 12, 1964) and the tendency of the infant to change the progression of states in the presence of stimuli from the environment. It is well recognized now that sleep-wake cycles change with age (see *Acta Paediatr.* 50:160, 1961). Infants small for gestational age may have difficulties because of their tendency to have only a short period of alertness (see *Dev. Med. Child Neurol.* 18:590, 1976).

4. **Interactive organization** includes auditory and visual orienting as well as responses to a caregiver's interventions. Most neonates visually fix on a face, light, or bright object, and can follow it 180° laterally and sometimes vertically if it is moved slowly enough and within close range. They can turn their head, or eyes, or both, toward a voice or the sound of a rattle or bell. The amount of intervention needed to console a crying newborn varies a great deal and soon becomes very important to the caregiver. Some babies are able to quiet themselves by sucking on their hands, while others need the assistance of a soothing voice, restraint of arms,

legs, or both, or rocking, cuddling, and a pacifier. Again, infants at risk are most likely to differ in this respect. It has been noted that infants small for gestational age may not cry easily, or, when they do, may be very difficult to console (see *Dev. Med. Child Neurol.* 18:590, 1976). Understanding of these qualities can greatly improve the pediatrician's ability to provide support for parents who have "difficult" infants.

7

Psychiatry in Pediatric Practice

The effective application of psychological principles enlarges pediatricians' understanding of their work and can be helpful in many aspects of his or her practice. Education and preventive techniques, as well as support for children and families as they deal with a variety of stresses, are integral aspects of a pediatrician's work. While pediatricians usually do not practice psychotherapy, much of their work can be psychologically therapeutic. They also face the difficult task of determining when and to what extent disturbances in behavior and adjustment should be explored. The extent to which pediatricians involve themselves in these problems is determined by their own interest, knowledge, and skill. However, they should be prepared to offer parents and children the opportunity to discuss their concerns in an orderly fashion and to provide an assessment.

I. ETIOLOGY Knowledge of **child development,** with emphasis on sequential developmental stages (see Table 7-1), provides the best framework for understanding disturbances. From this background, one assesses factors that nurture and support or impede and distort maturation. Disparities between the child's changing **needs,** growing **capacities,** and the stimulation from his or her **environment** are part of the child's life experience. Since the child has not reached maturity, the quality, quantity, and reliability of the **nurturing and supportive care** he or she receives from parents, family, and others must be understood. Growth and maturation occur when needs are satisfied, capacities supported and enlarged, conflict mastered and integrated, and the environment explored, understood, and accepted. Conflict for the child is derived from two sources:

A. Internal stress arises when the child's personality structure and capacities deal with his changing biological needs and desires.

B. External stress arises when environmental reality confronts the child's needs and his or her capacity to reconcile them.

II. EVALUATION Data include the physician's **previous experiences** with the child and his family; **historical data** derived from past and present contacts and enlarged upon as necessary during the assessment; and the physician's own **observations,** past and present, of the child and his or her family. In considering when and to what extent problems in behavior and development should be explored, the nature of the problems and the available data provide some guidelines. Parents often request advice about feeding difficulties, bedwetting, or school problems as though these are isolated events in their child's life. *The overt behavioral manifestation is not the problem but only a signal that something is wrong.* The physician should be prepared to evaluate such problems in a more detailed and orderly fashion when appropriate.

A **medical evaluation** is a wise place to begin. Somatic complaints are considered, keeping in mind that they may represent a focal point for a variety of

Table 7-1 Sequential Stages of Development and Behavior

Stage	Relationships	Developmental Tasks	Behavioral Characteristics
Birth–1 year	Parents or substitutes	Physiological stability Psychological dependence Attitudes toward self, world Trust, security, optimism	Dependence on mother Urgency of physical needs, e.g., eating, sleeping Responsive to mother's feelings, and sensory impressions
Preschool (1–4 years)	Parents or substitutes	Control of gross musculature, bowels, bladder, speech, temper, and behavior Early autonomy Learns meaning of "No"	Physically active Needs frequent limits Temper tantrums, stubborn, messy Separation fears
Nursery school and kindergarten (4–6 years)	Parents and siblings or substitutes	Curiosity, especially about sex differences Play, early social skills Tolerates brief separations Magical thinking	Imitative, imaginative questioning Tries to please Prefers parent of opposite sex Sexual exploration Some separation fears
Grade school (latency) 7–12 years	Family and others, especially of same sex	Learning and mastery in school, play, socialization, physical skills Explores world beyond family Concrete thinking	Friendships, especially with children of same sex Emphasizes rules, fairness Competitive organized play Secrets kept from adults
Junior and senior high school (adolescence) 13–18 years	Family and many others, especially of opposite sex	Sexual development Emancipation from family Concept of self, identity Further learning, mastery, skills Abstract thinking	Erratic, unpredictable, moody Falling in love Competitive, ambivalent, especially with adults Importance of peer groups Transient psychosomatic and psychological distress

other concerns. Undue attention to physical complaints or medical investigations can disguise important issues and may encourage hypochondriasis. The medical history can provide especially valuable information about births, deaths, illnesses, hospitalizations, or physical handicaps affecting the child or family members. Because physicians are frequently involved with families as they deal with stress, they have a unique opportunity to observe and understand constructive methods of coping with adversity as well as with areas of difficulty.

A. Parents The parents should be allowed to express their concerns in their own way. However, it is important to have a structure in mind to organize the data and ensure that important areas are covered.

1. The **physician's attitude** of calm, thoughtful understanding sets the proper tone and will be appreciated by the family. If he or she is defensive, hurried, or unsure as to how to proceed, the evaluation will not go well.

2. Though parents are usually eager for their physician to listen to their problems, untoward anxiety, defensiveness, or other poorly controlled feelings that interfere with communication and understanding should be dealt with as they arise. Support and reassurance can be helpful, but false reassurance, an overly friendly attitude, or excessive sympathy can be disruptive. With experience the physician can assure the parents that their feelings are not unusual and their problems can be understood.

3. Parents may sometimes feel guilty if their child has emotional problems and be fearful of criticism. The physician can cite their coming for help as evidence of their parental concern, defining the physician's role as **working with the parents** to enable them to better understand and help their child. While some parents may invite judgment or criticism, such responses should be avoided.

4. The **initial discussion** with the parents should be limited to outlining the problems and enlisting the parents' cooperation in discussing them in greater detail on another visit. A formal evaluation should not be attempted without the family's agreement and cooperation. Parents will often appreciate this consideration, utilize the time between appointments to discuss and consider the problem, and use their next appointment time more productively. Resistance on the parents' part to proceed further should be respected, and the door should be left open for them to return later when they are ready.

5. **Follow-up appointments** are scheduled so that interruptions are avoided and the family can have the physician's full attention. Twenty to thirty minutes is a reasonable length of time, and one should stay within the allotted time and schedule another appointment as necessary.

6. The mother ordinarily is considered the main source of historical material about her child and usually assumes the major responsibility for the child's physical care and comfort. However, **it is important that the father be included,** since his presence adds to the comprehensive understanding of the family and also involves him in considering his child's problems and participating in making plans to help. If it seems appropriate, the parents may be seen individually in subsequent visits.

7. It is unwise to allow the parents to discuss the child's problem while the child is present as it may cause him or her distress, shame, guilt, or embarrassment. It is preferable to see the parents for a follow-up visit without the child.

8. Advice, recommendations, referrals, or prescriptions should await completion of the evaluation.

9. History of the child

 a. The **chief complaint** is discussed by the parents in their own way and its history is elaborated. It is important to attend to the parents' exact words, their attitudes, and the degree of their understanding. One mother might angrily say that her child is "stubborn and hateful." Another might say that her child is fine but that "his father and his teacher can't handle him." The reason for seeking help is important to keep in mind as the evaluation proceeds. The duration of the symptom can be especially helpful: "He was always nervous but he seems to be getting worse this year." Circumstances at the onset of the symptom are elicited: "He has seemed upset since my operation." Details about the problem are ascertained: "How often does she wet the bed?" "Has she ever soiled herself in school?" Parents' efforts to deal with the problems should be determined and may include various forms of punishment, shaming, or visits to other physicians, social agencies, or psychiatrists.

 b. The child's **current functioning** is assessed by determining how he or she deals with the developmental tasks appropriate for age and family setting (Table 7-1). Fantasies, conflict, and symptomatic behavior are considered within the framework of relevant developmental issues and the child's ability to deal with them. The emphasis is on overall function, and the child's problems are placed in this perspective. Whatever framework is used should include relationships, work, play, and health.

  (1) Relationships with parents, brothers and sisters, friends, teachers, and other adults are assessed: "Does she have a best friend?" "Does he play with children his own age?" "Is she picked on by other children?" "Does he defend himself?" "How does she function in the family?" Observation will tell much here about parent-child relationships and parental attitudes toward the child. Changes in relationships with friends or family can be determined and compared with earlier relationships.

  (2) Work for the child usually includes school performance but also may include responsibilities assigned by the family or social setting. With younger children, one should know if they can do such things as dress themselves, bathe themselves, and sleep alone. School performance provides valuable data, and school attendance can be a sensitive indicator of difficulties. Frequent or prolonged absence from school may delay academic and social maturation and increase the child's dependency on the family. Earlier school experiences, functioning, and attendance should be determined and compared with present functioning. The age at which the child started school and changes in schools are important.

  (3) Play is an important index of the child's ability to derive pleasure and gratification from life. One asks about the child's interests, sports, and friends and determines their appropriateness in relation to family, peers, and social setting.

  (4) Physical health and the child's and parents' attitude toward it are assessed. Acute illness and hospitalization or surgery may result in prolonged concern with the body and cause regressive behavior. Chronic illness or handicaps may be complicated by social, emotional, and educational disability. Concerns about body functions such as appetite, bowel or bladder functions, acne, or weight problems are considered, as is overconcern about minor physical complaints such as frequent colds or vague stomachaches.

c. The **developmental history** is elicited, although much of these data may already be available from prior medical contacts. Emotional development is emphasized. Much information can be gathered from such open-ended questions as "What was she like as an infant?" and "How does he compare with his brothers and sisters?"

10. **History of the family** When the child's history has been obtained, the physician inquires into the general functioning of the parents and their background. Some parents may be initially defensive when asked questions about themselves and may wish to continue discussing their child. If this occurs, it should be explained that a general understanding of their functioning and that of other family members is important because of their relationship to their child.

   The ability of parents to identify their child's needs and to respond appropriately may be impaired by other problems or issues in the family and deficiencies in parenting ability. Although these factors are often interrelated, it is best to consider each separately for the purpose of the evaluation. Strengths within the family should also be assessed.

   a. **Problems** for families may include a variety of difficulties ranging from financial stress and marital discord to illness or death of one or more members. Issues that may preoccupy the parents but are not considered problems per se include the recent birth of a child, sibling rivalry, the mother's starting to work, or a recent move. Observations made during previous work with the parents may suggest appropriate inquiries. However, each parent should be given a clear opportunity to talk about problems or concerns they may have apart from their child.

   b. **Deficiencies** in parenting skills may simply represent a lack of knowledge. However, such difficulties are often attributable to the early upbringing of the parents themselves. General questions about the parents' early background can suggest areas for further elaboration: "What were things like when you were a child?" and "What was your mother (father) like?" One may discover that a mother who herself was too rigidly disciplined is now overindulging her child. One may also discover that one of the parents has had the same symptom their child is now displaying. It is wise to ask the mother and father about their past and present relationships with their own parents. They may fail sometimes to see the relevance of the maternal grandmother's death last year since their children did not see her often. However, if the mother continues to grieve for her own mother, this is of considerable relevance to the child.

   c. **Strengths** within the family should be ascertained. The ability of spouses, siblings, and grandparents to support and supplement one another is considered as the evaluation proceeds.

   d. **Other sources of information** may include school reports, other physicians, social agencies, courts, or other family members. These sources are no substitute for information from the parents, however, and it may be wise as well as timesaving for the physician to ask the parents to collect such outside information when possible.

B. Child Most pediatricians have considerable ability to engage and to enjoy children. The pediatrician's initial approach is that of a friendly adult who wishes to get to know the child. With the patience and composure to wait for children to approach in their own way, the physician is often rewarded with valuable interchanges. This also allows the physician to observe how the child relates to him or her as well as to others.

The **evaluation begins** when the child is first seen in the waiting room. Level of functioning is assessed by how the child deals with the developmental tasks appropriate for his or her age and social setting. The question is, "How is he doing?" and not "What is he doing wrong?" Special areas of function again include relationships, work, play, and health. Remember that children do not choose to come for help and may not be able to understand or put their concerns into words.

1. Preschool child Much of the evaluation of the preschool child is done with the parents present, and their ability to separate is assessed.

   a. Preliminary discussions of neutral topics and parts of the medical history may take place with parents and child together, while the child plays and becomes accustomed to the physician and office. If unusual behavior is observed, the parents can be asked about it later.

   b. The **physical examination** can provide valuable behavioral observations as well as an opportunity for the relationship with the physician to grow. Having the child draw pictures such as Draw-a-Person or Draw-a-Family can be helpful, as can play with simple toys. If a doll house is available in a playroom or waiting room, observations here can be useful. The time-honored question of three magic wishes usually provides valuable data.

   c. If the physician chooses to discuss the problem with the child, it should be done with care and understanding, so as not to distress the child unduly. Words such as *worries* or *troubles* can be used. With young children, observation is of more value than questions and answers.

2. School-age child The school-age child should be expected to separate from the mother and to be relatively verbal, especially in areas free from conflict. It is best to begin by inquiring about neutral areas or those of special interest and pleasure to the child: friends, fun, sports or games, likes and dislikes, and favorite television shows. School functioning, attitudes, and attendance are discussed. These children can usually make comments about family members and relationships, and their views concerning physical health can be discussed. When children's problems are discussed with them, a special sensitivity to a child's reactions to such a discussion is important in determining how to proceed.

III. DIAGNOSIS Diagnosis is an ongoing consideration of data obtained from historical information and the physician's own observations. It is a working formulation, always subject to review as new data accumulate.

When the findings are discussed, it should be kept in mind that the parents have also been thinking about their child during the evaluation if it has proceeded properly. Their conclusions about their child should also be considered. The pediatrician can often use the parents' own words and observations in presenting the findings. It is wise to frame explanations and findings in terms that invite the parents' understanding and agreement.

IV. TREATMENT

A. Preventive techniques

1. **Education** in early infant and child care practices, cognitive development, psychosexual development, somatic concerns, parental attitudes, management, and discipline is part of every pediatrician's practice. Other areas include parental education about such issues as preparation of the child for hospitalization and surgery, genetic counseling, chronic handicapping conditions, adoption, or helping the child to deal with divorce or death of a family member.

2. **Early identification** of and intervention in potential difficulties in behavior and development are regularly undertaken. Feeding problems, sleep disturbances, fears, breath holding, thumb-sucking, head banging, separation problems, enuresis, encopresis, and other somatic concerns are areas where the pediatrician's understanding and counsel are often helpful.

3. **Support in time of crisis** that often involves illness, debility, or death provides a special contribution. The pediatrician can listen to anxieties and misconceptions, provide accurate information, and support constructive methods of coping with adversity. Recuperation from illness is a time when parents and child can often use their physician's support to regain their former adjustment and return to their normal functioning.

B. A **comprehensive evaluation** provides the opportunity for child and parents to discuss their problems with the physician and to consider them in an orderly fashion. It provides the best framework for the family and physician should it become appropriate to consider additional help. It can also help the family and physician to provide medical care for a child who is emotionally disturbed. An effective evaluation is a most important therapeutic tool.

C. Parent counseling Many pediatricians reserve time each week for parent counseling, and patients are generally eager to have more of their physician's time. Most pediatricians have neither the time nor the training for psychotherapy with children but can use their knowledge of children to counsel parents. Empathy with the child underlies an understanding of what life is like for him or her, especially within the family. However, the pediatrician must be careful not to overidentify with the child to the detriment of work with the parents. Such work also requires knowledge of the adult personality, especially in parenthood.

1. **Treatment goals** should be determined on the basis of the evaluation. Unrealistic expectations are unfair to both patient and physician. The aim of treatment is not to change the personality of the child or to satisfy all the family's expectations.

   a. Factors to consider include the degree of psychological disability, the parents' ability to understand the problem and cooperate with the physician, and their motivation to improve the situation.

   b. It is important to determine what treatment resources are available in the community and for the physician to decide how much he or she is willing and able to undertake.

   c. Counseling should be an extension of the evaluation process, with the physician collaborating with the parents to see the problems more clearly and to attend to them competently.

2. The **extent of the pediatrician's involvement** should be given careful thought from the beginning.

   a. Clear definition of the **length** and **frequency** of interviews is important. A **contract** should be made with the parents for the number of interviews to be undertaken, with an agreement to meet several times or every 2 weeks for three or four visits and then determine whether further attention is indicated. Such structuring is of great importance, especially with highly troubled families whose needs are great and whose expectations may be unrealistic. Interviews that are unstructured, too long, or held too frequently can encourage dependency, regression, and unrealistic demands and reactions to the physician.

   b. A **short-term approach** that focuses on specific issues and can be reinstituted later if necessary is recommended.

3. The **best candidates** for this approach are troubled primarily by misconceptions or lack of knowledge about their child. Disturbed parents tend to deal with their physician in an unrealistic fashion and to transfer to him or her exaggerated feelings toward important people in their past. A common example of this phenomenon, called *transference*, is the patient who resents the physician because he has long resented anyone in authority. It is important that transference be recognized when it occurs, so that the physician's reaction to it can be more appropriate.

4. The **chief complaint** is the point of departure as the physician works with the parents to mobilize their own strengths and resources to improve their function as parents. The primary concern is to define and work on current reality issues. Knowledge gathered from experience with other families is used to support more constructive coping. The physician's active definition of problems, educational approach, suggestions, support, and encouragement mitigate parents' feelings of hopelessness and failure or overly dependent and regressive behavior.

5. **Restoration of function for the child** is sought and may sometimes be attained despite the persistence of complaints. Every effort is made to restore the child to full activity.

   a. **Clearly defined expectations** appropriate to mastery of relevant developmental tasks and overcoming symptomatic difficulties are outlined.

   b. The child's likes and dislikes, fears, and worries are heard while his active struggle with appropriate expectations is supported.

   c. The child's school attendance, school performance, ability to make friends, to play, and to have fun are usual important areas of function. Other relevant areas may include the ability to separate from parents, physical activities and development of motor skills, bowel or bladder control, control of aggression, and feeding problems.

6. **Problems of the parents** may well relate to difficulties the child is experiencing. If such issues need prolonged attention, the possibility of referring the parents for appropriate help should be discussed with them.

V. MEDICATIONS Medications are of well-established therapeutic value in treating emotional problems in adults, but their efficacy in childhood is less clearly established. Parents and schools may sometimes exert pressure on the physician to give medications to a child whose behavior is causing them difficulty. To sedate such children to a more manageable state does not solve the problem and may delay real attention to their difficulties. However, medication can be used as an adjunct to other measures that can produce more long-term benefits.

Hyperactive children with impulsivity, distractibility, and a short attention span may benefit from specific medication. This condition includes children with minimal brain damage as well as with emotional problems. A trial of methylphenidate (Ritalin) is indicated as part of the total management of some patients. Dextroamphetamine sulfate may be tried if methylphenidate is ineffective.

Phenobarbital may have a *paradoxical* effect in some children and infants, which may lead to increased agitation, hyperactivity, and confusion. **This effect is not always easily ascertained, and increasing dosage or prolonged use can lead to serious difficulty.** Diphenhydramine hydrochloride (Benadryl) has a calming effect, but its prolonged use may inhibit learning. Thioridazine (Mellaril) and chlorpromazine (Thorazine) are more potent but also have more side effects. Antidepressants are not effective with children but may be of use with some depressed adolescents.

VI. REFERRAL Referral is discussed with parents in the light of factors considered in the diagnostic assessment and the resources available. A comprehensive assessment may be discouraging for some parents and physicians because of the many factors that can contribute to a child's problems and the absence of some community resources. It should be remembered, however, that improvement in dealing with an important aspect of the problem usually supports a better total adaptation for both child and family. A comprehensive diagnostic and referral procedure increases opportunities for multilateral approaches to the problems. When **community resources** are considered, it is advisable for the pediatrician to have personal knowledge of the services provided as well as the people who provide them.

A. In spite of difficulties that are readily apparent to the physician, **a brief contact with the parents is rarely adequate to sustain a referral. Parents should feel that they have had an adequate hearing and have reached some understanding of their problems with their physician.** This mitigates the feelings of some patients who see referral as a criticism or rejection. The pediatrician should remember that the family chose to ask him or her for help with their child and quite likely will have established a relationship of considerable importance to them. Referral elsewhere means the loss of this important relationship; this fact alone accounts for the failure of many referrals. The sustained interest of the physician can often help the family to obtain additional assistance.

B. When referring a patient to a **psychiatrist,** the physician should not promise more than the psychiatrist can deliver, nor attempt to frighten the family by mentioning possible serious consequences if psychiatric help is not obtained. It is preferable to indicate that psychiatrists can be helpful with the kinds of difficulties the family has discussed and that it is worthwhile for the family to meet with the psychiatrist to obtain his or her opinion.

C. Pediatricians should also be aware that many of the children and families who consult them prefer to use **somatic symptoms** and concerns or physical explanations to express their psychic conflicts. Such families may have obvious emotional conflicts and may even discuss them to some extent, but they may not understand the implications, and their concerns remain fc cused on somatic issues. Referral of such patients may take considerabl preparation, and some may persist in their inability to deal with th psychological aspects of their difficulties.

VII. COMMUNITY RESOURCES

A. **Nursery schools and day care centers** can often be used by overburdene mothers or those wishing to return to work. Such a referral can be a god send when a mother and her 3- or 4-year-old child are locked into an u happy relationship at home. Some facilities are able to provide social wor services for mothers.

B. **School systems** provide a variety of services. These may include counseling social work services, psychological testing, individual tutoring, remedia classes for reading and mathematics, special classes for emotionally dis turbed or retarded children, speech therapy, and a variety of supervise activities and sports. Individual tutoring can be helpful for some childrer can provide a useful supportive relationship for the child, and reduc conflict between parents, school, and child.

C. **Visiting nurses and physical therapists** can sometimes help to share with th parents the care and rehabilitation of a chronically ill or physically hand icapped child who may also have emotional problems.

D. **Clergymen, lawyers, or legal services** can be helpful, especially when there i a death in the family or when divorce is contemplated or in process.

E. **Supervised group activities** such as scouting, recreational programs, Bi Brother and Sister services, and summer camps can be of use. In som areas there are summer camps that specialize in working with diabetic asthmatic, retarded, or emotionally disturbed children.

F. **Pediatric hospitalization** can relieve family crisis situations relating t emotional problems concerning the care of children with chronic o psychosomatic illnesses as well as undue anxiety about a child's physica health. For certain emotionally disturbed children, the pediatric ward of fers opportunities for assistance and observation by nurses, physica therapists, social workers, psychiatrists, and other personnel when parent are unable or reluctant to find help elsewhere.

G. **Institutions and agencies** such as child guidance clinics, drug treatmen centers, family service agencies, vocational rehabilitation services, adul psychiatric services and institutions, residential treatment centers, an homemaker services can sometimes be helpful.

H. A **clinical psychologist** has special training in the administration and inter pretation of psychological tests for evaluating learning problems, menta retardation, brain injury, or psychosis. Many psychologists are als qualified for psychotherapy with adults and children, and some can provid the same services a psychiatrist provides.

I. **Social workers** vary considerably in their training and in the kind of wor they do. A well-trained, skilled, psychiatric social worker can be of rea assistance, and some pediatricians are employing them to assist in thei practice. The psychiatric social worker can collect complete historical dat from the family, assist in providing information about sources of help i the community, coordinate and follow through on referrals, and provid casework services for selected parents; some are also trained in psyche therapy with children. However, they should not function in lieu of a psychiatrist when one is indicated and is available.

J. A **psychiatrist,** particularly one experienced in pediatric psychiatry, can be used as a **consultant** to the pediatrician. The psychiatrist can be of help with difficult diagnostic problems and may have suggestions regarding management, medications when indicated, and for future care. Collaboration with a psychiatrist is sometimes indicated in managing patients with interlocking physical and emotional problems. Illnesses such as anorexia nervosa and ulcerative colitis may be best managed by the psychiatrist and pediatrician working together. The psychiatrist can also be a source for referral to other agencies for some parents and children.

VIII. SYMPTOM PICTURES

A. Sleep disturbances

1. Fear of going to sleep

a. Etiology

(1) Age 1–3 Reluctance to go to sleep is common and may be aggravated by indulgent parents. The anxiety is from the fear of being left alone, a form of separation anxiety.

(2) Age 4–6 Children of this age may fear monsters or scary animals "getting them" at night. Aggressive feelings toward family or friends may appear before sleep as fears, hostility having been projected and displaced onto some object other than the one at which the child was angry.

b. Evaluation and therapy Support from the pediatrician may help parents not to overreact and become angry with their anxious children who are waking up at night.

(1) The pediatrician should tell parents that this behavior may be **transient** and **normal.** Often, reassurance by the parents that everyone is all right alleviates the child's anxiety.

(2) A night light and a favorite doll or toy are often a comfort to children at night.

(3) Sleep rituals alone can be of great help in regulating bedtimes. A snack or a story read to the child by the parents provides a "calming down" time, during which the child can express feelings. Most children will sleep 8–10 hr at night, but sleep requirements vary; parents should be helped to understand this.

(4) Sleep-related anxiety can be a clue to marital or other family stress.

2. Nightmares are common and generally mild. They are seldom reported by a 2-year-old, although it is not uncommon for a toddler to awaken at night and appear frightened. The peak incidence is between ages 4–6. Nightmares are often accompanied by some somatic expressions, even a sensation of suffocation.

a. Etiology Nightmares occur after the lowering of ego defenses takes place with sleep, and "forbidden" wishes can break through defensive structures. **Pavor nocturnus** is an extreme version of a nightmare, in

which it is difficult to wake and reorient the child to reality. Thi phenomenon appears to be associated with "reliving" a traumat early life experience, sometimes exposure to a primal scene if th child was in a crib in the parents' bedroom for a long period of tim

b. **Evaluation and therapy** If nightmares persist or are severe, a caref history of events surrounding the child's bedtime may sho anxiety-provoking arguing, marital discord, and lack of sleep ritual a outlined in **1.b.** These events can be assessed by the pediatricia **Sleep medication is not indicated.** If, despite pediatric attentio nightmares recur, psychiatric consultation should be sought.

B. **School phobia**   Common phobias in children include fear of school, dog and insects and may even involve transportation, leading to incapacitatio Children with school phobia usually dread one aspect of school, e.g., teacher. The phobia is often accompanied by a stomachache or a headach alleviated by school absence. School phobia occurs more frequently in gir and seldom coincides with learning disabilities.

1. **Etiology**   The fear of the child with school phobia emanates equally fro separation anxiety in both mother and child. Mothers of such childre often have poorly resolved dependent relationships and are unable t help their own children tolerate separation frustration at appropriat ages. It is difficult for such a mother to discipline her child withou experiencing excessive guilt. Fathers seldom play an active role in suc families.

2. **Evaluation and therapy**

a. If the anxiety about going to school occurs in a child 3–5 years o following a medical illness, it usually responds to support and gent firmness from the parents.

b. The pediatrician should consult school personnel for informatio about the child's pattern of behavior at school and should ask th parents' opinion about what could be wrong with their child. Th physician should not be critical either of the child or of the parent treatment of the child. It is helpful to meet with the parents and chi separately, so that there is less denial of the problem on either of thei parts.

c. If possible, arrange for the mother or father to accompany the child t school. Once the child is actually at school, he or she will generall stay.

d. The school nurse should be alerted prior to the child's return to scho to make arrangements to reduce further anxiety the child may e perience while in class.

e. **Medications are not indicated** in school phobia. The child with persi tent symptoms should be referred for psychiatric evaluation.

C. **Psychosomatic reactions**

1. **Emotional reactions to physical changes**

a. **Etiology**   Illness in children occurs against age-determined psych logical backgrounds (including body image, fantasies, and abiliti to articulate feelings).

(1) The sick toddler fears abandonment and messiness of diapers an bedclothes; anxiety for the child 4–6 years old may be related t

potential loss of or injury to body parts; latent anxiety concerns potential differences from peers.

(2) Children are concerned with the permanence of changes and may not understand that illness can be transitory, and they often experience guilty feelings about being sick.

b. Therapy

(1) Parents are usually sympathetic to the child's needs, especially if illness is self-limited and well understood, e.g., chickenpox. However, parents are seldom ready to cope with serious or prolonged illness and require considerable understanding of their own fears (e.g., anxiety over recovery, loss of the child's help, loss of prior life-style, financial loss). An explanation of the expected course of the child's regressive behavior reduces the parents' feelings of helplessness.

(2) Persistent physical illness requires adaptation by the family, which includes reevaluation of goals and recognition of, even grieving for, losses in life-style. Occasionally, this does not take place and the family may "extrude" and ostracize a sick child. If this occurs, psychiatric referral should be made.

2. Physical symptoms as a result of an emotional disturbance

a. Etiology Symptom formation is probably the product of a specific parent-child interaction, critical during the preverbal period when **somatization** is a primary outlet for emotions. Mothers who reject particular maternal functions concomitantly reject certain physiologic functions of the infant in the early months of life. Examples include asthma and ulcerative colitis. The emotional life of such children is severely constricted and altered with great difficulty.

b. Therapy

(1) Active intervention on the pediatrician's part might well constitute the best form of prevention of later psychosomatic illness. Regular visits and follow-up of such infants and mothers, perhaps even on a weekly basis, with careful listening and general advice about normal infant behavior may permit a mother to give her child the necessary "elbow room" in which to grow and behave normally. This can also be undertaken with parents who are not receptive to psychological approaches.

(2) Later in childhood, the chronic anger and frustration of such children may be taken out on themselves in masochistic fashion, in the form of psychosomatic illness. Therapeutic residences may be helpful, first, in allowing physical separation, then as a reworking, often through therapy, of the conflict between the wish to surrender to the fantasy of total care by the parent and the need for self-sufficiency.

D. Pica

1. Etiology Indiscriminate oral exploration is typical of the infant until near the end of the second year of life. Beyond that age, persistence in ingesting non-food substances constitutes pica. However, this disorder rarely lasts beyond the age of 5. Although malnutrition has been suggested as a cause, pica is largely unexplained. Psychologically, it may represent a wish to defy the mother's desire for the child to eat appropriate foods.

2. Therapy

a. Environments that neither stimulate nor furnish adequate care contribute to the general boredom of many children with pica. The child
day should be evaluated and restructured, so that supervision, pla
opportunities, and involvement with others are provided.

b. If there is parental neglect, the parents may respond to counselin
and support. If they do not, psychiatric referral or referral to an ap
propriate agency should be considered.

E. Anorexia nervosa, or "nervous loss of appetite," is usually seen in female
12–25 years old. **Symptoms** include amenorrhea, emaciation, constipation
loss of appetite, and lowered pulse rate and respirations. Behaviors includ
hiding and giving away food, including vomiting and stool passage (wit
laxatives and enemas). Untreated, anorexia nervosa is fatal.

1. Etiology

a. The patient may have parents with GI symptoms, or a history i
which food is central to a power struggle between adolescent an
parents, or resistance to heterosexual development.

b. Symptoms of anorexia can occur in an adolescent who is hysterica
(showing repression as a major defense) or even psychotic, using mor
primitive defenses, ranging from denial to hallucinations. The conflic
about eating for the hysterical patient is primarily sexual and ma
concern fantasies about impregnation and intercourse. An occasiona
patient may have regressive fantasies of killing. The schizophreni
patient may have fantasies related to refusal of contact with th
world and delusions that may be paranoid.

2. Diagnosis

a. Psychological criteria   More concern about weight loss than gai
(despite losses), unrealistic dieting, paradoxical "fat" body imag
bizarre food habits (induced vomiting, hiding food), and high activit
level.

b. Medical criteria   Weight loss of 20 percent of appropriate weight fo
height and age, amenorrhea, and decreased blood pressure, pulse
and respirations.

3. Evaluation and therapy

a. Evaluation must include all aspects of the patient (see **b**). A narrowe
approach is incomplete, does not lead to change, and consequentl
risks the patient's life. The mortality is considerable, not only from
suicide but also from association with peritonitis, hypoglycemia
pneumonia, and unexplained acute illness.

b. Commonly, the physician encounters the problem when parents as
what to do about their child's "crazy diet." Evaluation includes

(1) A **complete history** and a **physical examination, urinalysis,** and **CB**
help the anorectic patient feel that the physician takes her con
cerns seriously and initiate an alliance. It also clarifies the path
logic attitude of the patient toward weight gain and helps to de
termine whether or not she really believes herself to be fat despit
her thinness.

(2) Emphasizing to the patient that she is burning calories in excess of intake and attempting to plan with her (if she wishes to do so) a realistic program of weight gain.

c. While evaluating and making suggestions about dietary intake to parents, the pediatrician will observe how upset parents become in the struggle with the symptom of defiant weight loss.

(1) Initially, one must listen and form an alliance with angry parents and work toward lessening their expressions of frustration toward the child, lest the anorectic symptom be reinforced.

(2) Recognition of early maternal stress in coping with normal parenting enables early intervention by education and monitoring of feeding patterns that benefit from pediatric supervision. When children are already developing feeding problems in infancy and early childhood, nonjudgmental intervention by pediatricians and other professionals can be instrumental in effecting change (this is also useful with feeding problems that do not reach anorectic proportions).

(3) Specific answers to anxious or angry mothers' questions may not be as important as the willingness to listen to their complaints and the ability to help them tolerate their anxiety.

(4) Consultation with a psychiatrist can be useful to the pediatrician; is doubly important when referral for psychiatric help is impossible, as it often is with such patients. It is vital if later referral is to be made.

F. Obesity

1. Etiology The child who overeats often expresses an unconscious wish of the mother acted out through the child, despite a superficial struggle between mother and child over excess eating. Such mothers often have very hostile feelings about their children undertaking steps toward autonomy and growing up. Such children may enjoy being large and are gratified by meeting the mother's expectations that they remain dependent (orally). There is usually diminished self-esteem in children who are obese.

2. Therapy Obesity is difficult to treat successfully. Some families may be unaware of proper dietary planning and will benefit from education. Such families may also welcome the suggestion of exercise and be willing to cooperate in undertaking a program for a child.

a. Medications such as diet pills meet with little success, may foster dependency, and may work against the final outcome.

b. When the overeating is situational and secondary to family disturbances or events that bring about transient low self-esteem in children, such environmental situations can often be altered successfully.

c. Lifelong obesity and a predisposition to it is much more difficult to alter. Long-term regular relationships with such patients sometimes make it possible to find opportunities to intervene later in their lives.

d. Early detection of feeding problems and guidance is the most useful preventive. Satiation of excessive appetite in early childhood with food, instead of other healthy developing aspects of mothering, should alert the pediatrician that intervention and guidelines would help. When obesity persists, psychotherapy can be helpful in some patients.

G. Enuresis Onset is usually between 3–8 years of age. It usually occurs at night; daytime enuresis is rare and usually implies a more serious problem. Nighttime enuresis usually stops by 3–4 years of age, and daytime enuresis by 2½ years of age. Periodic enuresis occurs, but regular enuresis in school-age children, if not physiologically based, constitutes symptom formation. After a child has been able to remain dry, enuresis may occur transiently in response to an overwhelming stressful situation. Boys with enuresis outnumber girls 2 to 1. There is often a family history of enuresis.

1. Etiology

  a. Children who experience severe stress (e.g., a new sibling, loss of a parent) prior to bladder control often have unresolved hostile feelings about the stress. The symptom becomes a way to "eliminate" the feeling. They may fantasize something "broken" in their genitals.

  b. Traumatic sexual education and difficult early toilet training may result in enuresis.

  c. Enuresis that persists into adolescence is often related to unresolved feelings about masturbation; when masturbation begins, enuresis frequently stops.

2. Diagnosis and therapy

  a. Urinary tract infection, diabetes mellitus, and diabetes insipidus must be ruled out.

  b. Parents should be told that enuresis is not a willful symptom and should be advised to be as evenhanded as possible. Patience and tact are needed in explaining this symptom to the child's family.

  c. Conditioning with a buzzer or alarm to wake the child at night may be helpful and generally works within weeks or months if there already has been resolution of the underlying conflict. A brief course of imipramine (Tofranil) may help children who still have conflicts about underlying issues.

  d. It is often necessary to look for correctable situational disturbances in the family; psychiatric intervention is occasionally needed.

  e. Sometimes, regression in a child is brief; the pediatrician should so alert the family.

H. Encopresis is less common but more serious than enuresis, occurring in boys four times more frequently than in girls, generally after the age of 3–4 years.

1. Etiology The symptom may represent a regression in response to severe stress coincident with toilet training (e.g., birth of a new sibling). The conflict concerns learning to lose one's own body products, a difficult task for the toddler. In the more disturbed child, the symptom may represent a denial and rejection of the genital and anal areas.

2. Therapy Remember that parents are sensitive about their own failure in regard to their child's symptoms.

  a. First, assess the presence of adequate neuromaturational development.

  b. Encopresis evokes disgust in most parents, in excess of that evoked by other symptoms, making it difficult for the child to resolve the underlying difficulty in managing angry feelings. Symptoms commonly become a focus of struggle between parent and child. Pediatricians can be very helpful in defusing parental anger.

c. Mothers who pressure children in toilet training may elicit a continuous encopretic symptom; mothers who do not put enough emphasis on bowel control facilitate inconsistent symptoms. Careful guidance and retraining of the child can be very effective.

d. "Clean-out" techniques should be used judiciously and only if necessary. They probably are not needed in the "retraining" type of encopretic child and may reinforce the invasive, punitive style of the coercive parent.

e. Normal toilet training requires an accepting parent who is aware of the child's natural rhythm and able to help the child recognize his or her own cues to go to the toilet. Failure is seen when a parent overreacts to the cues or is unable or unwilling to be guided by them.

f. Children with consistent and persistent encopretic symptoms should be referred for psychotherapy.

I. Stuttering

1. Etiology   Most stuttering begins between the ages of 4–5 and is seen in approximately 15 percent of the population. It is more common in boys than in girls and is often familial. Forty percent of stutterers outgrow their symptoms.

Many classify incidents of stuttering as unconscious (patient is unaware of it) and conscious (the patient is painfully aware of it). Most feel that there is some constitutional predisposition to stuttering in addition to the functional determinants. The underlying conflict involves angry feelings toward the mother and fear of losing her.

2. Therapy

a. First, evaluate for family discord; the symptom may be secondary to it.

b. In families where the parents become angry and punish the child for stuttering, it can be helpful to explain to the parents that the symptom is secondary to the child's anxiety. Such children actually have aggravated symptoms of stuttering, even when the parents show only anxiety about the symptom. Therefore explanation of the natural evolution of speech patterns from the nonfluent state to the point where the infant begins stuttering is helpful in gaining the parents' understanding and cooperation.

c. Positive reinforcement of fluent periods of speech is important and consists of maintenance of eye contact with the child while speaking, encouraging speech during fluent periods, and being a patient listener. Negative reinforcement comes from admonitions to "take your time" or other inhibiting remarks, which make the child more aware of the stuttering. The entire family should be told not to give signals that indicate to the child that the stuttering is being noticed.

d. If it is found that the foregoing measures do not help within 3–4 weeks, both parent counseling and speech therapy should be undertaken.

J. School disturbances

1. Etiology

  a. Normal learning, like normal development, requires that the chil identify with the activity of the parents (versus the passive de pendency of infancy) to develop a positive orientation to life. If th child's curiosity is rewarded, it enhances acceptance of responsibilit and encourages enthusiasm toward further growth.

  b. Inability to learn may be secondary to traumatic events in the hom (e.g., marital strife, even beyond the "oedipal losses" of a 6-year-ol child). It may also represent guilty self-punishment for unexpresse aggressive feelings; a conflict about "intake" (feeding) from earl childhood; a retention of information based on conflicts at 2–3 years or it may represent the avoidance of growing up in general.

2. Therapy
If the symptom is a direct reaction to traumatic events in th home, counseling by the physician may be helpful. Pediatricians shoul meet with educators and counselors to inquire about the learning dis abilities in such children, and then to coordinate this information an any psychological intervention that the school or pediatrician may deen necessary. There should be a coordination of teaching efforts and an therapeutic effort. Sometimes, actual therapeutic tutoring is useful. It i most helpful to intervene with children during the first three grades.

K. Infantile autism
Characteristic behaviors include lack of eye contact an normal auditory and visual reactivity; absence of smile or pleasure in th presence of the parent; no special reaction to strangers on being left; n interest in game playing; failure of normal development of speech, inappro priate use of pronouns; greater facility with inanimate objects.

1. Etiology
May be an organic predisposition in addition to an inability o the infant and mother to overcome the undifferentiated state of th newborn.

2. Therapy
Parents are not prepared for the tasks involved in caring for a psychotic child and they need extensive help in planning therapeuti programs. They must be educated by their physicians about evaluatio procedures, available resources, care plans, and support systems. Choic of resource depends to a great extent on the parents' financial capacitie and the severity of the child's condition. Children dangerous to them selves or others or who are unmanageable may have to be placed i residential centers early in life. This is also true where the families o parents are unable to cope with the child because of internal disruptio (e.g., alcoholism, illness). Such children may have to be placed in an in stitution that is not therapeutic in style. Families willing and able t care for their children may be able to do so without placement, thougl placement may greatly enhance improvement. In such instances, a therapeutic setting is preferable. Medication may assist in managing a child at home. Psychiatric consultation should be implemented as soon a possible.

8

Fluid and Electrolytes

I. GENERAL PRINCIPLES

A. Renal function The glomerular filtration rate (GFR) is relatively depressed in infants and reaches a "normal" adult value (corrected for surface area) only at age 1½ to 2 years. Other functions similarly depressed include renal plasma flow (RPF), free-water clearance, acid excretion, phosphate excretion, and T_m glucose (Table 8-1).

B. Fluid and volume physiology At term the proportion of body water is 75–80 percent (the proportion in babies born by cesarean section tends toward the higher figure and falls to 60 percent in childhood. A rapid diuresis ensues over the first few days of life. During this period, 7 percent of body water is lost (5 percent in prematures).

1. Body fluids

a. Body water compartments

(1) Extracellular fluid (ECF) constitutes 35–45 percent of body water in infants and 20 percent in adults (15 percent interstitial and 5 percent intravascular).

(2) Intracellular fluid (ICF) constitutes 40 percent of body water in both infants and adults.

b. The **turnover rates** of ECF are one-half per 24 hr in infants and one-seventh per 24 hr in adults.

2. Regulatory mechanisms

a. The **kidney** regulates (1) water balance, (2) osmolarity of fluids by controlling free-water excretion, and (3) distribution of body water through sodium retention and excretion.

b. Principles

(1) Tonicity (concentration, osmolality) is conserved in preference to volume.

(2) The kidneys provide better protection against **dilution** of body fluids than against **dehydration.**

(3) ECF volume is controlled by **sodium,** and the intracellular compartment (cell volume, ionic content) is dependent on ECF. Hence, sodium control is the key to volume control and indirectly, to ICF regulation.

c. Osmolality refers to the number of osmotically active particles dissolved per unit volume (1 molal represents 1 gram molecular weight in a solvent to make 1000 ml; 1 gram molecular weight *added* to 1 liter (L) is a molar solution).

(1) ECF osmolality is somewhat higher than that of the ICF because of the contribution by plasma proteins.

Table 8-1   Normal Values of Renal Function*

Measurement	At Birth	1–2 Weeks	6 Months, 1 Year	1–3 Years	Adult
GFR (ml/min)	26 ± 2	54 ± 8	77 ± 14	96 ± 22	118 ± 1?
RPF (ml/min)	88 ± 4	154 ± 34	352 ± 73	537 ± 122	612 ± 9?
T_m PAH (mg/min)		13 ± 1	51 ± 20	66 ± 19	79 ± 1?
T_m glucose (mg/min)		17 ± 20			339 ± 5?

* Corrected to 1.73 M^2 surface area; mean ± S.E.

(2) Water flux follows ionic (osmolal) flux to equalize fluid concen trations.

(3) Osmolality is determined by freezing point depression of the solvent. As a rule of thumb:

$$\text{Osmolality} = 2(Na^+) + \frac{BUN}{2.8} + \frac{glucose}{18}$$

(4) Osmolar excretion is approximated by

$$V_{Osm} = 2(Na + K + NH_4 + urea)(\text{all values in mOsm/kg})$$

In calculating molal excretion, assume NH_4 excretion of 0.5–3.0 mOsm/kg/24 hr and conversion of all dietary protein to urea, which yields 5 mOsm urea/gm protein. Osmolar excretion depends on the concentrating ability of the kidney. To produce a minimal urinary volume requires a maximum osmolality; this ranges from 1,200 mOsm/L in the healthy child, down to 300 mOsm/L in the diseased kidney and 600–700 mOsm/L in the healthy infant.

d. **Volume** is a sine qua non for organ function. Factors include cardiac output, peripheral resistance, aldosterone, renin-angiotensin axis, prostaglandins, and catechol levels. Since the body's Na^+ content de termines ECF distribution, its adjustment is essential to volume reg ulation. By cation exchange, aldosterone operates in the distal tubul to conserve Na^+. Active transport of cation brings about passive water transfer, thereby restoring ECF volume. In addition, ADH re lease in response to hemoconcentration augments water retention and thereby aids volume repletion.

e. **"Third space"** accumulations occur in many disease states, trapping fluid, electrolytes, and drugs outside their normal boundaries and thus robbing the body of effective volume.

C. **Electrolyte physiology**

1. **Sodium (Na^+)**   1 mEq = 23 mg; 1 gm = 43.5 mEq; plasma concentration = 135–140 mEq/L. **Note:** 1 gm salt (NaCl) = 18 mEq Na^+.

a. Sodium is the principal volume regulator. Normally, Na^+ accounts for 90 percent of extracellular cationic osmolality. Sodium space is ap proximately 60 percent of body weight, but varies considerably with states of hydration.

b. Measurement of Na^+ by flame photometer is artifactually depressed in hyperlipemic and hyperglycemic states. **Rule of thumb:** Na^+ is depressed 5 mEq/L for every 200 mg/100 ml of glucose above 100 mg/100 ml.

c. Requirements for Na^+ vary. A typical daily requirement is 40–60 mEq/M^2, or 1½–2 mEq/kg. When excretory capacity is impaired (heart failure, renal compromise) or overwhelmed (salt poisoning), edema formation occurs.

   Symptoms of inadequate sodium include confusion, restlessness, seizures, and eventually coma and death. Hypotension and circulatory failure can result from acute, severe sodium depletion. (For a more complete discussion of sodium abnormalities, see p. 197.)

d. The administration of salt (PO, IV, or by clysis) results in uptake by the ECF. One-third enters the plasma space, while two-thirds is taken up by the interstitium.

e. In the **newborn,** the sodium and volume regulatory mechanisms are functionally limited. Excretory capacity is reduced by a relative concentrating defect (maximal urine osmolarity approximately 600–700), and therefore obligatory solute loads require extra free water for their elimination (see Table 4-2 for solute contents of various infant diets). Since infants cannot control their fluid intake, sufficient fluid must be provided to balance needs for solute excretion (see p. 197 for a discussion of the role of solute load in dehydration).

2. Potassium (K^+)   1 mEq = 39.1 mg; 1 gm = 25.6 mEq; plasma concentration 3.4–5.5 mEq/L (may be higher in neonates).

a. Potassium is the principal cation of the ICF (which contains 98 percent of the body potassium) and contributes to the maintenance of intracellular tonicity and cell membrane ECF, permitting electrical "discharge."

b. Measurement of serum K^+ provides only an indirect assessment of total body K^+ stores and may therefore be misleading (e.g., diabetic ketoacidosis). **No practical estimate of K^+ space can be given for therapeutic replacement purposes.**

c. A typical K^+ requirement is 30–40 mEq/M^2/24 hr, or 1–3 mEq/kg. There is an obligatory K^+ loss via the urine, since tubular resorption cannot lower U_{K+} below 10 mEq/L.

d. The limit of tolerance for IV potassium is 250 mEq/M^2/24 hr, or about 8 mEq/M^2/hr. An absolute maximal 1-hr IV dose is 1 mEq/kg, hand administered into a large vein.

e. The danger of **abnormal K^+** is exacerbated by abnormalities of Ca^{++} in the opposite direction.

f. Hypokalemia due to a renal tubular defect, starvation, chronic diarrhea or vomiting, diabetic ketoacidosis, hyperaldosteronism, chronic use of diuretics, or inadequate long-term IV replacement is usually accompanied by chloride depletion with metabolic alkalosis. Recently, carbenicillin has been reported to cause hypokalemia.

   (1) Symptoms include muscle weakness, cramps, paralytic ileus, decreased reflexes, lethargy, and confusion.

   (2) A urine K^+ concentration of 10 mEq/L or less suggests severe K^+ depletion. Acid urine in the presence of metabolic alkalosis (paradoxical aciduria) also indicates K^+ depletion. Hypokalemic metabolic alkalosis is usually accompanied by a K$^+$ deficit of at least 4–5 mEq/kg.

(3) Cardiac effects seen by ECG are low voltage T wave, presence of U wave, and prolonged Q–T interval.

(4) Chronic exposure to low potassium damages the kidney's concentrating ability, producing a vasopressin-resistant **diabetes insipidus.**

g. Hyperkalemia occurs with renal failure, hemolysis, tissue necrosis, Addison's disease, congenital adrenal cortical hyperplasia, certain diuretics, and overdose of K$^+$ supplements. A specific renal tubular defect with hyperkalemia, hypertension, and growth failure has been described.

(1) Hypocalcemia, hyponatremia, and acidosis all exacerbate dangerous effects of hyperkalemia.

(2) The toxic effects are mainly cardiac. Rising K$^+$ interferes with normal nodal and bundle conduction. ECG changes include peaked T wave, increased P–R interval and widened QRS, depressed S–T segment, and atrioventricular or intraventricular heart block. As serum K$^+$ rises beyond 7.5 mEq/L, there is grave danger of heart block, ventricular flutter, and ventricular fibrillation.

3. Chloride (Cl$^-$) 1 mEq = 35.5 mg; 1 gm = 28 mEq; 1 gm salt (NaCl) = 18 mEq Cl$^-$; plasma concentration = 99–105 mEq/L.

a. Chloride is the principal anion of both intravascular fluid and gastric juice. Although chloride may undergo active renal tubular transport, it can be considered to behave passively, in parallel to sodium.

b. Abnormal losses occur with vomiting, diuretic therapy, and cystic fibrosis (excess sweating) and tend to lead to metabolic alkalosis.
Paradoxical aciduria occurs when Cl$^-$ is in short supply in conjunction with dehydration. Avidity for Na$^+$ causes preferential retention of Na$^+$ and rejection of H$^+$ into the urine; the alkalosis is worsened. Cl$^-$ must be replaced as NaCl.

4. Calcium (Ca^{++}) 1 mEq = 20 mg; 1 gm = 50 mEq; plasma concentration = 9.5–10.5 mg/100 ml, except in the newborn and premature.

a. Ionized calcium constitutes about 40 percent of total serum calcium; 50 percent is protein bound (principally to albumin), and 10 percent remains complexed. A change in serum albumin of 1 gm/100 ml changes calcium by approximately 0.8 mg/100 ml. The calcium space is approximately 25 percent of body weight.

b. The ionized portion of Ca$^+$ carries out functions in enzyme regulation, stabilizing neuromuscular membranes, coagulation processes, and bone formation. Acidosis increases ionized calcium, while alkalosis decreases it even to the point of symptomatic tetany. In hypoproteinemic states, a lower total serum Ca^{++} is tolerated.

c. Calcium dynamics are active in the growing child, primarily under the control of vitamin D hormones. Even in states of hypocalcemia only about 50 percent of ingested calcium can be absorbed.

d. Hypocalcemia is most commonly seen in rickets, renal compromise, the hypoalbuminemic states of liver disease or nephrosis, and in the neonate who is fed cow's milk formulas. Other conditions producing lowered calcium are discussed in Chap. 12.

Drugs that cause hypocalcemia include furosemide, glucagon, calcitonin mithramycin, bicarbonate, and corticosteroids. Exchange transfusion with acid citrate–preserved blood can produce hypocalcemia (see Chap. 5).

(1) **Symptoms** of depressed ionized Ca^{++} include the Chvostek and Trousseau signs, carpopedal spasm, ECG changes and, occasionally, mental confusion. Neonates commonly become jittery and may have seizures with tetany of the newborn (see p. 135).

(2) Neonatal tetany occurs because a "relative" hypoparathyroid state in the normal infant is stressed by the excess phosphate found in cow's milk formulas (see Table 4-2).

(3) In hypocalcemia the ECG shows prolongation of the Q–T interval relative to the rate.

e. **Hypercalcemia** is seen with hyperparathyroidism, vitamin D intoxication, sarcoidosis, cancer, immobilization, thyroid disease, Addison's disease, hypophosphatasia, and the milk-alkali syndrome in those taking antacids. In the Williams syndrome, infantile hypercalcemia is associated with elfin facies and obstructive heart disease (especially supravalvular aortic stenosis). **Symptoms** of excess calcium include nausea, anorexia, vomiting, constipation, polyuria, dehydration, mental confusion, and eventually coma. Chronic elevation of calcium can lead to nephrocalcinosis, extraskeletal calcification, and renal calculi.

5. **Magnesium (Mg^{++})**   1 mEq = 12 mg; plasma concentration = 1–2 mEq/L.

a. Magnesium is located primarily in the intracellular compartment. In the serum, about one-third is protein bound, and the pH of plasma has an effect similar to that on calcium. A magnesium deficiency state may simulate hypocalcemia.

b. **Hypomagnesemia** occurs in patients on long-term parenteral nutrition, in parathyroid abnormalities and hyperthyroidism, and after mercurial diuretics.

c. **Hypermagnesemia** may be seen in the newborn following magnesium sulfate administration to the mother with eclampsia. Symptoms are seen when the Mg^{++} level exceeds 4 mEq/L. Hypotension and diminished responsiveness are early signs; at a level greater than 7 mEq/L, there is a loss of deep tendon reflexes. Coma occurs at levels of 12 mEq/L. Hypermagnesemia has occasionally developed in patients with renal failure who are treated with magnesium-containing antacids to lower phosphate. The ECG shows a prolonged Q–T interval, atrioventricular block, and, with extreme elevations, cardiac arrest.

6. **Bicarbonate (HCO_3)**   Plasma concentration = 23–25 mEq/L. The bicarbonate ion serves as part of the buffering system employed by the body in its pH regulatory mechanism. The role of bicarbonate is to maintain a normal plasma pH (see **D**).

D. Acid-base physiology

1. **General principles**   A shift of 0.1 pH units, at pH 7.40, represents a change of only 10 nanoequivalents (nEq)/liter in hydrogen ion concentration (Table 8-2). This delicate regulation comes about through blood buffering, respiratory activity, and renal compensatory mechanisms.

a. **Blood buffers** include erythrocyte hemoglobin proteinate, organic and inorganic phosphates, carbonate (from bone) and both plasma and red

Table 8-2   Values of H^+ with Varying pH

pH	$(H^+)(nEq/L)$*
6.70	200
6.80	159
6.90	126
7.00	100
7.10	80
7.20	63
7.30	50
7.40	40
7.50	30
7.60	29
7.70	20

* These values are easy to remember, since at pH 7.40, $(H^+) = 40$; moving upward in pH, subtract 10 nEq/L per 0.1 pH unit; moving downward in pH, add 15 nEq/L (H^+) per 0.1 pH unit.

cell bicarbonate. About half the buffering capacity derives from bicarbonate and roughly one-third from hemoglobin.

b. **Ventilation** removes thousands of milliequivalents of carbon dioxide per day, thus preventing buildup of the weak acid, H_2CO_3, formed when CO_2 remains dissolved in plasma.

c. Children ingest 1–2 mEq/kg/day of "fixed" acid in their diet as sulfate from amino acids, nitrate, and phosphate (from phosphoproteins) and from incomplete oxidation of fat and carbohydrate, yielding organic acids (e.g., lactic acid). **Blood chemical buffers** provide immediate defense against this tide of acid, but it remains to the kidney to maintain long-term pH homeostasis through (1) recovery of filtered plasma bicarbonate; (2) excretion of titratable acid (buffered by phosphate); and, (3) NH_4^+ production. The proximal tubules reabsorb 85 percent of filtered bicarbonate by bulk transfer, while the distal tubule H^+ gradient permits recovery of the last 15 percent of bicarbonate via H^+ excretion.

2. **Determination of acid-base status** requires measurement of blood pH and bicarbonate. Bicarbonate, total CO_2 content, and CO_2 combining power provide the same basic information, with total CO_2 (TCO_2) 1–2 mEq/L lower than combining power.

   Bicarbonate also can readily be calculated from pH and PCO_2 as follows, a method that is particularly handy for assessing acid-base status, since the apparatus for blood gas determination is now ubiquitous and requires only a few minutes for results.

a. $pH = pK + \log \dfrac{(base)}{(acid)}$, where $pK = 6.1$

b. $pH = 6.1 + \log \dfrac{(HCO_3^-)}{\text{dissolved } CO_2} =$

c. $6.1 + \log \dfrac{(HCO_3^-)}{0.03 \times PCO_2}$

This can be rearranged to

d. $PCO_2 = \dfrac{(H^+)(HCO_3^-)}{23.9}$

where pH is expressed in nEq H^+/L. Thus, knowing PCO_2 and H^+ (from pH), one can calculate bicarbonate. With pH and serum bicarbonate values, the extent of a patient's acid-base imbalance can be measured and the nature of the disturbance determined.

3. **Laboratory values** Ideally, arterial samples are obtained for the diagnosis of acid-base disturbances. Venous samples may prove inaccurate in patients with impaired peripheral circulation, local tissue damage, or blood stasis caused by a tourniquet. Normal values for arterial and venous blood are given in Table 8-3. A heparinized syringe minimizes collection errors in drawing blood. If a Vacutainer is used, it should either contain an oil film to seal the blood sample and prevent CO_2 diffusion or it should be a small (3 ml), heparinized tube, completely filled by the blood sample.

4. **Acid-base abnormalities** By convention, acid-base disorders are divided (Fig. 8-1) into the following categories: **respiratory** versus **metabolic**, **acute** versus **chronic**, **simple** versus **mixed**, and **pure** versus **compensated** and resulting in either **acidosis** or **alkalosis**, depending on pH. In pure imbalances of pH, the disequilibrium results from a deviation of either PCO_2 (respiratory) or HCO_3^- (metabolic) from the norm. As can be seen from Henderson-Hasselbalch equation **c** [see **(2)**], a rise in PCO_2 increases the denominator and pH falls; this constitutes **respiratory acidosis**. Conversely, a fall in PCO_2 diminishes the denominator and pH rises, leading to **respiratory alkalosis**. Similarly, retention of HCO_3^- causes **metabolic alkalosis**, and a drop in HCO_3^- results in **metabolic acidosis**.

These situations prevail only for brief periods. The change in the internal milieu brings compensatory mechanisms into play. Compensation is rarely sufficient to offset the primary disturbance completely, and the condition is usually only partially corrected, so that the patient has a compensated acid-base disorder (Table 8-4).

a. **Respiratory acidosis** results from retention of CO_2 and a consequent increase in H_2CO_2. Normally, the rise in PCO_2 stimulates a ventilatory effort to eliminate the hypercapnia. In the acute phase of respiratory acidosis, available buffering mechanisms are minimal, and pH falls rapidly as PCO_2 exceeds 50 torr (for a discussion of acute respiratory failure, see Chap. 2). Renal compensation functions very effectively in chronic respiratory acidosis via the induction of enzyme systems for ammonium production. By acidifying the urine, the kidney can raise ECF bicarbonate to 40 mEq/L or more to compensate for marked hypercapnia. Generally, the neonate is not capable of this adaptation, and will remain severely acidotic with respiratory distress syndrome.

Table 8-3 Normal Blood Values*

Blood Sample	pH	PCO_2	HCO_3^-	TCO_2
Arterial	7.38–7.45	35–45 torr	23–27 mEq/L	24–28 mEq/L
Venous	7.35–7.40	45–50 torr	24–29 mEq/L	25–30 mEq/L

* In infants, the normal range for TCO_2 is 20–26, and pH is lower by approximately 0.05.

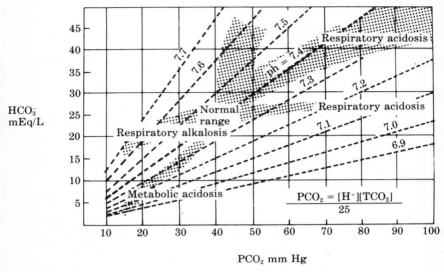

Figure 8-1 Acid-base nomogram.

b. Respiratory alkalosis is not a common pediatric problem. Hyperventilation (usually due to tachypnea rather than increased tidal volume alone) occurs in patients managed with mechanical ventilators (especially newborn infants with RDS) in the Reye syndrome, in the early phase of salicylate intoxication, in anxious or hysterical states (especially in teenagers), and in hypermetabolic states. Rapid correction of metabolic acidosis can result in respiratory alkalosis, since correction of the pH in the cerebrospinal fluid lags behind the ECF and continuing CNS acidosis stimulates the medullary ventilatory drive. Acute respiratory alkalosis can precipitate tetany (p. 180) and makes the patient feel light-headed. In psychogenic cases, symptoms of an acute anxiety state often dominate. Laboratory diagnosis rests on the triad of decreased PCO_2, elevated pH, and normal bicarbonate.

Table 8-4 Compensation in Acid-Base Disturbances

Acid-Base Disturbances	pH	HCO_3^-	PCO_2	Compensation
Metabolic acidosis	↓	↓	...	↓PCO_2; acid urine
Respiratory acidosis	↓	...	↑	Acid urine
Metabolic alkalosis	↑	↑	...	↑PCO_2; alkaline urine
Respiratory alkalosis	↑	...	↓	Alkaline urine

c. **Metabolic acidosis** results from increased blood H^+ with a concomitant fall in pH. Buffer base (bicarbonate and other blood buffers) is consumed, and TCO_2 falls.

(1) Accumulation of organic acids is reflected by a rise in the **anion gap.** Normally, the anion gap—$(Na^+ - [Cl + HCO_3^-])$—is ~12 mEq/L, but is somewhat higher in newborn infants. If metabolic acidosis results exclusively from bicarbonate loss, the anion gap changes little, since chloride rises proportionately. In lactic acidosis, the large anion gap reflects accumulation of an "unmeasured" anion.

(2) In response to the acidemic stress, both the kidney and lung undertake corrective measures. There is a prompt increase in minute ventilation, and PCO_2 falls (even more markedly than in primary respiratory alkalosis, in which PCO_2 usually remains above 25 torr), while urinary acidification maximizes over a few days within the limits of both reduced circulation and GFR.

(3) In children, chronic metabolic acidosis most commonly can be traced to a kidney abnormality, either parenchymal disease, obstruction, or a tubular disorder. Growth failure invariably accompanies chronic acidemia, and corrective therapy is necessary if severe impairment of normal development is to be avoided.

d. **Metabolic alkalosis** usually occurs as part of a generalized derangement in fluid and electrolytes. It necessarily involves either gain of a strong base or bicarbonate by the ECF or else a loss of fixed acid, which is analogous. Although the list of causes is long, the source of metabolic alkalosis in the majority of affected children is the GI tract. Most commonly, pyloric stenosis presents with metabolic alkalosis, due to the loss of HCl because of vomiting.

(1) **Potassium plays a central role in both the development and correction of metabolic alkalosis.** In acute alkalosis, K^+ moves from the ECF to the ICF to help maintain electroneutrality, since H^+ ion is lost. Although serum K^+ may then be low, total body K^+ remains normal.

(2) Conditions that produce K^+ depletion also stimulate aldosterone production. The kidney then becomes avid for sodium; as potassium depletion reduces available K^+, the distal tubule exchanges H^+ for sodium as it attempts to replete diminished circulating volume (due to a GI disturbance) by sodium resorption. The outcome is aciduria, coexisting with systemic alkalosis (paradoxical aciduria), and it tends to perpetuate the derangement.

Metabolic acidosis: $PCO_2 \downarrow 1–1.5 \times$ fall HCO_3^-

Metabolic alkalosis: $PCO_2 \uparrow 0.5–1.0 \times HCO_3^-$

Acute respiratory acidosis: $HCO_3^- \uparrow$ to maximum 30 mEq/L

Chronic respiratory acidosis: $HCO_3^- \uparrow 4$ mEq/L/10 mm $\uparrow PCO_2$

Acute respiratory alkalosis: $HCO_3^- \downarrow 2.5$ mEq/L/10 mm $\downarrow PCO_2$ (to minimum 18 mEq/L)

Chronic respiratory alkalosis: HCO_3^- falls to 15 mEq/L

e. **Mixed disorders** of acid-base homeostasis result from disturbances in both respiratory and renal function. Their diagnosis is simplified by reference to Fig. 8-1. Since the shaded areas in Fig. 8-1 represent the

95% confidence bands for each disturbance (including the normal compensatory response), any combination of values of PCO_2 and HCO_3^- that falls outside these areas represents a mixed disturbance.

II. DIAGNOSTIC PRINCIPLES   The data base for a therapeutic plan must include **vital signs** and **weight,** as well as the usual electrolyte and acid-base measurements. Significant data are readily obtained from urinary measurements —osmolality, sodium, potassium, urea nitrogen, and creatinine—which can produce a composite picture that greatly aids diagnosis. Table 8-5 lists typical blood and urine values for several disease states that lead to fluid and electrolyte disorders. These values cannot be absolute. They are intended only as diagnostic guidelines.

III. THERAPEUTIC PRINCIPLES   The contents of off-the-shelf IV solutions are listed in Table 8-6.

   A. Maintenance therapy   The figures given are for hospitalized children *without abnormal losses,* but whose activity level is decreased.

   1. Estimating fluid requirements

   a. Methods

   (1) Surface area   Levels of renal function and body fluid requirements correlate best with body surface area. Hence, the unit of measurement used is the square meter (M^2), and water needs are expressed as $ml/M^2/24$ hr. The nomogram (Fig. 8-2) correlates weight to surface area in children with normal body proportions. This system works well for children **weighing more than 10 kg** and has the advantage that a single formula can be used for all ages. The normal water requirement is about 1500 $ml/M^2/24$ hr (Table 8-7).

   (2) Calories expended   This method computes water requirements from metabolic expenditure. Figure 8-3 depicts energy use as a function of weight. To calculate fluid requirement, one allows 100–150 ml/100 cal metabolized.

   (3) Body weight   A rough rule of thumb for estimating fluids is 100 ml/kg, but this linear relationship provides a poor estimate for children, whether small or large.

   b. The fluid needs of the newborn

   (1) Maintenance needs are 60 ml/kg for the first 24 hr, advancing to 125 mg/kg/24 hr after the first week of life. A low solute load is better tolerated, so 0.2% saline in 5 or 10% dextrose, with added bicarbonate and calcium as needed, is a reasonable choice for uncomplicated cases (Table 8-8).

   (2) To provide the small volumes that newborns require, IVs should be run with constant infusion pumps. Frequent determination of blood chemistries (electrolytes, BUN, creatinine, calcium, phosphorus, pH, TCO_2, osmolality) is **mandatory.**

   (3) Phototherapy increases and mechanical ventilators with humidified oxygen substantially reduce insensible water loss.

   c. Urine output accurately reflects both circulatory status and adequacy of hydration. Although urine volume varies, about 50 ml/kg/24 hr is typical for the normal child. Infants excrete less urine in the first 24–48 hr of life but excretion increases thereafter. **An output less than 0.5 ml/kg/hr suggests pathologic oliguria and requires attention.**

Table 8-5 Diagnostic Guide for Serum and Urine Electrolytes

Condition	Serum Values					Urine Values			
	Na⁺ (mEq/L)	K⁺ (mEq/L)	Osm (mOsm/L)	BUN (mg/dl)	Creat.	Na⁺ (mEq/L)	K⁺ (mEq/L)	Osm (mOsm/L)	Urea (mg/dl)
Primary aldosteronism	140	↓	280	10	N	80	60–80	300–800	Low
Secondary aldosteronism	130	↓	275	15–25	↓	<20	40–60	300–400	800–1000
Na⁺ depletion	120–130	N or ↑	260	>30	N or ↑	10–20	40	600+	300
Na⁺ overload	150+	N	290+	N or ↑	N	100+	60	500+	300
H₂O overload	120–130	↓	260	10–15	↓	50–80	60	50–200	800–1000
Dehydration	150	↓	300	30 or N	N or ↑	40	20–40	800+	300
Inappropriate ADH	<125	↓	<260	<10	↓	90	60–150	$U > P_{Osm}$	300
Acute tubular necrosis									
Oliguric	135	↑	N or ↑	↑↑	↑	40+	20–40	300	300
Polyuric	135	N or ↑	275	↑	↑	20	30	300	100–300

187

Table 8-6 Solutions Available and Concentrations of Component (mEq/L)

Solution[a]	Glucose	Na$^+$	K$^+$	Cl$^-$	HCO$_3^-$	Lactate	Ca^{++}	NH$_4^-$
5% D/W	50							
10% D/W	100							
20% D/W	200							
0.85% saline (isotonic)		145		145				
0.9% saline		154		154				
3% saline		513		513				
5% saline		856		856				
1/6 M sodium lactate (1.9%)		167				167		
1/6 M NH$_4$Cl (0.9%)				167				167
2% NH$_4$Cl				374				374
Ringer's lactate		130	4	110		27	4	
Ringer's solution		147	4	156			5	
5% D/W in NS		145		145				
Multiple electrolyte solution[b]	50	40	35	40				

[a] *Additives:*
10% Ca gluconate = 100 mg/ml
7.5% KCl = 1 mEq/ml
K$_2$PO$_4$ = 2 mEq/ml
3.75% NaHCO$_3$ = 0.45 mEq/ml
7.5% NaHCO$_3$ = 0.90 mEq/ml
Tromethamine (THAM) 0.3 M = 0.3 mEq/ml
Mannitol 25% = 1 gm/4 ml
1 tsp salt/L fluid = 120 mEq/L Na and Cl
[b] Also contains 20 mEq acetate and 15 mEq phosphate.

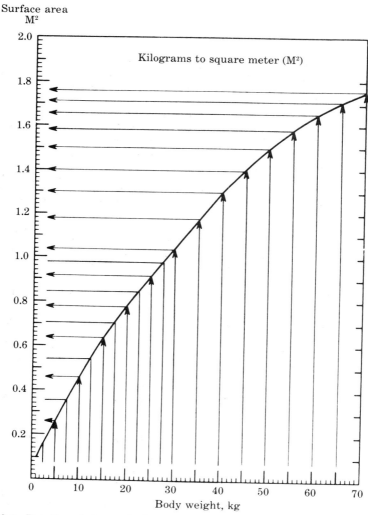

Surface area
M²

Kilograms to square meter (M²)

Body weight, kg

Figure 8-2 Relations between body weight in kilograms and body surface area. (Adapted from N. B. Talbot, R. R. Richie, and J. D. Crawford. *Metabolic Homeostasis*. Cambridge, Mass.: Harvard University Press, 1959. P. i.)

2. **Electrolyte requirements** are variable, with the excess intake readily excreted by the kidney (see Table 8-9).

3. **Calories**

   a. To reduce protein catabolism and avoid ketosis, 75–100 gm glucose/M²/day is required. However, this will *not* meet caloric needs. To do so requires 1200–1500 cal/M²/24 hr/L, not allowing for extra requirements imposed by illness.

Table 8-7 Fluid Balance in Children

Losses	
Insensible water	900 ml/M²/24 hr[a]
Gastrointestinal	100 ml/M²/24 hr
Urine	750 ml/M²/24 hr[b]
Total	1750
Sources	
Water of oxidation	250 ml/M²/24 hr
Net maintenance requirement	
Water	1500 ml/M²/24 hr

[a] Varies with size of child; e.g., 1200 ml/M² in a toddler versus 700 ml/M² at age 8–10 years.
[b] Based on excretion of isotonic urine, 300 mOsm/L, and minimal solute intake, e.g., dextrose in water.

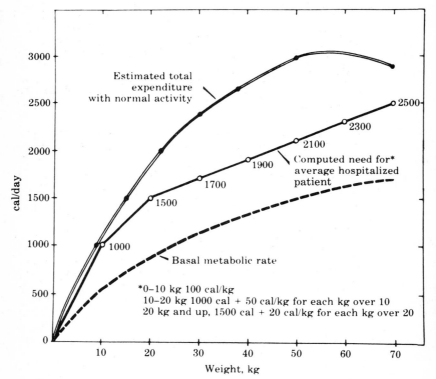

Figure 8-3 Comparison of energy expenditure in basal and ideal state. (Reproduced with permission from W. E. Segar, Parenteral fluid therapy. *Curr. Probl. Pediatr.* 3(2):4, 1972. Copyright © 1972 by Year Book Medical Publishers, Inc., Chicago.)

Table 8-8   Newborn Fluid and Electrolyte Therapy

Solute	Amount	Age
10% D/W	65 ml/kg/24 hr	Day 1
	80 ml/kg/24 hr	Day 2
	100 ml/kg/24 hr	Day 3
Sodium	Add 2–3 mEq/kg/24 hr	Day 3
Potassium	Add 1–2 mEq/kg/24 hr (if urine output adequate)	Day 2
Calcium	10 mg/kg elemental Ca^{++} IV push	
	30 mg/kg/24 hr IV maintenance	
Bicarbonate	1 mEq/kg (1 ml of 8% solution) IV	
	(may repeat for persistent acidosis)	

   b. Dextrose solutions of 5–10% are tolerated peripherally, whereas 15–30% sugar can be administered through a central IV line.

   c. For provision of high caloric content, **total parenteral nutrition** may be needed (see Chap 11).

4. Protein needs vary greatly with age and illness. The maintenance of positive nitrogen balance over long periods necessitates the use of protein hydrolysate (amino acid) solutions. Use of IV amino acids is best restricted to experienced units.

B. Correction and replacement of fluid balance distortions   (Dehydration is discussed in detail in Sec. **IV.**) A general guideline for **therapeutic priorities** includes maintenance of circulation, electrolyte, acid-base correction, cellular replacement, drug therapy, and calories.

   1. Abnormal fluid losses   Table 8-9 lists typical data on the composition of various body fluids; this information can be used to tailor IV solutions to replace losses accurately.

   a. Insensible water losses rise substantially with fever in children. Moderate febrile sweating in children can require a 10–25 percent increase in fluid requirement, best replaced with 5% D/W in ¼ NS. Increased insensible water losses also accompany rapid ventilation so

Table 8-9   Composition of Body Fluids

Source	Na^+ (mEq/L)	K^+ (mEq/L)	Cl^- (mEq/L)	HCO_3 (mEq/L)	pH	Osm (mOsm/L)
Gastric	50	10–15	150	0	1	300
Pancreas	140	5	50–100	100	9	300
Bile	130	5	100	40	8	300
Ileostomy	130	15–20	120	25–30	8	300
Diarrhea	50	35	40	50	Alk	
Sweat	50	5	55	0		
Blood	140	4–5	100	25	7.4	285–295
Urine	0–100*	20–100*	70–100*	0	4.5–8.5	50–1400

* Varies considerably with intake.

that fluid requirements will increase substantially in the febrile child with pneumonia, Kussmaul's respiration, or asthma.

b. Urinary losses become important in illnesses that impair concentrating ability or salt resorption. Measurement of urinary electrolytes helps to quantify such losses.

c. Third-space fluid collections, as in nephrotic syndrome, necrotizing enterocolitis, or pancreatitis, reduce the availability of body liquid stores for maintenance of fluid homeostasis, and these "internal losses" likewise need replacement.

2. Volume replacement

a. Attention must first be directed to the restoration of circulating volume. In the acute situation, isotonic fluid (e.g., Ringer's lactate, which mimics ECF) is safest to use; 10 ml/kg should be delivered into a large vein. If pulse and blood pressure fail to respond adequately, this should be repeated in 15 min and then again, if needed. This "priming dose" of 10–30 ml/kg should restore good circulation with resumption of capillary perfusion and (later) urine output. When hypoglycemia is a risk, use 5% D/W with Ringer's lactate. Plasma colloid expanders are used in shock, in protein loss.

b. The next phase of treatment continues until information is sufficient to suggest a diagnosis. Again, an isotonic solution is least likely to provoke complications while the patient's problem awaits better definition. Similarly, the child with moderate volume depletion should be started on IV Ringer's lactate until a biochemical profile permits specific tailoring of fluid therapy. An infusion rate of 300–400 ml/M²/hr over the first 1–2 hours will cover most contingencies, allowing the workup to proceed. Oral rehydration should be used only if (1) the child appears stable, (2) the GI tract is not contributing to ongoing losses, and (3) close observation for any deterioration is readily arranged. For details of fluid therapy for dehydration states, see p. 199.

c. If severe metabolic acidosis seems likely, a mixture of 5% D in ½ NS with ¼ normal bicarbonate added (i.e., 35 mM $NaHCO_3$ [35 ml of "stock" 8% solution] per liter 5% D in ½ NS) should be substituted for Ringer's lactate. See Chap. 14 for management of diabetic ketoacidosis.

d. Further replacement therapy should provide for

(1) Maintenance needs (see pp. 186 and 191).

(2) Correction of existing biochemical distortions.

(3) Restoration of normal hydration by the end of the first day's treatment, *except* in hyperosmolar dehydration.

e. Overhydration can result both from a disease process and from inappropriate medical management. Congestive heart failure, nephrosis, cirrhosis, and drowning may all result in excess ECF, manifested as edema or third-space fluid collections. Failure to restrict fluids *early* in several clinical conditions also can lead to excess volume, necessitating therapy aimed at its removal.

Treatment of excess volume depends on the cause. Diuresis is commonly used when renal function is intact. Osmotic diuresis usually is employed for CNS trauma with overhydration.

3. Treatment of electrolyte abnormalities   See also Sec. **IV.**

a. Sodium

(1) Hypernatremia results when water loss exceeds salt loss (hypertonic dehydration) or from inadvertent salt poisoning. Because the kidney can reject large amounts of sodium (urine Na^+ can exceed 200 mEq/L) when aldosterone is suppressed, it is rare to see hypernatremia from excess salt intake via the diet alone. However, in hypernatremic dehydration, aldosterone secretion remains high, with consequent exacerbation of the hypernatremia despite the presence of dehydration. Hypernatremia is also seen following x-ray contrast studies if high Na^+ content dyes are used. Hypaque contains 786 mEq Na^+/L and sodium iothalamate contains 1088 mEq/L.

(2) Severe hypernatremia The potential damage can be reversed by furosemide diuresis (1 mg/kg), replacing the urine output with 10% D/W solution, monitoring sodium values q4h, and repeating the administration of furosemide.

(3) Hyponatremia becomes clinically important at values less than 125 mEq/L. **If serum Na^+ acutely falls below 115 mEq/L, there is substantial danger of grand mal seizures.** Judicious use of 3% NaCl (513 mEq/L) can prevent or terminate seizures, but one should **never** attempt total correction, since severe circulatory overload may result. Raising serum Na^+ by 5 mEq, or at most by 10 mEq, will terminate the acute CNS disturbance. Much of the Na^+ administered in this fashion rapidly appears in the urine, so that the effect is transient. (Also note that the hypertonicity is very rough on veins and is quite painful.)

(a) Dilutional hyponatremia can occur from inappropriate ADH secretion (Schwartz-Bartter syndrome) [see **(d)**]; impairment of free-water clearance from rehydration using salt-free fluids; or from deficient mineralocorticoid production. Except for the crisis of adrenal insufficiency, these children are usually not total-body dehydrated, and the goal of therapy is to reduce excess water in relation to salt, which can be done most effectively by water restriction. **Beware of restricting fluid intake in hypoproteinemic patients, since this may lead to circulatory embarrassment.**

A rough estimate of **water excess** can be determined from

$$\text{Water excess (L)} = \text{measured body water}$$
$$- \text{normal body water volume} = 0.6 \times \text{wt (kg)}$$
$$- \frac{0.6 \text{ wt (kg)} \times \text{plasma Osm (mOsm/L)}}{\text{normal plasma osmolality (mOsm/L)}}$$

(b) Excess water intake leads to **water intoxication,** as seen in fresh-water drowning, psychogenic polydipsia, or inappropriate hydration. Treatment consists in (1) reducing further water intake, (2) loop diuretics, and (3) IV replacement therapy using an isotonic solution. In severe cases intravenous 3% NaCl may be necessary.

(c) Renal salt wasting can lead to hyponatremia. Treatment consists in chronic administration of oral salt supplements, titrated to needs (see **e**, p. 209).

(d) The syndrome of inappropriate ADH secretion (SIADH) occurs more commonly in children with CNS infections than in those with tumors. Diagnosis requires **simultaneous measurement** of serum and urine osmolality and electrolytes, which should demonstrate hyponatremia, and $P_{Osm} < U_{Osm}$ with high urinary sodium, despite the excess free water in the blood. To entertain the diagnosis, the clinical setting should exclude dehydration, and edema ought not be present. Treatment has been outlined in **(b)**.

b. Potassium See also p. 209.

(1) Hyperkalemia The best treatment for hyperkalemia is prevention. Most commonly, rapidly rising potassium occurs in the setting of acute renal compromise. Hence, the nephrologist's succinct commandment: "No P(ee), no K!"

False elevations of potassium are seen from heel-stick blood samples, thrombocytosis or marked leukocytosis as well as from hemolysis.

Rapidly rising serum levels make ECG monitoring mandatory and require therapy without delay. Four approaches are available: (a) remove K^+ from the body; (b) minimize the deleterious effects of hyperkalemia; (c) sequester the excess ion where it can do no harm; (d) drive K^+ into glycogen with insulin. Meanwhile one must identify the cause of and prevent further increase in potassium concentration.

Steps in the treatment of acute hyperkalemia are consonant with the danger. With serum K^+ above 7.5 mEq/L, the sequence includes

(a) Sodium bicarbonate, 2.5 mEq/kg IV; bicarbonate lowers potassium about 2 mEq/L (each increase by 0.1 pH units decreases K^+ by 1 mEq/L within minutes).

(b) Calcium infusion (except in digitalized patients), counteracts the cardiac effects of severe hyperkalemia.

(c) Cation exchange resins such as Kayexalate (Na polystyrene sulfonate) accumulate the K^+ ion in the gut, in exchange for Na^+. Kayexalate, 1 gm/kg, reduces the serum K^+ by 1 mEq/kg. **Excessive use may produce hypocalcemia.**

(d) The use of insulin–glucose has a limited role in pediatrics. In infants, profound hypoglycemia may result. This treatment can be used in older children, but only cautiously. It works in 20–30 min.

In the face of continuing likelihood of rising K^+, peritoneal dialysis should be initiated promptly, particularly if heart failure is part of the clinical picture, since the other therapies can convert impending cardiac failure to acute decompensation.

(2) Hypokalemia can often be treated by removing the cause (e.g., diuretic therapy, insufficient K^+ in parenteral fluids to replace losses, gastroenteritis).

(a) Oral therapy is necessary for chronic and irreversible causes such as renal tubular acidosis, Fanconi syndrome, Bartter syndrome (see Chap. 9).

(b) **IV therapy** becomes necessary if serum K^+ acutely falls below 2 mEq/L, or if the child cannot accept oral alimentation (e.g., in chronic vomiting). In nonemergent circumstances, allow 2–3 days to repair the deficit. IV solutions generally should not contain more than 40 mEq/L KCl (see Chap. 9).

c. **Chloride** is rarely the prime mover of metabolic disturbance, but reflects what has gone on before.

(1) **Hyperchloremia** is corrected as the patient's hypernatremia and acidosis come under control.

(2) **Hypochloremia** is seen with hyponatremic dehydration and in all the forms of dilutional hyponatremia and water intoxication. In hypokalemic alkalosis, two groups of patients are found: Those with low urinary chloride respond to saline infusion; in those with high urinary chloride (typically > 70 mEq/L and even > 200 mEq/L), a state of "saline resistance" occurs. To correct this, one must administer *both* K^+ and chloride. Saline resistance usually occurs after severe potassium depletion and may require enormous amounts of K^+, given over several days, to effect correction. The total potassium deficit has been reported to reach more than 1000 mEq in adults.

d. **Calcium**

(1) **Hypocalcemia**   Because of renal maturation, skeletal growth demands, and congenital abnormalities, the principles of treatment require a sensitivity to the practical limits involved in therapy in infants and children.

(a) **Symptomatic hypocalcemia** occurs most commonly in the nursery (tetany of the newborn), after exchange transfusion, and with hypoparathyroidism. Treat acutely with an IV calcium infusion, 10 mg/kg elemental Ca^{++} infused over 5–10 min, with ECG monitoring (see Chaps. 5, 9, and 12).

A 10% calcium gluconate solution = 18% Ca^{++}, or 9 mg/ml elemental Ca^{++}. Calcium lactate = 13% Ca^{++}, or 13 mg/ml elemental Ca^{++}. A 20% calcium gluceptate solution = 18% Ca^{++}, or 18 mg/ml elemental Ca^{++}. A 10% calcium chloride solution = 27% Ca^{++}, or 27 mg/ml elemental Ca^{++}. **$CaCl_2$ must not be delivered into tissue directly, since it causes local necrosis with slough.** It is unwise to run a $CaCl_2$ solution through a pump because of the danger from infiltration.

After the initial dose, treatment should continue, providing a total daily dose of about 40 mg/kg (25–50 mg) elemental Ca^{++} via IV infusion. Phosphate intake (especially milk or multiple electrolyte solution) must be halted.

(b) Management of **chronic hypocalcemia** depends on the underlying cause (see Chaps. 5, 9, and 12 for relevant discussions).

(2) **Hypercalcemia constitutes a medical emergency, when blood levels surpass 15 mg/100 ml acutely.** Treatment aims at reducing serum Ca^{++} to 12 mg/100 ml rapidly. The sequence of treatment is discussed on page 211.

e. **Magnesium**

(1) **Hypomagnesemia** may occasionally cause tetany, indistinguishable from hypocalcemic convulsions. IV therapy with magnesium sulfate should deliver 10 mg/kg elemental Mg^{++} over 2–3 hr. In babies, one can use 50% $MgSo_4$ IM, at the same dose.

(2) There is no specific drug therapy for **hypermagnesemia.** While awaiting dialysis, one should administer 10 mg/kg elemental Ca^{++} as a slow IV infusion, to minimize hypermagnesemic effects.

f. Phosphate

(1) Hypophosphatemia, as seen in vitamin D–resistant rickets and vitamin D–dependent rickets, responds to oral potassium acid phosphate (K-Phos; a 500-mg tablet = 115 mg phosphorus), and this form avoids the diarrhea inflicted by high-dose Neutrophos. The dose should be titrated, but may reach 10 mg/day in children with X-linked phosphate diabetes.

(2) Hyperphosphatemia in end-stage renal disease is discussed on page 210.

4. Treatment of acid-base disturbances

a. General comments

(1) The physician must attempt to ascertain the underlying cause of derangement. In short, never treat unless you have some idea of what you are treating.

(2) Make haste slowly in correcting "metabolic" pH disturbances. Attempts at abrupt and total restoration of normal values are poorly tolerated by the brain and other organs. **Exception:** At the extremes of pH abnormality—7.0 or less and 7.6 or greater—rapid treatment is required for survival, although only partial correction will suffice.

b. Respiratory acidosis While alkali is rarely indicated, extreme acidosis may require bicarbonate to bring the pH above 7. The key to effective therapy is improved gas exchange (see Chap. 20). In chronic respiratory acidosis, the compensatory metabolic alkalosis usually comes about via renal loss of potassium and chloride, and thus one must supply K^+ and Cl^- as pH correction gets under way.

c. Respiratory alkalosis in children is not common. In patients on mechanical ventilation, reduction of the rate setting or addition of dead space tubing will restore pH balance. When acute respiratory alkalosis is due to psychogenic or CNS hyperventilation, rebreathing CO_2 (breathing into a paper bag) is effective treatment.

d. Metabolic acidosis

(1) Acute therapy is needed for reduction of undue acidemia (pH < 7.20) or to correct a sudden onset of acidosis, e.g., following cardiac arrest. Calculate the bicarbonate deficit as follows: Deficit (mEq bicarbonate) = (TCO_2 normal − TCO_2 measured) × 0.4 × body weight (kg). The estimated bicarbonate space is 0.4 (closer to 0.5 in infants and toddlers). For therapy, half this estimated deficit is delivered over 6–8 hr, and the patient's chemical status is rechecked.

Once the patient's TCO_2 reaches 15 mEq/L, renal compensation usually is adequate to correct the remaining acidosis *if the source of acid is controlled.*

(a) Patients with congestive heart failure may not tolerate the large sodium load of $NaHCO_3$ therapy. Either slow the rate of infusion, or consider using THAM.

(b) THAM [tris(hydroxymethyl)aminomethane, tromethamine] has the advantage of raising the pH without adding excessive sodium and CO_2. It is available as a 3.6% (1/3 M) solution with a pH of 10.2. Since hypoglycemia has been reported with a rapid administration, 5% D/W can be used to prepare the solution (the osmolality is then equivalent to that of a 10% D/W solution). Infuse over 3–6 hr and give supplementary amounts (up to 25 percent of the total) over 5–10 min. The dose of THAM (in ml) should equal the base deficit times weight (in kg).

(c) The infusion of bicarbonate lowers serum K^+ by driving the ion into the intracellular space. Since patients with metabolic acidosis often carry a preexisting K^+ deficit, serum K^+ should be monitored frequently while administering bicarbonate.

(d) Infants with **hereditary amino acid disturbances** may present with seizures, chemical abnormalities, hyperammonemia, and severe acidosis. This combination may respond best to prompt peritoneal dialysis.

(e) Children with severe metabolic acidosis may suddenly **worsen** when placed on mechanical ventilation, since they are deprived of a compensatory respiratory drive.

(2) Chronic metabolic acidosis usually results from renal dysfunction. For specific treatment of renal tubular acidosis (see Chap. 9).

e. Metabolic alkalosis requires specific acid therapy only when severe. Most patients respond to correction of the underlying cause. When therapy is necessary, saline will correct the condition in the majority of patients.

If acid administration is required, one can use 0.1 N HCl solution (100 mEq/L) mixed with either 5% D/W or with added KCl, since hypokalemia generally will be present. Calculate the "base excess" (see **4.d**). Infuse the HCl into a central vein (but not over the atrium) over 8 hr. Calculate the dose needed to bring TCO_2 down to 30–25 mEq/L, but administer only half of this amount and recheck the patient. In cases of extreme alkalosis, adequate potassium replacement may require extraordinarily high IV concentrations of KCl (up to 100–150 mEq/L) which *must* be carefully monitored. NH_4Cl can also be used for correction of extreme alkalosis, but it imposes an added ammonia burden on the liver and should not be used in patients with impaired circulation or liver damage. NH_4Cl is supplied in 0.9% and 2% solutions.

IV. DEHYDRATION

A. General comments

1. The most useful way to consider dehydration is based on the amount of **sodium and potassium lost in relation to water.** Hence, we conventionally divide the dehydration states into isotonic (isonatremic), hypotonic (hyponatremic), and hypertonic (hypernatremic) for purposes of management.
   Hypotonic $Na^+ < 125$ mEq/L; ECF depletion with relative sparing of intracellular contents; hence, early vascular compromise.
   Isotonic Na^+ 130–150 mEq/L; balanced loss of water and ions.
   Hypertonic $Na^+ > 150$ mEq/L; intracellular fluid depletion; allows more chronic dehydration.

2. The best indicator of **short-term quantitative fluid loss** is change in body weight. Table 8-10 presents a rough clinical estimate of signs and degree of dehydration.

3. **Role of solute load** In understanding dehydration states, it is important to consider the contribution of **intake** in producing a negative bal-

Table 8-10   Estimation of Dehydration

Clinical Signs	Degree of Dehydration		
	Mild[a]	Moderate[b]	Severe[c]
Weight loss (%)			
Infant	5	10	15
Child	3–4	6–8	10–12
Behavior	Normal	Irritable	Hyperirritable to lethargic
Thirst	Slight	Moderate	Intense
Mucous membrane	May be normal	Dry	Parched
Tears	Present	+/−	Absent
Anterior fontanelle	Flat	+/−	Sunken
Skin	Normal	+/−	Increased
Urinary specific gravity	Slight change	Increased	Greatly increase with oliguria

[a] Assume present based on a history of GI losses.
[b] Objective clinical signs apparent.
[c] Impending circulatory collapse (unless dehydration is hypertonic).

ance as well as the role played by **output** via diarrhea or vomiting. Rena solute load hastens dehydration by causing obligatory urinary free water loss in the infant struggling to excrete an ingested solute load.

This means that the solute stress of a given feeding is different from the formula's measured osmotic load. Since infants cannot effectively concentrate urine much beyond 600 mOsm/kg, it is apparent that cow's milk causes free-water losses **three times greater** than those of human milk, while boiled skim milk imposes a fourfold free-water loss. Thus renal solute load should be minimized in infants with fluid losses to avoid hypertonic dehydration.

4. **Initial assessment** of the dehydrated child should include the following:

   a. **History**   Urine output, weight change, infectious disease contacts, estimate of stooling or vomiting frequency.

   b. **Clinical**   Urine output, skin turgor, mucous membrane moisture, eye turgor, fullness of fontanelle, mental state.

   c. **Laboratory**   Weight, CBC, serum and urine Na^+, K^+, Cl^+, pH, CO_2 BUN, creatinine, osmolality, glucose, calcium. Urinalysis, SG, pH glucose, ketones, amino acids (ferric chloride), appropriate cultures.

5. **Urinalysis** is particularly important. Electrolyte patterns are shown in Table 8-5. The specific gravity should be well above 1.015 **unless intrinsic renal disease** is contributing to the problem. Ketonuria often accompanies dehydration without diabetes. Trace or 1+ protein can be present along with cellular debris and a few hyaline casts. However, a very active sediment signals underlying primary renal disease. Alkaline urine should raise the question of renal tubular acidosis.

6. **Water and electrolyte losses**   Estimates of deficits in moderate to severe dehydration in these groups of patients are given in Table 8-11.

Table 8-11   Deficits in Moderate to Severe Dehydration

Type of Dehydration	Range of Na$^+$ (mEq/L)	Losses			
		Water (ml/kg)	Na$^+$ (mEq/kg)	K$^+$ (mEq/kg)	Cl$^-$ + HCO$_3^-$ (mEq/kg)
Isotonic	130–145	100–150	7–11	7–11	14–22
Hypotonic	<125	40–80	10–14	10–14	20–28
Hypertonic	>150	120–170	2–5	2–5	4–10

Modified from R. W. Winters. *Principles of Pediatric Fluid Therapy*, North Chicago: Abbott Laboratories, 1970. P. 56.

B. Acute fluid management and resuscitation

  1. Weigh the patient.

  2. If shock is present, or if no urine is produced in the first half hour, give 20–30 ml/kg Ringer's lactate, or 5% albumin IV until adequate circulation returns.

  3. After the first hour, give 10 ml/kg/hr of Ringer's lactate until shock is alleviated and actual fluid and electrolyte deficits can be accurately calculated.

  4. If the patient is asymptomatic and/or dehydration is hyponatremic or isotonic, one-half the fluids calculated for 24 hr should be administered in the first 8 hr. The remaining half should be administered in the remaining 16 hr.

  5. If hypertonic dehydration is present after correcting shock, correct the deficit slowly and evenly over 48 hr (see **E.2**, p. 201).

  6. Temperature will affect total maintenance needs; with fever, add 10% of the maintenance amount per degrees centigrade.

  7. Adequacy of therapy is indicated by urine output 40 ml/M^2/hr (1.5 ml/kg/hr), urine Na$^+$ ~ 40 mEq/L, normal circulation, and restoration of weight.

C. Hypotonic dehydration   In this condition, the fluid loss comes mainly from the intravascular and interstitial compartments rather than the intracellular reservoir. Hence, circulatory compromise appears early and there is marked loss of turgor. Patients arrive at this state when enteric losses are replaced with low-solute fluids (e.g., fruit juice, Coca-Cola).

  1. Clinically, infants present soon after the onset of illness because symptoms become apparent early. For a given weight loss, the clinical signs are more marked than in isotonic or hypertonic dehydration. Thus, estimates of weight loss should follow a 3, 6, 9 percent rule of thumb for mild, moderate, and severe, respectively. Seizures occur infrequently, even with marked hyponatremia, but generalized lethargy is common, and vascular collapse can occur early.

  2. Treatment   Since loss is mainly extracellular fluid, replacement therapy can advance rapidly, with volume and sodium restored by the end of 24–36 hr.

    a. Acute resuscitation   See **B.**

   b. **Symptomatic hyponatremia**   Regardless of the cause, whether Na
   loss or water excess, therapy is directed at raising the sodium concen
   tration quickly, to stop symptoms.

   (1) Use hypertonic saline (3% = 513 mEq Na^+/L) to deliver approxi
   mately 5 mEq/kg/hr. The sodium deficit (mEq) = (normal Na^+
   measured Na^+) × 0.6 × weight (kg).

   (2) Symptomatic hyponatremia may be seen with a serum Na^+ con
   centration of 130 mEq/L if the change in concentration has bee
   sudden. Thus, the patient's symptoms, if any, must be taken int
   account to determine the speed of correction of the serum sodiur
   concentration.

   (3) The following is a **sample calculation** for a 10-kg child with serur
   Na^+ of 120 mEq who manifests irritability and diminished con
   sciousness:

   (a) 10 kg × 0.6 × (15 mEq deficit) = 90 mEq (total Na^+ deficit = 9
   mEq)

   (b) To raise Na^+ by mEq acutely requires 5 mEq × 0.6 × 10 kg = 3
   mEq:

   $$\text{Dose of 3\% NaCl} = \frac{30 \text{ mEq Na}^+}{0.513 \text{ mEq Na}^+/\text{ml}} = 60 \text{ ml}$$

   $$\text{Dose of 5\% NaCl} = \frac{30 \text{ mEq Na}^+}{0.856 \text{ mEq Na}^+/\text{ml}} = 35 \text{ ml}$$

   Following acute correction, the patient's acidosis may worser
   Sodium bicarbonate (1 mEq/ml) may be mixed with the hyper
   tonic saline to supply one-fourth of the Na^+ dose while als
   providing bicarbonate as the anion.

   c. The therapy of **asymptomatic hyponatremia** requires gradual correc
   tion of the sodium deficit (see pp. 192 ff.) in increments of 10 mEq/L

   (1) The following is a **sample calculation** for a 10-kg child with 10%
   dehydration and serum Na^+ 125 mEq/L:

   (a) Volume deficit = 10% × 10 kg = 1.0 L

   (b) Volume maintenance = 100 ml × 10 kg = 1.0 L
   Total = 2.0 L

   (c) Na^+ needed = Na^+ deficit × 10 kg × 0.6
   $\qquad\qquad$ = (135 − 125) mEq × 6.0
   $\qquad\qquad$ = 10 × 6
   Deficit $\qquad$ = 60 mEq Na

   (d) Maintenance Na^+ = 3 mEq/kg × 10
   $\qquad\qquad\qquad$ = 30 mEq Na

   $$\text{Thus, } \frac{\text{total Na need} = 90 \text{ mEq}/24 \text{ hr}}{\text{total volume } 2.0 \text{ L}/24 \text{ hr}} = \frac{45 \text{ mEq Na}}{1.0 \text{ L}}$$

   $$= 1/3 \text{ normal saline}$$

   (2) Administer one-half of the total fluid in the first 8 hr and the res
   over the remaining 16 hr.

   d. **Potassium** deficit and **acidosis** both require specific therapy for co
   rection. Hemoconcentration and prerenal azotemia will resolve wit
   restoration of fluids.

e. A simplified approach to therapy is to use a multiple electrolyte solution, which contains (in mEq/L) Na^+ 40, K^+ 35, Cl^- 40, acetate 20,
phosphate 15, in 5% glucose after restoration of good circulation. **Do
not use for infants,** since they cannot tolerate the phosphate load, or
for patients unable to tolerate a high K^+ load (see Table 8-12 for restrictions on the use of multiple-electrolyte solution). Alternatively, one
can mix a "home brew" consisting of 5% D in ¼ NS with ¼ $NaHCO_3$
added (per 500 ml, add 17 ml of 8% $NaHCO_3$). Add to this an appropriate amount of K^+, e.g., 20 mEq/L.

D. Isotonic dehydration Children with enteric losses, taking an intermediate
solute load (e.g., breast milk), arrive at a balanced dehydration. The deficit
is lost both from ECF and ICF. For a given weight loss, symptoms will be
less dramatic than for hypotonic dehydration—assume a weight loss of 5,
10, or 15 percent for clinical estimation of mild, moderate, and severe involvement, respectively.

Treatment is similar to that for hypotonic dehydration (see **C.2**). However,
a more leisurely tempo in completing deficit repair is acceptable. Aim to
restore about two-thirds of the total estimated volume deficit during the
first day. During day 2, the emphasis should be on restoring both potassium
deficit and acid-base balance.

1. After acute therapy, supply **maintenance** at 1500 ml/M²/24 hr (or 100
ml/kg for infants weighing < 10 kg) plus deficit calculated from estimated
weight loss.

2. The fluid used can be either multiple electrolyte solution, or the "home
brew" described above, with exceptions as noted. Both these solutions
are hypotonic, but since the normal kidney needs only ⅛ N solution for
true maintenance, these ½ N solutions provide sufficient solute even for
correction of isotonic losses.

E. Hypertonic dehydration results when inappropriately high solute loads are
given as replacement fluid, or when a renal concentrating defect produces a
large free-water loss. Usually, hypernatremia represents the principal excess solute, but agents such as glucose, urea, and mannitol can produce the
same disturbance.

1. The **clinical presentation** in these infants can be deceptive. Shock is a late
manifestation. When it supervenes, one can be certain that fluid loss
exceeds 10 percent of body weight. Skin turgor does not exhibit the usual
tenting of advanced dehydration, but is a thick, doughy consistency.
Other findings include a shrill cry or mewling sound, muscle weakness,
tachypnea, and intense thirst in toddlers. In assessing these infants, be
sure to check *sugar* and *calcium*, since hyperglycemia is present in half
the patients, and calcium deficiency has been noted in 10 percent.

2. **Treatment** The total fluid deficit must be replaced slowly over 48 hr or
more, dropping serum Na^+ by 10 mEq/L/day. Rapid correction floods the
intracellular space with fluid, leading to cerebral (and sometimes pulmonary) edema. In general, the more dilute the solution being used to correct the deficit, the slower it should be infused.

a. If Na^+ is over 180 mEq/L, initiate emergency peritoneal dialysis.
Intravenous therapy cannot cope with this degree of derangement.

b. If shock is present, infuse 20 ml/kg of 5% albumin over 20–30 min.

c. **First hour** The goal is to reestablish urine flow. Give 10–20 ml/kg
Ringer's lactate to reduce the chloride load in favor of lactate (alkali).

d. Over the **next 4 hr** the goal is to ensure urine output and reduce the
serum Na^+ to about 165 mEq/L. There is no best regimen. The rate of

IV infusion is determined by the tonicity of the solution, i.e., isoton
solutions can be infused more rapidly.

Infuse 10 ml/kg/hr of 5% D/Ringer's lactate, Ringer's lactate, or
mixture of 2½% dextrose and ½ *N* saline to which is added ¼
bicarbonate (17 ml of 8% NaHCO$_3$/500 ml of solution), depending c
the degree of acidosis or hyperglycemia. This should establish
steady urine flow, which then permits addition of potassium to t
infusion.

e. The **next 48 hr** are utilized to replenish the volume lost; infusio
should proceed at a steady rate, based on calculated deficits. Th
deficit in a patient with severe hypernatremia will be approximate
10 percent of body weight, i.e., 1 L/10 kg.

Calculation of **water deficit:**

Water deficit (L) = normal body water volume

$$− \text{ measured body water}$$
$$= \frac{0.6 \times \text{body wt (kg)} \times \text{plasma Osm (mOsm/L)}}{\text{normal plasma Osm (mOsm/L)}} − 0.6 \times \text{wt (kg)}$$

Example: A 10-kg child with Na$^+$ 160 mEq/L and Osm of 340:

$$\text{Water deficit} = \frac{0.6 \times 10 \times 340}{290} − 0.6 \times 10$$

$$= 7.0 \text{ L} − 6.0 \text{ L}$$

$$= 1000 \text{ ml deficit, or 10 percent dehydration}$$

(1) Sodium should be supplied *only* for the deficit volume; maint
nance should be supplied as salt-free fluid. Assume that appro
mately 100–125 mEq Na$^+$/L of deficit was lost. After all the calc
lations, the final solution will be approximately ¼ *N* saline ov
the 48 hr. It is best to add 5% **dextrose** for calories and also
mEq/L **potassium** to replenish lost intracellular stores. Becau
of acidosis, part of the anion supplied should be basic, i.e., la
tate or bicarbonate. In short, the simplest infusion is **multipl**
electrolyte solution with 5% glucose.

(2) Do not allow the IV infusion to run rapidly. There is grave danger
CNS damage from acute osmotic shifts should fluid run in u
checked. It is also unwise to attempt rapid control of hyperglyc
mia, since the presence of the extra glucose acts as an "osmot

Table 8-12 Dangers of Multiple Electrolyte Solution

Case	Reason
Infant	Excess PO$_4$ load
Renal compromise	Excess K$^+$, PO$_4$
Acute resuscitation of dehydration	Hypotonic solution, excess K$^+$
Hypernatremic dehydration; acute manage- ment required	Same
Mineralocorticoid deficiency—Addisonian crisis; adrenogenital syndrome crisis	Excess K$^+$
Volume expansion	Hypotonic solution

Table 8-13 Conditions Requiring Special IV Therapy

System and/or Disorder	Correction
CNS	
Meningitis (SIADH)	½–⅔ maintenance
Trauma	½–⅔ maintenance
Tumor	½–⅔ maintenance
Renal	
Acute renal failure	No K^+
(except polyuric	350 ml/M^2/24 hr plus
acute tubular necrosis)	urine output
Chronic renal failure	No IV K^+
	Fluid limit
	Na^+ limit
Postobstructive diuresis (valves, etc.)	3500$^+$ ml/M^2/24 hr for at least first day
	Use ½ NS plus appropriate K^+
Tubular dysfunction	Supplemental
Renal tubular acidosis	$NaHCO_3$, 2–3 mEq/kg/24 hr
Fanconi syndrome/cystinosis	Na^+, 2–5 mEq/kg/24 hr
Bartter syndrome	K^+, 2–5 mEq/kg/24 hr
Osmotic diuresis (postangiography)	Replace urine output with ½ N saline
Endocrine	
Diabetes insipidus	3000–3500 ml/M^2/24 hr
Diabetes mellitus in ketoacidosis	4000 ml/M^2/24 hr
	Supplement K^+ after urine produced
Congenital adrenocortical (adreno-	No K^+
genital) with Na^+ loss	Supplement Na^+
Addisonian crisis	No K^+
	Supplement Na^+
Cardiac	
Congestive heart failure	Reduce Na^+
Gastrointestinal	
Liver compromise	Reduce Na^+
	May need K^+ supplement
Respiratory	
Pneumonitis (SIADH)	⅔ maintenance
Iatrogenic	
Postanesthesia	Reduce fluids
Posthypothermia	Supplement fluids
Postextracorporeal circulation	Close attention to central venous pressure and fluids
Postangiography or IVP	Replace obligatory diuresis with ½ NS
Diuretics	May need K^+ supplement
	Watch for alkalosis
Accidents	
Poisoning	See Chapter 3
Burns	Add to maintenance: 2 ml Ringer's lactate × % burn surface × weight (kg) up to 5% body surface
	Maintenance for $AgNO_3$ therapy: 3000 ml/M^2/24 hr NS + 40 mEq/L KCl + protein 25 gm/M^2/24 hr
Drowning	½ maintenance

buffer" under whose cover the necessary ion shifts can occur a
reequilibration proceeds. Slow sugar metabolism then provides
continuous source of free water, delivered at a gentle rate.

(3) Treatment of acute **salt poisoning** requires peritoneal dialysi
using a high glucose, low-solute dialysate. The potential damag
can be reversed by furosemide diuresis (1 mg/kg), replacing th
urine output with a 10% D/W solution, monitoring sodium value
q4h and repeating the administration of furosemide.

V. SPECIAL PROBLEMS

A. **Limits on the use of multiple-electrolyte solution** are given in Table 8-12.

B. The **special management of IV therapy** in certain conditions is outlined i
Table 8-13.

C. **Surgery in the neonate**

1. Elective surgery Avoid dehydration. Do not put the patient on NPO fo
more than 4–6 hr prior to surgery.

2. Emergency surgery

a. Administer fluids evenly over the day. Avoid large solute or free
water loads.

b. In the first month of life, use approximately 1/6 N solution (NaCl, 2
mEq/L) with added KCl (20 mEq/L).

c. For pyloric stenosis with vomiting, correct hypochloremic alkalosi
before surgery. The infant may require 3–5 mEq K^+/kg/24 hr.

d. **Postoperatively,** there is usually excessive retention of water, Na^+
and Cl^-, with augmented K^+ loss via the urine, *but the newborn doe
not manifest antidiuresis or hyponatremia.*

9

Renal Disorders

I. ACUTE RENAL FAILURE

A. Prerenal failure
All patients with apparent acute renal failure must be assessed for a prerenal cause.

1. Etiology Renal perfusion and intrarenal blood flow are reduced due to dehydration, hypovolemia, or hemodynamic factors.

2. Evaluation

   a. Review the history and physical findings for shock, dehydration, and left ventricular heart failure.

   b. Measure the blood pressure and central venous pressure (CVP).

   c. Insert an indwelling bladder catheter to ascertain the urine output (less than 0.5 ml/kg/hr indicates severe oliguria) and to obtain urine for urinalysis, Na^+, K^+, creatinine, and osmolality (see Chap. 8).

3. Diagnosis The diagnosis of prerenal failure is confirmed by

   a. Diuresis in response to an increase in intravascular volume and rehydration.

   b. Improved renal function with improved cardiac function.

   c. Urinary sodium < 15 mEq/L.

   d. Urinary potassium ≥ 40 mEq/L.

   e. A ratio of urine urea to plasma urea > 10:1, or of urine creatinine to plasma creatinine > 10:1.

4. Therapy The object of therapy is to restore urinary flow.

   a. Insert an IV line for infusion of fluids and solute and for the measurement of CVP.

   b. Reestablish an effective circulating blood volume (see Chap. 2).

   c. If after restoration of extracellular fluid volume, oliguria or anuria persists, mannitol, 0.5 gm/kg of a 20% solution, should be infused over 10–20 min. This should result in an increase in urine output of approximately 6–10 ml/kg over the next 1–3 hr. **If no increase in urine flow occurs, no further mannitol should be given.**

   d. A trial dose of furosemide, 1 mg/kg, IV, should then be administered **after** the extracellular fluid volume is restored. Note that this agent will cause changes in urine electrolytes and osmolality, making a distinction between prerenal and renal oliguria more difficult.

   e. If marked oligoanuria persists, assess the patient immediately for intrinsic renal or postrenal failure (see **B**).

B. Intrinsic renal failure

1. **Etiology** The causes are parenchymal injury due to acute tubular necrosis, severe or prolonged prerenal failure, vascular lesion, hemolytic uremic syndrome, or nephritis.

2. **Evaluation and diagnosis** First, be sure the patient does not have prerenal or postrenal failure (see rest of this section). A history of decreased renal perfusion suggests acute renal failure due to acute tubular necrosis. Acute renal failure may be associated with acute glomerulonephritis, hemolytic uremic syndrome, accelerated hypertension, uric acid nephropathy, or vasculitis.

   a. Stabilize the patient prior to any invasive diagnostic procedures.

   b. Obtain estimates of renal function (see Chap. 8).

      (1) Urine plasma creatinine

      (2) Creatinine clearance

      (3) Urinary sodium concentration

      (4) Fractional sodium excretion (FE_{Na})

   c. Obtain a radionuclide renal scan for estimate of renal perfusion and function when possible. Abdominal ultrasound will be helpful in ruling out obstruction.

3. **Therapy**

   a. The use of an indwelling catheter **should be discontinued** as soon as possible in a severely oligoanuric patient in whom intrinsic renal failure is established.

   b. Weigh the patient twice daily (or use a metabolic bed with a scale).

   c. Measure intake and output.

   d. **Fluid replacement**

      (1) Fluid and electrolyte replacement should be calculated as insensible losses (Table 8-7) plus urine output (if the patient is not edematous or does not have fluid overload).

      (2) As many calories as possible are given, orally if practical. A peripheral IV line can tolerate 20% glucose; a central line can tolerate more.

      (3) With fluid restrictions, weight should decrease by approximately 0.5 percent daily.

      (4) When diuresis begins, increasing urine volume must be replaced with a solution containing approximately the same electrolytes as are being excreted. If patient has been hyperkalemic, do not replace K^+ until the serum K^+ has returned to normal.

   e. **Nutrition** Optimal calories and protein nitrogen will help to decrease catabolism, lower BUN, ameliorate the uremic state, and improve healing and the immune response. With restricted fluids, little nitrogen and only 15–25 percent of calories can be given by a peripheral IV line.

      (1) If the patient can take fluids PO, add Polycose, which gives 2 kcal/ml in solution (600 mOsm/L) with cream. Add an oral amino acid mixture such as Aminade.

(2) If the patient will be npo for over a week and renal failure is profound, consider total parenteral nutrition (see Chap. 11).

f. Hyperkalemia

(1) If the serum K^+ is 5.5–7.0 mEq/L, Kayexalate at a dose of 1 gm/kg may be given PO or PR and repeated every hour until K^+ is lowered (see Chap. 8).

(2) If the serum K^+ is above 7 mEq/L, or ECG changes, or arrhythmias, or both, are present, the following immediate therapy is indicated:

(a) Sodium bicarbonate, 2.5 mEq/kg, as an IV push over 10–15 min.

(b) Calcium gluconate, 10%, 0.5 ml/kg IV over 5–10 min, with ECG monitoring.

(c) Glucose, 50%, 1 ml/kg. Follow with a 30% glucose IV infusion.

(3) If hyperkalemia persists, insulin, 0.5 U/kg IV, should be given while infusing 20% glucose. This dose may be repeated in 30–60 min if necessary. Prepare to dialyze the patient.

(4) Dialysis is usually necessary if K^+ is above 7.5, if the measures in **(2)** fail, or if **(3)** is needed.

g. Hypertension If hypertension is acute and severe (3 S.D. above the age-appropriate norms), treat as outlined for hypertensive emergencies in Sec. **III.A**, p. 215. Note that in acute renal failure

(1) Antihypertensive agents with rapid onset of action should be selected.

(2) Phlebotomy, or dialysis, or both, should be used when hypertension is severe and unresponsive to medical management.

h. Congestive heart failure See also Chap. 10.

(1) Congestive heart failure (CHF) can usually be prevented by proper **fluid restriction.**

(2) There is no place for diuretics in the anuric patient.

(3) Digitalis will not produce a dramatic effect.

(4) Digitalization must be done slowly and maintenance doses reduced as dictated by renal function. If CHF is severe, dialysis is indicated.

i. Acidosis can usually be alleviated by providing glucose for calories as well as 1–3 mEq/kg/day of exogenous bicarbonate, citrate, or lactate. **Warning:** A milliequivalent of bicarbonate contains 1 mEq of Na^+ or K^+. If acidosis is severe and treatment is difficult due to fluid overload, dialysis is indicated.

j. Seizures See Chap. 21.

C. Postrenal failure

1. Etiology Obstruction is usually due to congenital anomalies, urethral stricture, hematuria, or tumor.

2. Evaluation and diagnosis Obstruction is suggested by a history of genitourinary abnormalities, or lower abdominal trauma, or by the finding of flank masses or an enlarged bladder. Bilateral ureteral obstruction is suggested by absolute anuria.

   a. If creatinine is < 5 mg/100 ml or the urine-plasma creatinine ratio is > 15, an intravenous pyelogram (IVP) may be attempted. (Do a nuclide scan, and an ultrasonogram if facilities are available.)

   b. Urologic consultation should be obtained.

   c. Cystoscopy with a unilateral retrograde pyelogram may be considered if anuria and obstruction are suggested.

3. Therapy consists in surgical correction or bypass, as required.

II. CHRONIC RENAL DISEASE

A. Etiology   Almost half of chronic renal failure (CRF) is due to congenital causes—obstructive uropathy, renal dysplasia, juvenile nephronophthisis, or polycystic disease. About a third of CRF in childhood is due to glomerulopathy. As a cause of CRF chronic pyelonephritis is rare in the absence of an obstructive congenital lesion or marked reflux. Other causes include hemolytic uremic syndrome, malignant hypertension, interstitial nephritis, and renal vein thrombosis.

B. General therapeutic measures

1. Nutrition   Growth may be improved by appropriate dietary management. The limiting factor is the GFR.

   a. Fluid   The aim is to replace insensible losses and urine output (see Chap. 8). **For the patient in chronic renal failure, fluid restriction can be more detrimental than overhydration.**

   b. Calories   In fasting conditions, an obligatory loss of 25–35 cal/kg/day occurs. Since 50 percent is normally contributed by carbohydrates, the minimal administration of glucose necessary to avoid increased tissue breakdown is 400 gm/M^2 daily, or 3–4 gm/kg in the small child.

   c. Protein

   (1) The obligatory excretion of nitrogen through the kidney makes a progressive restriction of protein necessary. While the GFR remains above 25 percent of normal, any reasonable diet is usually tolerated.

   (2) The progression of renal disease decreases osmotic tolerance, and some protein restriction is necessary. (Each gram of protein contains 6 mOsm urea.) As the GFR decreases from 25 to 10 percent of normal, a decrease of urinary concentration ability from 900 to 300 mOsm/L occurs, forcing a restricted protein diet of 1.5–2.0 gm/kg/day. At these levels, proteins of high biologic value (egg, meat, milk) should be used in order to satisfy essential amino acid requirements.

   (3) For infants, the use of human milk or a human-like milk formula is lifesaving, and preferences for one could depend on the degree of renal failure (see Tables 5-2 to 5-5).

   (4) As renal function falls below 10 percent of normal and approximates zero, further restrictions are necessary until dialysis is started.

   (a) If hemodialysis is instituted on a schedule of 3 times a week, liberalization of the protein intake is then possible to a daily intake of 2–3 gm protein/kg (minimum), 2 gm Na$^+$/day, and 2 gm K$^+$/day.

(b) A gradual increase in protein intake to 2 gm/kg or more daily can produce growth in a substantial number of children in renal failure.

d. Multivitamins Daily administration of 1–2 standard multivitamin tablets or equivalent liquid preparations covers the basic requirements. Folic acid, 1–2 mg/kg/day, should be added as more severe renal failure supervenes.

e. Sodium

(1) To avoid arterial hypertension, sodium intake should be limited, except when significant osmotic diuresis produces renal sodium wasting. A "no-salt-added" diet is usually the maximal restriction needed under these circumstances or with the nephrotic syndrome. It provides 40–90 mEq Na^+/day (2–4 gm Na), depending on the amount used in cooking.

(2) If such a diet is not sufficient, it may be combined with antihypertensive drugs, diuretics, or both.

(3) If salt wasting occurs, free salt intake may be necessary (see Chap. 8). Daily requirements are estimated by monitoring urinary sodium excretion and by the appearance of pitting edema and hypertension, indicating excessive salt administration. If sodium bicarbonate must be used, careful monitoring is necessary.

f. Potassium

(1) Hypokalemia (See also Chap. 8.) Hypokalemia is a common complication in the management of the patient with edema and secondary hyperaldosteronism (especially in the nephrotic patient during spontaneous or corticosteroid-induced diuresis and the patient with polyuric renal disease complicated by an acute GI disorder). Unless renal failure supervenes, none of these patients will require any dietary potassium restrictions; rather, they will require potassium supplementation, as follows:

(a) Potassium chloride, 300-mg tablet with 4 mEq per tablet, or a 1 mM/ml solution. **Enteric-coated tablets should not be used** because of their intestinal insolubility. Of the available preparations, K-Lor (a pineapple-orange–flavored powder in a 25 mEq/packet) is the most palatable. If chloride is chosen because of alkalosis, K-Lor can be mixed in fruit juice and given in 3–4 doses over the day.

(b) Potassium bicarbonate, 300-mg capsules with 3 mEq per capsule, or Shohl's solution, 140 gm citric acid + 100 gm sodium citrate or potassium citrate dissolved in water to 1 L.

(c) The requirement may range from 1–2 to 2–5 mEq/kg/day and even higher in long-standing renal tubular disease.

(d) Triamterene (smallest available tablet = 50 mg) can aid in the prevention of urinary K^+ losses and works well for chronic conditions such as cystinosis or Bartter syndrome. (**Note:** In Bartter syndrome, inhibitors of prostaglandin synthetase [aspirin, indomethacin] have produced striking improvements in potassium balance.) Doses of 2–4 mg/kg daily or on alternate days can substantially reduce the need for K^+ supplements when urinary loss is a major factor.

(e) Prolonged hypokalemia will lead to secondary metabolic alkalosis and possible paradoxical aciduria if the patient also has a sodium deficit. If the hypokalemia is severe (less than 2 mEq/L serum), IV replacement should be given at 4–5 mEq/kg/day as potassium chloride (2 mEq/ml), at least in the first 24 hr, and continued according to the laboratory results and urinary output.

   (f) In renal tubular acidosis, cystinosis, postobstructive diuresis, and acute tubular necrosis, serum K^+ levels of less than 1 mEq/L may be found, and the required replacement may exceed the maximal recommended IV fluid potassium concentration of 40–80 mEq/L and reach 150–200 mEq/L. (Such a concentration may be extremely caustic to the vessel wall, but lifesaving.)

(2) Hyperkalemia   Conditions that usually lead to hyperkalemia are

   (a) The onset of severe renal failure or sudden oliguria due to vomiting, diarrhea, or both, or to GI bleeding.

   (b) The indiscriminate administration of aldosterone antagonists (spironolactone) or inhibitors of distal tubular sodium-potassium exchange (triamterene).

   (c) Drugs containing K^+, such as potassium penicillin.

   (d) Massive hemolysis or tissue destruction.

   (e) Treatment   Serum K^+ levels below 5.8 mEq/L are usually well handled by further restrictions in potassium intake, using the following guidelines:

   Fruits* high in K^+: Bananas, oranges (citrus), cantaloupe, watermelon, apricots, raisins, prunes, pineapples, and cherries.
   Vegetables* high in K^+: green leafy vegetables, potatoes, avocado, artichoke, lentils, and beets.
   Meats and fish high in K^+: All have K^+ content (lowest are chicken liver, shrimp, and crab).
   Breads and flours highest in K^+: Pumpernickel, buckwheat, and soy.
   Miscellaneous foods high in K^+: Chocolate, cocoa, brown (not white) sugar, molasses, nuts, and peanut butter.
      The potassium content of commonly used beverages is given in Table 9-1. Serum levels above 5.8 mEq/L must be treated with an exchange resin to remove K^+ from the body, or by temporizing measures until dialysis can be started (see I and Chap. 8).

2. Mineral metabolism in renal disease   Secondary hyperparathyroidism and metabolic bone disease occur in renal insufficiency (< GFR 25 percent of normal) unless vigorous measures are taken.

   a. Hyperphosphatemia   If the serum phosphatase level is over 5 mEq/L or if alkaline phosphate is elevated, dietary phosphate must be restricted and oral phosphate binders administered. Once phosphate is normalized, vitamin D (as dihydrotachysterol or actual D_3 analogues) and oral calcium supplements are used.
      Because of hypermagnesemia already present in patients with chronic renal failure, plain aluminum hydroxide (Amphojel, 300-mg and 600-mg tablets, 300 mg/5 ml liquid) is preferable as an **oral phos**

*Cooking bleaches out K^+; cook these foods.

Table 9-1   Potassium Content of Beverages

High K$^+$	mEq/L	Low K$^+$	mEq/L
Milk	36	Ginger ale	0.1
Cola	13	Pepsi-Cola	0.8
Orange juice	49		
Grape juice	31		
Tomato juice	59		

phate binder to magnesium-containing preparations such as Gelusil. The dose is 300–1800 mg/dose immediately after meals. Phosphate binders must be given with or just after all meals and snacks to bind the phosphate in the diet; otherwise, they are ineffective. Other acceptable preparations are Basaljel, Alu-Cap, ALternaGEL, Nephrox, and cookies or bread made from preparations. (ALternaGEL is especially tasty for young children, and is twice as potent as Amphojel.)

b. Calcium balance   In general, good control of serum phosphorus levels should precede the administration of calcium, but seizures or other complications make immediate treatment with calcium unavoidable.

   (1) Hypocalcemia   See Chap. 8.

      (a) Acute replacement is needed only if the patient is symptomatic, i.e., has hypocalcemic seizures or tetany. Then 10–15 mg calcium/kg is given IV q4h as 10% calcium gluconate or 22% calcium gluceptate. The correcting effects last only a few hours, and a new infusion or further PO administration is required.

      (b) Oral preparations   Calcium lactate is the oral preparation that is best tolerated. However, its low calcium content per weight (18 percent) requires ingestion of many tablets (each 300-mg tablet contains 54 mg of calcium) to provide the minimal allowance of 500–1000 mg/day. Concomitant administration of approximately 10–20 mg/kg/day of vitamin D will improve intestinal absorption.

   (2) Hypercalcemia   Although hypercalcemia is not common in renal disease it is a possible complication of indiscriminate use of vitamin D, severe secondary hyperparathyroidism, and inappropriate dialysate concentration of calcium (see Chap. 8). If acute hypercalcemia occurs and immediate treatment is necessary, the following measures should be carried out:

      (a) Reduce calcium intake   Special milk formulas are available with minimal calcium content (< 100 mg/day). Discontinue the administration of vitamin D in any form (as in multivitamins).

      (b) Administer IV saline   Use 1–2 L/M^2 in acute severe hypercalcemia if urine output is adequate.

      (c) Decrease the absorption of calcium   Decrease gut absorption by administration of corticosteroids (prednisone, 1–2 mg/kg/day). This takes days to act.

      (d) Phosphate salts are best reserved for patients unresponsive to the preceding measures. Because IV infusion of sodium phos-

phate is itself dangerous, often producing metastatic soft tissue calcification and an abrupt fall in calcium, the preferred
route of administration is PR. Sodium phosphate (Phospho
Soda contains 3.3 gm/5 ml) may be given as an enema or one
can simply administer a Fleet enema.

(e) **Hemodialysis** may be used to control severe hypercalcemia.

c. **Vitamin D**

(1) The use of dihydrotachysterol is recommended to improve intestinal resorption and increase the parathyroid hormone–end-organ
responsiveness, avoiding inappropriate hypertrophy of the parathyroid gland.

(a) Administration should start as soon as the GFR falls below
25–20 percent of normal and hyperphosphatemia is no longer
present; the initial dosage should be conservative (0.125 mg
M^2/day), and follow-up should include periodic urinary
calcium-creatinine ratio and serum calcium levels. These will
be needed as long as dihydrotachysterol is administered and
for 2–3 weeks thereafter.

(b) One milligram of dihydrotachysterol is approximately equivalent to 3 mg (120,000 U) of vitamin D_2.

(c) If vitamin D toxicity develops and is recognized early, the loss
in renal function will probably be reversible.

(d) Patients should be cautioned to decrease their vitamin D intake
when traveling or moving to areas with higher sun exposure.

(2) 1,25-Dihydroxycholecalciferol (1,25-hydroxy vitamin D, calcitriol,
Rocaltrol) is now available, though its safety and efficacy in young
children have not been established. The initial dose is 0.25 μg/
day for older children. Adult hemodialysis patients require 0.5 to
1.0 μg/day; the exact pediatric dose must be determined for
each child. The advantage of calcitriol may be a short half-life
with pharmacologic activity 3–5 days/dose.

3. **Anticonvulsant therapy**   See also Chap. 21.

a. The usual causes for seizures in the renal patient with preserved
renal function are hypertensive encephalopathy, severe metabolic alkalosis with relative hypocalcemia, or hypomagnesemia following
hyponatremia underlying CNS complications.

b. In chronic renal failure, the appearance of seizures is most probably
due to acute acid-base and electrolyte changes, and a careful evaluation of acid-base and electrolyte status should always be done to provide adequate therapy.

c. Disequilibrium following dialysis may cause convulsions, which are
best treated by a change in dialysis procedures.

d. Therapy depends on etiology. See Chap. 21 for appropriate management.

4. **Peritoneal dialysis**   The indications for dialysis in renal failure are intractable congestive heart failure, increasing acidosis, intractable
hyperkalemia, and continuing clinical deterioration. Every case should
be judged on its own merits. The decision to dialyze should not be made
on the basis of one isolated laboratory value.

a. Procedure

(1) Disposable catheter sets are now available for pediatric peritoneal dialysis.

(2) After it is certain that the bladder is empty, the skin of the abdomen is prepared in a sterile fashion.

(3) To make insertion easier and decrease the risk of perforation of intraabdominal contents, the abdominal cavity is distended by an initial load of dialysis fluid (approximately 20 ml/kg) introduced through an 18- or 20-gauge needle inserted at the potential catheter site.

(4) The catheter is inserted, usually in the midline, one-third of the distance between the umbilicus and the symphysis pubis. It can then be advanced to the left lower or right lower quadrant and connected to the tubing.

(5) The usual amount of fluid exchanged is 20 ml/kg initially, with a gradual increase to 40–50 ml/kg per exchange. (The initial loading fluid is not removed. The presence of such a reservoir will ensure that all the holes in the catheter are under water and will prevent air block.) The fluid is usually warmed to body temperature, then permitted to run in as fast as is tolerated, allowed to equilibrate for 15–20 min, and then drained (usual time is 15–30 min). At every sixth cycle the abdomen is allowed to drain dry, a specimen is sent for culture, and the patient is weighed, unless a constant read-out bed scale is available.

(6) The usual dialysis is carried on for 36–72 hr, depending on the indications and the patient's clinical status. The danger of infection increases after 48 hr.

b. Factors affecting dialysis

(1) Clearance Urea is cleared at the rate of 14–30 ml/min at 20°C. Creatinine is cleared at a slower rate of 10–15 ml/min.

(2) Temperature Warming the solution will decrease heat loss (especially important in small infants) and, more important, will increase urea clearance.

(3) Rate Increasing the flow of the dialysis fluid will shorten the time for dialysis, but is expensive and will increase protein loss and aggravate hyperglycemia.

c. Solutions

(1) Usually, 1.5% glucose and water with added electrolytes is used. Prepared solutions are available.

(2) Prepared solutions contain no potassium; K^+ should be added as required. In patients with hyperkalemia, except in those on digitalis, no K^+ needs to be added to the initial three to five exchanges; subsequently 2.5–3.5 mEq/L may be added to the dialyzing fluid (see Table 9-2 for the composition of a standard solution).

(3) The 1.5% glucose solution as used in dialysis is hyperosmolar (372 mOsm/L) and thus can cause appreciable fluid loss (up to 200–300 ml/hr). For removal of excess fluid, **glucose** can be added to increase the osmolality of the solution as desired. However, the use of solutions of higher osmolality can rapidly dehydrate infants and children (4.25% glucose = 525 mOsm/L; 7.5% glucose = 678

Table 9-2 Composition of a Standard Peritoneal Dialysis Solution (McGaw)

Sodium	140 mEq/L
Chloride	101 mEq/L
Calcium	4.0 mEq/L
Magnesium	1.5 mg/L
Acetate	45 mg/L

mOsm/L). Thus all patients being dialyzed should be weighed often and kept in fluid balance.

(4) Heparin (500–1000 U/L) should be added to the first liter of dialysate and continued if the fluid is not clear.

(5) When dialyzing for certain toxins, various additives such as albumin are useful in increasing removal.

d. **Infection** is usually due to *Staphylococcus aureus* and gram-negative organisms. Culture of fluid should be done every sixth cycle. Antibiotics are not advised for routine use, but treatment should be begun in a symptomatic patient even if culture results are not available (see Chap. 15). If intraperitoneal antibiotics are used, they must be given with extreme care, since high blood levels can result from peritoneal absorption.

e. **Hyperglycemia** is a special problem in diabetic patients, but it can also occur in nondiabetic patients and result in nonketotic hyperosmolar coma. The blood sugar must be monitored routinely in patients dialyzed with a 4.25% solution.

f. **Hypoproteinemia** can occur; about 0.5 gm/L of protein is lost in dialysis.

g. **Perforation** The risk of perforation of abdominal organs (e.g., bladder, bowel) can be reduced appreciably by distending the abdominal cavity with dialysate and emptying the bladder before catheter insertion [see **a.(3)**].

5. **Hemodialysis** Hemodialysis for childhood CRF is practical and should be available to all patients. It is more efficient than peritoneal dialysis, and children have been maintained by hemodialysis for years. Appropriate consultation should be obtained if the source is available.

6. **Transplantation** Transplantation is preferable to chronic dialysis for most children with CRF. Any child with CRF should be considered a transplant candidate. Though transplantation cannot be considered curative, long-term survival is the rule, and transplantation optimally offers the chance for rehabilitation from CRF. Referral to a transplant center should be made.

III. **HYPERTENSION** in CRF prior to need for dialysis should be treated with drugs (see below). In dialysis patients, hypertension is usually controlled with adequate ultrafiltration on hemodialysis.

Hypertension is suggested by blood pressure values (taken with a cuff of appropriate size covering two-thirds of the upper arm) that are 2 S.D. above the mean or above the 95th percentile for age. (Values for various age groups

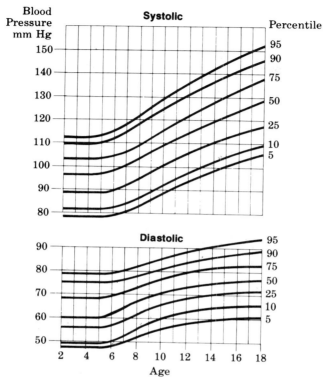

Figure 9-1 Percentiles of blood pressure measurement in boys (right arm, seated). (From *Pediatrics* 59:803, 1977, with permission.)

are depicted in Figs. 9-1 and 9-2.) *Any diastolic* blood pressure above 95 mm Hg in a small child or above 110 in a larger child requires immediate parenteral control. Such control is also necessary if blood pressure elevation has caused CNS or cardiac symptoms.

The curability of hypertension in children is greater than in adults. Primary (essential) hypertension in childhood has been identified in up to 30 percent in various series, but its natural history, both untreated and treated, remains to be delineated. Unless blood pressure is routinely recorded as part of the general physical examination, hypertension may be overlooked for considerable periods of time.

A. Hypertensive crisis In acute, severe hypertension, the immediate short-term goal is control of blood pressure. Simultaneously, there should be a program of medical or surgical investigation, or both, and treatment aimed at long-term control. The usual effective doses of antihypertensive medications are given in **1–6**; many patients require less, some more. Diuretics [see Sec. **B.2** and p. 240, Sec. **b(3)**] given concomitantly IV often will be helpful.

1. Diazoxide (Hyperstat) is the most practical effective drug for acute hypertension now available. A benzothiazide with no diuretic effect, it acts

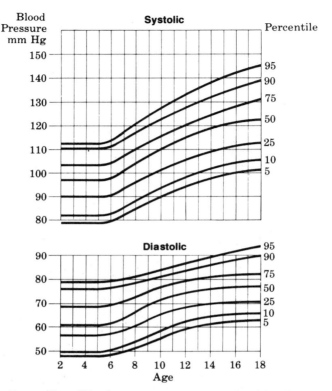

Figure 9-2 Percentiles of blood pressure measurement in girls (right arm, seated). (From *Pediatrics* 59:803, 1977, with permission.)

directly on the vessels' smooth muscles, promptly and effectively reducing muscle tone. Diazoxide does not reduce renal blood flow.

a. It is administered only IV (5 mg/kg/dose) **as fast as possible** to obtain minimal binding to serum protein and maximal action on the smooth muscle. The average fall in both systolic and diastolic pressures is 44 mm Hg, which occurs a few minutes after administration, and the effects last 3–15 hr. If the initial dose proves ineffective, a second can be tried after 15–20 min.

b. Disadvantages The effect of diazoxide cannot be titrated. It causes hyperglycemia and can cause sodium and fluid retention. Transient tachycardia often follows administration.

2. Sodium nitroprusside (Nipride) must be used as an IV drip with constant intensive care unit (ICU) monitoring. It is universally effective, since it causes immediate vasodilation and lowers pressure. The effects disappear when the IV drip is stopped.

a. The dose is 0.5 to 8.0 μg/kg/min. **Note:** The prepared solution (look at method every time to avoid error) is inactivated by light. Do not use with other drugs in same IV line.

b. Blood levels of thiocyanate must be checked daily, since nitroprusside is converted to thiocyanate by the hepatic enzyme rhodanase. **Caution** is necessary in the presence of hepatic insufficiency.

c. Advantages   The onset of action is instantaneous. Nitroprusside is effective when all other drugs have failed. The rate of infusion can be titrated against desired blood pressure.

d. Disadvantages   Nitroprusside requires constant supervision in the ICU. Discontinuance of the IV drip means instantaneous loss of the pharmacologic effect.

3. Hydralazine (Apresoline)   When hydralazine is given IM, the onset of action is within 15–30 min. Onset after IV administration is immediate.

   a. Dosage

   (1) Hydralazine is given parenterally at an initial dosage of 0.15 mg/kg, which is progressively increased q6h to up to 10 times the initial dose, according to the response.

   (2) When given with diazoxide or reserpine, the dose needed may be smaller than when given alone.

   (3) For the oral dose, see **B.3.**

   b. Advantages   Renal blood flow is not reduced; it is effective fairly rapidly; and it seldom produces hypotension. It can be used with diazoxide, propranolol, methyldopa, or reserpine.

   c. Disadvantages   The most important side effects are tachycardia, nausea, vomiting, headache, diarrhea, and positive lupus erythematosus (LE) and rheumatoid factor (RF) reactions (very rare in children). The drug should be avoided in patients with arrhythmias and heart failure. It is not consistently effective.

4. Propranolol (Inderal) is a beta-adrenergic blocker and is most safely given PO. It also has antirenin action. For discussion, see Chap. 10, Sec. **II.C.3.**

5. Methyldopa (Aldomet) is an inhibitor of dopa decarboxylase, and is metabolized to alpha-methyl norepinephrine, a weak pressor that displaces norepinephrine at nerve endings.

   a. Dosage

   (1) IV dosage is from 10–50 mg/kg daily, administered in 4 divided doses q6h, beginning with 10 mg/kg/24 hr and doubling each subsequent dose until the desired effect is obtained. It is recommended that it be diluted in 5% D/W and be given over 30–60 min. A paradoxical rise in blood pressure can be seen with too rapid injection.

   (2) Oral dose   See **B.3.**

   b. Advantages   Gradual lowering of blood pressure. The renin level is also lowered.

   c. Disadvantages   Side effects are minimal but include drug fever and hemolytic anemia with a positive Coombs test, positive LE cell reaction, positive RF, granulocytopenia, and thrombocytopenia. Methyldopa is not recommended for patients with pheochromocytoma. Both methyldopa and its metabolites produce false-positive blood and urine tests for pheochromocytoma.

6. Reserpine   The rauwolfia alkaloids deplete stores of catecholamines and

5-hydroxytryptamine in many organs. Depletion starts 1 hr after administration and becomes maximal by 24 hr. Tissue catecholamines are slowly restored, and repeated doses have a cumulative action even at intervals of a week or longer.

   a. Dosage   In acute hypertensive crisis, the recommended IM dosage is 0.07 mg/kg/dose q4–6h (in patients weighing over 25 kg, an initial dose of 1–2 mg should be given and subsequent doses based on the response) followed by an oral maintenance dose of 0.02 mg/kg/day. As the cumulative effect of the drug takes place, this dose usually can be reduced to 0.1–0.5 mg/day, given in 1 dose.

   b. Advantages   Consistent and gradual lowering of blood pressure.

   c. Disadvantages   Somnolence; mental depression is almost never seen in children; night terrors may occur. Nasal stuffiness is common and is generally well tolerated. However, reserpine should not be used in the neonate who is an obligate nose breather.

B. Mild and/or chronic hypertension   Symptomatic therapy should consist of

   1. Diet   If blood pressure elevation is mild, a low-salt diet alone may be tried first.

   2. Diuretics   (Table 10-1) may be used if mild hypertension fails to respond to diet.

   3. Antihypertensive agents should be added if **1** and **2** do not control blood pressure *or* if hypertension is moderately to severely elevated (see **A**). The doses are as follows:

   a. Hydralazine   1 mg/kg/24 hr initially, up to 200 mg/day PO in 3–4 doses. Increase at intervals of 3–4 days.

   b. Propranolol   See p. 232.

   c. Methyldopa   10 mg/kg/24 hr PO initially. Increase the dose to a maximum of 40 mg/kg/24 hr PO. Increase at intervals of 3–7 days.

   d. Reserpine   0.25–0.5 mg PO/day initially, up to a maximum of 2 mg.

   e. Clonidine (Catapres) is a central alpha-adrenergic stimulator.

      (1) Available only PO in 0.1-mg and 0.2-mg tablets, clonidine may be used at starting dose of 0.1 mg.

      (2) It works well with a diuretic, or propranolol, or both.

      (3) An important side effect is severe rebound hypertension if doses are missed, even for as short a time as 16 hr. **The drug must be tapered if discontinuation is planned.**

   f. Guanethidine sulfate is an adrenergic neuron-blocking agent with a tissue catecholamine–store depletion effect. It is a long-acting medication with a cumulative effect.

      (1) Dosage is 0.2 mg/kg/24 hr in a single dose PO, increasing by the same dose at weekly intervals until the desired effect is achieved.

      (2) Postural hypotension is a serious and common complication. Muscle weakness and diarrhea are less often seen. A rise in BUN thought to be secondary to decreased cardiac output and edema without heart failure can also occur.

   g. Minoxidil, a potent vasodilator, may be used in hypertension that is extremely difficult to control. This drug is still investigational.

h. Prazosin (Minipress), a smooth muscle relaxant, is available for children over age 12. The initial dose is 1 mg tid. The maximum dose is usually 20 mg/day.

IV. RENAL TUBULAR ACIDOSIS (RTA)
This syndrome consists of hyperchloremic acidosis associated with normal or slightly decreased glomerular function and inappropriately alkaline urine.

A. Proximal renal tubular acidosis

1. Etiology A tubular defect producing an abnormally low threshold for $NaHCO_3$ is present.

2. Evaluation and diagnosis

   a. Growth failure is usually present.

   b. Arterial blood gases and serum electrolytes reveal a hyperchloremic acidosis with normal K^+ and Ca levels.

   c. Urine pH varies with the degree of acidemia. **All urine for pH should be collected under oil and measured while fresh.** A urine pH of less than 5.5 and a serum $NaHCO_3$ below the patient's renal threshold are seen in severe acidemia.

   d. A bicarbonate titration test may be done by infusing $NaHCO_3$ slowly (e.g., 1–2 mEq/kg over 1 hr) when the patient is acidotic and measuring serum HCO_3^- levels, urine pH, titratable acidity, and ammonium excretion. The renal threshold for HCO_3^- resorption in proximal RTA will be below the norms for children of comparable age.

3. Therapy

   a. Large doses of bicarbonate (10–15 mEq/kg/day) are required to maintain serum pH. In primary proximal RTA the dose is decreased after 6 months to determine if the threshold is still abnormal, in which case acidosis will redevelop when therapy is stopped.

   b. A repeat bicarbonate titration test should be performed, since it appears that the disorder improves spontaneously after 2–3 years and some children will recover.

B. Distal renal tubular acidosis

1. Etiology A defect in the distal tubule is present, resulting in an inability to establish a hydrogen ion gradient between blood and tubular fluid.

2. Evaluation

   a. The presenting symptoms are usually growth failure, polyuria, and polydipsia.

   b. Arterial blood gases and serum electrolytes reveal a hyperchloremic acidosis, with hypokalemia seen in a number of patients.

   c. The urine pH is rarely below 6.5, even in the face of severe existing acidemia.

   d. Concentrating ability is markedly impaired, with maximal urine osmolalities of less than 450 mOsm.

   e. Urinary calcium excretion is elevated (above 2 mg/kg/day).

   f. The GFR may be decreased.

   g. Ammonium chloride loading test If the urine pH is spontaneously 5 or less even in an acidemic patient this test is not necessary as the patient has proximal RTA. To distinguish disease of the proximal from the distal tubule, an ammonium chloride loading test may be done (Table 9-3). The test is done by administering 75 mEq/M² ammonium chloride followed by measurement of the urine pH, titratable acidity, and ammonium excretion. The serum HCO_3^- concentration should fall to 17 mEq/L or less. If it does not, a larger dose of ammonium chloride (150 mEq/M²) should be given cautiously on a second testing day.

h. X-rays will reveal nephrocalcinosis in many patients.

3. The **diagnosis** is confirmed by performing an ammonium chloride loading test. There is an inability to acidify the urine below 6.5, with depressed rates of excretion of titratable acid and ammonium.

4. Treatment

a. Sodium and potassium bicarbonate and citrate in daily doses of 1–3 mEq will correct the acidosis, improve growth, and normalize the GFR. However, they will not reverse nephrocalcinosis or improve concentrating ability.

b. There is no indication at present that children will recover spontaneously from distal tubular acidosis, and therapy must be continued for life.

c. The dose of sodium and potassium bicarbonate and citrate should be adjusted according to the blood pH, and daily urine calcium excretion should be kept below 2 mg/kg. Plasma K^+ must be monitored, and some patients require all their bicarbonate as potassium bicarbonate.

V. DISORDERS WITH PROTEINURIA

A. Etiology   Increased protein excretion occurs with or without renal pathology; massive proteinuria (> 2 gm/M²/day) always indicates renal disease.

1. Mild to moderate proteinuria (200–500 mg/day) may be seen with fever, dehydration, exercise, cold exposure, hypermetabolic states, heart failure, constrictive pericarditis, or lower urinary tract disease. **Orthostatic proteinuria** occurs without signs of renal disease.

2. Casts or altered renal function may be seen with either minimal or massive proteinuria.

a. Minimal proteinuria **with** hematuria suggests a focal nephritis, vascular disease, or an infectious process. **Without** hematuria, it suggests tubulointerstitial disease, "inactive" nephritis, congenital abnormalities of the kidneys, or drug toxicity.

Table 9-3 Ammonium Chloride Loading Test (Normal Values)

Age	Urine pH	Titratable Acid (μEq/min/1.73 M²)	Ammonium Excretion (μEq/min/1.73 M²)
1–12 months	5.0	62 (43–111)	57 (42–79)
4–15 years	5.5	52 (33–71)	73 (46–100)

Adapted from C. Edelmann et al., *Pediatr. Res.* 1:452, 1967; *J. Clin. Invest.* 46:1309, 1967. Although current data are sparse, normal values for ages 1–4 years appear to approximate those of older children.

b. **Massive** proteinuria **with** hematuria suggests renal vein thrombosis, significant glomerulopathy (with or without systemic disease), or malignant hypertension. **Without** hematuria, it suggests minimal lesion nephrotic syndrome, membranous nephropathy, and is consistent with the presence of amyloid, diabetic nephropathy, or myeloma.

B. **Evaluation and Diagnosis** In healthy adults protein excretion is 30–100 mg/day; in children, it is 100 mg/day; in infants (1 month of age), 240 mg/M^2/day.

1. Note how sample was collected; look for fever, metabolic stress, etc., which might cause proteinuria. Recheck for protein on two more occasions to be certain that the patient is proteinuric.

2. Look for orthostatic (postural) proteinuria: (a) Check A.M. and P.M. urines with dipstick; A.M. should be negative. Obtain 12-hour daytime (active) urine and 12-hour night-time (recumbent) urine collections. The recumbent urine collection should have **completely normal** protein excretion.

3. **Urinalysis** and **culture** are necessary. Watch for false-positive reactions caused by tolbutamide, penicillins, sulfonamides, radiologic contrast material, or zephiran. Recheck patient after a suitable interval.

4. Evaluation of history, clinical features, and laboratory results suggests diagnostic category.

5. Persistent, constant (seen in all postures) proteinuria may require referral to a nephrologist for further evaluation and possible renal biopsy.

C. **Treatment** No therapy is needed for orthostatic proteinuria; therapy of proteinuria due to other causes depends on the diagnosis (Fig. 9-3).

VI. **NEPHROTIC SYNDROME** The nephrotic syndrome is characterized by proteinuria, edema, hypoproteinemia, and hyperlipidemia. The incidence is 1.0 per 100,000 among whites and 2.8 per 100,000 among nonwhites under 16 years of age. The peak incidence is between 2–3 years (75 percent of cases occur in children under 5 years of age).

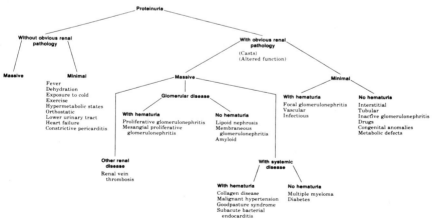

Figure 9-3 Proteinuria with and without obvious renal pathology.

A. Etiology   The nephrotic syndrome can occur as part of the clinical course of any progressive glomerulonephritis, but the pathogenesis is unknown.

B. Evaluation

   1. History   A history of infection or nephritis is sought.

   2. Physical examination   A careful assessment should include weight, blood pressure, sites and extent of edema, and cardiac status.

   3. Laboratory evaluation includes 24-hr urinary protein, serum protein and A/G ratio, urinary serum protein electrophoresis, serum lipid, BUN, electrolytes, creatinine clearance, C3, and selective protein index (ratio of IgG-transferrin clearances with selectivity [as opposed to nonselectivity] ≤ 0.2).

   4. The presence of gross hematuria, a low C3, unselective proteinuria, an age of presentation below 2 months or over 10 years, a failure to respond to steroids, elevated BUN, or elevated blood pressure should cast doubt on the diagnosis of lipoid nephrosis, and a renal biopsy should be performed.

C. Diagnosis   A combination of the defined clinical features with proteinuria in excess of 1 gm/M^2/24 hr confirms the diagnosis. **However, all features need not be present,** especially early in relapse.

D. Treatment

   1. Drugs   (generally for minimal lesion nephrotic syndrome only)

   a. Steroids are the treatment of choice, usually 2 mg/kg/day of prednisone PO in divided doses (maximum dose of 80 mg should not be exceeded). This regimen is continued until the urine is protein free for 3–10 days, or for up to 4–8 weeks if the urine fails to become protein free. (Lack of response by 8 weeks suggests steroid resistance.) Following this, a further alternate-day regimen is generally given in a reduced dose (1.0 to 1.5 mg/kg/day as 1 dose q48h) for a month, after which it is tapered over 2–3 weeks and discontinued.

   b. Immunosuppression   In patients who fail to respond to prednisone, a trial of immunosuppressive therapy may be indicated. Such therapy appears to be more effective in patients who are frequent "relapsers" and require many or prolonged courses of prednisone; it appears less effective in those who show no response to corticosteroids. **Immunosuppressive therapy should only be undertaken after renal biopsy and consultation with a pediatric nephrologist.**

   c. Diuretics and albumin   See **(3)**, p. 240.

      (1) The use of a diuretic alone can be hazardous in the presence of a low serum albumin, since this can aggravate an already existing contraction of the circulating blood volume. However, diuretics may be used alone in the following circumstances:

         (a) Orally in patients who have problems with recurrent edema. Use furosemide, 1–2 mg/kg/day, adding triamterene, 0.7 mg/kg/24 hr, or thiazides, or both, if need be.

         (b) Intravenously to mobilize edema fluid and alleviate symptoms from ascites, to help control infections while the patient is edematous, and to alleviate the aggravation of edema, which can occur when steroids are first begun. **Caution:** If diuresis is ineffective, if pulse rate increases, or if blood pressure drops or goes up precipitously, discontinuation or use only with albumin is indicated.

(2) When accumulation of edema fluid is severe, or when diuretics alone fail, salt-poor albumin may be given in a dose of 1 gm/kg IV slowly q12h, to be followed by IV furosemide, 1 mg/kg. **Caution:** Too rapid administration of salt-poor albumin may cause pulmonary edema and congestive heart failure.

2. General measures

a. Diet There is no need for dietary restriction other than a low-salt diet (1–2 gm/M²) during period of edema. Fluid restriction will be self-imposed if salt is restricted. Prior to diuresis fluid may be restricted to insensible losses plus urine output (or a bit less).

b. Activity No restriction of activity is required.

c. Infection Early and vigorous treatment of **bacterial** infection is important, since it can lead to relapses and was the leading cause of death prior to the advent of antibiotics.

d. Instruction of family Parents and child should be well informed about nephrosis and should be taught to test urine for albumin with dipsticks.

E. Prognosis

1. In the usual type of minimal change nephrotic syndrome 90–95 percent of children show an initial response to corticosteroids. Of these, 85 percent will have a further relapse. These relapses are more common in the first year than later, but thereafter can occur up to 15 years later.

2. The rate of relapse in a group of children tends to decrease after the first 10 years. If a child remains free of a relapse for up to 3–4 years, there is a 95 percent chance he or she will remain free of relapses thereafter. However, after one relapse, the subsequent course cannot be predicted, and the number of relapses per se does not affect the ultimate outcome.

VII. HEMATURIA

Hematuria is defined as the presence of more than five red blood cells per high-power microscopic field on at least two properly performed urinalyses. Red urine and urine dipstick test results have a high false-positive rate. Thus red urine, or a positive urine dipstick test, or both, mandate microscopic examination of the urine. The absence of red cells on microscopic examination suggests free hemoglobinuria or myoglobinuria (Table 9-4). Both pigments, hemoglobin and myoglobin, may be nephrotoxic, and full evaluation, with attempts at forced diuresis and urine alkalinization, should proceed.

A. Evaluation Normal children excrete 200,000–500,000 red blood cells every 24 hr through the urinary system. High fever and vigorous exercise cause a transient, benign increase in red cell excretion rate. Based on average urinary volumes, it is abnormal to see more than a few red blood cells per high-power microscopic field on routine urinalysis.

The first step in evaluation is a complete history, physical examination, and baseline laboratory profile.

1. History Any possible precipitating event is noted.

a. Particular attention is focused on symptoms of *cystitis* or renal colic.

b. The **past medical history** focuses on any previous hemorrhagic tendencies and details of any drug or travel history.

Table 9-4   Hemoglobinuria Versus Myoglobinuria

Observation	Myoglobin	Hemoglobin
Color of serum	Clear	Pink
Level of serum haptoglobin	Normal	Decreased
Mix urine with 80% (NH_4) S_2O_4 and filter	Pink	Clear
Muscle tenderness and elevated serum creatinine phosphokinase	Present	Absent
Clinical setting	Crush injuries, trauma, infection, rhabdomyolysis	Transfusion, disseminated intravascular coagulation

    c. Any **family history** of tuberculosis, renal failure, or deafness is delineated.

    d. **Review of systems** includes recent rashes, arthralgias, arthritis, and abdominal pain and notes fevers, malaise, anorexia, or weight loss.

  2. A thorough **physical examination** is performed, with careful attention to height, weight, blood pressure, rashes, and edema. Anomalous features on abdominal or perineal examination are noted.

  3. **Baseline laboratory profile**   Basic laboratory tests include a complete blood count, ESR, platelet count, prothrombin time, partial thromboplastin time, urinalysis with complete microscopic examination, urine culture, and a PPD skin test for tuberculosis.

B. Differential diagnosis (See Fig. 9-4.)   The baseline investigations may provide the diagnosis **without further evaluation.** If not, all other causes of hematuria may be separated into the following distinct categories: Symptomatic hematuria; hematuria associated with serious underlying systemic disease; asymptomatic hematuria; and complicated hematuria with significant proteinuria.

  1. Etiology suggested by baseline evaluation

    a. Multiple telangiectasias and characteristic mucous membrane lesions indicate **hereditary hemorrhagic telangiectasia** (Rendu-Osler-Weber disease).

    b. An abdominal mass with hematuria requires exclusion of **Wilms tumor** or **hydronephrosis.**

    c. Perineal excoriation or meatal inflammation implicates **local factors.**

    d. Hematuria occurs in association with sickle cell trait and S-C hemoglobin.

    e. A family history of asymptomatic hematuria suggests **benign familial hematuria,** while a family history of hematuria, deafness, and renal insufficiency suggests **Alport's hereditary nephritis.**

  2. Symptomatic hematuria

    a. A clinical picture of **cystitis** accompanied by hematuria, mild proteinuria (trace to 1+ unless hematuria is gross), and leukocyturia is

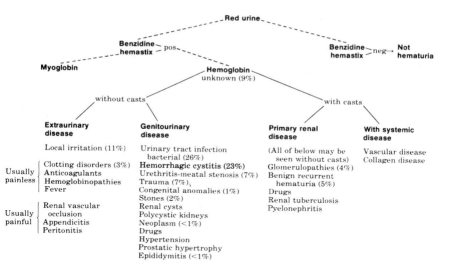

Figure 9-4 Differential diagnosis of red urine. The percentages indicate hematuria.

diagnostic of bacterial, viral, or traumatic involvement of the bladder or lower urinary tract. A **Gram stain** of the unspun urine and culture are done. When bacterial infection is documented, an **IVP** and **voiding cystourethrogram** are performed 4–6 weeks following successful antimicrobial therapy [see **(5)**, p. 379].

b. Culture-negative cystitis may be secondary to **viral infection.** Adenoviruses 11 and 21, influenza virus, and a papovalike virus have been implicated. Viral cystitis with resolution of hematuria and normal findings on urinalysis at follow-up requires no further investigation.

c. Culture-negative cystitis may also be caused by **tuberculosis** and **schistosomiasis** and should be suspected in appropriate clinical and endemic settings.

d. In addition to **gonococcal** or **nongonococcal urethritis,** vigorous masturbation and mechanical trauma to the urethra may also cause symptomatic hematuria with urethritis.

e. In younger children with apparent cystitis, particularly in girls ages 2–6, urethral or vaginal foreign bodies may be present.

f. Hematuria accompanied by moderate to severe abdominal pain is characteristic of **nephrolithiasis.** True renal colic is rare in the pediatric age group.

g. Microscopic hematuria following abdominal or flank trauma is common and often benign. However, following gross hematuria, when persistent, or with hematuria following seemingly minor trauma, an IVP should be obtained to determine the extent of renal damage as well as structural abnormalities that might cause bleeding with minor trauma.

3. **Hematuria in systemic disease** (See Fig. 9-4.) Attention should be focused on the evaluation and therapy of the **primary disorder.** The hematuria requires no further evaluation per se.

    a. Hematuria occurs with casts and protein in the critically ill child with catastrophic vascular diseases such as acute tubular necrosis, renal infarction, renal cortical necrosis, and renal vein thrombosis.

    b. In subacute bacterial endocarditis and neurologic shunt infection, hematuria is immunologically mediated and represents focal areas of glomerulonephritis.

4. **Asymptomatic hematuria**

    a. Glomerulonephritis should be the first consideration in asymptomatic hematuria. Microscopic hematuria may be a manifestation of active subclinical disease or reflect a resolving, clinically apparent case.

        (1) Further evaluation consists of

            (a) Antistreptolysin O (ASLO) titer and/or **anti-DNase B titer** in an attempt to document a group A β-hemolytic streptococcal infection.

            (b) Measurement of the **third component of complement,** which is depressed for 4–8 weeks in acute poststreptococcal glomerulonephritis and more persistently in most cases of membranoproliferative glomerulonephritis.

    b. Family members should be screened with urinalyses to rule out benign **familial hematuria,** inherited as an autosomal dominant trait.

    c. Extraglomerular hematuria may be asymptomatic; anatomic lesions can be detected by an IVP.

    d. Repeated episodes of gross hematuria with a normal IVP should be followed with a **voiding cystourethrogram** and cystoscopy.

    e. In a large group of patients, hematuria may persist without serologic or radiologic abnormalities. Such patients should be followed closely, with periodic examinations and urinalyses. During the follow-up period, the appearance of proteinuria, active urinary sediment with casts, deterioration in renal function, or development of hypertension suggests the need for renal biopsy.

    f. Asymptomatic microscopic hematuria that persists undiagnosed is regarded as **idiopathic.** Follow-up of such children has shown to deterioration in renal function. With careful longitudinal follow-up there is no indication for renal biopsy or invasive urologic investigations.

5. **Complicated hematuria** is asymptomatic hematuria in the presence of hypertension, active urinary sediment with casts, or proteinuria. All such patients should have the following laboratory studies: BUN and serum creatinine, ASLO titer, anti-DNase B titer, and serum complement level.

    a. Acute poststreptococcal glomerulonephritis is easily recognized. Evidence of antecedent group A β-hemolytic streptococcal infection in the previously well child who has an acute onset of malaise, edema, hypertension, hematuria with RBC casts, proteinuria, and serum hypocomplementemia is diagnostic. No radiologic studies are indicated, and biopsy is reserved for atypical cases or for persistent hypocomplementemia suggesting membranoproliferative glomerulonephritis or *SLE* nephritis.

b. Similarly, **acute anaphylactoid purpura** should be clearly apparent. Biopsy is reserved for atypical cases.

c. When glomerulonephritis is present, an **antinuclear** antibody test should be performed to delineate the subgroup with SLE nephritis. Renal biopsy is usually indicated to identify the histopathologic lesion and provide prognostic information.

  (1) IgG-IgA mesangial nephropathy (Berger's disease) is characterized by recurrent episodes of macroscopic hematuria associated with respiratory illnesses on a background of persistent microscopic hematuria and proteinuria.

  (2) Focal sclerosing glomerulonephritis, membranoproliferative glomerulonephritis, and **mesangial proliferative glomerulonephritis** are all chronic renal diseases. They are characterized by occasional clinical remissions, but generally progress to varying degrees of chronic renal failure.

VIII. ACUTE POSTINFECTIOUS GLOMERULONEPHRITIS

A. Etiology A nephritogenic strain of group A β-hemolytic streptococci is the most common preceding infection. Other agents include influenza A, coxsackievirus B4, echovirus type 9, mumps, Epstein-Barr virus, and bacterial infections due to staphylococcal species (in infected shunts) and pneumococcus.

B. Evaluation Edema, initially periorbital, hematuria, and hypertension are usually present either singly or in combination. Some children present with abdominal pain, and hypoalbuminemia and hyperlipemia may occasionally be seen early in the course of the disease. Hypertension, hypertensive encephalopathy, and congestive heart failure are the common complications and should be sought in the initial evaluation.

C. The **diagnosis** is suggested by the finding of urine sediment containing red cell casts and protein, elevated BUN and creatinine, decreased C3, and evidence of preceding streptococcal infection. (The antistreptolysin O level may not rise if the initial infection is treated early with appropriate antibiotics.) A search for other agents should be undertaken if suggested by the clinical history.

D. Treatment is entirely symptomatic.

  1. Appropriate antibiotics are given to eradicate the streptococcal infection (see Chap. 15, Sec. **IV**).

  2. A 1–2-gm salt diet is prescribed until the patient is asymptomatic, when a normal diet is resumed. There is no need for protein restriction in the usual case.

  3. Bed rest is maintained until there is clinical improvement. Normal activity is resumed within a few weeks in most instances.

  4. Hypertension See Sec. **III**.

E. Prognosis The usual course ends in complete recovery. Up to 5 percent of patients who appear clinically to have acute poststreptococcal glomerulonephritis may have a continuously downhill course and progress to renal insufficiency. Renal biopsy in such patients usually reveals evidence of preexisting underlying chronic glomerular disease. The urine sediment may remain abnormal for a prolonged period; the proteinuria often clears up before the hematuria, which can persist for up to 2–3 years following the illness. However, even these patients make a complete recovery.

IX. **HEMOLYTIC UREMIC SYNDROME (HUS)** The triad of acute nephropathy, hemolytic anemia with fragmented red cells, and thrombocytopenia constitutes one of the most common syndromes of acute renal failure seen in childhood. It is endemic in Argentina, California, South Africa, and the Netherlands. It is often preceded by gastroenteritis or upper respiratory tract infection (URI).

A. **Etiology** No discrete causes are known for the syndrome. Familial clustering has suggested that genetic predisposition is important.

B. **Evaluation** Evaluate as for acute renal failure.

1. Do a CBC with a smear in any patient with acute renal failure.

2. Suspect HUS if preceding viral gastroenteritis or URI is found in a patient with renal failure of if marked pallor is present.

3. Separate into mild or severe category as follows:

a. **Mild** No single 24-hr period of anuria. The patient may have oliguria, hypertension, or convulsions, but not all.

b. **Severe** Anuria or oliguria plus hypertension or convulsions is present.

C. **Diagnosis**

1. There is a history of prodromal illness.

2. Microangiopathic hemolytic anemia is found, including low hematocrit, burr cells, helmet cells on smear, low platelets, and consumption coagulopathy.

D. **Treatment** is as for acute renal failure. In addition, note the following:

1. Early dialysis may be lifesaving.

2. Transfusion with only frozen glycerolated white cell–poor blood, since these patients may be renal transplant candidates in the future.

3. Control hypertension (see Sec. **III.A**).

4. Do not use heparin or streptokinase, since studies to date indicate no benefit from either.

5. Antiplatelet agents are probably not indicated.

E. **Prognosis** Mildly affected patients tend to do well, with little or no long-term proteinuria, hypertension, or azotemia. At least 20 percent of those with severe HUS will have long-term sequelae, such as hypertension, proteinuria, and/or progressive renal insufficiency.

10

Cardiac Disorders

For particular attention to management of cardiac disease in the newborn, see Chap. 5.

I. CARDIAC ARRHYTHMIAS

A. General considerations

1. Cardiac arrhythmias are uncommon in children, especially in comparison with their incidence in adults. Without associated heart disease arrhythmias are almost always benign, and care should be exercised lest any therapy undertaken becomes more of a hazard than the underlying arrhythmia.

2. Arrhythmias themselves are not diseases but may be the manifestation of serious cardiac or metabolic disorders. Arrhythmias may be seen in the following clinical settings:

   a. Congenital or acquired heart disease.

   b. Procedures such as cardiac catheterization, surgery, or general anesthesia.

   c. Hypothermia.

   d. Electrolyte disturbances, including sodium, potassium, calcium, and magnesium imbalance.

   e. Systemic disorders of the musculoskeletal, endocrine, pulmonary, hematopoietic, or neurologic systems; in association with inherited disorders of metabolism, collagen diseases, or infectious diseases.

   f. Drug toxicity or poisoning.

   g. Neoplasia.

B. Evaluation
The accurate diagnosis of an arrhythmia is usually possible from a careful analysis of the surface ECG, including atrial and ventricular activity and the relationships between them. Occasionally, noninvasive studies such as carotid sinus massage, exercise electrocardiography, or ambulatory tape (Holter) monitoring are useful. Invasive procedures such as esophageal ECGs, His bundle electrograms, and atrial or ventricular pacing may be necessary in difficult cases.

C. Drug treatment

1. Digitalis

a. General considerations

(1) Digitalis is the most important single drug for the treatment of congestive heart failure (CHF) and may be exceedingly useful in the treatment of arrhythmias. It is the best agent for slowing the

heart rate in atrial flutter and fibrillation and may be effective in the treatment of paroxysmal atrial tachycardia.

(2) Although many preparations are available, digoxin is the drug of choice in pediatrics.

(3) A relatively narrow gap exists between optimal therapeutic doses and toxicity. In addition, variability in absorption, metabolism, excretion, and intracellular electrolyte concentrations makes the titration of each patient's correct dose an individual experiment.

(4) Care must be taken to make certain that the correct dose has been ordered and given. **Avoidable deaths have occurred because of a misplaced decimal point.**

b. **Mechanism of action**

(1) **Inotropic effects** Digitalis appears to interfere with the adenosinetriphosphatase (ATPase) involved in the sodium pump that removes sodium from the myocardial cell. The accumulation of sodium at the inner surface of the cell membrane allows for increased influx of calcium into the myofilament, thus potentiating myocardial contractility.

(2) **Antiarrhythmic effects** The cholinergic effects of digitalis slow the sinus rate, prolong the atrioventricular (AV) node refractory period, and slow AV conduction. Additionally, digitalis results in hyperpolarization of atrial conducting cells and decreases the slope of phase 4 depolarization, thus slowing or suppressing atrial ectopic impulse formation.

(3) **ECG changes** Digitalis prolongs the P–R interval, shortens the Q–T interval, and depresses the S–T segment.

c. **Route of administration, absorption, and metabolism** Digoxin can be given PO, IM, or IV. Orally, approximately 70–90 percent of the drug is absorbed, with peak levels within 1–3 hr. The half-life is about 2–3 days. About one-third of the drug is excreted daily, and a steady state will be achieved when this amount is replaced. Approximately 25 percent of the drug is bound to protein. Digoxin is excreted primarily by the kidney.

d. **Dosage**

(1) Before administration, a baseline ECG, electrolyte determinations (especially serum potassium), and some estimation of renal function are required.

(2) The therapeutic plasma concentration is 1.0–2.4 ng/ml. However, individual variations in response can occur; children with inflammatory disease of the myocardium may have enhanced sensitivity.

(3) Dosages should be calculated carefully and written in milligrams and milliliters to avoid errors.

(4) Digoxin is usually administered in two stages: Initial digitalization establishes the body stores; thereafter, one-fourth to one-third the total digitalizing dose (TDD) is given daily (usually in 2 divided doses 12 hr apart) to replace losses.

(a) **Variation of TDD with age**

i. **Prematures** 0.035 mg/kg PO over 24 hr. Usually, one-half the TDD is given, followed by one-fourth q12h twice (see also Chap. 5).

ii. Newborn   0.05 mg/kg (see also Chap. 5).

iii. Under 2 years   0.05–0.07 mg/kg PO.

iv. Over 2 years   0.03–0.05 mg/kg PO.

Parenteral doses should be about 75 percent of the oral dose.

(b) Maintenance digoxin should be 25–33 percent of the TDD. In children with renal disease, decreased excretion may be present, and maintenance should be calculated by using the following equation to determine the percent digoxin excreted per day.

$$\frac{14 + (\text{creatinine clearance})}{5} = \%\text{ digoxin excreted/day}$$

e. Toxicity

(1) Cardiovascular   Virtually any arrhythmia may be a manifestation of digitalis toxicity, but in children, supraventricular arrhythmias predominate, while in adolescents and adults, ventricular arrhythmias are more common. The vagal actions may result in sinus node depression and AV conduction disturbances.

(2) Gastrointestinal   GI complaints, such as anorexia, nausea, vomiting, diarrhea, and abdominal pain, are not uncommon.

(3) Neurologic   Fatigue, muscle weakness, and psychic disturbances are occasionally seen.

(4) Visual   Hazy vision, perceptual color (red and green), photophobia, and diplopia are occasionally seen in adults but are rare in children.

(5) Treatment

(a) Stop the drug.

(b) Check electrolytes. The administration of potassium may correct digitalis-induced arrhythmias but is contraindicated in the presence of AV block.

(c) Lidocaine, phenytoin sodium, and propranolol have been used for digitalis-induced arrhythmias.

(d) A temporary pacemaker may be necessary for high-grade AV block.

(e) Cardioversion should be used only as a last resort, since it may exacerbate rather than help and occasionally induces ventricular fibrillation.

2. Lidocaine is an effective drug for ventricular arrhythmias and is the drug of choice for the acute treatment of premature ventricular contractions and ventricular tachycardia. It is less effective against atrial or junctional arrhythmias. **It should not be used in the presence of complete heart block.**

a. Mechanism of action   Lidocaine depresses the automaticity of the heart and slows conduction. There are no effects on the surface ECG.

b. Route of administration, absorption, and metabolism   Lidocaine should not be given PO, since the liver eliminates most of the drug before it reaches the systemic circulation. When it is given as an IV bolus, effective blood levels can be achieved in 5 min and last up to 2 hr, with a peak concentration at 30 min. Since lidocaine is almost entirely metabolized in the liver, **it should be used with care in children with liver disease.**

   c. **Dosage**   As a bolus, give 0.5–1.0 mg/kg IV; this may be repeated in 30–60 min. As a constant infusion, the dosage is 0.5–1.0 mg/kg/hr. The therapeutic plasma concentration is 1–5 μg/ml.

   d. **Toxicity**

   (1) Lidocaine is the least cardiotoxic of the commonly used antiarrhythmic agents. However, at very high levels, hypotension and cardiovascular collapse can occur.

   (2) At serum levels of over 5 μg/ml, CNS disturbances such as drowsiness, lethargy, paresthesias, slurred speech, and double vision can occur. At over 9 μg/ml, convulsions and coma have been reported.

   (3) Discontinuation of the drug is the usual treatment for toxicity.

3. **Propranolol** is effective against a wide variety of atrial and ventricular arrhythmias. **It must be used with great care in patients with a compromised cardiac status,** since its beta-blocking effects may result in a significant decrease in contractility and may precipitate or exacerbate CHF. Asthma is also a contraindication.

   a. **Mechanism of action**   Propranolol is a beta-adrenergic blocking agent and works by reducing adrenergic tone and by depressing impulse formation and membrane responsiveness in the myocardial cell.

   b. **Route of administration, absorption, and metabolism**   Propranolol may be given PO or IV. Oral administration is accompanied by variable GI absorption, with a maximal blood level within 1–2 hr and a half-life of 2.5 hr. The therapeutic plasma concentration is 20–150 mg/ml. With IV administration the onset of action is within 2–5 min. Most of the drug is protein bound and is metabolized in the liver.

   c. **Dosage**   The oral dose is 0.2–4.0 mg/kg/day in 4 divided doses. The IV dose is 10–20 μg/kg over 10 min.

   d. **Toxicity**

   (1) Propranolol may be extremely deleterious in patients with a compromised cardiac status who depend on high circulating levels of catecholamines to maintain cardiac contractility. Hypotension or exacerbation of heart failure may result. Sinus bradycardia with resting rates below 50 are not uncommon.

   (2) Other signs of toxicity include GI symptoms (nausea, diarrhea, cramps) bronchospasm, and hypoglycemia.

   (3) Treatment includes stopping the drug. Bradycardia can be treated with atropine, and hypotension with large doses of isoproterenol, a beta agonist.

4. **Quinidine,** a stereoisomer of quinine, is effective against a variety of atrial and ventricular arrhythmias, especially atrial premature beats, atrial fibrillation, and ventricular premature beats. It has also been used to maintain normal sinus rhythm in hearts converted from atrial fibrillation or flutter.

   a. **Mechanism of action**   Quinidine depresses automaticity and refractoriness in the cardiac cell and slows conduction. On the surface ECG these are manifested by an increase in the P–R, QRS, and Q–T intervals.

b. **Route of administration, absorption, and metabolism** Quinidine has been given parenterally in adults, but there is little experience with this route in children. Oral absorption of quinidine sulfate is almost complete, with a peak plasma level in less than 2 hr and a half-life of approximately 6 hr. Approximately 80 percent of quinidine is bound to plasma protein. It is metabolized in the liver and excreted via the kidney. Thus, blood levels are dependent on the integrity of both these systems.

c. The **dosage** is 15 to 60 mg/kg PO in 4 divided doses. The therapeutic plasma concentration is 2–6 μg/ml.

d. **Toxicity**

   (1) **Cardiovascular**

      (a) Quinidine is a myocardial depressant, and the negative inotropic effect and decreases in systemic vascular resistance may produce severe hypotension.

      (b) By altering phase 4 depolarization, serious arrhythmias, such as ventricular tachycardia and ventricular fibrillation, may be induced.

      (c) ECG changes associated with quinidine toxicity include an increase in the QRS duration of more than 50 percent and an increase in the QT interval of more than 0.10 sec.

   (2) **GI toxicity** is common, with diarrhea the usual manifestation.

   (3) **Cinchonism** (blurred vision, tinnitus, altered color perception) is not uncommon.

   (4) **Other toxic manifestations** include thrombocytopenia and CNS symptoms, such as headaches, confusion, delirium, and psychosis.

   (5) Treatment is symptomatic after stopping the drug.

5. **Procainamide** is effective against the same arrhythmias and has the same mechanism of action as quinidine, but its metabolism and toxicity differ.

   a. **Route of administration, absorption, and metabolism** The most common route is PO, although IV administration has been used in adults. When it is given PO, 75–95 percent is absorbed, with peak levels appearing about 60 min later. The half-life is 3–4 hr. Metabolism is primarily in the liver, with approximately half being excreted unchanged by the kidney.

   b. The **dosage** is 15–50 mg/kg/day in a q6h schedule. Since the half-life is only 3–4 hr, a q4h schedule may be necessary in some patients. The therapeutic serum level is 3–10 μg/ml.

   c. **Toxicity**

      (1) The **cardiovascular effects** are the same as those for quinidine, but are less pronounced.

      (2) A lupuslike syndrome has been described. Antinuclear antibodies (ANA) develop in more than 80 percent of adults after 3–6 months of procainamide, but usually disappear when therapy is discontinued.

(3) Thrombocytopenia, Coombs-positive hemolytic anemia, and GI symptoms occur occasionally.

6. Phenytoin sodium is an effective drug for treating digitalis-induced arrhythmias, but is less effective in other situations.

    a. Mechanism of action Some of the antiarrhythmic effects of phenytoin sodium may be mediated, at least in part, by the CNS. It decreases automaticity in the specialized conducting system and also decreases the effective refractory period. ECG changes include shortening of the P–R and Q–T intervals.

    b. Route of administration, absorption, and metabolism Orally, absorption is slow, with a maximal plasma level in 8–12 hr and a half-life of 15–24 hr. Without a loading dose, it takes 6–7 days to achieve a therapeutic plasma level. The drug is metabolized in the liver and excreted into the GI tract. Resorption occurs, with only 5 percent excreted in the urine unchanged. IV use should be reserved for emergencies and should be accompanied by **constant ECG monitoring.** The therapeutic plasma level is 5–18 μg/ml.

    c. The **dosage** is 2–5 mg/kg/day in 2–3 doses PO and 3–5 mg/kg in 5 min IV.

    d. Toxicity

        (1) Cardiovascular Mild hypotension, bradycardia, transient AV block, and ventricular fibrillation have been reported after IV use.

        (2) CNS toxicity includes ataxia, vertigo, drowsiness, confusion, respiratory depression, and even respiratory arrest.

        (3) Other signs of toxicity include hypersensitivity reactions such as leukopenia, thrombocytopenia, morbilliform rashes, and serum sickness.

        (4) Gingival hyperplasia, megaloblastic anemia, and GI upset occur occasionally.

D. Electrical cardioversion

    1. General considerations Electrical cardioversion is the use of a synchronized direct current shock applied to the heart to convert certain arrhythmias to normal sinus rhythm. **Electrical cardioversion can be dangerous or fatal in the presence of digitalis toxicity.** It is indicated as the initial method of therapy in severe CHF, hypotension, or shock and when drug therapy has been unsuccessfully attempted. Arrhythmias requiring cardioversion include atrial flutter, atrial fibrillation, paroxysmal atrial or junctional tachycardia, and ventricular tachycardia.

    2. Techniques One must be prepared for complications, and the procedure should be done only **in an intensive care setting.**

    a. Analgesia should be obtained with IV administration of a short-acting barbiturate such as sodium pentobarbital or thiopental or diazepam.

    b. The cardioverter should be synchronized on the R wave to avoid the atrial and ventricular vulnerable period. **For treating ventricular fibrillation the synchronizing switch must be turned off.**

    c. The electrode paddles should be liberally covered with conductive paste and placed in the 2nd right intercostal space and 5th left interspace at the anterior axillary line in older children and adults or in the 3rd space in the parasternal area and below the left scapula in younger children.

d. Low energy levels should be tried, especially with atrial arrhythmias. Levels above 1.2 watt-sec/lb are not recommended routinely.

e. Postconversion arrhythmias are not uncommon and include atrial or ventricular premature beats and delayed function of the sinoatrial (SA) node, manifested by slow junctional rhythm or sinus bradycardia. Occasionally, these must be treated.

E. Specific arrhythmias

1. Sinus mechanisms

a. Sinus tachycardia is a normal response to exercise, fever, or fright, but may be associated with anemia, myocarditis, shock, CHF, or thyrotoxicosis.

  (1) Diagnosis A normal P wave is present, and AV conduction is normal. Although the heart rate normally varies with age, tachycardia is present when the heart rate exceeds 170 in a neonate, 140 in an infant, or 100 in a child.

  (2) Treatment consists in management of the underlying condition, if any. Propranolol may be useful for the tachycardia of hyperthyroidism while the underlying disease is being treated.

b. Sinus bradycardia is associated with increased vagal tone. It may be a normal finding in athletic children, but can also be a manifestation of hypothyroidism, hypothermia, hypopituitarism, typhoid fever, or hyperkalemia.

  (1) Diagnosis A normal P wave and normal AV conduction are present, with a heart rate less than 100 in neonates (see Chap. 5) and less than 60 in children and adolescents.

  (2) Treatment is unnecessary unless there is evidence of a low cardiac output. Atropine, 0.01–0.02 mg/kg IV, will increase the rate by reducing vagal tone.

c. Sinus arrhythmia is a normal finding and is a manifestation of peripheral and central circulatory reflexes.

  (1) Diagnosis The P waves are normal, as is AV conduction, with varying P–P intervals. The heart rate usually increases during inspiration and slows down during expiration.

  (2) Treatment is not necessary.

2. Supraventricular mechanisms

a. Premature atrial contractions (PACs) may be an incidental finding in infants or children without other evidence of heart disease. When repetitive in groups of two or three, they may be a precursor to atrial flutter or fibrillation.

  (1) Diagnosis PACs are characterized by a premature P wave, usually of a different configuration than the sinus P wave, followed by a QRS that is similar or identical to the normal QRS.

  (2) Treatment is unnecessary.

b. Escape beats are usually a protective mechanism when a higher pacemaker slows for any reason. They are commonly seen with a marked sinus arrhythmia, but may be seen occasionally with the sick sinus syndrome.

(1) Diagnosis   The QRS is usually of normal configuration. The P waves may be normal, with a short P–R interval (nonconducted) that is completely or partially obscured by the QRS or absent. In sinus arrhythmia with nodal escape, the escape rhythm is usually phasic with respiration.

(2) Treatment is unnecessary.

c. Atrial flutter may occasionally be seen in newborns or infants without other evidence of heart disease. In older children it is often associated with rheumatic heart disease or other diseases causing atrial dilatation.

(1) Diagnosis   There is a rapid, regular atrial rate of 250–350 beats/ min, with P (flutter) waves having a sawtooth pattern in leads II, III, VF, and VI (but usually not in I). Conduction to the ventricles may be 1:1, 2:1, 3:1, or 4:1.

(2) Treatment   Digoxin (see **C.1**) is useful in controlling the rate by increasing block at the AV node. DC cardioversion at very low energy is almost always successful in converting atrial flutter to normal sinus rhythm (see **d.(2)**).

d. Atrial fibrillation is usually associated with significant heart disease and atrial dilatation. It may also be seen with hyperthyroidism or the Wolff-Parkinson-White (W-P-W) syndrome.

(1) Diagnosis   Irregular "f" waves are present at a rate of 400–600/ min, with an irregular ventricular response. The QRS usually appears normal, but some aberrant beats may be present.

(2) Treatment   Digitalis is effective in slowing the rate (see p. 230); while quinidine has been used in children in the past to convert sinus rhythm, electrical conversion is now used instead (see **D**). Patients with atrial fibrillation for more than 1 month should be given anticoagulants to decrease the risk of embolism during cardioversion. Long-standing atrial fibrillation is likely to recur.

e. Paroxysmal atrial tachycardia is seen in association with cardiac catheterization or surgery, W-P-W syndrome, emotional stress, or hyperthyroidism. An idiopathic form occurs in male infants.

(1) Diagnosis   The rhythm is regular, at a rate of 160–260 beats/min, with a normal or slightly widened QRS. P waves, if present, are usually of a different configuration than sinus P waves.

(2) Treatment

(a) Reflex stimulation of the vagus by a Valsalva maneuver, gagging, eyeball pressure, or unilateral carotid sinus massage may occasionally be effective in converting the heart to normal sinus rhythm.

(b) Digoxin or propranolol are the drugs of choice.

(c) In desperately ill patients or those resistant to drug therapy, electrical cardioversion may be effective.

(d) Rarely, increasing vagal tone by increasing systemic blood pressure using alpha-adrenergic drugs such as phenylephrine

(0.005–0.01 mg/kg IV), or directly increasing vagal tone with edrophonium (0.1–0.2 mg/kg/IV) has been used in children.

3. Ventricular mechanisms

a. Premature ventricular contractions (PVCs) are commonly found in children without other evidence of heart disease. They may also occur secondary to myocardial inflammation or ischemia, hyperkalemia, sympathomimetic drugs, digitalis toxicity, and cardiac tumors or with mitral valve prolapse.

(1) Diagnosis   There is usually a wide QRS with opposite polarity of the T wave and a full compensatory pause before the next QRS complex. A preceding P wave is not seen.

(2) Treatment

(a) Most PVCs in patients without heart disease are benign and require no treatment. Characteristically, benign PVCs are unifocal, unassociated with other evidence of heart disease, disappear with exercise, and have a fixed coupling interval.

(b) Significant PVCs are usually associated with heart disease, are multifocal with a variable coupling interval, and are accentuated by exercise. A prolonged resting Q–T interval may be present.

 i. The best treatment is to remove the cause if possible.

 ii. For the acute problem, lidocaine, 1 mg/kg IV in a bolus, is the drug of choice.

 iii. In the absence of significant myocardial failure, oral propranolol should be tried for long-term suppression. If CHF is present, quinidine or procainamide is preferable, although these drugs are also myocardial depressants.

(c) Ambulatory testing, either with exercise stress or 24-hr tape recordings may be useful in assessing the significance of the PVCs or in judging the efficacy of treatment.

b. Ventricular tachycardia is almost always associated with severe congenital or acquired heart disease.

(1) Diagnosis

(a) Intermittent   Runs of three or more consecutive ventricular ectopic beats.

(b) Sustained   A wide QRS and a rate of 140–200 beats/min are present. There may be evidence of separate atrial activity, such as AV dissociation and intermittent ventricular capture, or fusion beats. The configuration of the QRS is often similar to that in isolated PVCs observed before the onset of the tachycardia.

(2) Treatment

(a) Acute   For the intermittent form, a bolus of lidocaine, 0.5–1.0 mg IV, is usually effective. For the sustained variety, a sharp blow to the anterior chest wall should be tried. If this fails, DC cardioversion (1–2 watt sec/lb) should be attempted.

(b) Chronic   Treatment is same as for PVCs.

c. Ventricular fibrillation

(1) Diagnosis Ventricular fibrillation is characterized by low-amplitude, rapid, irregular depolarizations with no identifiable normal electrical activity.

(2) Treatment is the same as that for sustained ventricular tachycardia.

4. Heart block

a. First-degree heart block is associated with increased vagal tone, inflammatory diseases affecting the conduction system, and congenital heart disease, especially atrial septal defects, endocardial cushion defects, and Ebstein's anomaly.

(1) Diagnosis First-degree heart block is defined as a P–R interval longer than rate and age corrected normal. A P–R interval greater than 0.14 sec in an infant, greater than 0.18 in a child, or greater than 0.20 in an adult represents first-degree heart block.

(2) Treatment None is necessary.

b. Second-degree heart block

(1) Diagnosis

(a) Mobitz type I (Wenckebach) block consists of regular P waves with progressive prolongation of the P–R interval. The R–R interval becomes progressively shorter until a QRS is dropped.

(b) In **Mobitz type II** block, a normal P wave, P–R interval, and QRS are followed by a P wave with no QRS. The next P wave is conducted normally. The dropped beats can occur every second, third, or fourth beat.

(2) Treatment is unnecessary, but progression to third-degree block may occur.

c. Third-degree (complete heart block) may be congenital or may be acquired in children with an otherwise normal heart. It also may be associated with congenital heart disease (corrected transposition of the great vessels) or acquired heart diseases, such as rheumatic fever, cardiac tumors, or endocardial fibroelastosis. Acquired heart block following cardiac surgery now occurs less often than previously.

(1) Diagnosis Complete AV dissociation with the ventricular rate slower than the atrial rate is diagnostic. A wide QRS suggests block below the bundle of His.

(2) Treatment

(a) The need for therapy is dependent on the ventricular rate, the presence or absence of symptoms, and the stability of the inherent pacemaker.

(b) Congenital or acquired heart block in children without associated heart disease needs no therapy unless syncope or unremitting heart failure is present. Block acquired after cardiac surgery should always be treated with a pacemaker.

(c) Transvenous pacemakers in older children or epicardial pacemakers in young children or those with right-to-left shunts constitute the treatment of choice when raising the heart rate is necessary.

(d) Atropine, 0.01–0.02 mg/kg IV, or isoproterenol, 0.1 µg/kg/min, may be effective in increasing ventricular rate while awaiting insertion of a temporary or permanent pacemaker.

II. CONGESTIVE HEART FAILURE (CHF)   Congestive heart failure is a clinical syndrome in which the heart is unable to supply an output sufficient to meet the metabolic requirements of the tissues.

A. Etiology

1. Congenital diseases of the heart, usually with large left-to-right shunts or obstructive lesions of the left or right ventricle.
2. Acquired diseases of the heart, including myocarditis, acute or chronic rheumatic heart disease, and infectious endocarditis.
3. Arrhythmias, including paroxysmal atrial tachycardia, atrial fibrillation or flutter, or complete heart block.
4. Iatrogenic causes, including damage to the heart at surgery (ventriculotomy), fluid overload, or doxorubicin (Adriamycin) therapy.
5. Noncardiac causes, such as thyrotoxicosis, systemic arteriovenous fistula, anemia, acute or chronic lung disease, glycogen storage disease, or connective or neuromuscular disorders.

B. Clinical manifestations   The signs and symptoms of CHF fall into the following three categories:

1. **Signs of impaired myocardial performances**   These include growth failure, sweating, cardiac enlargement, gallop rhythm, and alterations in peripheral pulses, including pulsus paradoxus and pulsus alternans.
2. **Signs of pulmonary congestion**   These include tachypnea, dyspnea with effort, cough, rales, wheezing, and cyanosis.
3. **Signs of systemic venous congestion**   These include hepatomegaly, neck vein distention, and peripheral edema.

C. Treatment

1. General supportive treatment

a. **Sedation** with morphine or chloral hydrate may be needed in the anxious, fretful, agitated child or the irritable infant.

b. **Cool, humidified oxygen** by tent, mask, or nasal prongs.

c. **A sitting or semirecumbent position** is favored for older children and may be achieved in infants by the use of a "cardiac chair."

2. Increasing the efficiency of the heart

a. **Digitalis** increases cardiac output by increasing the force of contraction and thus increasing stroke volume (for dosage, see p. 230).

b. Infusion of **Isoproterenol**, 0.1 µg/kg/min, or, more recently, **dopamine**, 5–10 µg/kg/min, has been used in some children who failed to respond to other methods. The use of these agents is not without risk, but may be helpful in carefully selected patients preliminary to emergency surgery.

3. Reducing the work of the heart

a. **Bed rest** is advisable in infants and older children. In toddlers and younger children, quiet play in a playroom may be preferable to leaving the child screaming in bed.

b. Reduction in volume overload

(1) Diet   No-added-salt diets are used in children. Infants should receive high-calorie, low-volume, low-sodium diets.

(2) Fluids are moderately restricted to 50–90 ml/kg/day. If salt is being restricted, stringent fluid restriction is not necessary. In general, IV fluids should be low in salt or salt free.

(3) Diuretics   The effectiveness of a diuretic is dependent on renal perfusion and electrolytes and acid-base balance. Diuretic agents may cause profound changes in electrolyte composition, and frequent electrolyte evaluations made be made. In the presence of shock or acute renal failure they will have little effect. Potassium depletion, especially in the digitalized patient, is dangerous and may be lethal.

The characteristics of commonly used diuretics are given in Table 10-1.

(a) Mercurial diuretics are no longer used.

(b) Thiazides are sulfonamide derivatives that share moderate potency and low toxicity. Those most commonly used in pediatrics are chlorothiazide (Diuril) and hydrochlorothiazide (Hydro-DIURIL).

  i. Mechanism   The thiazide diuretics inhibit resorption of sodium and chloride in the ascending loop of Henle. The nature of the chemical interaction between the thiazides and specific receptors is unknown.

  ii. Route of administration, absorption, and metabolism   The thiazides are rapidly **absorbed** from the GI tract and begin to have a diuretic effect within 1 hr. The duration of action of chlorothiazide is about 6–12 hr, while that of hydrochlorothiazide is 12 hr or more. **Excretion** is via the kidney, with some subsequent resorption.

  iii. Dosage
Chlorothiazide, 20–40 mg/kg/day
    PO in 2 divided doses,
      or
Hydrochlorothiazide, 2–5 mg/kg/day
    PO in 2 divided doses.

  iv. Toxicity   Potassium depletion may occur with long-term use. Alternate-day therapy, intake of foods high in potassium, administration of liquid potassium, or the addition of a potassium-sparing diuretic such as spironolactone or triamterene may protect against potassium depletion. However, periodic measurements of serum potassium are necessary, especially early in therapy. **Allergic reactions** such as thrombocytopenia, leukopenia, or vasculitis are rarely seen. **Hyperglycemia** and **aggravation of preexisting diabetes or hyperuricemia** may occur.

(c) Furosemide (Lasix) and ethacrynic acid (Edecrin)   These potent diuretics are different structurally, but have similar diuretic effects. Because of the massive diuresis that may be produced, they should be used rarely in previously untreated children unless careful observation of electrolytes, especially serum potassium, and blood volume is possible.

Table 10-1 Dosages and Characteristics of Various Diuretics

Drug	Dosage	Action Onset	Action Peak	Action Duration	Contraindications	Adverse Reactions	Mechanism of Action
Furosemide (Lasix)	IV: 1.0 mg/kg/dose (over 1–2 min) PO: 2–3 mg/kg/day	5 min 1 hr	30 min 1–2 hr	2 hr 4–6 hr	Anuria	Hypovolemia Hypokalemia Hyperuricemia Ototoxicity	Blocks resorption of Na+ in ascending loop of Henle
Ethacrynic acid (Edecrin)	IV: 1 mg/kg/dose PO: 2–3 mg/kg/day	5 min 30 min	45 min 2 hr	3 hr 6–8 hr	Hypersensitivity Women of childbearing potential		
Chlorothiazide (Diuril)	PO: 20–40 mg/kg/day in 2 doses	2 hr	4 hr	6–12 hr	Anuria, progressive renal insufficiency	Hypokalemia	Blocks resorption of Na+ in ascending loop of Henle
Hydrochlorothiazide (Hydro-DIURIL)	PO: 2–4 mg/kg/day in 2 doses	2 hr	4 hr	6–12 hr	Hypersensitivity to this or other sulfonamide-derived drugs	Hyperuricemia Hypersensitivity Dermatitis Photosensitivity	
Spironolactone (Aldactone)*	PO: 1–3 mg/kg/day in 2 doses		Several days		Renal insufficiency	Headaches Gynecomastia Nausea and vomiting Rashes	Blocks aldosterone exchange of K+ for Na+
Acetazolamide (Diamox)	PO: 5 mg/kg/day	1 hr	2 hr	24 hr	Hypokalemia Anuria Renal insufficiency Hyperchloremia acidosis	Drowsiness Paresthesias Drowsiness Hypersensitivity	Carbonic anhydrase inhibitor

*Spironolactone is rarely given alone, but its potassium-sparing effect makes it useful in combination with other agents.

241

i. Mechanism Both furosemide and ethacrynic acid increase renal excretion of sodium and chloride and an accompanying volume of water by inhibiting resorption in the ascending loop of Henle. The biochemical mechanism is not known.

ii. Route of administration, absorption, and metabolism Both drugs are well absorbed PO or may be given IV. Orally effects can be expected within 30–60 min. Parenterally, the onset of action is within 5 min for furosemide and within 15 min for ethacrynic acid. Duration of action for the parenteral dose is 2–3 hr and, when given orally, 6–8 hr. Both drugs are bound to plasma protein with approximately two-thirds excreted by the kidney.

iii. Dosage
Ethacrynic acid, 1 mg/kg/dose IV over
  1–2 min IV; 2–3 mg/kg/day PO,
    or
Furosemide, 1 mg/kg/dose over
  1–2 min IV; 2–3 mg/kg/day PO.

iv. Toxicity Both drugs are potent, and clinical toxicity is usually manifested by **hypovolemia** or **hypokalemia.** Both drugs competitively inhibit urate secretion in the proximal tubule and may cause **hyperuricemia** and, in susceptible persons, **gout.** Transient or even permanent **deafness** has been reported, especially with ethacrynic acid (possibly due to electrolyte changes in the endolymph). **GI disturbances, bone marrow suppression, skin rashes,** and **paresthesia** have been reported occasionally.

(d) Spironolactone (Aldactone) is a weak diuretic by itself but may be useful as an addition to the diuretics previously discussed both because of its different site of action and because of its potassium-sparing effects.

i. Mechanism The diuretic properties of spironolactone result from its structural similarity to aldosterone. It is competitive inhibitor of the mineralocorticoids that normally stimulate sodium resorption and potassium excretion in the distal tubules.

ii. Route of administration, absorption, and metabolism Spironolactone is absorbed orally but the diuretic effect may not be manifested for 2–3 days. Its effects may persist for 2–3 days after cessation of therapy.

iii. Dosage 1–3 mg/kg/day PO.

iv. Toxicity The major complication is **hyperkalemia,** resulting from inhibition of potassium secretion with normal or increased potassium intake. Careful monitoring of serum potassium will avoid this problem. Spironolactone has been shown to be **oncogenic** in chronic toxicity studies in rats. **Gynecomastia** may be seen in adolescents.

(4) Afterload reduction may be used in patients without intracardiac shunts who fail to respond to digitalis and diuretics. Vasodilator drugs, by decreasing peripheral resistance and reducing ventricular filling pressures, may improve cardiac output. Sodium nitroprusside, 0.5–10 mEq/kg IV, has been used acutely with careful monitoring of arterial pressure; thiocyanate levels should be measured if the drug is to be used for an extended period. For chronic treatment, isosorbide dinitrate, 0.25–1.0 mg q4–8h, and/or hydralazine, 0.75–3.0 mg/kg/day q6–8h, have been used.

III. ACUTE RHEUMATIC FEVER

A. **Etiology** Acute rheumatic fever (ARF) is a sequel of pharyngeal infection with a group A streptococcus, but the exact pathogenesis is still unknown. It has been proposed that the disease may be (1) a direct reaction to streptococcal extracellular or cellular substances; or (2) an immunologic process stimulated by *Streptococcus*; or (3) persistent infection by *Streptococcus* or one of its variants.

B. **Evaluation** should include the following:

1. A **history,** with emphasis on antecedent infections, fever, arthralgia, and previous RF, as well as a familial and social history.

2. **Physical examination,** with attention to joints, skin (rashes and subcutaneous nodules), and the cardiovascular system.

3. **Laboratory studies** should include acute phase reactants, ESR, C-reactive protein (leukocytosis), ECG, x-ray, streptococcal antibodies (antistreptolysin O, anti-DNase B, anti-NADase, antihyaluronidase), and throat culture.

C. **Diagnosis**

1. No single laboratory test, symptom, or sign is pathognomonic, although several combinations are suggestive of ARF.

2. According to the revised Jones criteria, RF is likely in the presence of one major and two minor criteria (see **4, 5**), or two major criteria plus evidence of a preceding streptococcal infection. Chorea alone may be sufficient for a diagnosis, *but*

3. **Acute rheumatic fever may not fulfill the revised Jones criteria,** especially early in the disease. Conversely, other diseases, such as rheumatoid arthritis, systemic lupus erythematosus, Schönlein-Henoch purpura, serum sickness, sickle cell hemoglobinopathy, and septic or postinfectious arthritis may occasionally fulfill the criteria at certain points in their natural history.

4. **Major criteria**

   a. **Carditis**

   b. **Polyarthritis** Tenderness, usually with heat, swelling, and redness, involving more than one joint especially, but not exclusively, and involving the larger joints, especially the knee, ankle, elbow, wrist, and hip.

   c. **Subcutaneous nodules** usually occur only in children with severe carditis of several weeks' duration.

   d. **Erythema marginatum** is an uncommon finding in RF and is not specific to the disease.

   e. **Chorea** is often associated with emotional instability.

5. **Minor criteria**

   a. **Fever** Rarely above 104°F, or associated with shaking chills.

   b. **Arthralgias** Joint pain without objective findings.

    c. Prolonged P–R interval on the ECG (not in and of itself diagnostic of carditis).

    d. Increased ESR, C-reactive protein, leukocytosis.

    e. Previous history of ARF or rheumatic heart disease.

  6. Other criteria include epistaxis, abdominal pain, and rheumatic pneumonia.

D. Treatment

  1. Eradication of streptococci See Table 15-2.

  2. Antiinflammatory agents

    a. Aspirin is indicated for arthritis without carditis and possibly in children with mild cardiac involvement. The dosage of acetylsalicylic acid is 100 mg/kg/day in 4–6 divided doses for 3–4 weeks. The optimal serum level is about 20–25 mg/100 ml. Although salicylates undoubtedly give symptomatic relief, there is no proof that they alter the course of the myocardial damage.

    b. Corticosteroids have been controversial in the therapy of ARF since their introduction.

      (1) Steroids are almost mandatory in patients with severe carditis and CHF. Prednisone, 2 mg/kg/day for 4–6 weeks, is given, with tapering over the next 2 weeks. Steroids reduce inflammation promptly, but there is no conclusive evidence that they prevent residual valvular damage.

      (2) In patients with carditis without cardiomegaly or CHF, the use of steroids instead of salicylates remains controversial and more a matter of personal preference.

  3. Anticongestive measures, including digitalis (p. 229), should be used in patients with ARF in the same fashion as in other patients with CHF despite possible increased sensitivity in the inflamed myocardium.

  4. Bed rest is accepted during the acute phase when CHF is present. In the absence of objective data, we think it is prudent to keep children on limited activity, if not on bed rest, until the ESR returns to normal.

  5. Children with chorea should be moved to a quiet environment with understanding nurses and should be protected against self-inflicted injury due to uncontrollable movements. Drug treatment with phenobarbital, chlorpromazine, diazepam, and haloperidol has been tried, with varying success.

  6. Prevention of rheumatic recurrences

    a. All children with documented RF with or without carditis—and all those with rheumatic heart disease—should receive prophylaxis against a second attack.

    b. Any of the following approaches are acceptable, provided that compliance is assured. If severe residual heart disease is present or the patient is unreliable, the first alternative is preferable.

      (1) Benzathine penicillin, 1.2 million U every 28 days.

      (2) Penicillin G, 0.2 million U PO bid.

      (3) Sulfisoxazole (Gantrisin), 0.5 mg/day for those weighing under 60 lb; 1 gm/day for those weighing over 60 lb.

c. The most recent recommendation of the American Heart Association is for **lifetime prophylaxis, whether or not the patient has residual heart damage.**

IV. HYPOXIC OR CYANOTIC SPELLS

Paroxysmal dyspnea with marked cyanosis often occurs in infants and young children with tetralogy of Fallot. Rarely, it may occur in other types of cyanotic congenital heart disease. It is characterized by increasing rate and depth of respirations with increased cyanosis, progressing to limpness, loss of consciousness and, in the more severe cases, convulsions, cerebrovascular accidents, and even death.

A. Etiology

1. Although cyanotic spells are due to an acute reduction of pulmonary blood flow, increased right-to-left shunting, and systemic hypoxemia, the mechanism that triggers these events has not been completely elucidated.

2. The usual explanation is "spasm" of the infundibulum of the right ventricle. Other explanations include inadequate systemic venous return, decreased systemic vascular resistance, and a vicious cycle of arterial hypoxemia due to hyperpnea.

3. Anemia, either absolute or relative to the child's oxygen saturation, may predispose to cyanotic spells.

B. Diagnosis

1. Signs and symptoms

a. Reduction in intensity or disappearance of the pulmonary ejection murmur.

b. Hyperpnea.

c. Increased cyanosis.

d. Irritability, often leading to unconsciousness and occasionally to convulsions due to cerebral anoxia.

2. Laboratory findings

a. Hypoxemia and acidosis.

b. Diminished pulmonary blood flow on x-ray.

c. Increased voltage of the P wave on the ECG.

C. Treatment

1. Place the child in a knee-chest position.

2. Give oxygen by hood or mask at 5–8 L/min.

3. Give morphine sulfate, 0.1–0.2 mg/kg IM or SQ.

4. If the spell is severe, give sodium bicarbonate, 1 mg/kg IV.

5. If the hemoglobin is less than 15 gm/100 ml, a transfusion (5 ml/kg) should be given.

6. Propranolol, 0.1 mg/kg IV, may be tried in a protracted spell that does not respond to the preceding measures.

7. Surgery (corrective or palliative) may be necessary to increase pulmonary blood flow.

11

Gastrointestinal Disorders

I. GENERAL PRINCIPLES

A. Nutrition Maintenance of adequate nutrition is recognized as one of the most important aspects of medical therapy in acute and chronic disease. Even in the absence of disease, nutritional deficiencies are not limited to underdeveloped countries but occur in Western society as well.

Varying sources of calories are continually being sought, and the introduction of total parenteral nutrition without oral supplementation has reemphasized the importance of daily calorie, protein, fat, carbohydrate, vitamin, and trace metal requirements (see Chap. 1, Sec. **III.A**, p. 17).

The primary therapeutic goal in the management of GI disease is restoration of adequate nutrition. This should be considered in diseases of other organ systems as well.

1. Diets Diets prescribed at the Children's Hospital Medical Center for the management of specific nutritional deficiency may be obtained by writing to the Nutrition Department at the Center.

2. Total parenteral nutrition (TPN) The instillation of hyperosmolar glucose protein hydrolysate fluid into central high-flow veins can maintain and may surpass usual nutritional requirements.

a. Nitrogen sources are generally provided as either protein hydrolysate or a mixture of pure crystalline amino acids. The usual requirements of either of these is 2–4 gm/kg/day in infants and children. The bulk of the caloric content of hyperalimentation fluid is derived from glucose. The amount required in most infants is 25–30 gm/kg/day. The remainder of the metabolic needs, i.e., water, electrolytes, minerals, and vitamins are provided in customary amounts (see Chaps. 1, 4, and 8).

b. Intralipid (soybean oil) is a fat emulsion that provides 1.1 cal/ml and can provide a low-volume source of calories as well as preventing essential fatty acid deficiency. Intralipid should not provide more than 60 percent of total calories.

c. Indications for TPN Any patient unable to maintain nutrition adequate for metabolic needs is a candidate for TPN. Specific disease states in which TPN is employed include

(1) Chronic diarrheal states

(2) Inflammatory bowel disease with growth failure or fistulas

(3) Postoperative status

(4) Chronic pancreatitis

(5) Short-bowel syndrome

(6) Esophageal injury

3. Management of hyperalimentation program

a. A central venous catheter is placed and its position checked radiographically.

b. A 10% glucose solution is given IV at a rate 1½ times maintenance fluid as tolerated (see Chap. 8). Adequate electrolytes should be provided. Continue the infusion for 12–24 hr.

c. A 20% glucose–amino acid solution is then given at ¾ maintenance fluid requirement for 12 hr.

d. The infusion rate is increased approximately 10 percent every 12 hr until fluid intake is 135 ml/kg/day, irrespective of age. An infusate with 20% glucose and 3 gm/100 ml protein provides the equivalent of 110 cal/kg/day. Generally, no more than 200 ml/kg/day is used in infants. It may be necessary to decrease the protein content of the infusate at such rates.

e. Intralipid infusion

    (1) Intralipid is administered via a peripheral vein and does not require "breaking" the central venous circuit for administration.

    (2) The initial rate of intralipid infusion via a peripheral vein should provide 15 ml/kg/day given over 6–12 hr. If the patient's serum is not lipemic, the infusion is increased by 5 ml/kg/day until 30–40 ml/kg/day is attained.

4. Monitoring the patient receiving TPN

a. Daily weights should be measured.

b. Intake and output is charted and qualitative sugar and acetone measured on all urine specimens.

c. Na, K, Cl, BUN, and glucose are determined daily while increasing fluid and then weekly when fluid requirements have been reached.

d. Mg, Ca, P, and total protein are measured initially and then weekly.

e. SGOT, SGPT, LDH, alkaline phosphatase, bilirubin, and creatinine are measured initially and then weekly.

f. Copper, zinc, and iron levels are measured at the beginning of therapy and then monthly.

5. Complications of TPN

a. Infection is the most serious complication of TPN.

    (1) The incidence of this complication increases dramatically if less than scrupulous care is applied to maintaining the integrity of the central venous line.

    (2) Unexplained glycosuria may be the first clue. Fungi (usually *Candida albicans*) and bacteria are the infecting agents. Several blood cultures should be obtained from the patient and from the line. When sepsis is documented, the central venous line should be withdrawn if possible. Although appropriate antibiotics (see Chap. 15) should be used for documented sepsis, chemotherapy may not be necessary for *Candida* infection.

b. Hepatic complications Abnormalities in liver function test results are common during the course of TPN. Hepatomegaly with elevations of serum transaminases (often to high levels, with prolongation of prothrombin time (PT) and partial thromboplastin time (PTT) may be seen, and liver biopsy reveals a fatty liver. Cholestatic liver disease frequently develops in premature infants.

c. Metabolic complications

   (1) Hyperglycemia is common in septic patients, premature infants, and patients with renal disease.

   (2) Hypoglycemia is a common and severe complication *if TPN is stopped abruptly.*

   (3) Acidosis occurs in patients with renal compromise or prematurity when large (4 gm/kg/day) protein loads are administered.

   (4) Hypomagnesemia may occur in patients with low endogenous magnesium stores (e.g., those with chronic diarrhea).

   (5) Hyperlipemia occurs with excess Intralipid administration.

d. Trace metal deficiency

   (1) Copper deficiency is not uncommon and is manifested by anemia, neutropenia, and rash.

   (2) Zinc deficiency is common and is manifested by an erythematous, maculopapular rash (acrodermatitis enteropathica) (see Chap. 22) involving the face, trunk, metacarpophalangeal joints, and perineum. *Low* serum alkaline phosphatase is common.

e. Mechanical complications

   (1) Arrhythmias may occur with an improperly placed catheter.

   (2) Venous thrombosis is rare.

   (3) Air embolus occurs only after accidental coupling of the IV line.

f. Local complications   Skin sloughs may occur from infiltration of peripheral venous infusions.

g. Complications of Intralipid administration

   (1) Pulmonary   May decrease oxygen diffusion at the alveolar-capillary junction.

   (2) Bilirubin   Intralipid displaces bilirubin from albumin and is contraindicated in jaundiced infants.

   (3) Eosinophilia may be present.

h. Contraindications to the use of Intralipid include hyperlipemic states and severe liver disease.

B. Evaluation of gastrointestinal disease   See later in this chapter for a discussion of vomiting (p. 271).

1. Examination of the stool

   a. Examine the stool for consistency, odor, blood, or mucus. The presence of gross blood and mucus indicates colitis.

   b. Clinitest to detect the presence of reducing substances

   (1) Mix 1 part *fresh* stool in 2 parts water (to detect sucrose intolerance, hydrolyze with 1 N HCl).

   (2) Centrifuge and add 15 drops of supernatant to Clinitest tablet.

   (3) The test is positive if 0.5 percent or more of reducing substance is present. The presence of reducing substance is always abnormal and indicates sucrose or disaccharide intolerance, or both.

c. pH

(1) Normal stool pH is 7–8.

(2) A decreased pH suggests the presence of organic acids, as seen in disaccharide intolerance.

d. Hemoccult or **guaiac test** for blood.

e. Sudan stain for fat. A positive stain indicates steatorrhea.

f. Fecal leukocytes

(1) Stain with methylene blue or Wright's stain.

(2) The presence of many polys, or bands, or both suggests inflammatory colitis. However, in typhoid fever, only lymphocytes are seen.

(3) Viral enteritis usually inflames the small bowel, and in this condition the finding of neutrophils is unusual.

g. Ova, parasites, and cultures   See Chaps. 15 and 16.

2. Fecal fat excretion   Although often distasteful to patient and clinician, this is the best method for detecting steatorrhea.

a. All stools are collected for 72 hr.

b. Since fecal fat excretion is expressed as a percentage of intake, the patient must keep a diary of food intake during this period, so that the amount of fat in the diet can be estimated.

c. Normal values   (Values for breast-fed infants are lower but are not precisely known.)

Premature infants: 15–30 percent of intake
Full-term infants: up to 15 percent until 10 months of age
After 1 year of age: less than 5 percent of intake

3. D-Xylose excretion   This test reflects enteric mucosal absorption.

a. Give 14.5 gm/M^2 after an overnight fast.

b. Measure serum xylose at 1 hr; > 25 mg/100 ml is normal.

c. Delayed gastric emptying is a variable that may cause falsely low levels. The reliability of this test for detecting mucosal disease is controversial. However, it remains a useful screening test.

4. Breath tests include three stages: delivery of a substrate; enzymatic metabolism of the substrate by bacteria, or body cells, or both; and the measurement of the products. A number of different breath tests are in current use or trial. The **breath hydrogen test** for lactose and sucrose malabsorption is well studied.

a. After an overnight fast, the patient is given a loading dose of the disaccharide to be studied.

b. A nasal prong is inserted and 3–5 ml of expired air is collected in a syringe at 30-min intervals for 3 hr.

c. H_2 excretion is measured; excretion of 11 ppm H_2 indicates disaccharide malabsorption.

d. False-positives and false-negatives may be seen due to natural or antibiotic-induced changes in bacterial flora. No antibiotics should be administered within 1 week prior to the test.

5. Jejunal biopsy is a safe, well accepted, and invaluable tool for the diagnosis of intestinal mucosal disease.

   a. All patients must have a platelet count, PT, and PTT prior to the procedure.

   b. After an overnight fast, patients over 6 months of age and under 6–7 years are premedicated with chlorpromazine (Thorazine), 1 mg/kg IM, and pentobarbital, 4 mg/kg. Older patients require no premedication; instead, an anesthetic spray (e.g., tetracaine [Pontocaine] or Cetacaine) is used to anesthetize the pharynx.

   c. The biopsy specimen is sent for histologic examination and assay of small-intestine disaccharidases. The values at Children's Hospital Medical Center (normal values vary from laboratory to laboratory) are

   Lactase 30.5 ± 16.6 U/gm protein
   Sucrase 62.8 ± 26.7 U/gm protein
   Maltase 203.6 ± 75.2 U/gm protein

6. Duodenal fluid should be obtained by a nasogastric tube or at the time of biopsy. The fluid is examined for parasites, especially *Giardia lamblia*, and sent for bacterial culture.

7. Sweat test Pilocarpine iontophoresis for sweat electrolytes diagnoses cystic fibrosis in 99 percent of cases. Sweat weight should be greater than 100 mg. A chloride level above 60 mEq/L or a sodium level above 60 mEq/L is positive.

C. Malabsorption The three phases of digestion and absorption are shown in Table 11-1. Because fat absorption depends on all the phases of digestion, the presence of steatorrhea (fat malabsorption) is the best indicator of a malabsorptive defect. Further tests (see Sec. **I.B.3–7)** will permit the localization of specific sites of abnormality.

D. Gastrointestinal bleeding

1. Etiology See Table 11-2. The probable cause varies with age.

2. Evaluation and diagnosis

   a. The patient should first be stabilized as described under treatment (see **3**).

   b. Initial assessment requires a thorough history and physical examination. A very careful, detailed drug history must be taken, especially with respect to the use of aspirin. The nasopharyngeal and oral cavity should be carefully inspected.

   c. Hematemesis indicates a pathologic condition proximal to the ligaments of Treitz. **Melena** usually indicates bleeding above the ileocecal valve, although the lesion may occasionally be in the colon in the presence of a slow transit time. **Bright red blood per rectum** usually is colonic in origin; however, massive bleeding proximal to the ileocecal valve may also present in this fashion.

   d. The following approach to diagnosis may be helpful:

   (1) Initial laboratory tests in all patients should include the following: hematocrit, WBC, differential, peripheral smear, reticulocyte

Table 11-1 Mechanisms of Digestion and Absorption

Diet	Intraluminal Phase		Mucosal Phase	Removal Phase
	Pancreatic	Biliary		
Fat				
Triglycerides →	Monoglycerides (MG) Fatty acids (FA) →	FA, MG Bile acids → Micelle →	Chylomicrons	Lymphatics
Medium-chain triglycerides	→	→		Portal vein
Protein →	Small peptides Amino acids	→	Amino acids	Portal vein
Carbohydrate →	Oligosaccharides Disaccharides	→	Monosaccharides	Portal vein

Table 11-2 Causes of Gastrointestinal Bleeding

Upper Gastrointestinal Tract	Lower Gastrointestinal Tract
Swallowed blood	Anal fissure
Esophagitis	Meckel's diverticulum
Esophageal varices	Intussusception
Gastritis	Polyps
Peptic ulcer	Volvulus
	Duplications
	Hemangiomas
	Hemorrhoids
	Foreign body
	Infectious colitis
	Allergic colitis (milk, soy)
	Ulcerative colitis
	Crohn's disease
	Schönlein-Henoch purpura
	Hemolytic-uremic syndrome
	Necrotizing enterocolitis
	Coagulation disorders

count, platelets, PT, PTT, BUN, creatinine, and urinalysis. Type and crossmatch blood.

(2) Insert a nasogastric tube and aspirate the gastric contents.

(a) If the aspirated material is **positive** for blood, lavage the stomach with iced saline until the return is clear. Endoscopic evaluation of the esophagus, stomach, and duodenum is an extremely valuable tool and should be performed next. An elective upper GI series is done the next day. Should the rate of bleeding be too severe to permit endoscopic examination, selective arteriography is indicated. Therapy should be initiated as discussed in **3.**

(b) If the aspirated material is **negative** for blood (this only excludes bleeding above the pylorus), sigmoidoscopy is indicated. If the findings are positive, follow by a barium enema; if they are negative, proceed with a Meckel's scan, barium enema, and upper GI series in that order, depending on the age of the patient. If these studies are unproductive, endoscopy, colonoscopy, and arteriography may be necessary.

3. Treatment

a. Stabilize vital functions. Insert a large-gauge IV catheter and begin intravascular replacement as necessary with saline, Ringer's lactate, or plasma.

b. Transfuse fresh whole blood in an actively bleeding patient, packed cells in a stable patient who has stopped bleeding (see Chap. 1, Sec. **2,** p. 13).

c. Specific treatment depends on the cause of the bleeding.

d. If peptic ulcer disease, gastritis, or esophagitis is found, neutralize gastric acid. Hourly antacids in a dose of approximately 1 ml/kg, up to a maximum of 30 ml/dose, should be administered. Magnesium hydroxide antacids (Maalox, Mylanta) may be alternated with aluminum hydroxide mixtures (Amphojel) to prevent diarrhea or constipation. Cimetidine, a gastric (H^+) receptor antagonist, is very effective in diminishing gastric acid secretion. The adult dose is 300 mg PO or IV q6h. The gastric pH should be maintained at 5.0. Children over 12 are given 20–40 mg/kg/day in 4 divided doses. *(This drug is not yet approved by the FDA for use in children under 12 years of age.)*

II. SPECIFIC ENTITIES

A. Diarrheal disease Diarrhea is among the most common symptoms in pediatrics, and in underdeveloped countries it is the most common cause of morbidity and mortality in childhood.

Evaluation of chronic diarrhea includes a history, with particular attention to blood or mucus in the stools, weight loss, failure to thrive, associated symptoms (fever, recurrent infection), drugs taken, particularly antibiotics, GI surgical procedures, family history, travel, age, and race.

A **physical examination** should be done, with attention to nutritional status, hydration, edema, protuberant abdomen, abdominal masses, muscular habitus, rectal prolapse, and affect, particularly irritability. The cardiopulmonary system and neurologic status should be carefully evaluated.

Laboratory studies include a CBC, ESR, urinalysis, serum protein analysis (SPA), stool examination (see Sec. **I.B**), and sweat test. If the results of malabsorption screening are positive, the steps listed in **I.B** should be followed.

1. Acute nonspecific gastroenteritis

a. Etiology This common condition has many causes. These are listed in Table 11-3.

b. Evaluation This condition is often manifested by a sudden onset of vomiting, followed by diarrhea. It is most often self-limited. Fever may or may not be present, but with a reduction of fluid intake and abnormal losses, dehydration may occur, especially in children under 3 years of age.

(1) History In evaluating the patient with gastroenteritis, record the following: weight loss, duration, presence of blood or mucus, type

Table 11-3 Common Causes of Acute Diarrhea in Childhood

Viral enteritis (reovirus)

Bacterial enteritis

    Enterotoxin associated (*E. coli*, cholera, *Clostridium perfringens*, *Staphylococcus*)

    Nonenterotoxin associated* (*Salmonella*, *Shigella*, *E. coli*, *Yersinia*)

Parasitic enteritis (amebiasis,* giardiasis)

Extraintestinal infection (e.g., otitis media, urinary tract infection, sepsis)

Antibiotic induced*

Hemolytic-uremic syndrome*

Inflammatory bowel disease* (ulcerative colitis, Crohn's disease)

* May be associated with blood in the stool.

and frequency of stools, type and amount of feedings, frequency of urination, presence or absence of tears, associated symptoms (e.g., fever, vomiting, localized abdominal pain), and current family illnesses.

(2) Physical examination should include a description of the skin turgor, mucous membranes, fontanelles, eyes, presence or absence of tears, activity state, irritability, and associated rashes.

(3) Laboratory tests can be minimized in the milder clinical states, but stool cultures and Wright's stain for neutrophils may be helpful, and urinary specific gravity is a useful sign of early dehydration. (For further workup in cases of diarrhea, see Sec. **II.B**, p. 261.)

c. Therapy

(1) Children with acute diarrheal disease and minimal dehydration are treated most effectively with clear fluids, including water, Coca-Cola, or ginger ale *with the bubbles shaken out*, apple juice, diluted tea, and Jell-O. In the initial vomiting stage in infants or small children, large-volume feedings should be avoided. Small amounts (1–2 oz qh) as tolerated are sufficient initially.

(2) Water may be sweetened with sugar, or a 5% glucose solution can be used.

(3) Oral electrolyte solutions (Table 11-4) may be administered for up to 24 hr.

(4) Boiled skim milk has a very high solute load and can cause hypernatremia.

(5) Frequent large feedings stimulate the gastrocolic reflex and may aggravate the problem.

(6) Clear fluids alone should not be continued more than 48 hr, or reactive loose stools may be passed. Bland solids can then be added, such as rice cereal, banana flakes, applesauce, saltines, Ritz crackers, dry cereal, or toast with jelly for older children.

(7) The value of drugs such as kaolin and belladonna-containing compounds remains unproved, and their use should probably be discouraged. In the rare case when an **antispasmodic** is considered, diphenoxylate (Lomotil)* or camphorated opium tincture (paregoric, 0.2 ml/kg/dose) may be used sparingly. Even when spasm is reduced, fluid losses continue to occur into the lumen of the gut, but are not measurable and give a false sense of security. In toxogenic diarrhea the elimination of the toxin is also delayed by these agents.

(8) Antiemetics such as promethazine (Phenergan) or dimenhydrinate (Dramamine) (6–12 years, 12.5–25.0 mg tid) suppositories or capsules in 1 or 2 doses are useful adjuncts when simple gastroenteritis is established as the cause of vomiting. The side effects of these drugs preclude their long-term use. If vomiting persists, more vigorous evaluation and management is indicated.

(9) Close follow-up, including daily weights, is imperative, particularly in smaller infants, who may rapidly become dehydrated.

(10) Avoid milk products for 2-3 days after diarrhea ceases

---

* Diphenoxylate should not be used in children *under* 2 years of age. The dosage is as follows: 2–5 years, 6 mg/day; 5–8 years, 8 mg/day; 8–12 years, 10 mg/day.

Table 11-4 Approximate Electrolyte Content for Fluid Replacement or Oral Administration of Electrolytes

Solution	Calories per Ounce	Carbohydrate Source	Carbohydrate (gm/100 ml)	Milliequivalents per Liter			Osmolarity	Osmolality	Estimated Renal Solute Load (mOsm/L)
				Na$^+$	K$^+$	Cl$^-$			
Lytren (Mead Johnson)	9	Glucose	7.6	30.0	25.0	25.0	440	536	106
Pedialyte (Ross)	6	Glucose	5.0	30.0	20.0	30.0	405	(Estimated)	116
5% Glucose	6	Glucose	5.0				278	293	
10% Glucose	12	Glucose	10.0				562	625	

Table 11-5 Causes of Chronic Diarrhea

Chronic nonspecific diarrhea (irritable bowel syndrome)
Chronic infections: *Salmonella, E. coli, Giardia*
Cystic fibrosis
Gluten-sensitive enteropathy (celiac disease)
Disaccharide deficiency (particularly lactose intolerance)
Inflammatory bowel disease
Immunodeficiency states
Anatomic causes
  Short-bowel syndrome
  Malrotation
  Hirschsprung's disease
Endocrine
  Hyperthyroidism
  Addison's disease

2. Chronic gastroenteritis Diarrheal symptoms lasting more than 2 weeks are chronic. The causes of chronic diarrhea are listed in Table 11-5.

  a. Nonspecific diarrhea is the most common cause of chronic diarrhea in childhood.

    (1) The **etiology** is unknown. Psychosocial and family stress is often implicated.

    (2) Evaluation and diagnosis The classic history is of profuse, watery diarrhea with multiple formula and dietary changes in age group 1–5 years. On close questioning, parental discord or another social stress is often revealed. The physical findings and growth are normal. The findings of routine urinalysis and stool cultures are negative. The diagnosis is based on exclusion of other causes of diarrhea.

    (3) Therapy The goal of therapy is to stop diarrhea.

      (a) The family should be reassured that the illness is not too serious.

      (b) Often, past dietary manipulations may have contributed to the production of symptoms and correction of the diet may result in relief of diarrhea. A decrease in the intake of fructose and sucrose-containing drinks or changing the diet may function as a placebo.

      (c) Should reassurance and dietary adjustment fail, hospitalization may be necessary. The disappearance of diarrhea during hospitalization will help convince the family of the absence of significant disease and permit the examination of psychosocial factors.

      (d) Antidiarrheal medication is not indicated.

      (e) X-ray contrast studies should be done when it is necessary to rule out anatomic abnormalities.

  b. Cystic fibrosis

    (1) Etiology This is an inherited autosomal recessive condition with a gene frequency of 1:20 and an incidence of 1:1600.

(2) Evaluation and diagnosis   The pulmonary aspects of the disease are discussed in Chap. 20.

(a) Pancreatic insufficiency occurs in 85 percent of patients with cystic fibrosis. These patients usually present with a history of chronic diarrhea with foul-smelling stools and failure to thrive. There are many GI manifestations of cystic fibrosis, and the disease should always be excluded in patients presenting with these features.

(b) Meconium ileus presents with intestinal obstruction, often associated with ileal atresia, in the immediate neonatal period (see Chap. 5) in 15 percent of patients. The sweat test is often not diagnostic in the first week of life, and thus the diagnosis may not be definitive until later.

(c) Rectal prolapse is a common presenting feature.

(d) Meconium ileus equivalent (intestinal obstruction in the older child or adult) presents with abdominal pain and may be associated with intussusception.

(e) Cirrhosis of the liver develops in 15–20 percent of patients. An elevated alkaline phosphatase is often the first sign of liver involvement. Subsequent development of portal hypertension is common.

(f) Diabetes mellitus   Overt diabetes occurs in 1 percent of patients with cystic fibrosis. Ketoacidosis is rare.

(g) Gallstones occur in nearly one-third of all cystic fibrosis patients, although acute cholecystitis develops in only a few.

(3) Treatment

(a) Pancreatic preparations   All patients with cystic fibrosis who have steatorrhea (85 percent) require pancreatic enzymes. Although fat absorption improves with these agents, it does not return to normal even with massive doses.

Various pancreatic preparations are available. The dosage can be established only by trial. Excessive dosage may result in the "meconium ileus equivalent," i.e., recurrent abdominal pain, palpable fecal masses, and obstruction. Rough dosage schedules for various pancreatic preparations are as follows:

i. Viokase (powder and tablets) is given in the following dosages:

Newborn, ¼–½ tsp/bottle
1–2 years, ½–1 tsp/meal, ¼ tsp/snack
After age 3, 2–4 tablets/meal
Adolescents, 8–12 tablets/meal

ii. Cotazyme   The dose is roughly ½ that for Viokase. Cotazyme can be taken before meals. The dose is titrated on stool frequency, degree of steatorrhea, and growth.

iii. Pancrease   The dose is roughly ¼ that of Viokase.

(b) Diet   A low-fat diet (about 30–40 gm fat/day in older children) is indicated. Medium-chain triglycerides (MCT), which are more readily absorbed than long-chain fats, are an important source of calories. MCT supplementation is indicated in patients with poor weight gain.

Infant formulas such as Pregestimil and Portajen supplemented with MCT are utilized for infants with cystic fibrosis.

(c) **Vitamins** Multivitamins are given daily. Vitamin E and vitamin K are given as follows:

Vitamin E, until age 2–3 years, 50 IU/day; over age 3, 100 IU/day

Vitamin K, until age 1, 2.5 mg biweekly; over age 1, vitamin K is indicated only if liver disease is present, or when the PT is prolonged.

(d) **Salt supplementation** In hot weather, supplementary sodium chloride, 3–5 gm/day, should be given.

c. **Shwachman-Diamond syndrome** (congenital hypoplasia of the pancreas) is a rare disease characterized by pancreatic insufficiency and neutropenia or pancytopenia. After cystic fibrosis it is the commonest cause of pancreatic insufficiency in childhood.

(1) **Etiology** This condition is probably hereditary.

(2) **Evaluation** The history includes failure to thrive, chronic diarrhea, and recurrent infection. Physical examination reveals a small, malnourished child. Laboratory investigation includes a sweat test, stool examination, CBC, platelets, 72-hr stool fat test, pancreatic function test, bone x-rays, and bone marrow examination.

(3) **Diagnosis**

(a) The findings of a sweat test are normal.

(b) A blood count reveals cyclic or constant neutropenia. Some patients have anemia and thrombocytopenia as well.

(c) A stool examination reveals positive Sudan stain.

(d) A 72-hr stool fat test reveals steatorrhea.

(e) The bone marrow shows maturation arrest of the neutrophils.

(f) A bone x-ray reveals metaphyseal dysostosis in 10–15 percent of patients.

(4) **Treatment**

(a) Replace pancreatic enzymes [see **b.(3)**].

(b) Give antibiotic therapy for recurrent infections.

d. **Gluten-sensitive enteropathy** (GSE, celiac disease) is manifested clinically by malabsorption and morphologically by a flat intestinal lesion. Both improve on a gluten-free diet and are reexacerbated by the reintroduction of gluten into the diet. It is a lifelong disease that presents most frequently between 9 and 18 months of age (earlier in formula-fed infants), but can be seen at any age.

(1) **Etiology** The mechanism of gluten sensitivity is unknown. Genetic factors play an important role. It is more common in Ireland (1:200) than in the rest of the world (United States estimate is 1:3000). Theories as to its cause include immune mediation of gluten toxicity and an enzymatic defect.

(2) **Evaluation**

(a) Relevant features in the history may include a family history of GSE, failure to thrive, irritability, anorexia, and chronic diarrhea.

(b) The physical examination classically reveals an irritable, malnourished child with a pot belly and proximal muscle wasting, characteristically including the buttocks. However, some patients present atypically with features only of a selective malabsorption, i.e., only growth failure, anemia, and rickets.

(c) Laboratory investigations should include a blood count, serum albumin, immunoglobulin, folate, iron, iron-binding capacity, stool examination, and sweat test. **Jejunal biopsy is mandatory for the diagnosis of GSE.**

(3) Diagnosis

(a) The finding of a **stool examination,** including culture, ova, and parasites, is negative. Clinitest findings are variable. Sudan stain and a 72-hr stool fat test reveal steatorrhea.

(b) D-Xylose absorption test results are abnormal.

(c) Jejunal biopsy reveals a flat, villous lesion. This is not a pathognomonic finding.

(d) **Clinical and morphologic improvement on a gluten-free diet** and **exacerbation on a gluten challenge** confirm the diagnosis.

(4) Treatment

(a) A gluten-free diet is begun immediately. Rye, oats, and barley should also be excluded.

(b) Lactose should be omitted for the first 6 weeks to ameliorate the secondary disaccharide intolerance that is usually associated with GSE. Pregestimil or a soy-based formula will accomplish this purpose in infants (see Chap. 4, Sec. I).

(c) Irritability is the first symptom to respond to therapy; diarrheal symptoms may linger for up to 6 weeks. If diarrhea persists, it may be necessary to alter the sugar base of the formula prescribed.

(d) Vitamins and minerals should be replaced according to specific losses. A multivitamin preparation and iron are usually administered for 2–3 months, after which resolution of malabsorption permits normal dietary replacement. Common specific deficiencies are vitamin D, folic acid, vitamin K, and iron.

(e) **A gluten-free diet is maintained for life.** For this reason, confirmation of the diagnosis must be as clear as possible. It is presently accomplished by **gluten challenge.** This is done after the patient has returned to a normal growth pattern and is symptom free, usually a minimum of 1 year after the initial diagnosis.

    i. A jejunal biopsy is performed to demonstrate return to normal morphology.

    ii. Gluten-containing foods are reintroduced using at least two slices of white bread each day.

    Parents are often reluctant to reintroduce gluten, remembering their child's previous symptoms. On the other hand, once the child (*particularly* older children) tastes previously restricted foods, he or she may resist a return to gluten restriction. To obviate this problem, gluten powder, where available, may be sprinkled into food in a dose of 10 gm/day. In the absence of this material (presently unavailable in the United States) gluten-rich flour may be substituted. In any case, the clinician must be resourceful, since a positive gluten challenge is the only available confirmatory test for GSE.

(f) The challenge is done for up to 6 weeks, at which time (or earlier if symptoms recur) a third jejunal biopsy is done. It is *unusual* for overt diarrheal symptoms to occur during the challenge period. If the biopsy demonstrates evidence of active enteritis, the diagnosis is confirmed. If the biopsy findings are negative, celiac disease is almost certainly not present. A subsequent biopsy may yet be needed after 1 year on the normal diet if symptoms recur.

(5) Prognosis

(a) On adequate gluten restriction, patients achieve normal life expectancy and fertility.

(b) Spontaneous remission does not occur.

(c) Recent reports indicate an increased incidence in the subsequent development of GI malignancy in patients with GSE.

B. Disaccharidase deficiency may be primary (genetic) or secondary to intestinal mucosal damage. The most clinically relevant disaccharidases are lactase and sucrase.

1. Lactose intolerance (primary) Primary lactase deficiency is extremely common and an important cause of recurrent abdominal pain in childhood.

a. Etiology The condition is genetic.

b. Evaluation

(1) Lactase deficiency usually presents in blacks over 3 years of age and Caucasians over 5 years of age. Detection of lactase intolerance prior to these ages indicates a secondary lactase intolerance.

(2) The history includes recurrent abdominal pain and flatulence or diarrhea, or both.

(3) The physical examination usually reveals no abnormality.

(4) Laboratory tests include a stool examination, lactose intolerance test, and lactose breath test. Jejunal biopsy is usually not indicated.

c. Diagnosis

(1) The stool may be positive for reducing substances.

(2) The results of the lactose tolerance test are usually, but not always, positive.

(3) Jejunal biopsy shows a normal morphologic picture and normal disaccharidase levels except for lactase.

(4) The **lactose breath test** is an easy, reliable, noninvasive test for the diagnosis of lactase deficiency.

(5) There is usually a dramatic response to milk withdrawal in both primary and secondary lactase deficiency. It does not distinguish one from the other.

d. Therapy

   (1) A lactose-free diet is begun immediately.

   (2) A calcium supplement may be needed for long-term therapy (see Food and Drug Administration requirements). This can be supplied in patients over 5–6 years of age by commercially available calcium containing antacid tablets (e.g., Tums, Rolaids).

   (3) Lactase deficiency persists for life. However, patients may reintroduce lactose in small amounts until symptoms supervene. Lact-Aid, a commercially available lactase, appears to be of value in some patients who wish to try a limited amount of lactose.

2. Sucrase-isomaltase deficiency

   a. Etiology   This is a rare autosomal recessive disorder.

   b. Evaluation

   (1) History   These patients present with chronic diarrhea that starts with the introduction of sucrase-containing foods.

   (2) The physical findings are usually normal. Failure to thrive is not a feature of this disease.

   (3) Laboratory tests include stool examination, sucrose tolerance and breath tests, and jejunal biopsy.

   c. Diagnosis

   (1) The stools may be positive for reducing substances.

   (2) Sucrose tolerance test findings are usually positive.

   (3) The sucrose breath test is a reliable indicator of the presence of sucrase-isomaltase deficiency.

   (4) Jejunal biopsy shows a normal histologic picture and, except for low to absent sucrase-isomaltase, normal disaccharide levels.

   d. Treatment

   (1) A sucrose-free diet is instituted immediately, usually with a dramatic response.

   (2) Sucrose-isomaltose restriction is lifelong.

   (3) Dietary supplements are not indicated.

C. Food sensitivity (see also Chap. 19)   The commonest food sensitivities associated with GI disease are cow's milk and soy protein.

   1. Cow's milk protein sensitivity   The incidence of cow's milk protein sensitivity is estimated at 0.5–1.0 percent of infants under 6 months of age.

   a. Etiology   Systemic sensitivity (e.g., anaphylaxis, wheezing) to cow's milk appears to be mediated by immediate hypersensitivity (IgE) whereas GI disease *appears not to be mediated in this manner.* Gastrointestinal involvement is usually limited to the upper GI tract or to the colon.

   b. Evaluation   Sensitivity to cow's milk usually presents in infants 6 months of age.

(1) The history may include pallor, edema, irritability, vomiting, diarrhea, colic, and failure to thrive.

(2) Physical examination may reveal a pale, edematous child. Some infants may present with a colitislike picture with profuse, bloody diarrhea.

(3) Laboratory tests include CBC, serum albumin and immunoglobulins, serum iron, iron-binding capacity, IgE, RAST (Chap. 19) to milk sensitivity, gastric and intestinal biopsy, sigmoidoscopy, and rectal biopsy (if patient has grossly bloody diarrhea). *Occult blood is always present in the stool.*

c. Diagnosis

(1) The CBC shows iron deficiency anemia and eosinophilia.

(2) SPA reveals low serum albumin and immunoglobulins.

(3) IgE levels are normal and the RAST is negative in GI disease alone, but usually not in systemic allergic disease.

(4) Gastric biopsy may reveal a gastritis with eosinophilic infiltration.

(5) Small-intestine biopsy reveals a patchy, flat, villous lesion.

(6) In patients with colonic involvement, sigmoidoscopy reveals colitis.

(7) Withdrawal of milk protein (not lactose) produces a dramatic clinical and morphologic response. Reintroduction of milk protein after remission produces exacerbation of clinical and morphologic abnormalities. Unlike GSE, this disease is transient, and milk protein can be tolerated after the age of 2. A **milk challenge should not be attempted in patients with history of milk anaphylaxis.** In patients with GI disease who have negative skin tests and normal serum IgE, mild challenge is a safe technique.

d. Therapy

(1) A milk-free diet is instituted immediately.

(2) In view of associated secondary disaccharidase deficiency, a disaccharide-free formula or diet is introduced.

(3) An iron supplement should be provided.

2. Soy protein sensitivity The incidence of isolated soy sensitivity is unknown. It is estimated that 10 percent of patients with milk sensitivity have associated soy sensitivity.

a. Etiology The cause is unknown.

b. Evaluation The history, physical examination, and laboratory investigations are similar to those carried out in patients with cow's milk sensitivity. The syndrome is usually seen in infants for whom soy formulas have been prescribed.

c. Diagnosis

(1) The CBC shows iron deficiency anemia and eosinophilia.

(2) SPA reveals low levels of serum albumin and immunoglobulins.

(3) IgE levels are normal. The RAST reaction is negative in GI disease alone but positive in systemic allergic disease.

(4) Gastric biopsy may reveal a gastritis with eosinophilic infiltration

(5) Small-intestine biopsy reveals a patchy, flat, villous lesion.

(6) Sigmoidoscopy reveals colitis.

(7) Withdrawal of soy protein produces a dramatic clinical response

(8) Rechallenge after remission will reproduce abnormalities in a manner similar to that occurring with milk challenge.

(9) It is unknown whether this lesion is transient or permanent.

d. Therapy

(1) A soy protein–free diet is instituted.

(2) An iron supplement is indicated.

3. Eosinophilic gastroenteritis

a. Etiology   The cause is unknown.

b. Evaluation

(1) The history reveals the onset of systemic allergy (usually asthma and abdominal pain.

(2) Growth failure is a prominent part of the syndrome. The physical finding may also include pallor and edema.

(3) Laboratory investigations include a stool guaiac test, CBC, SPA IgE, serum iron, and skin and RAST test reactions to various foods (see Chap. 19).

c. Diagnosis

(1) The CBC reveals peripheral eosinophilia and iron deficiency anemia.

(2) SPA reveals hypoalbuminemia and hypogammaglobulinemia.

(3) Serum IgE is elevated.

(4) RAST and skin test reactions to many foods are positive.

(5) Gastric biopsy reveals gastritis with eosinophilic infiltration.

(6) Jejunal biopsy reveals a patchy, flat, villous lesion.

d. Treatment

(1) Dietary manipulations may alleviate acute symptoms (anaphylaxis) but have no effect on the chronic course of disease.

(2) Initially, prednisone in a dose of 1–2 mg/kg/day is used. Then alternate-day steroids may be used.

(3) Vitamins and iron supplements are indicated.

(4) Unlike cow's milk sensitivity, eosinophilic gastritis (like GSE) appears to be a lifelong condition.

D. Inflammatory bowel disease

1. Ulcerative colitis

a. Etiology   Ulcerative colitis is an inflammatory disease of the colon of unknown etiology. Genetic, environmental, psychological, infectious and immunologic mechanisms have been implicated.

b. Evaluation

(1) The history usually includes bloody diarrhea and recurrent abdominal pain.

(2) Systemic manifestations, including arthritis, erythema nodosum, uveitis, episcleritis, and liver disease, may precede or accompany the GI symptoms.

(3) The findings on examination of the abdomen are usually benign, unless local complications of toxic megacolon or perforation have occurred. Growth failure may be present. Laboratory tests include CBC, stool examination, cultures, ova and parasites, SPA, sigmoidoscopy, rectal biopsy, barium enema, and upper GI series.

c. Diagnosis

(1) Stool examination reveals blood and fecal leukocytes.

(2) Sigmoidoscopy reveals colitis, confirmed by rectal biopsy.

(3) Stool cultures are negative, and ova and parasites are not present.

(4) The CBC reveals anemia, leukocytosis with left shift, thrombocytosis, and elevated ESR.

(5) Serum albumin levels may be low or normal.

(6) A barium enema reveals colitis (the findings may be normal in the early stages of the disease). An upper GI series reveals nothing abnormal.

d. Treatment depends on the severity of the symptoms and signs.

(1) Sulfasalazine (Azulfidine) is usually the drug of choice in mild to moderate cases. Therapy is begun at 500 mg/day and increased over 4–5 days to 2–3 gm/day in 3 divided doses. Under the age of 5 years, 50 mg tid should be sufficient. Side effects include leukopenia, agranulocytosis, hemolytic anemia, arthralgia, headache, rash, and, rarely, lower GI bleeding.

(2) Corticosteroids are the mainstay of therapy in inflammatory bowel disease. In the moderate case where sulfasalazine alone is inadequate, prednisone, 1–2 mg/kg/day in a daily dose, is given. In patients requiring IV therapy, methylprednisolone sodium succinate (Solu-Medrol), 1–2 mg/kg/day in 2–4 divided doses is indicated.

(3) Parenteral alimentation (see p. 247) should be used in all patients requiring IV therapy.

(4) Psychiatric consultation may be required to assist the patient, or the parents, or both to cope with chronic ulcers.

(5) Surgery   Colectomy is curative. The indications are

(a) Perforation.

(b) Toxic megacolon.

(c) Massive bleeding.

(d) Severe steroid side effects that preclude further use.

(e) Malignancy   There is a definite risk of the development of colon cancer in patients with long-standing ulcerative colitis. Appropriate screening, such as colonoscopy and rectal biopsy, should be performed annually for more than 10 years on patients with the disease. Any sign of dysplasia on biopsy is an absolute indication for colectomy.

2. Crohn's disease

a. Etiology   This is an inflammatory disease of unknown etiology that can affect any part of the GI tract from mouth to anus.

b. Evaluation

   (1) The history commonly includes growth failure, recurrent fever, abdominal pain, and diarrhea. Systemic symptoms include arthritis and erythema nodosum.

   (2) Physical examination may reveal evidence of malnutrition, localized abdominal signs or perianal disease on rectal examination, and blood and mucus. Laboratory tests include a CBC, ESR, SPA, electrolytes, iron, iron-binding capacity, folate, sigmoidoscopy, barium enema, and upper GI series.

c. Diagnosis

   (1) Stools   Cultures are negative for bacteria, ova, and parasites. Leukocytes are present. The guaiac test findings are positive if colitis is present.

   (2) A CBC reveals anemia, leukocytosis with left shift, and thrombocytosis. The ESR is elevated.

   (3) Serum iron and folate are low, and iron-binding capacity is increased.

   (4) SPA reveals a serum albumin that may be low.

   (5) Sigmoidoscopy may show colitis (if the colon is involved).

   (6) A barium enema, or upper GI series, or both, may show involvement.

   (7) Growth failure   Severe growth failure occurs in 30 percent of patients with Crohn's disease. Less than 5 percent of patients have malabsorption. The cause of growth failure is believed to be lack of caloric intake.

d. Treatment

   (1) Sulfasalazine and corticosteroids are given for ulcerative colitis.

   (2) IV hyperalimentation with a normal dietary intake has been used with good success in prepubertal patients to promote growth and initiate puberty in those who fail to respond to corticosteroids.

   (3) Psychiatric consultation is useful for the patients and their families in managing this chronic, often debilitating, disease.

   (4) The **indications for surgery** are less clear-cut than for ulcerative colitis because of the chronic nature of this disease. They include

   (a) Perforation.

   (b) Obstruction.

   (c) Extensive perianal or rectal disease unresponsive to other therapeutic modalities.

   (d) Severe growth failure, in which a localized segment may be

Table 11-6   Clinical, Pathologic, and Radiographic Features of Ulcerative Colitis and Crohn's Disease

Features	Ulcerative Colitis	Crohn's Disease
Diarrhea	Severe	Moderate or absent
Rectal bleeding	Common	Rare
Abdominal pain	Frequent	Common
Weight loss	Moderate	Severe
Growth retardation	Mild	Severe
Extraintestinal man- ifestations	Common	Common
Percentage with bowel involvement		
Anus	15	85
Rectum	95	50
Colon	100	50
Ileum	0 (except for backwash ileitis)	80
Distribution of lesions	Continuous	Skip areas
Pathologic features	Diffuse mucosal disease	Granulomas; focal disease
Radiographic features	Loss of haustra	Thumbprinting
	Superficial ulcers	Skip areas
	No skip areas	String sight
Cancer risk	High	Less than with ulcerative colitis but still increased

removed. (See Table 11-6 for a comparison of the features of ulcerative colitis and Crohn's disease.)

E. Hirschsprung's disease (congenital, aganglionic megacolon)   Congenital absence of the intrinsic ganglionic plexus of Auerbach and Meissner, which involves varying lengths of the rectum and colon. The incidence is estimated at 1 in 5000. A family incidence exists in 10 percent of cases.

1. Etiology   The cause is unknown.

2. Evaluation   The neonatal history includes failure to pass meconium in the first 24 hr of life or bile-stained vomiting in the first week of life. In late infancy and childhood the history is of increasing constipation. Rectal examination classically reveals an empty rectum followed by an explosive gush of stool and gas. In the neonatal period abdominal distention is a prominent feature, whereas in the older child, fecal masses are palpable. Laboratory investigations include a kidney-ureter-bladder (KUB) study, barium enema, rectal manometry, and rectal biopsy.

3. Diagnosis

    a. X-rays of the abdomen reveal dilated loops of bowel on an anteroposterior film. Rectal air is absent.

    b. The barium enema is usually diagnostic, revealing a narrow aganglionic segment with a dilated colon above. In the immediate neonatal period this typical pattern may be absent. An important clue will be a 24-hr film showing that the barium is still present. Rarely, in "low segment" Hirschsprung's disease, the barium enema findings may be normal or nondiagnostic.

    c. Rectal manometry may reveal absence of the normal relaxation reflex of the internal sphincter.

    d. Rectal biopsy is the definitive method of diagnosis. If a suction biopsy does not reveal ganglion cells, a full-thickness surgical biopsy is necessary. Rarely, if symptoms persist when laboratory findings are normal, a second or even a third biopsy may be needed.

4. Treatment

    a. The neonate is often extremely ill, with entercolitis, shock, and sepsis.

        (1) A vasogastric tube is passed for decompression.

        (2) Urgent rehydration is begun.

        (3) Antibiotics are indicated.

        (4) An emergency colostomy is performed in an area of the colon where ganglion cells are seen.

        (5) Resection of the aganglionic segment is delayed for 6 months to 2 years.

    b. In infants and children who are relatively well, the definitive surgery may be performed with a diverting colostomy.

    c. Surgical management   Three types of operations have been in vogue.

        (1) Swenson   Aganglionic colon is resected, and the ganglion-containing bowel is anastomosed to the rectal stump.

        (2) Duhamel   A longer piece of rectum, usually 5–7 cm, is left and closed proximally. Ganglionic bowel is pulled down retrorectally to 1 cm from the mucocutaneous junction, leaving part of the internal sphincter intact. Colorectal anastomosis is achieved by clamping the posterior wall of the rectum to the anterior wall of the colon.

        (3) Soave   Ten to twenty cm of rectal stump is left. The mucosa is stripped and the ganglionic bowel pulled through.

    d. Surgical complications

        (1) Following colostomy

            (a) Circulatory collapse resulting in severe enterocolitis may occur following colostomy for decompression. Treatment is supportive, i.e., fluid and electrolyte replacement and antibiotics.

            (b) Persistent diarrhea, which is often due to disaccharide deficiency, may occur. A Clinitest is positive, and a change in the type of sugar in the formula will alleviate symptoms.

        (2) After definitive surgery   Segmental obstruction with overflow incontinence is often a problem, especially in the first few months after surgery.

III. HEPATIC FAILURE

    A. Etiology   Acute hepatic failure is a clinical syndrome resulting from severe hepatic dysfunction or massive hepatic necrosis. The causes are listed in Table 11-7.

Table 11-7   Causes of Hepatic Failure in Childhood

Infections
  Viral hepatitis, particularly hepatitis B, non-A, non-B hepatitis (rare in type A)
  Leptospirosis
  Adenovirus
  Coxsackievirus
  Infectious mononucleosis
  Q fever
  Disseminated herpes simplex virus
  Clostridium perfringens
Metabolic abnormalities
  Reye syndrome
  Wilson's disease
Drugs, chemicals, poisons
  Acetaminophen
  Salicylates
  Tetracycline
  Carbon tetrachloride
  Ethanol
  Phosphorus
  Anesthetic agents
    Halothane (fluothane)
    Methoxyflurane (penthrane)
  Mushrooms (*Amanita phalloides*)
Ischemia and hypoxia
  Acute circulatory failure
  Acute Budd-Chiari syndrome
  Acute pulmonary failure
  Ligation of hepatic artery
  Heat stroke

B. Evaluation

1. The **history** may reveal evidence of a previous viral infection; exposure to blood products, drugs, or chemicals; circulatory collapse; preexisting liver disease, or a family history of liver disease.

2. The physical examination reveals progressive jaundice (except in Reye syndrome), asterixis ("liver flap"), fetor hepaticus, mental confusion, or coma.

3. **Laboratory investigations** include urinalysis, CBC, platelet count, reticulocyte count, monospot test, PT, PTT, BUN, electrolytes, glucose, creatinine, ammonia, SGOT, SGPT, alkaline phosphatase, bilirubin, blood gases, serum albumin, serologic tests for hepatitis B, slit lamp examination for Kayser-Fleischer rings, serum copper, ceruloplasmin, 24-hr urine copper, alpha₁-antitrypsin level, and toxic screen.

C. Diagnosis

1. The blood count may reveal leukocytosis, or hemolytic anemia, or both. (Always rule out Wilson's disease when liver disease and hemolytic anemia occur.)

2. PT and PTT are prolonged. Serum albumin may be low. These parameters reflect impaired liver synthetic function.

3. SGOT and SGPT are increased and reflect liver structural damage, with leakage of enzymes from hepatocytes.

4. Alkaline phosphatase may be normal or increased.

5. Serum bilirubin is usually increased except in Reye syndrome. The increase is usually both in direct and indirect bilirubin fractions.

6. Blood glucose may be low.

7. BUN and electrolytes may reflect electrolyte imbalance, especially hypokalemia and hyponatremia.

8. Blood gases may reveal a metabolic alkalosis or, less commonly, acidosis.

9. Serologic tests for hepatitis B (Hb_sAg, Hb_sAb, Hb_cAg, Hb_cAb) may be positive.

10. Serum copper may be low. Ceruloplasmin is low, with increased 24-hr urinary copper excretion. These findings may suggest Wilson's disease, and further diagnostic tests (e.g., slit lamp examination for Kayser-Fleischer rings and liver copper) are needed.

11. The findings of a toxic screen may be positive if ingestion has occurred.

D. Treatment The purpose of therapy is to alleviate the systemic effects of liver failure and promote liver cell regeneration.

1. Prepare a flow sheet to record laboratory data and daily intake and output.

2. Give a 10–15% glucose solution IV at a rate dependent on renal function. Monitor blood glucose.

3. Give vitamin K, 5–10 mg/day IV for 3 days or while PT remains prolonged. If therapy is needed for more than 3 days, reduce the vitamin K dose to 1–2 mg daily. Fresh frozen plasma may be required to control bleeding.

4. To decrease ammonia production

   a. Initially, give 10 gm protein/day if the patient is able to take food orally.

   b. Give lactulose, 1 ml/kg q6h, or neomycin, 50 mg/kg/day q6h, or both, to reduce activity of endogenous flora.

   c. Prevent constipation with magnesium citrate (4–8 gm).

5. Pass a nasogastric tube to identify GI bleeding and as a route for medication.

6. A central venous pressure line is needed to maintain fluid balance.

7. Avoid all sedatives, especially those metabolized by the liver (e.g., barbiturates).

8. Always culture urine, blood, and ascitic fluid.

9. Treat GI bleeding vigorously. If gastritis or peptic ulcer disease is present, start cimetidine, 300 mg IV q6h (children under 12 years, 5–10 mg/kg q6h). Monitor gastric pH > 5. If bleeding is due to varices use a Sengstaken-Blakemore tube, or a vasopressin infusion may be necessary. In certain circumstances, emergency surgery may be undertaken.

10. Monitor serum and urinary electrolytes daily. Characteristically, low urinary sodium and high urinary potassium with urine osmolarity

Table 11-8 Differentiation of Renal Disorders Associated with Hepatic Failure

Feature	Renal Circulatory Failure	Acute Tubular Necrosis	Preexisting Renal Disease
Liver function	Severely impaired	Variable	Variable
Ascites	Usually	Sometimes	Sometimes
Encephalopathy	Usually	Sometimes	Sometimes
Precipitating factors	Diuretics Paracentesis GI bleeding	Hypotension	Variable
Course	Slow	Rapid	Slow
Hypotension	Late	Early	None
Oliguria	Gradual	Acute	Variable
Urine sediment	Normal	Abnormal	Abnormal
Urine osmolarity	Greater than plasma	Low, fixed	Low
Urine sodium	Very low	Moderate	Moderate
Kidney size	Normal	Normal or large	Small
Renal pathologic findings	None	Often	Yes

Adapted from W. P. Baldus, *Prog. Liver Dis.* 4:251, 1972.

greater than plasma osmolarity are found. (See Table 11-8 for the differential diagnosis of renal impairment in severe hepatic failure.)

11. If intravascular volume and serum albumin are low, give albumin, 1.75 gm/kg. This dose of albumin will increase serum albumin 1 gm/100 ml.

IV. **VOMITING** Vomiting is one of the most common complaints brought to the attention of the pediatrician. It is a nonspecific symptom and thus must be evaluated in the context of a medical history. The causes of vomiting in different age groups are listed in Table 11-9.

   A. **Infancy** A careful history will determine the nature and quantity of the vomitus, its relation to meals, and the general health of the infant.

   1. **Infection** **Viral gastroenteritis** is the most common cause of vomiting in the first year of life. The peak incidence is in the winter months. Usually, diarrhea and fever are also seen. The course may be protracted, but the disease normally lasts 3–4 days.

      Parenteral infection may present as vomiting in infancy. Sepsis, meningitis, otitis, pyelonephritis, and pneumonia must be considered.

   2. **Neuromuscular incoordination** Cricopharyngeal incoordination may be expressed as vomiting, nasal regurgitation, and aspiration.

   3. **Esophageal dysfunction** Chalasia, or lower esophageal incompetence, is common in infancy. Up to 50 percent of all newborn infants will show regurgitation at fluoroscopy. The condition usually resolves by age 1 year. However, a small number of infants will have enough vomiting to cause poor weight gain. In addition, chronic gastroesophageal reflux may lead to *esophagitis* or *aspiration pneumonia*. The **diagnosis** is generally made by x-ray, although lower esophageal pH probes and endoscopy are being used increasingly.

Table 11-9 Causes of Vomiting According to Age Group

Causes of Vomiting	Age Group
Neuromuscular incoordination	Infants
Formula intolerance	Infants
Rumination	Infants
Adrenal insufficiency	Infants
Inborn error of metabolism	Infants
Uremia	Infants
Cyclic vomiting	Children
Heavy metal poisoning	Children
Pregnancy	Adolescents
Inflammatory bowel disease	Adolescents
Neurosis	Adolescents
Food poisoning	Children, adolescents
Drug ingestion	Children, adolescents
Infection	
Bacterial	Infants, children, adolescents
Viral	Infants, children, adolescents
Esophageal dysfunction	Infants, children, adolescents
Peptic ulcer	Infants, children, adolescents
Intestinal obstruction	Infants, children, adolescents
Increased intracranial pressure	Infants, children, adolescents
Reye syndrome	Infants, children, adolescents

4. **Formula intolerance** Either the sugar or protein component of milk may be responsible for vomiting (see Chap. 4). Lactose intolerance is usually secondary to gastroenteritis. Rarely, milk protein allergy may present with vomiting alone.

 The **diagnosis** is often empirical, made after elimination and reintroduction of the milk protein. Approximately 10–15 percent of children intolerant to cow's milk protein are also intolerant to soy.

5. **In rumination,** previously digested food is regurgitated, rechewed, and reswallowed. It is believed that this action is an attempt to provide oral gratification in an emotionally deprived infant. Severe **failure to thrive** may be seen.

6. **Peptic ulcer** Vomiting is seen in nearly all infants with ulcer disease. Ulcers are not rare in infants. Gastric ulcers are more frequent than duodenal ulcers in this age group and may present with melena and hematemesis. **Diagnosis** is by barium x-ray examination. Endoscopy will detect the 10–20 percent of ulcers missed radiologically.

7. **Intestinal obstruction** Vomiting and abdominal distention in the neonatal period should suggest obstruction. Conditions to consider include tracheoesophageal fistula, intestinal atresia, stenosis, or a web, malrotation, volvulus, meconium ileus, or Hirschsprung's disease. An abdominal mass and projectile vomiting in a first-born male infant is the classic, but not usual presentation of **hypertrophic pyloric stenosis.**

 In the first 6 months of life an **incarcerated umbilical hernia** is the most common cause of obstruction. After this age, **intussusception** assumes primary importance. Sudden and remittent vomiting, abdominal pain, and currant-jelly stool in a previously well infant should suggest the diagnosis. X-ray examination will reveal intestinal obstruction.

8. **Adrenal insufficiency** may cause vomiting in an infant 1–2 weeks old, most usually secondary to the **adrenogenital syndrome** (see Chap. 12). Although hypokalemia is usually found in protracted vomiting, hyperkalemia is noted in this syndrome.

9. Multiple **inborn errors of metabolism,** notably phenylketonuria, maple syrup urine disease, galactosemia, fructose intolerance, and glycogen storage disease may present with vomiting. Peculiar odors, organomegaly, and unexplained acidosis should suggest these diseases.

10. **Increased intracranial pressure** In the presence of intractable vomiting, careful measurement of head circumference, fundoscopy, and inspection of suture may suggest increased intracranial pressure.

11. Rarely, the **Reye syndrome** may present in the first year of life. Protracted vomiting and stupor, with a previous history of viral illness, now resolving, may signal Reye syndrome.

12. **Uremia** Rarely, uremia in the infant may present with vomiting, pallor, and failure to thrive.

B. Causes of vomiting in childhood

1. Infection

a. **Viral gastroenteritis** is the leading cause of vomiting in this age group. **Acute viral hepatitis** is not uncommon in children, and jaundice and hepatomegaly should be looked for.

b. **Bacterial infections,** particularly involving the middle ear, pharynx, lung, or urinary tract infection may cause vomiting.

2. **Esophageal dysfunction** Chalasia and achalasia may be seen during childhood. The **diagnosis** is evident on barium swallow.

3. **Peptic ulcer** Vomiting, abdominal pain, and melena are seen in the majority of children with peptic ulcer disease. Over the age of 6, males with ulcer disease outnumber females 3 to 1. The **diagnosis** is confirmed by the methods described in **A.6.**

4. **Intestinal obstruction** In addition to the causes of intestinal obstruction listed in **A.7** one should consider **ruptured viscus** or **spleen, pancreatitis,** or **duodenal hematoma;** appendicitis may present with vomiting in addition to abdominal pain and tenderness and fever. Intestinal pseudo-obstruction also presents with vomiting.

5. **Increased intracranial pressure** Vomiting, headache, a change in mental state, and neurologic impairment suggest this entity.

6. **Reye syndrome** See **A.11.**

7. **Cyclic vomiting** is characterized by recurrent episodes of nausea and vomiting, often accompanied by abdominal pain. The child is usually 6–11 years old, is well between attacks, and may suffer from periodic headaches. Migraines will develop in as many as 75 percent of these children in later life. EEG abnormalities may be seen.

8. **Food poisoning** Food poisoning that is usually due to either coagulase-positive *or* coagulase-negative *Staphylococcus aureus* usually presents 6–12 hr after ingestion of the tainted food. Other organisms include *Clostridium perfringens,* and *Clostridium botulinum.*

9. **Heavy metal poisoning** Acute and/or chronic ingestion of heavy metals may cause vomiting. In children under 6, it is a common presentation of lead poisoning (see Chap. 3, Sec. III).

10. **Drug ingestion** Any child capable of coming in contact with drugs or chemicals should be suspected of ingesting them (see Chaps. 2 and 3).

C. Causes of vomiting in adolescence

1. **Infectious** In addition to the viral and bacterial disorders previously mentioned, pelvic inflammatory disease should be considered in the vomiting febrile adolescent girl (see Chap. 13).

   Viral hepatitis (hepatitis A) is common in this age group. Parenteral drug abuse should suggest the possibility of hepatitis B, and liver function tests should be done, even in the absence of icterus.

2. **Esophageal dysfunction** A history of vomiting in addition to heart burn or vomitus on the pillow seen on arising should suggest **gastroesophageal reflux**. The **diagnosis** is best made by a barium swallow, esophageal manometry, Tuttle test (acid reflux measurement with pH probe), and esophagoscopy with esophageal biopsy.

   Vomiting and dysphagia should suggest **achalasia** or **hiatus hernia**.

3. **Peptic ulcer** See **A.6** and **B.3**.

4. **Intestinal obstruction**

   a. The **superior mesenteric artery syndrome** is seen particularly in adolescence. This disorder should be suspected in thin children who are often recumbent for long periods of time. **Diagnosis** is by fluoroscopy and occasionally by angiography.

   b. Rarely, **intraluminal objects** may cause intestinal obstruction.

   c. **Cholecystitis,** both acute and chronic, may present with vomiting. It is more common in females than in males.

5. **Increased intracranial pressure** See **B.5**.

6. **Reye syndrome** See **A.11**.

7. **Food poisoning** See **B.8**.

8. **Drug or heavy metal ingestion** See **B.9** and **B.10**.

9. **Pregnancy** should be suspected in the adolescent girl who gives a history of chronic nausea and vomiting, often in the morning (see Chap. 13).

10. **Inflammatory bowel disease** Rarely, chronic vomiting, usually with abdominal pain and weight loss, may be seen as a presenting manifestation of Crohn's disease.

11. **Neurosis** The emotionally ill adolescent may present with chronic vomiting. The vomiting usually occurs just after meals, may be self-induced, and rarely causes severe weight loss unless the patient also has anorexia nervosa. Psychiatric referral may be indicated.

12

Disorders of the Endocrine System

I. GENERAL APPROACH TO ENDOCRINE DISORDERS The evaluation of a child with a suspected endocrine disorder requires a thorough pediatric interview and examination. Especially relevant considerations are the past history (including the mother's pregnancy), a review of the child's body systems, the family history, the child's social history, a comprehensive physical examination, and laboratory evaluations.

A. Evaluation

1. The value and necessity of compiling past growth data into a **growth curve** cannot be overemphasized. Vigorous attempts should be made to obtain any available measurements from records of physicians, schools, camps, baby books, or even wall markings. These data are inexpensive to obtain, noninvasive, and may save a patient from a needless workup or indicate an urgent need for evaluation.

2. **Past serial photographs** may document the onset and progression of subtle changes incurred by disease.

3. **Bone age of the left hand and wrist** reflects a composite of biologic growth. Comparison of bone age to height age, as well as to chronological age, may differentiate normal from pathologic conditions.

4. **Twenty-four-hour urine collections** should be obtained from 8 A.M. to 8 A.M. the following day. Since most hormones are subject to cyclic secretion, a 24-hr interpretation of their metabolites minimizes temporal variation. Adequacy of collection may be estimated by measuring the milligrams of creatinine per total volume. (Normal ranges of urinary creatinine excretion are between 10 mg/kg/day in infants and 20–22 mg/kg/day in adults.)

B. Therapy

1. Since most endocrine disorders are chronic diseases, **parent and patient education (and reeducation)** are essential if life-styles are to be as normal as possible. The social effects of an often highly visible condition must be approached with concern and support. The importance of relating the child to his or her chronological age, despite size or sexual development, should be emphasized.

2. Hormonal therapy is at best an artificial replacement, is not as sensitive as endogenous secretion, and is always dependent on compliance.

3. Personality and behavior may be affected directly by hormonal excess or deficiency. It may be difficult to determine the relative contributions of organic factors and psychological problems incurred because of a chronic disease.

4. **Medic Alert bracelets** or **necklaces** should be worn by patients with diabetes mellitus, diabetes insipidus, congenital adrenogenital hyperplasia, and adrenal insufficiency.

II. DISORDERS OF GROWTH

A. Short stature

1. Etiology See Table 12-1.

2. Evaluation

 a. In general, patients in whom short stature is due to endocrine conditions are overweight for height, whereas patients with severe gastrointestinal, genitourinary, cardiac, or pulmonary disease are un-
derweight. A change in height velocity (increments of increase per
unit time) is highly suggestive of an organic condition and merits
full investigation.

 b. The **history** should focus on the perinatal period (gestational age, birth
weight, birth length, complications), onset of short stature, intellectual, social, and motor development, CNS abnormalities, diet, and
past illness. Heights of members of the immediate family should be
recorded.

3. Diagnosis

 a. The **past growth pattern, or rate,** is of critical importance. Once
growth velocity is ascertained, the differential diagnosis is narrowed
down.

 b. **Screening tests** may include CBC, erythrocyte sedimentation rate
(ESR), urinalysis with specific gravity, bone age, T_4, RT_3, Na, K, Cl
CO_2, BUN, creatinine, calcium, P, alkaline phosphatase (AP), total
protein (TP), urinary amino acids, and stool for fats.

 c. **Constitutional short stature** is a diagnosis of exclusion and is supported
by a normal history, normal physical findings and growth velocity,
bone age equal to or greater than height age, and, often, a family
history of short stature.

4. Treatment Normal growth velocity may be restored if the underlying
cause is treated effectively. No treatment is currently available that
increases the mature height of children with constitutional short stature.

B. Tall stature

1. Etiology

 a. **Organic causes** include growth hormone–producing tumors (see Sec
III–VII), cerebral gigantism, Beckwith, XXYY, Klinefelter, and
Marfan syndromes, homocystinuria, lipodystrophy, neurofibromatosis, and hyperthyroidism. Patients with sexual precocity may
have accelerated growth velocity.

 b. **Constitutional tall stature** is the most frequent diagnosis.

2. Evaluation and diagnosis

 a. The probable diagnosis should be established following a history and
physical examination.

 b. Past growth data and bone age are necessary to evaluate velocity and
predict mature height. Skull x-rays, fasting growth hormone, insulin
blood glucose determinations, and karyotyping may be indicated.

3. Treatment

 a. Treatment of a pituitary tumor follows the guidelines outlined in Sec
IV.B.4.

Table 12-1 Causes of Short Stature

Familial factors
  Constitutional*
Congenital factors
  Prader-Willi syndrome
  Male Turner, or Noonan, syndrome*
  Progeria
  Laurence-Moon-Biedl syndrome*
Chromosomal disorders
  Down syndrome*
  Trisomies 13, 18
  Turner syndrome
Intrauterine growth retardation
  Infection
  Placental insufficiency
  Congenital anomalies (Russell-Silver, Seckel, Bloom syndromes)
  Congenital without associated anomalies
Skeletal disorders
  Achondroplasia*
  Osteogenesis imperfecta*
  Rickets
  Osteochondrodystrophy*
  Metaphyseal dysostosis*

Nutritional factors
  Low caloric or protein intake
  Persistent vomiting
  Malabsorption, celiac disease, cystic fibrosis*
Endocrine factors
  Hypothyroidism*
  Psychosocial deprivation
  Growth hormone deficiency*
  Corticosteroid excess
  Androgen or estrogen excess
  Diabetes insipidus*
  Somatomedin deficiency*
Metabolic disorders
  Acidosis
  Unavailability of glucose
  Altered mineralization
  Fanconi syndrome
  Galactosemia*
  Aminoacidurias*
  Glycogen storage disease*
  Mucopolysaccharidoses*
  Mucolipidoses*
  Sphingolipidoses*
  Pseudohypoparathyroidism*
  Pseudopseudohypoparathyroidism*

CNS disorders
  Microcephaly
  Mental retardation
  Diencephalic syndrome
Hematologic disorders
  Chronic anemia
  Fanconi's anemia
  Blackfan-Diamond anemia
Cardiovascular abnormalities
  Cyanotic congenital heart disease
Pulmonary conditions
  Asthma,* bronchiectasis, tuberculosis, cystic fibrosis*
Gastrointestinal disease
  Regional enteritis or ulcerative colitis
Renal disease
  Renal acidosis
  Chronic renal failure
Chronic infection
Immune deficiencies

* May have genetic transmission.

277

    b. Attempts to decrease mature height should be restricted to patients who are significantly disturbed about their stature, understand the questionable efficacy of treatment, and accept the potential risks of therapy. For those who are adamant,

        (1) Treatment should begin as early as possible, preferably at 8–10 years of age and certainly prior to menarche.

        (2) **A conjugated estrogen** is employed, e.g., Premarin, beginning at 0.3 mg/day to minimize side effects, then increasing the dosage gradually to 10–15 mg/day. A progestational agent, e.g., Provera, 5–10 mg/day, is added on days 1–5 of each month after the first year of therapy to effect withdrawal bleeding. Treatment is continued until epiphyseal fusion is documented by bone age of the hand, wrist, and knee.

            Side effects include nausea, vomiting, areolar pigmentation, metrorrhagia, and transient amenorrhea after discontinuation of therapy.

        (3) **Diethylstilbestrol is contraindicated** in view of its carcinogenic potential.

C. Obesity

  1. Etiology

    a. Idiopathic (exogenous) obesity is characterized by excessive food intake for caloric requirements, inadequate activity for calories consumed, abnormally balanced diet, and/or food consumption as a response to psychological stress. The family history is often positive for obesity, but the relative contributions of genetic and environmental factors are controversial.

    b. Organic conditions associated with obesity include hypothyroidism, pseudohypoparathyroidism, the Cushing, Turner, Prader-Willi, and Laurence-Moon-Biedl syndromes, and hypothalamic lesions.

  2. Evaluation

    a. A person who is at least 10 percent overweight for his or her height is considered obese.

    b. Most children with idiopathic obesity are of normal or tall stature. Patients with organically caused obesity are usually short or have a deceleration in height velocity.

    c. The **history** should elicit the age of onset of obesity, a complete dietary history (preferably of a 3-day diet with a calorie count), unusual eating or drinking patterns, food preferences, exercise habits, history of past CNS injury or disease, intellectual ability, and symptoms suggestive of hypothyroidism, tetany, or the Cushing syndrome.

    d. The **severity of obesity** should be assessed.

Kg overweight = current weight − ideal weight

$$\% \text{ Overweight} = \frac{\text{no. kg overweight}}{\text{current weight}} \times 100$$

    e. Particular attention should be directed to the distribution of body fat, muscle and bone, facial abnormalities, fundoscopic changes, presence of a goiter, abnormal sexual development, tetany, skin texture, short 4th metacarpal, and polydactyly. Striae and a buffalo hump may be present in patients with either idiopathic or organic obesity.

3. **Diagnosis** of organic conditions should be made primarily by clinical evaluation, with confirmation pursued as indicated.

   a. **Growth data** should be obtained in all cases.

   b. Documentation of bone age, T_4, RT_3, and fasting and 8 P.M. cortisol may be a helpful screen.

   c. Elevated insulin levels, a "diabetic" response to glucose challenge, impaired growth hormone release, and elevated urinary 17-hydroxycorticosteroids may be observed in the obese state, but may revert to normal when normal weight is attained.

4. **Treatment**   Obesity usually resolves after successful treatment of hypothyroidism or Cushing syndrome. In obesity from other causes, therapy must be directed to decreasing caloric intake and increasing caloric expenditure.

   a. **Dietary intake** should be realistically restricted, if possible to 1000 cal/day. Physical activity is encouraged, particularly swimming (which alleviates the handicap of weight), and biking.

   b. **Psychological support and frequent visits** are essential to reinforce reduction efforts and offer counsel.

   c. Medications are ineffective, potentially dangerous, and **should be avoided.**

   d. **Hospitalization** or **intestinal bypass** may be necessary for **severely obese patients.**

   e. **Goals** include **long-term weight reduction** and **continual weight surveillance,** even if ideal weight is attained.

III. DISORDERS OF SEXUAL DEVELOPMENT

A. Ambiguous genitalia

1. Etiology

   a. **Female pseudohermaphrodites** have 46 XX karyotypes and signs of virilization. **Causes** include prenatal exposure to androgens or progestational agents, congenital adrenal hyperplasia, or androgen-producing tumors. The severity of virilization may vary from subtle clitoromegaly to male-appearing external genitalia.

   b. **Male pseudohermaphrodites** have 46 XY or mosaic chromosomes and incomplete masculinization of the external genitalia. The spectrum of abnormality ranges from mild hypospadias to testicular feminization. Causes include (1) genetic defects in testosterone biosynthesis or metabolism, e.g., Reifenstein syndrome (hereditary familial hypogonadism); (2) congenital malformation syndromes, e.g., Smith-Lemli-Opitz and Ullrich-Feichtiger; and (3) certain chromosomal anomalies, e.g., X/XY mosaicism.

   c. **True pseudohermaphrodites** have varying karyotypes (most are chromatin positive) and both ovarian and testicular tissue.

2. Evaluation and diagnosis

   a. The **history** includes documentation of maternal hormone ingestion or production, family history of ambiguous genitalia, infant deaths, sexual precocity, amenorrhea, or infertility.

b. The size and configuration of the phallus, urethral position, degree o labioscrotal fusion, amount of rugation, measurement of gonads presence of a uterus or inguinal mass, and stigmata suggesting a syndrome should be described.

c. Serum cortisol, 17-hydroxycorticosteroids, progesterone, electrolytes buccal smear or karyotype, and 24-hr urine for 17-ketosteroids should be obtained. Retrograde x-ray studies, laparoscopy, gonadal biopsy, o surgical exploration may be appropriate.

3. Treatment

a. An **accurate determination of the cause** of ambiguous genitalia is criti cal to sex assignment in the newborn period in order to maximize the potential for sexual and reproductive function. In general, designing a vagina is less complicated than reconstructing an adequate phallus and penile urethra. However, each case should be considered indi vidually.

b. Operations on the female genitalia are usually performed early in the first year; second-stage vaginoplasty is completed at adolescence.

c. Reconstruction of the penis and correction of hypospadias may re quire four to six operations from infancy to age 9–10. To preserve valuable tissue for reconstruction, **circumcision is contraindicated.**

d. Intraabdominal or inguinal testes should be sought and removed t avoid future malignant degeneration or virilization of a phenotypi female at adolescence.

e. **Growth and sexual development** should be monitored closely and **hor monal therapy** instituted as indicated (see **B.4.b**).

f. The diagnosis and prognosis for sexual and reproductive functior should be discussed frankly with the parents and later with the pa tient. Psychological support, guidance, and repeated explanations especially when the patient has reached adolescence, are of critica importance.

B. Delayed puberty

1. Etiology

a. **Constitutional (idiopathic) delay** occurs more commonly in males thar in females and at an increased frequency in patients with constitu tional short stature.

b. **Genetic delay** Occasional patients with "constitutional" delay ma have striking family histories of moderately to extremely late de velopment.

c. **CNS abnormalities** Luteinizing hormone (LH) or follicle-stimulatins hormone (FSH) deficiencies may be associated with hypothalamic o pituitary tumors, congenital vascular anomaly, CNS trauma, psy chosocial deprivation, ichthyosis (males), or Kallmann or Laurence Moon-Biedl syndromes.

d. **Systemic conditions,** such as anorexia nervosa, severe cardiac, pulmo nary, renal, or GI disease, malabsorption syndromes, weight loss o weight gain, sickle cell anemia, thalassemia, chronic infection, hypo thyroidism, or Addison's disease, are associated with an increasec incidence of delayed or incomplete sexual development.

    e. Primary gonadal insufficiency may be caused by the following: Turner, Noonan, Klinefelter, Reifenstein, and Sertoli-cell-only syndromes; testicular feminization, pure or mixed gonadal dysgenesis; cryptorchidism and anorchism; trauma, infection, pelvic radiation, and surgical castration.

2. Evaluation Although there are normal variations in the time of onset of puberty, differential diagnosis of delayed puberty should be considered when a girl over 14 or a boy over 15 lacks any secondary sexual characteristics, or when an adolescent has not completed maturation over a period of 5 years.

    a. The **history** should concentrate on the details and chronology of any sexual development, previous growth pattern, CNS symptoms, including anosmia, and nutrition. Any **family history** of abnormal puberty, amenorrhea, infertility, or ambiguous genitalia should be elicited.

    b. The **physical examination** should include all growth measurements (height, weight, span, upper-lower ratio), sexual staging, careful observation of the genitalia for ambiguity, palpation for inguinal masses, a pelvic examination (or at least a rectal), and a search for stigmata suggesting a syndrome. Signs of virilization in the female or incomplete masculinization in the male strongly imply an underlying pathologic cause that must be pursued.

    c. Review of past growth data is mandatory; a subtle growth spurt may be the first indication of impending sexual development. Conversely, abnormal deceleration may be a sign of active disease.

    d. Screening tests may include CBC, ESR, serum LH, FSH, and estrogens or testosterone, 24-hr urine for 17-ketosteroids, gonadotropins, bone age, skull films, and possibly a buccal smear and karyotype.

    e. In females, a vaginal smear for cytologic indexes, laparoscopy, or laparotomy may be indicated. Males may require a semen analysis, or testicular biopsy, or both.

    f. A single or 4-day LHRH (luteinizing hormone-releasing hormone) stimulation test or other tests of hypothalamic-pituitary function may be indicated.

    g. Evidence of a CNS lesion requires specific definition.

3. Diagnosis A specific diagnosis of the cause of delayed puberty is essential to ensure maximal realization of sexual and reproductive function, to provide genetic counseling, and to protect the patient against potential malignancy.

    a. The diagnosis of constitutional or hereditary delay in an otherwise normal patient is always tentative, since it can be confirmed only after normal sexual development has evolved.

    b. Patients with hypothalamic or pituitary deficiencies have low (usually prepubertal) levels of LH, or FSH, or both. An LHRH test may differentiate hypothalamic from pituitary lesions.

    c. In systemic conditions, an absence of cyclic levels of FSH-LH is sometimes observed.

    d. In primary gonadal failure, gonadotropins are usually elevated by age 12–13 years. A precise diagnosis of the gonadal abnormality requires clinical acumen and appropriate investigation.

4. **Treatment**   Before therapy is begun the patient's height, growth potential, emotional needs, and the risks of treatment must be considered.

   a. **Constitutional and genetic delay**   The patient and family should be reassured that no abnormalities are apparent, that normal development is anticipated, but that continued surveillance is important. Progression of development should be monitored and emotional support offered. For certain patients, temporary hormone replacement therapy may be justified.

   b. **CNS abnormalities**

      (1) Therapy is first directed to the indicated surgical or radiation treatment of the lesion.

      (2) **In females,** the replacement regimen includes an oral conjugated estrogen, e.g., Premarin, 0.3 mg/day, with the dosage gradually increased to 1.25 mg/day over 9–12 months; Provera, 10 mg/day on days 1–5 of each month, is then added to induce cyclic bleeding.

      (3) **In males,** ideal therapy consists of human chorionic gonadotropin (HCG), 1000–2500 IU IM q5 days. Serum testosterone may be helpful in monitoring dosage needs.

   c. **Systemic conditions**   Improvement of the underlying medical condition may be followed by normal puberty. Replacement therapy as outlined in **b** may be necessary, but its efficacy varies in different conditions.

   d. **Primary gonadal insufficiency**

      (1) **In females,** treatment consists of estrogens and progesterone (see **b**).

      (2) **In males,** a therapeutic trial of HCG should be attempted if there is a possibility of testicular function. If no response is demonstrated, testosterone enanthate, 100–200 mg IM q2–4 weeks, may be prescribed. Testicular prostheses should be offered if necessary. The prognosis for fertility should be evaluated and discussed frankly.

C. **Sexual precocity**

1. **Etiology**   See Table 12-2.

2. **Evaluation** should focus on the points emphasized in **B.2.** In addition, a careful search should be made for an abdominal or testicular mass (if necessary, under anesthesia), galactorrhea, and hyperpigmentation. A kidney-ureter-bladder film (KUB), adrenal photoscan, serum HCG, dehydroepiandrosterone (DHA), and androstenedione determinations, or a dexamethasone-suppression test may be indicated. Hormonal levels should be interpreted in relation to the stage of sexual development and age.

3. **Diagnosis**

   a. **Isosexual precocity** refers to an abnormally early onset (girls less than 8 years of age, boys less than 9 years of age) of sexual characteristics appropriate to the child's sex, with eventual attainment of full sexual maturation. In girls, isosexual precocity is usually idiopathic; organic and often malignant conditions are responsible in males. Inappropriate precocity, i.e., masculinization in the female or feminization in the male, is always pathologic and requires investigation.

Table 12-2   Causes of Sexual Precocity

Idiopathic (constitutional)

Familial

Central nervous system

  Tumor (teratoma, astrocytoma, ependymoma, pinealoma, craniopharyngioma, optic glioma, hamartoma, other)

  Infection (tuberculosis, meningitis), postencephalitic scarring

  Hydrocephalus

  Neurofibromatosis

  Tuberous sclerosis

Androgen and/or estrogen-producing tumors

  Ovarian (granulosa or theca cell tumor, theca-lutein or follicular cyst)

  Testicular (Leydig cell, adrenal rest tumors)

  Adrenal (adenoma, carcinoma, hyperplasia)

Gonadotropin-producing tumors

  Ovarian (chorioepithelioma, teratoma, dysgerminoma)

  Testicular

  Teratoma (CNS, presacral)

Endocrine dysfunction

  Hypothyroidism

  CAH

Exogenous hormones

  Birth control pills

  Estrogens (cosmetics, poultry, cattle)

  Androgens

  HCG

Syndromes

  Russell-Silver

  Polyostotic fibrous dysplasia (McCune-Albright syndrome)

---

      b. Precocious adrenarche (pubarche) consists of the early appearance of pubic hair, axillary hair, and/or apocrine odor, which are effects of adrenal androgens.

      c. Precocious thelarche refers to the premature development of one or both breasts in females, without vaginal estrogenization or any other signs of sexual development.

      d. The **differential diagnosis** should be narrowed down by determining the source(s) of hormone (e.g., CNS, adrenal or gonadal) and intensifying investigation of that limited area.

    4. Treatment   Unless eradication of the specific cause of the precocity is possible, no satisfactory treatment to prevent progression of sexual changes is currently available. Patients should be followed closely to monitor growth and development, to examine for treatable lesions, and to offer psychological guidance.

  D. Gynecomastia

    1. Etiology

      a. Idiopathic (benign)   Some degree of unilateral or bilateral gynecomastia occurs commonly during male pubertal development.

   b. **Iatrogenic sources** may be estrogens, androgens, HCG, desoxycorticosterone acetate (DOCA), isoniazid, digitalis, reserpine, spironolactone, phenothiazines, meprobamate, and amphetamines.

   c. **Organic conditions** include true or male pseudohermaphroditism (e.g., Klinefelter or Reifenstein syndromes), estrogen-producing tumor, hypothyroidism, hyperthyroidism, acromegaly, diabetes mellitus, hepatic disease, nephritis, paraplegia, primary testicular failure, and testicular tumors.

2. **Evaluation**

   a. The **history** should concentrate on measures of sexual development and function, symptoms of pain, tenderness, galactorrhea, hair loss, iatrogenic sources, and systemic illness.

   b. The size and configuration of ductular tissue, color of the areolae, presence of galactorrhea (best elicited with the patient in the sitting position), dimensions and consistency of the testes, and stage of sexual development should be noted.

3. **Diagnosis** If abnormalities are present, measurement of FSH, LH, estrogen, testosterone, buccal smear and/or karyotype, and cortisol and/or 24-hr urinary 17-ketosteroids and 17-hydroxycorticosteroids may be indicated.

4. **Treatment** Spontaneous regression occurs in most normal boys after 1–3 years. Removal of the hormonal or pharmacologic agent usually results in disappearance of ductular tissue. If the gynecomastia is unusually severe or contributing to significant psychological problems, mammoplasty may be warranted.

IV. DISORDERS OF THE PITUITARY

A. Hypopituitarism

1. **Etiology**

   a. Tumor (especially craniopharyngioma), neurofibromatosis, trauma, hemorrhage, infarction, previous irradiation, psychosocial deprivation, or hypothalamic deficiencies may cause isolated or multiple pituitary hormone deficiencies. In time, an "idiopathic" diagnosis often proves to be organic.

   b. Isolated growth hormone deficiency may be inherited as an X-linked, recessive disorder.

   c. Isolated FSH or LH deficiencies, or both, may occur in Kallmann and Laurence-Moon-Biedl syndromes and in males with ichthyosis (see Sec. **III.B.1.c**).

   d. Isolated TSH deficiency has been reported.

   e. Rarely, isolated ACTH deficiency may occur.

2. **Evaluation** Systematic investigation of all anterior and posterior pituitary hormones is necessary to determine the status of current function and establish a baseline for future alterations.

   a. The **history** should cover past growth, CNS symptoms (anosmia, visual changes, symptoms of increased intracranial pressure), and previous head or neck illnesses or therapy.

b. The **physical examination** should include precise growth measurements, staging of sexual development, a neurologic survey, including visual fields and fundoscopy, and a search for the signs of hypothyroidism and hypoadrenalism.

c. **Laboratory evaluation** should consist of plotting of the growth curve, determination of bone age and levels of serum growth hormone, FSH, LH, testosterone or estrogen (if the patient is an adolescent), T_4, RT_3, and TSH, metyrapone test, serum osmolarity, and urinary specific gravity.

d. **CNS evaluation** should include skull films and may require an electroencephalogram, computer tomography, or pneumoencephalography.

3. Diagnosis

a. Patients with isolated growth hormone deficiency have a normal birth weight and length; growth velocity begins to decrease at 6–12 months of age.

(1) Signs of growth hormone deficiency may include a weight age greater than height age; high-pitched, thin voice; small immature facies; protuberant abdomen with "hammered-silver" appearance.

(2) The growth rate is usually less than 4 cm/year.

(3) No significant response of serum growth hormone is detectable following stimuli known to provoke growth hormone release (fasting, exercise, stress, third-stage rapid eye movement sleep, hypoglycemia, arginine, propranolol, glucagon).

b. Deficiencies of FSH or LH may not be diagnosed until the patient presents with delayed puberty (see **III.B**).

c. Deficiency of TSH may be responsible for mild to severe clinical hypothyroidism without a goiter. Thyroid function tests, including tests for TSH, reveal low levels.

d. Patients with ACTH deficiency often have a relatively mild form of adrenal insufficiency that may go undetected until they are under stress. These patients are differentiated from patients with Addison's disease by the lack of hyperpigmentation or salt craving. Serum cortisols may be low or even within normal range, but a significant response to metyrapone or in diurnal variation of adrenocortical activity is absent.

4. Treatment

a. Surgical or radiation treatment of the underlying condition should be carried out as indicated.

b. Growth hormone, 2–3 mg IM 3 times a week, may be given, but it is available only in limited supply.

c. FSH and LH deficiency are treated as outlined in Sec. **B.4**.

d. TSH deficiency is treated with oral thyroid hormone replacement.

e. ACTH deficiency may not require long-term therapy. For the stress of illness, trauma, or surgery, however, glucocorticoid treatment may be lifesaving. Mineralocorticoid function is not affected by ACTH deficiency.

B. Hyperpituitarism

1. Etiology Excessive levels of growth hormone, TSH, ACTH, or prolactin result from autonomous hormone production by a primary pituitary tumor or by altered regulation at a hypothalamic level.

2. Evaluation

   a. Clinical states reflecting hypersecretion may be a result of elevated serum levels of the hormone or of uninterrupted secretion within a "normal" range.

   b. Evaluation consists in documenting the onset of observed changes (serial photographs are very helpful), determining current CNS and pituitary function, and measuring the ability of pharmacologic stimuli to suppress pituitary secretion.

3. Diagnosis

   a. Gigantism in children is characterized by accelerated growth velocity.

   b. After epiphyseal closure has occurred, signs of **acromegaly,** if present, include disproportionate enlargement of the hands, feet, and face.

   c. Abnormalities include severe headaches, weakness, thickened skin, excessive perspiration, hypertrichosis, and joint pains.

   d. Growth hormone levels may be elevated or fail to be suppressed by glucose administration, and *glucose tolerance* may be mildly or overtly that of a diabetic person.

   e. Excess TSH results in a clinical picture of hyperthyroidism, with elevated thyroid hormone levels and elevated TSH.

   f. Cushing's disease in which the basic defect is hypercortisolism secondary to excessive or inappropriate secretion of ACTH presents with the clinical picture of the Cushing syndrome as a result of a CNS tumor (see Sec. **VII**).

   g. Patients with **hyperprolactin states** usually present with galactorrhea, oligomenorrhea, or amenorrhea.

4. Treatment

   a. Complete eradication of the tumor is often difficult and may require two approaches. These are surgery (transphenoidal or frontal approach) and cryosurgery plus radiation (x-ray, proton beam, isotope implantation).

   b. Since the effect of radiation may not be maximal for months to years following therapy, pituitary function must be monitored at intervals of 3–6 months.

   c. Replacement therapy is instituted as required.

C. Diabetes insipidus

1. Etiology Hypothalamic or posterior pituitary antidiuretic hormone (ADH) deficiency, or both, may be idiopathic or a result of CNS tumor (especially Hand-Schüller-Christian disease or postoperative craniopharyngioma), infection, infarction, trauma, or familial (autosomal dominant, ADH deficiency, or X-linked dominant) nephrogenic diabetes insipidus.

2. Evaluation

   a. Although the onset of symptoms may be abrupt, a cycle of polyuria-polydipsia may allow the older child to remain well compensated. Infants, however, may present with severe failure to thrive and dehydration. Evidence of CNS or pituitary abnormalities may not be present.

b. Polyuria is investigated by a record of 24-hr urine input and output, urinalysis with specific gravity, serum Na, K, BUN, creatinine Ca, P, and AP, concomitant serum and urine osmolality (random or following a defined fast), and 24-hr urine tests for Na, K, and Ca creatinine.

3. Diagnosis

a. The patient should be observed carefully during a trial of water deprivation to ensure safety and compliance. Patients with neurogenic or nephrogenic diabetes insipidus are unable to concentrate urine above a specific gravity of 1.010 and usually do not concentrate above 1.002–1.004; serum Na and osmolarity rise, and weight decreases. Patients with psychogenic diabetes insipidus concentrate urine appropriately.

b. Administration of aqueous or depot vasopressin (Pitressin) will cause an increase in urinary specific gravity in ADH deficiency, but not in nephrogenic diabetes insipidus.

4. Treatment

a. Neurogenic diabetes insipidus is very effectively treated with **vasopressin tannate in oil,** 5 units IM q48–72h; frequency of administration is titrated to the degree of polyuria and polydipsia. To ensure full efficacy, the vial must be shaken vigorously to mix the contents, and the vasopressin is then injected deeply with a 1-in., 22-gauge needle.

b. A **nasal spray (Diapid),** 2–3 squirts in each nostril q4–6h, may be used for convenience between vasopressin injections. The disadvantages of nasal irritation and short duration of action limits its use as the sole long-term treatment. Longer-acting synthetic nasal sprays, when available, may eliminate the need for vasopressin injections.

c. Chlorpropamide may enhance the ADH effect in patients with partial ADH deficiency, but the side effect of hypoglycemia is frequently observed in children.

d. Treatment of nephrogenic diabetes insipidus consists of a low-solute diet. Some patients have benefited from chlorothiazide.

V. DISORDERS OF THE THYROID

A. Neonatal hypothyroidism

1. Etiology

a. Endemic.

b. Embryonic errors in development (thyroid dysgenesis).

c. Idiopathic, with the majority of cases remaining unexplained.

d. Maternal hyperthyroidism Administration of iodides, radioactive iodine, or propylthiouracil during pregnancy may be the cause of inadequate fetal thyroid hormone production.

e. Inherited inborn errors of thyroid hormone production are usually transmitted as an autosomal recessive trait. Abnormal thyroid function may begin in the neonatal period or in early childhood.

2. Evaluation In view of the significant neurologic sequelae, the possibility of hypothyroidism should be considered in an infant with any suggestive signs or symptoms.

   a. The **history** may include postmaturity, unusually placid behavior (e.g., "a good baby who never cries"), somnolence, hypotonia, feeding difficulties, constipation, and prolonged jaundice.

   b. **Physical features** may include hypothermia, abnormal movement (as if in slow motion), hypotonia, enlarged anterior and posterior fontanelle, macroglossia, coarse facial features, umbilical hernia, and cool, dry, mottled skin. The thyroid may be enlarged or absent.

3. Diagnosis

   a. The **infant's age** must be considered in interpreting the results of thyroid function tests.

   b. A **thyroid scan** may document the absence of functioning thyroid tissue.

4. Treatment is begun as soon as the diagnosis is made.

   a. **L-Thyroxine** (Synthroid), 0.025 mg/day, is employed initially, and the dosage is gradually increased over the following 1–2 months, with monitoring of clinical and laboratory findings. Most infants require 0.05 mg/day until they are 1 year of age.

   b. If a goiter is present, the risk of **respiratory obstruction** must be assessed and thyroid treatment instituted as soon as evaluation has been completed.

B. Neonatal hyperthyroidism

1. Etiology

   a. Women with **Graves' disease** may have offspring with hyperthyroidism, presumably secondary to transplacental passage of long-acting thyroid stimulation.

   b. Patients with "idiopathic" disease may have a family history of thyroid disease.

2. Evaluation A goiter is usually present.

3. Treatment

   a. When the mother has Graves' disease, the possibility of **respiratory obstruction secondary to fetal goiter** should be anticipated prior to delivery. Resection of the thyroid isthmus or tracheostomy may be necessary.

   b. If **significant toxicity** persists, treatment with phenobarbital, propranolol, and/or propylthiouracil may be indicated.

   c. The hyperthyroid state is usually transient, but may require long-term therapy into childhood, especially if idiopathic.

C. Acquired hypothyroidism

1. Etiology

   a. **Idiopathic.**

   b. **Thyroiditis** Many cases of thyroiditis may go undiagnosed in the inflammatory or hyperthyroid phase and later present as "idiopathic."

  c. **TSH deficiency** may be secondary to a pituitary or hypothalamic defect.

  d. **Exogenous causes** include thyroidectomy, radioactive iodine, iodine excess or deficiency, fluorine, lithium, cobalt, perchlorate, thiocyanate, para-aminosalicylic acid, propylthiouracil, phenylbutazone, resorcinol (in skin creams), and certain foods in large amounts (e.g., cabbage, turnips, cauliflower, rutabaga, soybeans).

  e. Rarely, **thyroid carcinoma** may produce hypothyroidism.

2. **Evaluation and diagnosis**

  a. Iodine goiters are very hard. Goiters associated with thyroiditis may be moderately firm, granular, and suggested by a Delphian node. A discrete, hard mass (or masses) may be a malignant tumor or adenoma. Absence of a goiter suggests TSH deficiency or, rarely, ectopic thyroid tissue.

  b. **Titers of thyroid antibodies** are often elevated in thyroiditis but are not diagnostic. **Protein-bound iodine** may be more than 1 μg/100 ml above the level of T_4 or butanol-extractable iodine. Since therapy would not be altered by a specific diagnosis of thyroiditis, biopsy is usually not justified.

  c. A **thyroid scan** may be useful if carcinoma or ectopic thyroid is suspected. If a cold nodule is detected, open biopsy or excision is indicated.

3. **Treatment**

  a. Treatment with L-thyroxine is begun with 0.025 mg/day, with the dosage gradually increased by 0.025 mg every 1–2 weeks until the appropriate dosage is attained. Most children require 0.1 mg/day from age 1–9 and 0.15 mg/day from age 10 to adolescence. Adults usually require 0.15–0.2 mg/day.

  b. **Thyroid function tests** may be done to monitor the appropriateness of the dosage, or compliance, or both. TSH may be the most sensitive guide to the adequacy of therapy.

  c. Striking alterations in personality and behavior may be observed initially, but such problems eventually resolve as the patient and family adapt to the euthyroid state.

D. Acquired hyperthyroidism

1. **Etiology**

  a. Elevated thyroxine (T_4) may be seen in Graves' disease (hyperthyroidism with exophthalmos), diffuse toxic goiter, thyroid adenoma, thyroiditis, or, very rarely, hyperfunctioning thyroid carcinoma or a TSH-producing tumor.

  b. In T_3 toxicosis, only triiodothyronine is excessive, while T_4 is normal.

2. **Evaluation and diagnosis** Patients with T_3 toxicosis or pheochromocytoma may seem hyperthyroid yet have a normal T_4 level.

3. **Treatment**

  a. **Temporary restrictions on sports or strenuous activity** may be indicated until the severe toxicity resolves.

  b. **Oral medication** A chemical block of T_4 is effected by propylthiouracil, 100 mg tid, or by methimazole (Tapazole), 10 mg tid.

(1) **Side effects** may include rashes, arthritis, jaundice, hepatitis, a lupuslike syndrome, or leukopenia.

(2) The dosage is titrated by the clinical and laboratory finding, and therapy is continued until the hyperthyroid process has remitted; seemingly tiny doses may be required to maintain a euthyroid state.

(3) Remissions may be temporary or permanent, or the patient may progress to a hypothyroid state.

   c. **Surgery is the treatment of choice of an adenoma or carcinoma** and may be considered in recalcitrant cases of hyperthyroidism. Complications include recurrent hyperthyroidism, permanent hypothyroidism, hypoparathyroidism, recurrent laryngeal nerve(s) paralysis, hemorrhage, and keloid formation.

   d. Radioactive iodine may be appropriate for patients with poor compliance or at surgical risk. Its safety in children remains debatable.

VI. DISORDERS OF THE PARATHYROIDS

A. Hypoparathyroidism

1. **Etiology**

   a. **Neonatal hypoparathyroidism** is described in Chap. 5.

   b. **Idiopathic hypoparathyroidism,** thought to occur as an "autoimmune" process, may be associated with endocrine deficiencies and other conditions (thyroiditis, Addison's disease, diabetes mellitus, primary gonadal insufficiency, pernicious anemia, alopecia, vitiligo, candidiasis).

   c. **DiGeorge syndrome,** a congenital condition, is characterized by developmental defects of midline structures arising from the third and fourth pharyngeal pouches; partial or incomplete parathyroid hormone (PTH) deficiency occurs.

   d. **Iatrogenic hypoparathyroidism** may occur transiently or permanently following thyroid or neck surgery.

   e. **Pseudohypoparathyroidism** or **pseudopseudohypoparathyroidism** are X-linked dominant conditions in which end-organ response to PTH is inadequate.

2. **Evaluation**

   a. The **history** should include symptoms of hypocalcemia, large milk intake, cramps, paresthesias, carpopedal spasm, laryngospasm, seizures, headaches, photophobia, susceptibility to infections, diarrhea, and psychomotor development. The family history should be pursued for members with subtle signs of pseudohypoparathyroidism, autoimmune diseases.

   b. Pertinent **physical findings** may include hyperreflexia, a positive Chvostek's or Trousseau's sign, cataracts, papilledema, unusual facies, dental or nail abnormalities, short 4th metacarpal, mental retardation, or signs of autoimmune processes.

   c. Diagnostic **laboratory studies** should include serum Ca, P, AP, total protein, magnesium, pH, BUN, 24-hr urinary Ca-creatinine ratio, and bone age. PTH stimulation tests, antibody studies, immune evaluation, and psychometric testing may be necessary to determine the specific cause.

3. Diagnosis

  a. Hypoparathyroidism is characterized by an elevated P, low or normal Ca, and normal or slightly low alkaline phosphatase level. Urinary Ca and P excretion are low. Soft tissue or basal ganglia calcifications may be seen on x-ray examination. Electroencephalograms are frequently abnormal.

  b. Differential diagnosis of the causes of hypoparathyroidism may be facilitated by a PTH stimulation test. PTH, 100–200 IU, is infused IV over 1 hr or administered IM (25–50 IU q8h) for 3 days. A positive response is indicated by a rise in serum Ca, a decrease in serum P, a tenfold increase in urinary P excretion, and an increase in urinary cyclic AMP.

   (1) Patients with **PTH deficiency** have low-normal to nondetectable serum PTH and a positive response to PTH stimulation.

   (2) Patients with **pseudohypoparathyroidism** have normal to elevated PTH levels and no response to PTH by the criteria in **b.**

  c. Patients with **idiopathic hypoparathyroidism** may have clinical or laboratory evidence of autoimmune disease. Antibodies to thyroid, adrenal, parietal cell, ovary, or testis may be detected.

  d. DiGeorge syndrome is recognized by abnormal facies, cleft palate, abnormal cardiac vasculature, congenital heart disease, mental retardation, and defects in delayed hypersensitivity immune mechanisms.

  e. Pseudohypoparathyroid patients have slight to moderate mental retardation, short stature, weight age above height age, short 4th and 5th metacarpals, increased incidence of hypothyroidism, and no candidiasis. Bone age may be advanced for chronological age, and TSH may be elevated, even in an apparently euthyroid state.

  f. Pseudopseudohypoparathyroid patients show the same somatic stigmata as those with pseudohypoparathyroidism, but may have normal serum chemistries intermittently.

4. Treatment

  a. Acute hypocalcemia is treated with 15 mg/kg elemental calcium IV over 4 hr. Serum calcium may be expected to increase by 2 mg/100 ml/4 hr of treatment, but the effect will disappear in 4 hr if no other therapy is instituted. ECG monitoring is essential during the infusion.

  b. Long-term therapy consists of the lowest dose possible of vitamin D_2 (ergocalciferol, 25,000–50,000 U/day, or dihydrotachysterol, 0.25–0.5 mg/day).

   (1) Evidence of **vitamin D excess** includes CNS symptoms (ataxia, seizures), polydipsia, polyuria, anorexia, nausea, vomiting, constipation, and urinary calculi.

   (2) In view of the potential toxicity of vitamin D, the clinical response and urinary Ca-creatinine ratios should be monitored closely. Supplemental calcium, up to 1 gm/day of elemental Ca^{++}, may also be necessary. Most patients tolerate borderline serum Ca levels and are thereby protected from potential vitamin D toxicity.

B. Hyperparathyroidism

1. Etiology

   a. Primary hyperparathyroidism, due to parathyroid adenoma or hyper-plasia, is extremely rare in children.

   b. Secondary hyperparathyroidism may occur in response to low calcium in chronic renal disease, vitamin D–resistant rickets, malabsorption, or sprue.

   c. Tertiary hyperparathyroidism is a state in which autonomous secretion of PTH persists despite resolution of the condition causing secondary hyperparathyroidism and correction of hypocalcemia.

2. Evaluation

   a. The **history** should investigate anorexia, personality changes, CNS symptoms (headache, confusion, hallucinations), nausea, vomiting, abdominal pain, constipation, weight loss, polyuria, polydipsia, ulcer, pancreatitis, renal colic, or hematuria. A **family history** of other endocrine tumors (pheochromocytoma, medullary thyroid carcinoma, Zollinger-Ellison syndrome, pituitary tumors) should be elucidated.

   b. The **physical findings** may include hypertension, nail changes, alopecia, and band keratitis.

3. Diagnosis

   a. The diagnosis is confirmed by an elevated Ca, low P, normal or increased AP, normal or low magnesium, increased Cl, increased PTH, and increased 24-hr urinary Ca and P.

   b. X-ray studies may show subperiosteal bone resorption, demineralization, bone cysts, or nephrocalcinosis.

   c. Angiography and PTH sampling from parathyroid veins may localize the adenoma(s).

4. Treatment

   a. In **primary hyperparathyroidism,** removal of the hyperplastic gland(s) is indicated.

   b. In **secondary hyperparathyroidism,** therapy is directed to the primary disease. The goals are to correct acidosis, increase the absorption of calcium with vitamin D, and decrease serum phosphorus with phosphorus binders or a low phosphorus diet, or both (see Chap. 9).

   c. If **tertiary hyperparathyroidism** does not resolve in time, partial or complete parathyroidectomy may be necessary.

VII. DISORDERS OF THE ADRENALS

A. Adrenocortical insufficiency (Addison's disease) may appear abruptly (adrenal crisis) or insidiously. The deficiency may be temporary or permanent.

1. Etiology

   a. Idiopathic atrophy, with or without evidence of autoimmune disease, is the most common cause in children.

   b. Trauma, tumor, or fulminating infections may cause adrenal hemorrhage or necrosis. The meningococcus is the most frequent pathogen (Waterhouse-Friderichsen syndrome). Tuberculosis is now a rare cause of Addison's disease.

c. Other causes are congenital adrenal hypoplasia or aplasia, diffuse cerebral sclerosis (Schilder's disease), primary familial xanthomatosis with adrenal involvement (Wolman's disease), and congenital adrenal hyperplasia (patients with the latter may have a positive family history).

d. Glucocorticoid deficiency may occur in patients with **ACTH deficiency** or **familial unresponsiveness to ACTH.** Transient glucocorticoid insufficiency may occur in patients treated with **long-term steroids** or, rarely, in infants born to mothers with iatrogenic or endogenous Cushing syndrome.

e. Addison's disease may be **familial** and has been described in association with diseases such as hypoparathyroidism, candidiasis, diabetes mellitus, and Hashimoto's lymphocytic thyroiditis.

2. Evaluation

a. Personality changes, increased pigmentation, salt craving, hypotension, anorexia, nausea, vomiting, diarrhea and weight loss, menstrual abnormalities, and hypoglycemia may be present for months before the diagnosis is made. GI symptoms may mimic those of influenza or simulate an acute abdominal condition.

b. In adrenal crisis, often precipitated by mild stress, vomiting, dehydration, hypoglycemia, and hypotension may lead to coma and shock.

3. Diagnosis

a. Decreased Na, increased K, hypochloremic acidosis, hypoglycemia, increased urinary Na, decreased urinary K.

b. Eosinophilia and relative neutropenia may be documented, depending on the severity of the illness.

c. Serum cortisol and aldosterone may be low or within normal range, but ACTH levels are significantly elevated in primary adrenal insufficiency, especially if they are obtained at the time of maximal stress.

d. Urinary 17-hydroxycorticosteroids are usually less than 3.0 ± 1.0 mg/m^2/day.

e. The findings of metyrapone and water-loading tests are abnormal, but do not distinguish primary from secondary glucocorticoid deficiency.

f. The diagnosis is confirmed when serum cortisol and aldosterone and 24-hr urinary 17-hydroxycorticosteroids and 17-ketosteroids do not respond adequately to exogenously administered ACTH.

4. Therapy

a. **Shock** must be treated by rapid volume expansion (20 ml/kg of normal saline IV stat). If hypoglycemia is suspected (or documented with a Dextrostix), 1–2 gm/kg of dextrose solution is given IV. Hydrocortisone sodium succinate (Solu-Cortef), 25–50 mg, should be given IV stat; the equivalent of 150 mg/m^2/day should be given IV in divided doses q4–6h and continued over the next 24 hr. Pressor agents usually are not necessary if adequate fluids are administered.

b. For patients with **mild symptoms,** 1½–2 times the amount of maintenance fluids (see **c**) may be sufficient to equilibrate the electrolytes and allow diagnostic tests to be carried out.

   c. **Maintenance therapy** consists in the equivalent of 13 mg/m²/day of hydrocortisone in divided doses tid, or fludrocortisone (Florinef), 0.05–0.1 mg/day, and table salt ad lib, especially in the summer.

   d. **During periods of stress,** the hydrocortisone dosage should be doubled or trebled and the frequency of administration increased to q6h. Patients, or parents, or both, should know how to use cortisone acetate, 25–50 mg IM, in emergencies. Patients should wear a Medic Alert identification tag.

B. Congenital adrenogenital hyperplasia

1. **Etiology** Congenital adrenogenital hyperplasia (CAH, adrenogenital syndrome) is an inherited lack or deficiency of an enzyme required for adrenocortical hormone synthesis. It is inherited as an autosomal recessive trait. Each defect is genetically specific. If one form occurs in a family, subsequently affected infants will have the same type of defect and, usually, a defect of equal severity.

   a. Five distinct types of enzyme deficiencies in the synthesis of cortisol have been described: 21-hydroxylase (90–95 percent of CAH patients), 11-β-hydroxylase, 3-β-hydroxysteroid dehydrogenase, 20,22-desmolase defect, and 17-hydroxylase deficiency.

   b. In compensation for inadequate levels of cortisol, the pituitary secretes large amounts of ACTH, resulting in adrenocortical hyperplasia and accumulation of cortisol precursors. A sixth defect, 18-hydroxylase deficiency, is manifested by inadequate mineralocorticoid activity, but sexual development and cortisol synthesis are normal.

2. **Evaluation and diagnosis** See Table 12-3.

   a. Prenatal exposure to large amounts of androgen result in various degrees of virilization of the external genitalia in the newborn female (21-hydroxylase, 11-β-hydroxylase, 3-β-hydroxysteroid dehydrogenase deficiency), but often with subtle signs of virilization in the male (21-hydroxylase, 11-β-hydroxylase). The diagnosis may not be made in the neonatal period (often the case in non-salt-losing males), but signs of sexual precocity will appear later.

   b. Inadequate androgen synthesis (17-hydroxylase, 3-β-hydroxysteroid dehydrogenase, 20, 22-desmolase) results in incomplete masculinization in the male, but normal genitalia in the female. In CAH, the uterus, fallopian tubes, and ovaries in the female and testes in the male are normal. With successful treatment, the prognosis for fertility is good.

   c. Enzymatic blocks in the synthesis of mineralocorticoid hormones (21-hydroxylase, 3-β-hydroxysteroid dehydrogenase, 20,22-desmolase) are manifested by salt losing within the first 3 weeks of life. Anorexia, vomiting, polyuria, and weight loss lead to dehydration and eventually to circulatory collapse. Hyponatremia, hyperkalemia, and hypochloremic acidosis are usually documented.

   d. Hypertension develops in infants with excess mineralocorticoids (11-hydroxylase, 17-hydroxylase deficiency).

   e. The diagnostic workup should include a family history (unexplained deaths in infancy, excessively tall children with sexual precocity, dwarfed adult stature), buccal smear, plasma cortisol level, ACTH, serum electrolytes, and measurement of urinary 17-ketosteroids and

Table 12-3 Evaluation and Diagnosis of Congenital Adrenogenital Hyperplasia

Enzyme Deficiency	External Genitalia		Symptoms	Diagnostic Abnormalities	
	Female	Male		Urine	Serum
21-Hydroxylase	Virilized	Virilized	1/2–1/3 have salt losing	Increased 17-ketosteroids Increased pregnanetriol	Increased 17-OHP
11-β-Hydroxylase	Virilized	Virilized	Hypertension	Increased 17-ketosteroids Increased pregnanetriol	Compound S (11-deoxycortisol compounds)
3-β-Hydroxysteroid dehydrogenase	Mildly virilized	Incompletely masculinized	Salt losing	± increased 17-ketosteroids	Increased dehydro-epiandosterone
20, 20-Desmolase	Normal	Incompletely masculinized	Salt losing	Normal or decreased 17-ketosteroids	
17-Hydroxylase	Normal	Incompletely masculinized	Hypertension	Increased pregnanediol	

17-hydroxycorticosteroids (24-hr 17-ketosteroids should be less than 2 mg/24 hr in the newborn period).

3. **Treatment**

   a. **Salt-losing crisis** is treated vigorously with volume and salt replacement, 0.9% NaCl in 5% D/W. Newborns usually require at least 150 ml/kg/day. Intake and output, weight, and electrolytes should be monitored closely while serum and urine collections are obtained for diagnosis. When oral intake is established, 2–4 gm of salt can be added to the diet and discontinued when the child is old enough to titrate salt needs by ad lib intake. **Long-term therapy** consists of fludrocortisone acetate, 0.05–0.1 mg/day. DOCA, 1–2 mg IM, may be given in the acute situation or in pellet form for long-term treatment. The latter can be used in infancy, but may cause hypertension.

   b. **Initial glucocorticoid therapy** may require 3–4 times the maintenance dosage to suppress ACTH levels, especially during stress. Newborns may be treated with 5 mg of hydrocortisone q8h for 3 days. The dosage is then tapered to 2.5 mg q8h and continued for the first 6–12 months. Patients with CAH seem to require 15–20 mg/M²/day of hydrocortisone or its equivalent, given tid to provide adequate glucocorticoid replacement, to suppress ACTH, and to allow for normal growth and development. DOCA may also be needed. Optimal dosage timing may vary among patients.

   c. Females with virilization may require an operation on the clitoris, or vagina, or both. If necessary, this procedure should be performed as early in infancy as is feasible.

   d. Patients should be followed at intervals of 3–4 months to monitor growth, urinary 17-ketosteroids, and bone age. The medication should be adjusted as necessary.

C. **Cushing syndrome**

1. **Etiology**   Glucocorticoid excess may be caused by adrenal tumors, adrenal hyperplasia, an ACTH-producing tumor of the pituitary (Cushing's disease), or prolonged treatment with corticosteroids.

2. **Evaluation**

   a. **Manifestations** of glucocorticoid excess include an initial increase then a decrease in appetite, weight gain, slowing or arrest of height velocity, weakness, fatigue, and personality changes.

   b. Fat deposition occurs in the facial, nuchal, shoulder, and abdominal areas producing the characteristic "moon" facies and "buffalo hump." The extremities often appear thin, the result of muscle wasting.

   c. Hypertension, plethora, purplish red striae, ecchymoses, and weakness may be present.

   d. Signs of excess adrenal androgens (acne, pubic hair, enlarged clitoris or phallus) may indicate a mixed tumor or hyperplasia secondary to excess ACTH.

3. **Diagnosis**

   a. Serum F (cortisol) and urinary 17-hydroxycorticosteroids and free cortisol are usually increased. Serum androgens and urinary 17-ketosteroids may be increased in the virilized patient, but the most specific diagnostic feature is the **absence of the normal diurnal varia-**

tion of cortisol level. Serum ACTH should be low in primary adrenal tumors and inappropriately elevated in CNS or ectopic ACTH-producing tumors.

b. Glucocorticoid excess may be accompanied by a hypokalemic hypernatremic alkalosis, polycythemia, eosinopenia, and abnormal glucose tolerance with hyperglycemia, or glucosuria, or both. Bone age may be less than height age and chronological age. Osteoporosis may be present.

c. Dexamethasone suppression and metyrapone tests, CNS evaluation, an intravenous pyelogram, and an adrenal arteriogram may be necessary to determine the cause of the syndrome.

4. Treatment

a. Resection of an adrenal tumor may be complicated by the patient's clinical state (hypertension, obesity, poor wound healing). When a demonstrable pituitary tumor, especially with visual field changes, is demonstrated, surgery, radiation, or both, must be considered.

b. Recently, metyrapone (which blocks the synthesis of cortisol), or mitotane (Lysodren) (an adrenolytic drug), or both, have been used to eliminate the effects of glucocorticoid excess, either to prepare for surgery or to perform a "medical" adrenalectomy, with preservation of mineralocorticoid activity.

D. Pheochromocytoma

1. Etiology   The adrenal medulla is derived from the ectoderm of the neural crest and secretes the catecholamines epinephrine and norepinephrine. Overproduction of the catecholamines may be due to tumors of the adrenal medulla or of accessory chromatin tissue. In children, as many as 20–30 percent of pheochromocytomas are extramedullary in location, and, in 25 percent of patients, more than one tumor may be found.

2. Evaluation   The **clinical manifestations** most commonly noted are hypertension, headache, tachycardia, weight loss, visual changes, palpitations, nervousness, abdominal or chest pain, hyperhydrosis, anxiety, fatigue, facial pallor, polydipsia, polyuria, and tremors. A **family history** of autoimmune disease, neuroectodermal dysplasias, medullary carcinoma of the thyroid, and parathyroid tumors should be explored.

3. Diagnosis   Typically, symptoms and signs are intermittent. The diagnosis is usually made by the detection of an increased concentration of epinephrine, norepinephrine, or metanephrine in the urine or blood, or of increased urinary vanillylmandelic acid. Localization of the tumor(s) may be difficult, and surgical exploration may be necessary.

4. Treatment   The hypertension should be brought under control with dibenzamine prior to invasive diagnostic procedures or surgery. Blood pressure must be monitored carefully during surgical resection.

13

Prepubertal and Adolescent Gynecology

Pregnancy and venereal disease are common among adolescents. Pediatric and adolescent gynecologic complaints should be investigated and initially treated in the familiar setting of the pediatrician's office. This setting may eliminate much of the emotional and physical discomfort otherwise associated with these procedures.

I. GYNECOLOGIC EVALUATION

A. The **pelvic examination** should be carefully explained before it is begun, with no surprises in store for the patient. The use of plastic models of pelvic organs is helpful in demonstrating the procedure. As the examination proceeds, each step should be reexplained. Alert the patient to expect mild discomfort, e.g., on insertion of the speculum. Show the instruments to be used and allow the patient to touch them. This will be especially helpful with the younger child and may allay many of the parent's fears as well. Whether or not a parent remains in the room depends on the parent-child relationship. Little girls usually prefer to have the mother readily accessible. The adolescent, however, should be examined alone if the examiner is female, or with a chaperon present if the examiner is male.

1. Examining the young child

a. Inspecting the external genitalia The child is told that the procedure will not hurt. She is placed on her back, with the knees wide apart and the soles of the feet touching each other. As the external genitalia are inspected, the patient is asked to help by holding the labia apart. This allows her to participate and have a sense of control.

Note the presence or absence of pubic hair, clitoral size, character of the introitus, and perineal hygiene. The premenarcheal clitoris should not exceed 3 mm in length and 2 mm in transverse diameter.

b. Visualizing the vagina Placing girls over 2 years old in the knee-chest position allows the examiner to view the vagina and cervix without instrumentation. The patient is told to "lie on her tummy with her bottom in the air." She is reassured that the examiner is only going to look with the help of the otoscope light. She is allowed to see and touch the light. As the child takes a few deep breaths and allows her spine and stomach to "sag like an old horse," the vaginal orifice falls open. The otoscope provides the necessary light and magnification needed to visualize the cervix.

c. Rectal-abdominal examination While the child is lying on her back, a gentle rectal-abdominal examination is carried out. The index or fifth finger of one hand is inserted into the rectum. The other hand is placed on the abdomen for bimanual palpation. The example of a rectal thermometer can be used to explain how the examining finger will feel.

The examiner will feel only a "button" of a cervix. The ovaries are not palpable in the prepubertal child; hence, if an adnexal mass is felt, a cyst or tumor should be suspected.

2. **Examining the adolescent** The psychological implications of a pelvic examination in a teenager warrant taking the time to establish a trusting relationship before proceeding.

   a. **Preparations** The patient is given an examining gown and told to remove all her clothes and put the gown on while the physician is out of the room. Respect for the patient's privacy is essential, and the procedure should be explained. She is then placed on the table in stirrups and draped. Older adolescents often prefer no draping and appreciate watching the examination with the help of mirrors.

   b. **Inspecting the external genitalia** The Tanner staging of pubic hair is noted, along with size of the clitoris (the normal glans is 2–4 mm in width; 10 mm indicates significant virilization) and the appearance of the introitus.

   c. **Speculum examination** Two types of specula are available for use in the adolescent age group (Table 13-1).

      (1) The appropriate speculum, once selected, is shown to the patient. If possible, the speculum is warmed and touched to the patient's thigh before insertion.

      (2) Before the speculum is inserted in the virginal teenager, a slow, one-finger examination is done to demonstrate the size of the introitus and location of the cervix.

      (3) With a finger, the introitus is gently depressed and spread, and the speculum is slowly slipped into the vagina. After a moment's pause the speculum is carefully opened, the cervix located, and the speculum secured in place.

      (4) Note the appearance of the cervix and vaginal mucosa. Cultures and smears may be taken at this time. The speculum is then removed.

   d. **Bimanual examination** After the speculum is removed, lubricant is applied to the index and middle finger before insertion into the vagina.

      (1) The fingers are placed just under the cervix, and with the other hand on the abdomen, the uterine size and location are determined. The adnexae are then checked.

      (2) In tense or obese patients it may be difficult to identify ovarian tissue by touch. A confirmatory rectovaginal examination is done by placing the index finger in the vagina, the middle finger in the rectum, and the other hand on the abdomen. The patient is

Table 13-1 Specula for Use in the Adolescent Age Group

Type of Speculum	Usage
Huffman (½ × 4½ in.)	Small hymeneal opening
Pederson (1 × 4½ in.)	Sexually active adolescent
Graves (⅝ × 3 in.)	Sexually active adolescent

warned that she will feel as though she is having a bowel movement.

(3) When the examination is completed and the patient has dressed, the examiner's findings are discussed with her.

B. Breast examination Breast cancer will develop in 1 in 13 women. Adolescents should be taught how to do a breast self-examination and should become familiar with their breasts, so that when an unusual lump is noted, they will seek prompt medical attention. Cancer of the breast is extremely rare in children and adolescents. In girls with a strong family history of breast cancer, particularly in the maternal line, the importance of self-examination should be stressed.

1. Methods of self-examination

a. Supine Lying on her back, she places the left hand under the head. The fingertips of the right hand are placed on the left breast at 12 o'clock. The breast is gently palpated clockwise. The examination is repeated for the right breast, using the left hand for palpation, with the right hand under the head.

b. Upright The procedures described above are repeated in a standing position (usually in the shower, since the wet skin is easier to manipulate).

The breasts should be examined each month, just at the *end* of the menstrual flow. If periods are irregular, an arbitrary day each month is selected, e.g., the first Monday of the month.

2. Findings

a. Some evidence of **benign cystic change** is found in 85 percent of women.

b. Mild **asymmetry** of the breasts is normal. However, when the unequal size results in an obvious cosmetic deformity, plastic surgery may be indicated.

c. Lack of development may be secondary to a congenital absence (amastia) or to a systemic disorder, e.g., malnutrition, congenital adrenal hyperplasia, gonadal dysgenesis, or hypogonadotropic hypogonadism. In Western society, where breast size is often used as a measure of femininity, girls with normal, small breasts may need reassurance. (You might remind them that there would not be so many size 32A bras to choose from if they were the only ones who need that size!)

d. Accessory nipples or breasts occur in 1–2 percent of healthy patients. No therapy is indicated.

e. Nipple discharge is rare. Galactorrhea is seen in patients on phenothiazines, reserpine, methyldopa, and oral contraceptives. Amenorrhea with galactorrhea requires evaluation to rule out a CNS tumor. A periareolar follicle may drain brownish fluid for several weeks; no treatment is needed.

f. Periareolar hair is not uncommon in healthy adolescents. No treatment is indicated.

C. Diagnostic studies

1. A **Papanicolaou smear** should be done on all young women who have a speculum examination.

a. With the speculum in place, an Ayer wooden spatula is scraped around the cervix, and the collected material is spread on a slide. In addition, a cotton-tipped applicator moistened with saline is swirled in the endocervical canal (¼ in. through the cervical os) and streaked on the frosted side of a glass slide.

b. The slide is then placed in a bottle of Papanicolaou fixative or sprayed with fixative and sent to the cytology laboratory.

c. The results are classified as follows:
  I. Negative
  II. Benign aplasia (also negative)
  IIR. Atypical cells
  III. Dysplasia
  IV. Suspicious cells, probably carcinoma in situ
  V. Definite tumor cells

d. Treatment

  (1) Class I or II Annual Papanicolaou smears should be done.

  (2) Class IIR The atypical cells seen may be secondary to infection (*Trichomonas, Candida albicans*) or endometrial cells (present when the smear was taken at the end of the menstrual period). Treat the vaginitis and repeat the smear in 2–3 months at midcycle.

  (3) Class III, IV, V Refer the patient to a gynecologist.

2. In the absence of infection, a **vaginal smear for estrogen** (see Chap. 12) is useful for evaluating the patient's hormonal status. When the speculum is in place, the side wall of the vagina is scraped with a tongue depressor or a Q-tip moistened with saline. When the speculum is not used, a Q-tip is inserted directly through the introitus. The material obtained is streaked on a glass slide and placed in Papanicolaou fixative.

3. The **cervical mucus** can be used to evaluate the patient's estrogen status. First, swab the cervix with a large, cotton-tipped applicator. Then obtain a small sample of cervical mucus with a long forceps or saline-moistened Q-tip. On day 8–9 of the menstrual cycle the mucus is scant and watery. On day 14–16 it is profuse, clear, and elastic. On day 20 it is thick and sticky.

Spread the collected cervical mucus on a glass slide, allow it to air dry for 10 to 20 min, and examine it under the microscope. The late proliferative phase of the menstrual cycle is characterized by *ferning* of the cervical mucus. The presence of ferning in sexually active patients with secondary amenorrhea indicates a persistent proliferative phase suggesting an anovulatory cycle, not pregnancy. Ferning will not occur when progesterone is present.

4. Wet preparations are used in determining the cause of a vaginal discharge.

  a. In the prepubertal child, the sample is collected with a saline-moistened Q-tip or eyedropper while the patient is supine.

  b. In the adolescent, the specimen is collected from the vaginal pool while the speculum is in place. The Q-tip is taken from the vaginal pool to a slide, where it is mixed with one drop of saline, and then is placed on another slide, where it is mixed with one drop of 10% potassium hydroxide (KOH).

c. A coverslip is promptly applied, and the slides are examined under the microscope (low and high dry power).

  (1) *Trichomonas* infection is indicated by the presence of lively. flagellated organisms.

  (2) In *Haemophilus vaginalis* infection, refractile bacteria, large epithelial cells ("clue cells"), and leukocytes are seen.

  (3) In *Candida albicans* infection, budding hyphae and yeast forms are present.

5. Gram stain (see Chap. 15)   In symptomatic gonorrhea the smear may reveal gram-negative intracellular diplococci. However, because saprophytic *Neisseria* organisms are present in the vagina, only a positive culture establishes the diagnosis.

6. Cultures (see also Chap. 15)   Sexually active adolescents should have routine cervical culture for gonorrhea every 6 months. The sites of culture in the symptomatic patient or a contact are the urethra, cervix, rectum, and pharynx.

  a. Swab the area to be cultured with a Q-tip and streak directly on a slide, using a Transgrow, modified Thayer-Martin-Gembec, or Thayer-Martin medium.

  b. To confirm yeast vaginitis, swab the vagina and streak on Nickerson's medium.

  c. Leave the cap of the bottle with the medium partially unscrewed and incubate the tube in your office at room temperature. The appearance of brown colonies in 3–7 days confirms the diagnosis.

7. Progesterone test   Progesterone is used as a diagnostic test in the evaluation of primary and secondary amenorrhea; it is not a test for pregnancy. Medroxyprogesterone (Provera), 10 mg PO is given for 5 days, or progesterone-in-oil, 50–100 mg, is given IM. If the endometrium is estrogen primed and the patient is not pregnant, withdrawal bleeding will result in 3–10 days.

8. Pregnancy tests

  a. Several 2-min urine pregnancy tests (Gravindex, Pregnosticon Accuspheres, Pregnosis, and the UCG Slide test) are available. These tests detect human chorionic gonadotropin (HCG) 10–14 days after the first missed period. Tube tests done in commercial laboratories and hospitals require 2 hr and become positive 1 week earlier than the 2-min tests.

  b. Blood test   The Biocept G test measures HCG in serum and is positive one day after a missed period.

  c. False-negative and false-positive tests

   (1) Urine   False-negative tests occur when the patient is less than 6 weeks pregnant and in ectopic pregnancies. False-positive tests are seen with detergent residue on the glassware, significant proteinuria, and some drugs (e.g., methadone, phenothiazines, and progestational agents).

   (2) Blood   False-negative tests are obtained very early in pregnancy when HCG is less than 0.2 IU/ml serum. The presence of choriocarcinoma or hydatidiform mole may result in false-positive tests in young women.

9. **Buccal smear**   The patient rinses her mouth with water, and a tongue depressor is then scraped along the buccal mucosa.

   a. The material is streaked on a glass slide and placed in Papanicolaou fixative or a 3:1 methanol–acetic acid solution.

   b. The chromatin-positive material (Barr body) represents the second X chromosome. Normal Barr-body counts vary from 10–49 percent. The absence of Barr bodies indicates XO or XY; a low count suggests a mosaic; XXX or XXXY causes two Barr bodies per cell.

10. The **basal body temperature chart** is used primarily for infertility patients, although it is also helpful in determining when ovulation occurs in a patient with oligomenorrhea or a mosaic Turner syndrome. Instruct the patient to keep a thermometer by the bedside, place the thermometer in her mouth as soon as she awakens, and record the temperature on a chart. There is a drop in the basal body temperature at the time of ovulation.

II. COMMON GYNECOLOGIC COMPLAINTS OF CHILDREN AND ADOLESCENTS

A. Vulvovaginitis in the prepubertal child

1. **Etiology**   Poor perineal hygiene is likely after the age of 3, when mothers are not directly involved with toileting.

   a. Pinworm infestation with the subsequent anal scratching can contaminate the vaginal area; an adult pinworm may migrate to the vagina and produce vaginal irritation and discharge.

   b. Bubble bath and harsh soaps cause vulvitis and secondary vaginitis.

   c. Tight-fitting nylon underpants worn in hot weather cause maceration and secondary infections, usually yeast.

   d. *Trichomonas, Neisseria gonorrhoeae,* group A beta-hemolytic streptococci, and pneumococci are specific agents causing vulvovaginitis.

2. **Evaluation**

   a. A careful history should be traced, questioning the child about the etiologic factors listed in **1.** Ask about the quantity, duration, and type of discharge. Determine the direction in which the child wipes the anal area, ask about the use of bubble baths, the type of soap used, symptoms of anal pruritus, and whether or not there is exposure to an infected adult through sexual contact or indirectly by sharing a bed, towels, and so on.

   b. Examine the child in the knee-chest position to rule out the presence of a foreign body.

   c. A vaginal discharge that is persistent or purulent should have gram stains, wet preps, and cultures. If the amount of discharge is scant, use brain-heart broth and Thayer-Martin-Gembec as a medium. If the discharge is copious, use Thayer-Martin-Gembec and either brain-heart infusion or send swab to the laboratory for culture on blood, McConkey, and chocolate agar.

   d. Do a wet preparation for yeast and *Trichomonas.* Yeast infection is rare, but when found, check the urine for glucose to rule out diabetes. Do the Scotch-tape or pinworm paddle test to confirm the presence of pinworm infestation.

3. **Diagnosis** A **history of exposure** to offending agents, the presence of **symptoms** (itching, discomfort, vaginal discharge), the **character of the discharge**, and the **physical findings** aid in establishing the diagnosis of vulvovaginitis.

4. **Therapy**

   a. **Nonspecific vaginitis** (culture shows *E. coli*, other gram-negative enteric organisms, or normal flora) The following measures are recognized:

      (1) Instruct the child to

         (a) Improve perineal hygiene.

         (b) Wear white cotton underpants.

         (c) Avoid bubble baths and harsh soaps.

         (d) Take sitz baths tid in plain warm water. Wash the vulvar area with mild soap (Basis, Oilatum, Castile) and pat dry. Allow for further drying by lying on the back with the legs spread apart for 10 min.

      (2) If there is no improvement in 3 weeks, treat the child with oral antibiotics (such as amoxicillin, ampicillin, or cephalexin) for 10–14 days.

      (3) If improvement still does not occur, treat the child with an estrogen-containing cream for 2–3 weeks (reversible breast tenderness and vulvar pigmentation may occur).

   b. **Acute severe edematous vulvitis**

      (1) Sitz baths should be taken q4h, without soap and with air drying.

      (2) Witch hazel pads (Tucks) should be used instead of toilet paper.

      (3) After 2 days, sitz baths should be alternated with painting of the vulva with a bland solution, e.g., calamine lotion.

      (4) For *pruritus*, hydrocortisone cream 1%, Neo-Cortef Cream 1%, or Vioform-Hydrocortisone cream should be applied to the vulva.

   c. **Specific vaginitis**

      (1) **Gonococcus** See Chap. 15.

      (2) For **group A beta-hemolytic streptococci or pneumococci:**

         (a) Penicillin, 125–250 mg PO qid for 10 days, or

         (b) Erythromycin, 30–50 mg/kg/day PO tid.

      (3) For *Trichomonas* Metronidazole (Flagyl), 125 mg tid PO for 5 days, or 1–2 gm PO in 1 dose, is recommended.

      (4) **Pinworms** See Chap. 16, p. 408.

      (5) *Candida albicans* Nystatin cream (for moist lesions) or ointment (for dry scaly lesions) should be applied to the vulva tid for 2 weeks. For persistent yeast infections, nystatin, 100,000 units PO qid for 2 weeks, or 1 ml in the vagina tid for 2 weeks is recommended.

      (6) **Condyloma acuminatum** is often seen in association with *Trichomonas* vaginitis. Examine the lesions by biopsy to establish a definitive diagnosis, and treat with podophyllin (see Sec. **B**).

(7) Labia adhesions can occur in girls 2–6 years of age. The cause is unknown. In mild cases, no treatment is required. When vaginal or urinary drainage is impaired, Premarin cream is applied bid for 2 weeks and lubrication with K-Y Jelly should be continued for several months to prevent the adhesions from re-forming. **The labia should not be forced apart.** This is traumatic to the child and leads to further adhesion formation.

B. Vulvovaginitis in the adolescent

1. **Etiology**   Unlike prepubertal vaginitis, which is nonspecific most of the time, vaginitis in the adolescent usually has a specific cause and is often related to sexual contact, e.g., *N. gonorrhoeae*, *Trichomonas*, *Candida*, *Haemophilus vaginalis*, or herpesvirus. However, the most common cause of discharge in the adolescent is physiologic leukorrhea (normal desquamation of epithelial cells).

2. **Evaluation and diagnosis**   A pelvic examination is required, with wet preparations and cultures.

   a. *Trichomonas*   A wet preparation (saline) reveals flagellated organisms dancing under the microscope. Small punctate hemorrhagic spots may be seen on the cervical and vaginal cells.

   b. *Candida*   A wet preparation (KOH) reveals budding hyphae. Nickerson's medium is used for culturing.

   c. **Nonspecific vaginitis**   A wet preparation reveals large epithelial cells coated with small refractile bacteria (clue cells). To identify *H. vaginalis*, the discharge is streaked on chocolate agar and incubated under increased CO_2 tension.

   d. **Gonorrhea**   The discharge should be cultured.

   e. **Leukorrhea**   A wet preparation reveals epithelial cells only.

   f. **Condyloma acuminatum**   Wartlike growths are inspected.

   g. **Herpes vulvitis** (see Chap. 15, Sec. **V**)   The vesicles are inspected and the base of the lesion is scraped and stained with Wright's stain. A smear reveals multinucleated giant cells and inclusions. Viral cultures are impractical in practice.

   h. **Pediculosis pubis (crabs)**   Firmly attached flakes will be seen on the pubic hair. (The flakes are adult leci or nits.)

   i. **Pinworms**   See Chap. 16.

   j. **Foreign body**   Inspect the patient for the presence of a foreign body. In the adolescent, this is often a forgotten tampon.

3. **Treatment**

   a. For *Trichomonas* vaginitis, give metronidazole, 2 gm PO, all in 1 dose or 250 mg tid for 10 days. Treat sexual partners at the same time. Instruct the patient not to drink alcohol while on metronidazole, since vomiting often results.

   b. For **candidal (monilial) vaginitis,** miconazole (Monistat) vaginal cream 1 applicatorful intravaginally for 7 nights, or Mycostatin vaginal suppository, 1 bid for 14 days, is recommended.

   c. For nonspecific vaginitis, therapy is still controversial. Recent studies suggest Flagyl 500 mg bid PO for 7 days for patient and partner.

Alternate but less effective treatment is ampicillin 500 mg qid for 10 days.

d. Gonorrhea See Chap. 15.

e. Leukorrhea Reassure the patient and recommend good perineal hygiene and the wearing of *white* cotton underpants.

f. Condyloma acuminatum Treating the associated vaginitis often results in spontaneous regression of the lesions. If the associated vaginitis is not treated, the warts will recur.

(1) Apply podophyllum resin (25%) in tincture of benzoin to the lesions. Do not touch the normal skin. Tell the patient to wash the lesions 2 hr later.

(2) If burning occurs, use petrolatum (Vaseline) or lidocaine (Xylocaine) 2% jelly topically.

(3) Treat the lesions once a week. If they are larger than 1 cm in diameter, refer the patient for excision, fulguration, or cryocautery.

g. Herpes vulvitis Soothing relief may be obtained with Betadine (1%) Solution and/or Xylocaine 2% Jelly plus sitz baths. Urinating in the shower or tub may be necessary for patients with severe pain.

h. Pediculosis pubis Kwell shampoo should be used on all hairy areas. Repeat in 24 hr. Clothing and bedding should be washed.

i. Pinworms See Chap. 16.

C. Delayed sexual development See Chap. 12.

D. Secondary amenorrhea

1. Etiology

a. The most common causes are pregnancy and stress caused by fever, emotional turmoil, weight change, change in environment (camp, boarding school, college).

b. Also consider anorexia nervosa, obesity, Stein-Leventhal syndrome, thyroid disease, ovarian tumor, and diabetes.

2. Evaluation

a. Pregnancy When a sexually active patient's period is 2 weeks late, the patient should have a pelvic examination and a pregnancy test.

b. Stress The history will elicit areas of stress in a patient's life.

c. Anorexia nervosa No specific laboratory test is available. Psychiatric evaluation is essential.

d. Obesity Determine whether or not weight gain (often rapid) is correlated with cessation of periods.

e. Stein-Leventhal syndrome A pelvic examination will determine the size and characteristics of the ovaries. If the syndrome is present, serum testosterone and LH are usually elevated. The FSH is normal. Urinary 17-ketosteroids are normal to moderately elevated. The diagnosis is confirmed by laparoscopy.

f. Thyroid disease See Chap. 12.

g. **Ovarian tumor**   Pelvic examination should be done.

h. **Diabetes mellitus**   See Chap. 14.

3. **Diagnosis**

   a. **Pregnancy** is indicated by an enlarged uterus and a soft, blue cervix and is confirmed by a positive pregnancy test.

   b. **Stress**   A stressful situation in the patient's life is identified and correlated with the onset of amenorrhea.

   c. **Anorexia nervosa**   The classic history of prolonged weight loss secondary to poor intake, coupled with excessive activity, amenorrhea and emotional problems, confirms the diagnosis of anorexia nervosa.

   d. **Obesity**   Documentation of excessive weight gain with resultant amenorrhea is required.

   e. **Stein-Leventhal syndrome**   The diagnosis is considered in a patient with a history of oligomenorrhea, the physical findings of hirsutism, obesity, and enlarged cystic ovaries on pelvic examination, and abnormal hormonal levels. It is confirmed at laparoscopy when the ovaries demonstrate the typical findings of a thickened capsule and multiple cysts.

   f. **Thyroid disease**   See Chap. 12.

   g. **Ovarian tumor**   The presence of an adnexal mass on pelvic examination is confirmed by direct visualization and histologic study of sections in estrogen-deficient patients.

   h. **Diabetes mellitus**   See Chap. 14.

4. **Therapy of secondary amenorrhea**   Identify the cause and when possible eliminate it.

   a. **Stress**   Provera 10 mg PO for 5 days. Withdrawal bleeding will result in 3 to 7 days after completing the medication.

   b. **Anorexia nervosa**   Regaining sufficient weight is critical for the individual's hypothalamic suppression to cease. Interestingly, the final weight at which menstruation spontaneously recurs is usually higher than what the patient weighed at menarche. If the youngster insists on having a period she can be cycled with Premarin 1.25 mg qd from day 1 through day 21 and Provera 10 mg qd from day 17 to day 21.

   c. **Obesity**   Loss of excessive weight initiates spontaneous periods. Provera in the usual dose is effective in producing withdrawal bleeding.

   d. **Stein-Leventhal syndrome**   Provera, 10 mg qd for 5 days monthly, is given to prevent endometrial hyperplasia. In patients with enlarged ovaries and elevated testosterone, birth control pills are the treatment of choice. Clomiphene citrate and/or wedge resection are reserved for patients desirous of becoming pregnant.

   e. **Thyroid disease**   See Chap. 12.

   f. **Ovarian tumor**   Surgical removal of the tumor mass when feasible. If a bilateral oophorectomy is done, cycle the patient on Premarin and Provera as described above (see **b**).

   g. **Diabetes mellitus**   See Chap. 14.

E. Dysfunctional uterine bleeding

1. **Etiology**   One of the most common gynecologic complaints in the adolescent is irregular, prolonged menstruation.

    a. In the **young adolescent** the cause is anovulatory cycles (unopposed estrogen) with incomplete shedding of the proliferative endometrium.

    b. In the **older adolescent** it is secondary to anovulatory cycles from stress or illness.

2. **Evaluation**

    a. Pelvic examination

    b. Complete blood count with platelet estimate

    c. Cultures for gonorrhea

    d. Tine test

    e. Pregnancy test

    f. Drug ingestion (warfarin), birth control pills

3. **Diagnosis**   A past history of painless irregular periods occurring every 2–3 weeks suggests anovulatory bleeding. Any positive findings in the evaluation procedures suggest specific diagnoses.

4. **Treatment**

    a. For irregular periods of short duration with normal hemoglobin and if patient is not bleeding at the time of the visit, Provera 10 mg bid for 7 days. Repeat in 1 month.

    b. For **persistent vaginal bleeding** without significant anemia or no response to **a**:

       (1) Ortho-Novum 2 mg once or twice daily for 20 days.

       (2) The bleeding should stop in 2–4 days, followed by withdrawal flow in 2–4 days after the last pill.

       (3) Then cycle the patient with Provera, 10 mg daily PO for the first 5 days of the month for 3–6 months.

    c. For **heavy vaginal bleeding** with anemia:

       (1) Ortho-Novum, 2 mg q4h, until bleeding stops, or

       (2) Enovid-E, 2.5 mg q4h, until bleeding stops.

       (3) Once bleeding stops, 1 tablet is taken bid until the package is gone. Withdrawal flow follows the last tablet in 2–4 days.

       (4) Then cycle the patient with Ortho-Novum, 2 mg, or Enovid-E, 2.5 mg, for 2–3 months.

       (5) If bleeding does not stop in 36–48 hr, consult a gynecologist.

F. Dysmenorrhea

1. The etiology is unclear. It is theorized that prostaglandins released during the menstrual flow stimulate the contractility of the endometrium.

2. **Evaluation**   Review the menstrual history, premenstrual symptoms, timing of cramps, and how the patient deals with cramps. In a virginal girl of 13–14 years, inspect the genitalia to rule out a hymenal abnor-

mality. Patients with severe dysmenorrhea require a pelvic examination.

3. **Diagnosis**   Cramping lower abdominal pain usually starts 1–4 hr before a period and lasts up to 24 hr. Some girls experience dysmenorrhea days before the onset of menstrual flow, and the pain can last 4–6 days. Nausea and vomiting may accompany the cramps. Dysmenorrhea is functional in 95 percent of patients. Organic lesions associated with dysmenorrhea include chronic pelvic inflammatory disease, vaginal agenesis, rudimentary uterine horn, paramesonephric cysts, and endometriosis.

4. **Treatment** is directed at symptomatic relief.

   a. **Pain**

   (1) Aspirin, 300–600 mg q4h

   (2) Naprosyn, 250 mg bid

   (3) Empirin Compound with Codeine, 15–30 mg q4h

   (4) Motrin, 400 mg tid

   b. **Nausea and vomiting**

   (1) Prochlorperazine (Compazine), 5–10 mg 1 q4h

   (2) Chlorpromazine (Thorazine), 25 mg PR q6h

   c. Bed rest, use of a heating pad, and clear fluids can be helpful.

   d. See the patient every 3 months to evaluate the effectiveness of therapy and foster the physician-patient relationship.

   e. If analgesics fail, give a 3–6-month course of birth control pills, which eliminate or substantially reduce cramps.

   f. If the cramps persist despite oral contraceptives, refer the patient for a laparoscopy to rule out endometriosis.

G. **Mittelschmerz** is the pain experienced at the time of ovulation.

1. **Etiology**   It is thought to be secondary to spillage of fluid from the rupturing follicular cyst, which irritates the peritoneum.

2. **Evaluation**   The patient usually complains of midcycle, unilateral dull and aching lower quadrant abdominal pain lasting from a few minutes to 6–8 hr. Rarely, the pain can be severe, mimicking appendicitis, torsion or rupture of an ovarian cyst, or an ectopic pregnancy. Refer the patient for laparoscopy to rule out these diagnoses.

3. **Diagnosis**   The midcycle nature of the pain and absence of significant disease establish the diagnosis.

4. **Treatment**   Explain the benign nature of the pain to the patient. A heating pad and mild analgesics are helpful.

H. **Diethylstilbestrol exposure in utero**

1. **Etiology**   Diethylstilbestrol (DES) was given as an antiabortant to women during the 1950s and 1960s. The development of clear cell adenocarcinoma in girls exposed to DES in utero was reported in 1970. Adenosis (glandular epithelium of müllerian origin) of the vaginal wall has been described in 36–90 percent of girls exposed to DES. Although adenosis is a benign condition because of its cytologic similarity to adenocarcinoma, regular follow-up is required. Abnormal uterine shape

and incompetent cervix are associated with an increased miscarriage rate among DES-exposed offspring.

2. Evaluation

  a. Obtain a history of all drugs taken by the girl's mother during pregnancy.

  b. Refer known DES-exposed patients at age 14 to a gynecologist.

  c. Stress the importance of gynecologic follow-up.

3. The **diagnosis** must be made by a gynecologist.

4. Treatment Patients with adenosis should be followed up every 6–12 months.

III. ADOLESCENT SEXUALITY The care of adolescents includes dealing not only with their physical and emotional well-being, but also with their emerging sexuality. The spectrum of adolescent sexual concerns ranges from homosexual fears to an unwanted pregnancy. To be able to allay these concerns, the pediatrician must establish a confidential trusting relationship with the teenager, which requires time and patience. Most adolescents are reluctant to initiate sexual discussions. However, sexuality introduced in the context of the system review eliminates the mutual embarrassment often felt by both physician and patient.

A 15-year-old male experiencing spontaneous erections while roughhousing with a male friend fears he is a homosexual. A 14-year-old girl missing her period after a session of heavy petting is convinced she is pregnant. A 16-year-old boy has been taught that masturbation is a sin, yet he continues, convinced he is beyond redemption. A 16-year-old girl is having unprotected intercourse in the belief that she is too young to use any type of birth control.

These are but a few of the issues adolescents will raise as they progress in their normal psychosexual development. By not patronizing them because of their lack of sexual expertise and sophistication, but providing respectful reassurance, the pediatrician can correct most sexual misconceptions.

The decision whether or not sex becomes a part of a teenage relationship rests ultimately with the persons involved. Young people are influenced in such a decision by the family standards, religion, society's expectations, peer pressure, internal needs, drug and alcohol usage, and partner availability. The pediatrician's role is not to judge the patient's behavior, but to provide sufficient information to permit the teenager to make a responsible decision.

The issue of whose obligation it is to educate adolescents about sexuality has not been resolved. The young person has three readily available sources of information: parents, peers, and school. Some parents are uncomfortable discussing sexuality with their children. An equal number of children cannot tolerate discussing sex with their parents. Parents who hand their child a book on sex and say "Read it" have not fulfilled their role in educating their child. As important as the mechanisms of sex are, the feelings involved are of equal value. To understand sexuality, the "why" of sex must be explored, and this is not available in a book. It is during frank discussions between parent and child that the psychology of sex is taught.

Peers as an information source are often a cause of confusion. Why then do children turn to their friends? They are available, approachable, willing to listen, and rarely make moral judgments. Their lack of expertise is rarely seen as a drawback.

Schools in general cannot provide the subtle sensitivity needed to explore adolescent sexuality. Most sex education classes are limited to the mechanics of intercourse. Many states still prohibit the schools from teaching the available methods of birth control. The feelings involved in a sexual experience, the expectations, fantasies, fulfillment, and disappointments are virtually ignored.

The dilemma of adolescent sexuality has not been resolved, which is one reason why teenage pregnancy has reached epidemic proportions in this country. Pediatricians have the opportunity and responsibility to educate and counsel their patients on sexual issues.

IV. BIRTH CONTROL   Statistics clearly show that more than half of all first sexual encounters among teenagers are unprotected. Despite the availability of contraceptives, adolescents often refrain from using them because they detract from the spontaneity of the act. Question your patients on their sexual activity (teenagers rarely volunteer this type of information). If asked in a direct, nonjudgmental manner, most adolescents are willing to share this information and to request a method of birth control that is most appropriate for them.

A. Oral contraceptives   The "pill" is viewed by some as the salvation of women, liberating them from the fear of pregnancy. Others see it as consisting of dangerous chemicals that poison those who use it. There is some truth to both points of view. The pill, taken as prescribed, will prevent pregnancy with over 99 percent efficiency. This is not achieved without complications, however.

   1. The **complications and side effects** of oral contraceptive use include the following:

      a. Nausea, bloating, and weight gain.

      b. Breakthrough bleeding.

      c. Headaches.

      d. Hypertension.

      e. Thrombophlebitis.

      f. Fluid retention, which may increase frequency of epileptic seizures.

      g. Scanty or absent periods.

      h. Depression.

      i. Dry eyes secondary to lack of tearing or corneal edema.

      j. Birth control pills containing 50 μg or more of estrogen produce abnormal results on glucose tolerance tests in some patients. Diabetic patients on the pill may have increased insulin requirements.

      k. The pill has produced positive LE preparations and arthralgias in normal patients. Both of these findings disappear when the pill is stopped.

   2. Contraindications   The pill is contraindicated in patients with lupus erythematosus, chemical diabetes, and cholestatic jaundice of pregnancy.

   3. Indications for estrogen-dominant pill

      a. Hirsutism

      b. Acne

      c. Scanty periods (on or off the pill)

      d. Increased appetite and weight gain on the pill

      e. Early-cycle spotting on the pill

Table 13-2   The Hormonal Content of Commonly Used Oral Contraceptive Pills

Product	Estrogen	Progestin
Combination pills		
Enovid-E	Mestranol 0.1 mg	Norethynodrel 2.5 mg
Enovid 5 mg	Mestranol 0.075 mg	Norethynodrel 5 mg
Ortho-Novum 1/50, Norinyl 1 + 50	Mestranol 0.05 mg	Norethindrone 1 mg
Ortho-Novum 1/80, Norinyl 1 + 80	Mestranol 0.08 mg	Norethindrone 1 mg
Ortho-Novum 2 mg, Norinyl 2 mg	Mestranol 0.1 mg	Norethindrone 2 mg
Norlestrin 1/50, Zorane 1/50	Ethinyl estradiol 0.05 mg	Norethindrone acetate 1 mg
Norlestrin 2.5/50	Ethinyl estradiol 0.05 mg	Norethindrone acetate 2.5 mg
Ovulen	Mestranol 0.1 mg	Ethynodiol diacetate 1 mg
Demulen	Ethinyl estradiol 0.05 mg	Ethynodiol diacetate 1 mg
Ovral	Ethinyl estradiol 0.05 mg	Norgestrel 0.5 mg
Ovcon-50	Ethinyl estradiol 0.05 mg	Norethindrone 1 mg
Ovcon-35	Ethinyl estradiol 0.035 mg	Norethindrone 0.4 mg
Zorane 1.5/30, Loestrin 1.5/30	Ethinyl estradiol 0.03 mg	Norethindrone 1 mg
Zorane 1/20, Loestrin 1/20	Ethinyl estradiol 0.02 mg	Norethindrone 1 mg
Brevicon	Ethinyl estradiol 0.035 mg	Norethindrone 0.5 mg
Lo/Ovral	Ethinyl estradiol 0.03 mg	Norgestrel 0.3 mg
Ortho-Novum SQ	14 white: 0.08 mg mestranol 6 blue: 2 mg norethindrone, 0.08 mg mestranol	
Mini-pills		
Nor-Q.D. & Micronor		Norethindrone 0.35 mg
Ovrette		Norgestrel 0.075 mg

Modified from Emans, S. J. H., and Goldstein, D. P., *Pediatric and Adolescent Gynecology.* Boston: Little, Brown and Company, 1977.

4. Indications for progesterone-dominant pill

   a. Mucorrhea

   b. Cervical erosion

   c. Nausea or bloating on pills

    d. Fibroids

    e. Fibrocystic breast disease

    f. Cyclic weight gain

    g. Dysmenorrhea

    h. Hypermenorrhea

    i. Late-cycle spotting on the pill

5. Changes in common laboratory values

    a. T_4 is increased, and resin T_3 is decreased. Free T_4 is unchanged.

    b. There is a slight increase in coagulation factors II, VIII–X, and XII and a moderate increase in factor VII.

    c. Triglyceride, cholesterol, and phospholipid levels are increased in some patients.

    d. Serum folate is decreased in some patients and is rarely associated with megaloblastic anemia.

    e. The ESR is increased slightly.

6. Prescribing the pill

    a. Patient evaluation requires the following:

        (1) A complete history and physical examination, including a pelvic examination.

        (2) Laboratory studies Hemoglobin and Papanicolaou smear. In patients with a family history of arteriosclerotic heart disease or stroke, cholesterol and triglyceride levels should be determined. In sexually active patients, test for syphilis once a year and culture for gonorrhea every 6 months.

    b. Choice of pill See Table 13-2.

        (1) A medium-dose pill (e.g., Norinyl 1+50, Ortho-Novum 1/50) can be prescribed for girls with regular periods and no special indication for an estrogen-dominant or progesterone-dominant pill.

        (2) A low-dose pill (e.g., Brevicon, Lo/Ovral, Loestrin) can also be given. Although girls on low- to middle-dose pills often experience midcycle breakthrough bleeding, the elimination of weight gain secondary to fluid retention is considered worth the aggravation. However, if the bleeding persists for more than three cycles the next higher dose pill is prescribed. Because of the higher incidence of breakthrough bleeding in the low-dose pill, many girls prefer the medium-dose pill.

        (3) Pills for 21-day and 28-day cycles are available. Since, with the latter, the teenager is taking a pill *every* day, the chances that she will forget to take it are reduced.

    c. Follow-up The patient should be seen in 3 months for a blood pressure and weight check. At this visit, any problems she may be having can also be explored. Thereafter, she is seen every 6 months.

    d. The mini-pill is a progestogen-only pill. The pregnancy rate on this pill is higher than on combination pills (1.5–3.0 pregnancies/100 woman-years), and irregular menstrual bleeding occurs.

B. Intrauterine devices (IUDs) that are available include the Cu_7 (copper), Lippes Loop, Saf-T-Coil, and Progestasert. Because of the risk of infection the IUD should be considered only in nulliparous patients who cannot or will not use other means of contraception.

1. Complications

   a. Irregular bleeding and cramps.

   b. Expulsion (most common in the first month after insertion).

   c. Infection (increased risk of pelvic inflammatory disease).

   d. Pregnancy The rate is 1.1–2.5 pregnancies/100 woman-years.

   e. Perforation occurs in less than 1/2000 insertions.

   f. Mortality is 2/100,000 insertions.

2. Patient evaluation

   a. Check the strings attached to the IUD once a week for 1 month, then after each period.

   b. Have the patient return in 6 weeks, then every 6 months–1 year. Replace the Cu_7 in 36 months.

C. Diaphragms The use of a diaphragm should be limited to adolescents who are highly motivated, feel comfortable with their bodies, and are not offended by inserting a mechanical device into the vagina in anticipation of intercourse.

1. Fitting Fitting rings of various sizes are inserted into the vagina to determine the appropriate size. A correctly fitting diaphragm covers the cervix snugly without discomfort to the patient.

2. Instructions The following written instructions are given to the patient on the use and care of the diaphragm:

   a. Put 1 tbsp of contraceptive cream in the cup of the diaphragm.

   b. Insert the diaphragm no more than 2 hr prior to intercourse, checking that the cervix is covered.

   c. If more than 2 hr have passed since insertion, place an applicatorful of contraceptive cream in front of the diaphragm.

   d. Leave the diaphragm in place at least 6 hr after intercourse.

   e. After removing the diaphragm, wash it with a mild soap (cornstarch may be used after washing).

   f. Check the diaphragm once a week for holes by holding it up to the light.

   g. A weight change of 10 lb requires a refitting.

D. Foam is a readily available form of birth control that requires no prescription. The adolescent is given the following instructions:

   1. Insert the contraceptive foam into the vagina 1 hr or less *before* intercourse. It is not effective after intercourse.

   2. Do not douche for 6 hr after intercourse.

   3. When possible, have the partner use a condom with foam to lessen the risk of pregnancy.

E. Condoms are the only birth control devices that lessen the risk of venerea disease dissemination. Condom usage allows the male to participate ac tively in birth control.

F. Administration of the **"morning-after" pill**   High-dose estrogens (DES) afte unprotected intercourse is an effective means of lowering the risk of preg nancy. However, it should be used only in cases of rape and after firs intercourse because of possible risk of uterine carcinoma. Because of th risk of giving it to a patient who is already pregnant by previous exposure estrogen therapy should be prescribed only to those patients who woul have an abortion if already pregnant at the time of unprotected intercourse.

1. **Administration**   DES is taken within 24–72 hr after intercourse.

2. **Dosage**   DES, 25 mg bid for 5 days
   Premarin, 25 mg bid for 5 days
   Estinyl (ethinyl estradiol), 2 mg bid for 5 days

3. **Complications**

   a. **Nausea**   All high-dose estrogens are associated with nausea an vomiting. Prochlorperazine, 5–10 mg PO, given 2 hr prior to estroger reduces the nausea.

   b. Fluid retention.

   c. Headache, dizziness.

   d. Menstrual irregularities.

   e. Breast soreness.

V. PREGNANCY   Each year, more than 1 million girls 15–19 years of age becom pregnant. Unfortunately, the "it can never happen to me" philosophy stil prevails. The majority of pregnant teenagers are neither emotionally dis turbed nor promiscuous, but psychological issues often precipitate the preg nancy. The baby is seen as a love object and is used to replace a recent loss b death, separation, or divorce. The baby is expected to love the teenager an provide the stability needed to maintain the relationship with her boyfriend Threatened with punishment if she becomes pregnant, an adolescent ma become pregnant to test her parents' love. Thus, pregnancy is a plea for some one to care. Unless these complex emotional issues are resolved, anothe pregnancy is likely to follow the first.

A. Diagnosis

1. Many girls cannot bring themselves to express concern over a misse period, and many will deny that the possibility of pregnancy even exists Every girl should be questioned about her menstrual cycles and sexua activity.

2. A pregnancy test is given to confirm the suspected diagnosis (see Sec I.C).

3. Pelvic examination and sizing of the uterus

   a. An 8-week pregnant uterus is the size of an orange.

   b. At 12 weeks, the uterus is the size of a grapefruit at the symphysi pubis.

   c. At 16 weeks, the uterus is felt midway between the umbilicus an symphysis pubis.

   d. At 20 weeks, the uterus is palpable at the umbilicus.

B. Mortality and morbidity complications

1. The **death rate** from the complications of pregnancy, delivery, and the postpartum period is 60 percent higher for girls who become pregnant before the age of 15 years than for those who became pregnant at a later age.

2. **Causes of death** include the following:

   a. **Toxemia,** resulting from

   (1) An immature endocrine system

   (2) Emotional stress

   (3) Poor nutrition

   (4) Inadequate prenatal care

   b. **Hemorrhage**

   c. **Infection**

3. Pregnancy is a common cause of school dropout; 9 of 10 girls whose first delivery occurs at age 15 or younger never complete high school.

4. Couples who marry because of pregnancy have a higher divorce rate than that of the general population.

C. Abortion

1. **Methods**

   a. **Suction curettage** is done before 12 weeks (in many hospitals to 15 weeks) under local or general anesthesia. **Complications** include perforation and hemorrhage (secondary to incomplete removal of the products of conception), and infection.

   b. **Saline or prostaglandin infusion** is done at 16–24 weeks of pregnancy. **Contraindications** to saline infusion are chronic renal disease, cardiac disease, and severe anemia. **Complications** include infection, retained products of conception, coagulopathy, and mortality.

2. **Counseling**   Explore thoroughly with the pregnant teenager the options of abortion, adoption, or keeping the child. She must participate in the decision-making process. Once she has reached a decision, it should be supported by the health professionals caring for her.

VI. RAPE   By definition, rape is the introduction of the penis within the genitals of the victim by force, fear, or fraud. Statutory rape is intercourse with a female below the age of consent (usually 16 years). Sexual molestation is non-coital sexual contact without consent.

A. Patient evaluation

1. Carefully collect and record the medical data.

2. The history should include the time, place, circumstances, and witnesses, if any, as well as efforts to resist the attack.

3. Inquire if the patient has bathed, douched, or urinated since the attack.

4. Record the patient's menstrual history and the type of contraceptive used, if any.

5. Consent forms for all procedures should be signed and witnessed.

6. Physical examination

   a. The patient's appearance (e.g., torn, bloody clothing) and emotional state should be noted and recorded.

   b. The physical examination should include inspection for evidence of trauma.

   c. In the pelvic examination, the vulvar area, urethra, and anus should be carefully inspected. A water-moistened speculum should be used (do not use a lubricant).

7. Laboratory tests

   a. Swab the vaginal pool and vulvar area (place the swab in a test tube and give to the police if an officer is investigating).

   b. Swab the vaginal pool and streak on slides labeled with the patient's name and the date and numbered 1 and 2.

   (1) #1 Slide   No. 1 is placed in Papanicolaou's fixative for hematoxylin and eosin staining (permanent record).

   (2) #2 Slide   No. 2   Mix 1 drop of saline with the swab on the slide and cover with a coverslip. Using high dry power on the microscope, check for red blood cells or motile sperm. Motile sperm indicate sexual contact within 28 hours; nonmotile sperm persist in the vagina up to 48 hours. (If the smear is positive, place it in Papanicolaou's fixative.) **The absence of sperm does not eliminate the possibility of rape**; ejaculates contain no sperm in men with primary azoospermia or who have had a vasectomy.

   c. Endocervical, urethral, rectal, and pharyngeal cultures for gonorrhea and a serologic test for syphilis should be done.

   d. A pregnancy test should be done to detect a preexisting pregnancy.

   e. A CBC should be done.

B. Treatment

   1. If the patient agrees to be treated prophylactically for syphilis, gonorrhea, and pregnancy, treat with

   a. Procaine penicillin G, 4.8 million U IM. Give probenecid, 1 gm PO, immediately before the injection.

   b. Give diethylstilbestrol or conjugated estrogen (Premarin) (see Sec. **IV.G**).

   c. A follow-up visit should be made 1 week later to assess healing. In the second visit, at 6 weeks, repeat the serologic test for syphilis, the pregnancy test, and the cervical culture (if obtained automatically at the time of pelvic examination).

   2. The patient should be counseled by health professionals skilled in **rape management**.

14

Diabetes Mellitus

I. GENERAL FEATURES OF DIABETES Diabetes mellitus is characterized by a metabolic derangement secondary to partial or complete insulin deficiency. In mild cases of insulin lack, the metabolic consequence is a decreased capacity to assimilate ingested foodstuffs, resulting in glucose intolerance. In severe failure of the insulin-producing system, there is hyperglycemia, ketogenesis, and protein wasting.

The most recently reported (1977) prevalence of diabetes in the United States is 1.9/1000 population ages 5–18 years. In about 5 percent of the total diabetic population, the diagnosis is made before 16 years of age.

Diabetes in the young is considered to be hereditary. The mode of inheritance is probably polygenic.

II. CLINICAL COURSE

    A. The **initial phase** begins from the onset of clinical symptoms to the time of diagnosis, lasting anywhere from 1 day to several weeks. It is often precipitated by infection, emotional upset, or physical trauma.

    B. The **recovery phase** usually occurs a few days following therapy, when the stress is controlled and tissue sensitivity to insulin increases.

    C. The **remission phase** is typical of juvenile diabetes. It usually occurs 1–3 months following the introduction of insulin therapy. The duration is variable, lasting anywhere from weeks to months.

    D. The **intensification phase** follows the remission phase and occurs about 6–18 months after the initial diagnosis. Endogenous insulin is depleted. About one-third of the total juvenile diabetic population bypasses the remission phase.

III. DIAGNOSIS

    A. Clinical presentation The possibility of diabetes is usually brought to medical attention by one or more of the following situations:

        1. Family history First-degree relatives of a juvenile-onset diabetic patient have a 5–10 percent risk of the development of the disease.

        2. Symptoms Polydipsia, polyuria, weight loss with polyphagia, enuresis, recurrent infections, and candidiasis.

        3. Glycosuria on routine examination. Screening is best performed during the stress of infection.

        4. Ketoacidosis and coma.

    B. Diagnostic tests It would be easy to make the diagnosis in the situations in **A.3** and **A.4**, but in the asymptomatic patient the diagnosis of diabetes mellitus, particularly of the prediabetic, subclinical, or chemical type, is

Table 14-1   Normal Oral GTT Percentiles for Children (Whole Blood) (mg/100 ml)

Time Sampled (hr)	Percentile		
	3rd	50th	97th
0 (fasting)	56	83	111
½	80	131	183
1	66	110	172
2	64	100	140
3	48	82	126

dependent on the demonstration of carbohydrate intolerance. A series of carbohydrate function tests, namely, the oral glucose tolerance test(OGTT), the IVGTT, and the tolbutamide test, may be necessary to make the definite diagnosis. For the standardization of testing conditions the patient should be on a diet high in carbohydrates for 3 days prior to the test and should then be tested in a fasting and basal state.

1. The **OGTT** is still generally accepted as a standard test for the initial workup in asymptomatic diabetes mellitus.

   a. A loading dose of 1.75 gm glucose/kg of body weight is given (maximum dose, 100 gm).

   b. Blood samples are obtained at 0, ½, 1, 1½, 2, and 3 hr for glucose determination by the Somogyi-Nelson or ferrocyanide method and for insulin by immunoassay. When possible, urine is obtained simultaneously for glucose determination. **"Whole blood" sugars are 10–15 percent lower than serum values.** Normal OGTT percentiles for children (whole blood) are given in Table 14-1.

2. **IVGTT**

   a. A loading dose of 0.5 gm glucose/kg of body weight at 0 time is given by IV push.

   b. Blood samples are obtained at −30, 0, 1, 3, 5, 15, 30, 45, 60, 90, 120, 150, and 180 min for the determination of sugar and immunoreactive insulin (IRI). The result of blood sugar is expressed by the glucose disappearance rate (K-rate). A K-rate higher than 1.2%/min is usually suggestive of carbohydrate intolerance. A blunted and decreased insulin response is suggestive of the early diabetic state.

3. **Tolbutamide stimulation test**

   a. Tolbutamide, 25 mg/kg of body weight (maximum dose, 1 gm), is given by IV push at 0 time.

   b. Blood samples are obtained at −30, 0, 1, 3, 5, 10, 15, 30, 45, 60, 90, and 120 min for the determination of sugar and IRI. Asymptomatic diabetes is usually found to produce a blunted and decreased IRI response.

4. **Individual variations in tolerance and response to carbohydrate function tests**   The carbohydrate tolerance in the same person may vary from time to time. Also, different responses may be elicited from different tests. Some patients are thus required to go through multiple and repeated tests in order to elicit carbohydrate intolerance.

5. The **glycosylated hemoglobin test (hemoglobin A₁)** provides an index of blood glucose concentrations during the weeks prior to sampling. Values

are found to be elevated in virtually all patients with newly diagnosed diabetes. The test is unreliable in hemolytic states and hemoglobin variants, including fetal hemoglobin.

IV. THERAPY

A. General objectives in management

1. Maintenance or establishment of optimal physical and emotional growth and development.

2. Education of the patient, family, and school personnel to a full understanding of diabetes and their role in its management.

3. **Short-term goals**

   a. Control of insulin-deficient metabolic alterations (hyperglycemia, glycosuria, infections, weight loss, ketoacidosis).

   b. Control of effects of insulin therapy: hypoglycemia, lipodystrophy.

4. The **long-term goal** is to prevent or delay the onset of complications (which usually are not clinically evident for 10 years).

   a. Control of blood sugar to **as normal a level as can be obtained** within the limits of available therapy. Hyperglycemia may be responsible for microangiopathic complications resulting from glycosylation and thickening of capillary basement membranes and neuropathy.

   b. Avoidance of other cardiovascular risk factors: hyperlipemia, obesity, and cigarette smoking.

B. Management of diabetic acidosis and coma

1. The basic principles of management of these conditions are

   a. Maintaining an adequate insulin administration program.

   b. Proper handling of precipitating factors (e.g., infection).

   c. Prompt correction of dehydration and the prevention and control of complications such as shock, oliguria, cardiac arrhythmias, and potassium deficiency.

2. There is no rigid guide for insulin or fluid and electrolyte therapy. The clinical response and the improvement of biochemical status dictate subsequent management in the individual patient.

3. **Guidelines for the treatment of severely acidotic and dehydrated comatose children** include the following:

   a. Thoroughgoing **history,** particularly of the event leading to the onset. Recent weight and the last insulin administration in the known diabetic patient should be noted. A **physical examination** (for signs of infection and physical trauma) should be done.

   b. **Accurate body weight.**

   c. **Baseline studies**   Venous blood glucose; serum acetone (serial dilutions on Acetest tablets, which detect acetoacetic and *not* beta-hydroxybutyric acid); pH; total CO_2; BUN; electrolytes; CBC; urinalysis; ECG (T waves); appropriate cultures.

   d. Urine bagging for constant collection to avoid catheterization except in the comatose patient. Urine samples should be collected q1–2h for sugar and acetone determination.

   e. Determination of **blood sugar** q1–2h and **venous pH, TCO$_2$, electrolytes,** and **acetone** q2–3h until the patient is out of danger.

   f. A **flow sheet** containing hourly intake and output, insulin administered, urinary sugar and acetone, blood chemistries, body weight (q12h), and mental status.

   g. An **IV infusion** (cutdown or central venous catheter if the patient is in shock) (see Chap. 2, Sec. **II.C**).

   h. Serial ECG monitoring (lead II), to detect T wave changes of hyperkalemia and hypokalemia.

   i. Administration of regular (crystalline) insulin Various methods are effective (Table 14-2). Low dose (IV and IM) methods require hourly monitoring and immediate reporting of blood glucose. The half-life of insulin injected IV is only 8 min in new diabetics.

   j. Treatment of infection if present.

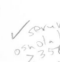

   k. Alertness to signs and symptoms of acute cerebral edema, a rare (1% incidence) but ever-present risk, especially in hyponatremic patients. It often occurs *after* a semicomatose patient becomes alert. The prognosis is grim; see Chap. 2, Sec. **V**.

4. Fluid and electrolyte program for the first 24 hr (see also Chap. 8, Sec. **E**)   The fluid deficit in severe diabetic acidosis is about 10–15 percent of ideal body weight (100–150 ml/kg). The deficit consists of equal amounts of extracellular (ECF) and intracellular (ICF) fluid.

   a. The amount of fluid replacement for the first 24 hr consists of 75 percent of the total deficit (100% of ECF lost; 50% of ICF lost) plus maintenance and continuing losses (NG tube drainage, etc.).

   b. First hour   Main goal is treatment and prevention of hypovolemic shock. Give 20 ml/kg/hr of normal saline and continue at this rate until patient is out of shock.

   c. Hours 2–8   Replace the remainder of ECF loss (50% of total deficit) as *N* saline. Switch to 5% dextrose in ½ *N* saline when blood sugar falls to 250 mg/100 ml.

   d. Hours 9–24   Give the remainder of the calculated requirement (50% of ICF lost, plus maintenance and continuing losses which are increased by hyperpnea and osmotic polyuria). 5% Dextrose in ⅓–½ *N* saline. 2.5–10% Dextrose may be necessary to **maintain** blood sugar at 200–250 mg/100 ml.

5. Potassium   When urinary output is established, give K$^+$, 40–80 mEq/L, as equal amounts of potassium chloride and potassium phosphate (Table 14-3). (Phosphate replaces erythrocyte 2,3-DPG and improves tissue oxygenation.) Overzealous phosphate replacement can produce hypocalcemia, and thus serum calcium levels and the ECG (Q–T interval) must be monitored.

6. Sodium   Assume a loss of 7–8 mEq/kg in the typically isotonic dehydration of ketoacidosis (70–80 mEq/100 ml of fluid loss).

7. Bicarbonate should be administered **only** when the pH is ≦ 7.10, since infused bicarbonate increases plasma osmolality and may *increase* tissue hypoxia (via a shift of the O$_2$–hemoglobin dissociation curve), hypo-

Table 14-2 Methods of Regular Insulin Administration

Method and Dose	Advantages	Disadvantages
SQ		
0.5–1.0 U/kg (½ IV push and ½ SQ), then 0.25–0.5 U/kg SQ q2–4h	Most physicians and hospitals familiar with method	Delayed absorption in markedly dehydrated or poorly perfused patient Late hypoglycemia and sudden hypokalemia common
Low-dose IV		
0.1–0.5 U/kg IV push, then 0.1 U/kg hr. IV drip or pump (mix with albumin or preflush 25% infusate to prevent adherence of insulin to glassware and tubing). Discontinue infusion; give SQ insulin when acidosis improving and blood glucose $\cong$ 300 mg/100 ml	Steady reduction in blood glucose and serum hypertonicity Less risk of sudden hypokalemia Total ability to adjust rate of insulin	Accurate infusion pump necessary Infiltrated IV yields negligible dose to patient Low dose may be insufficient in severe infection Hourly monitoring of blood glucose essential
Low-dose IM		
0.1–0.5 U/kg IV push, then 0.1 U/kg/hr IM. (When blood glucose 300 mg/100 ml, give SQ insulin.)	As effective as IV in reducing blood glucose and reversing acidosis *if* IV priming dose given Do not use infusion pump	Repeated injections necessary Less ability to discontinue insulin in case of "overshoot"

kalemia, and cerebrospinal fluid acidosis. For replacement, 0.7 mEq $NaHCO_3$/kg raises the CO_2 content (TCO_2) 1 mEq/L. Give 0.3 mEq/kg sodium bicarbonate IV stat, then give 20 mEq in each 500 ml of IV solution until the pH reaches **7.10. Then stop.**

C. Insulin

1. **Insulin preparations** are divided into three categories according to promptness, duration, and intensity of action following SQ administration. They are classified as fast, intermediate, and long-acting types (Table 14-4).

2. **Insulin selection** In general, NPH is preferred as the intermediate-acting insulin. New diabetic patients should use the U-100 strength (100 U/ml). Smaller syringes (0.5 ml capacity) are also available for patients on small doses.

   a. While some new diabetic patients can be controlled on a single daily dose of intermediate-acting insulin, most require combinations of intermediate and regular (⅔–¾ intermediate, ¼–⅓ regular).

   b. Better control is achieved in most patients, particularly adolescents, with twice-daily injections; with ⅔–¾ of the total daily dose given

Table 14-3 Potassium Replacement*

Initial K$^+$ (mEq/L)	Clinical Status	Replacement Rate (mEq/kg/24 hr)
<4	No signs, symptoms, or ECG changes	5
<4	Positive signs, symptoms, or ECG changes	6–8
4–5		3
>5		None until K$^+$ $\leqq$ 5

* Monitor ECG continuously for T wave changes if infusate contains >40 mEq/L K$^+$.

before breakfast, the remainder before supper. Each dose may contain a combination of intermediate and regular, as outlined in **a**.

c. Regular insulin is required during acidosis and other acute situations in which the patient's food intake is variable.

d. Long-acting insulin (Ultralente) is not recommended in pediatric patients. Hypoglycemic reactions following its administration often occur during sleeping hours and hence may be prolonged and severe.

3. Insulin therapy The administration of insulin therapy is based on the various phases of the clinical course of diabetes mellitus.

a. Initial phase (newly diagnosed patient with moderate to severe ketoacidosis or coma) The administration of adequate quantities of rapidly acting insulin (regular) is essential for recovery from diabetic ketoacidosis.

(1) Initial dosage See Table 14-2.

(2) After ketoacidosis is reversed

(a) Give regular insulin SQ q4–6h, the amount depending on the clinical and chemical response. Each dose should be specifically ordered, rather than preprogrammed by a sliding scale. The two-drop Clinitest method is preferable, since it registers up to 5 percent glucosuria, equivalent to a 10+.

(b) As a rule of thumb, the maximum dose administered (for 5 percent sugar and high acetone) is ¼–½ U/kg dose.

(3) The insulin dosage is adjusted until the total daily requirement can be estimated moderately well, which is usually after 48 hr of initial therapy. Then ⅔ of the total daily requirement is given as a single dose of an intermediate preparation (or in a split dose as outlined in **2.a**).

(4) Further adjustments in dosage will be necessary, based on the results of blood sugars obtained preprandially and before bedtime.

(5) In mild to moderate ketoacidosis, insulin therapy should be less vigorous (initial dose, 0.25–0.5 U/kg) because of the danger of inducing hypoglycemia in these glycogen-depleted patients.

(6) For patients presenting with mild or moderate diabetes without significant ketosis, treatment may be started with an arbitrary amount (0.25–0.5 U/kg/day) of an intermediate preparation; further adjustments are made as dictated by the response.

Table 14-4 Insulin Preparations

Type	Appearance	Action	Peak Activity (hr)	Duration (hr)	Composition*	Compatible in Use with Regular Insulin
Regular (crystalline)	Clear	Rapid	2–4	5–7		
NPH (neutral protamine Hagedorn)	Turbid	Intermediate	6–12	24–28	Protamine, zinc, insulin	Yes
PZI (protamine zinc)	Turbid	Prolonged	14–24	36+	Same as NPH	No
Semilente	Turbid	Rapid	2–4	12–16	Zinc, acetate buffer, insulin (no protein modifier)	
Lente (30% Semilente, 70% Ultralente)	Turbid	Intermediate	6–12	24–28	Same as Semilente	Yes
Ultralente	Turbid	Prolonged	18–24	36+	Same as Semilente	No

* Available as 40 and 100 U/ml (U-40 and U-100).

   b. The **remission phase** usually occurs after the patient's discharge from the hospital. At this stage the insulin requirement decreases, and the patient should be on a gradually decreasing dosage to avoid hypoglycemia. If there is no glycosuria, consider maintenance on a minimum dose of intermediate-acting insulin (2–4 U/day), and prescribe a dietary regimen to avoid the emotional trauma of discontinuing and then reintroducing insulin.

   c. Stabilized (intensification) phase

     (1) In general, the range of the average requirement for exogenous insulin as the patient approaches the stage of "total" diabetes usually rises slowly and unevenly, eventually stabilizing between 0.6–1.0 U/kg/day.

     (2) Sexual maturation and the adolescent growth spurt increase the requirement for insulin in many children, up to 0.8–1.2 U/kg/day. There is a variable decline in the requirement for exogenous insulin after attainment of full growth and sexual maturation.

4. Insulin regulation

   a. Preprandial second-voided urines and 24-hr fractionated urine glucose measurements assist in the adjustment and dosage of insulin during follow-up care.

   b. Generally, preprandial urine sugar tests are maintained at negative to 0.5 percent. If the 24-hr urine sugar falls between 5–10 percent of the daily carbohydrate intake, regulation is accepted as good, provided that the patient is free of frequent or severe reactions.

   c. Glycosylated hemoglobin tests may help to evaluate overall blood glucose regulation over a period of weeks.

5. Problems in insulin therapy

   a. Hypoglycemia is a major and common complication of insulin therapy and may be manifested acutely by behavioral changes (inattention, confusion, or hyperactivity), headaches, perioral pallor, or "glassy stare," diaphoresis, anxiety, or tremor and may progress to convulsions and coma if untreated. Hypoglycemia may result from

     (1) Excessive dosage of insulin due to visual failure, mismatched insulin and syringe, inappropriate site of injection, or deliberate overdose.

     (2) A reduced need for insulin, resulting from increased exercise (insulin is absorbed more quickly from an injection site that is exercised); diminished caloric intake; development of concomitant endocrinologic or systemic disease; recovery from "stress states" (infection, ketoacidosis, surgery); and the use of drugs with a hypoglycemic effect.

     (3) Treatment

       (a) Simple sugars such as orange juice and soft drinks should be given if the patient can swallow. If not, glucagon (0.03 mg/kg body weight SQ maximum, 1 mg), is useful for raising the blood sugar temporarily at home. Nausea often follows its administration, however.

       (b) Carbohydrate input should be continued until sugar appears in the urine. In severe cases, it is necessary to administer 50% glucose IV (0.5 gm/kg or 1 ml/kg 50% D/W).

b. Lipodystrophy Fat atrophy at the site of injections develops in about one-third of juvenile diabetic patients. Injection of commercially available "single peak" insulins or highly purified "monocomponent" insulin (obtainable from manufacturer) into the atrophic areas has been beneficial.

c. Allergic reaction Transient, localized urticarial lesions may occur during the first few weeks of insulin therapy and later disappear. Generally, no change in regimen is needed. Occasionally, pure pork insulin may be useful.

d. The **Somogyi phenomenon** is the establishment of a pattern of inapparent hypoglycemia, followed by reactive hyperglycemia and ketonuria. It results from administration of excessive insulin.

   (1) The mechanism of the hyperglycemia and ketonuria is increased concentration of hormones (catecholamine, glucocorticoid, growth hormone) with actions antagonistic to insulin, so that insulin hyposensitivity develops.

   (2) The Somogyi phenomenon should be suspected when continual increases in the dosage of insulin do not produce beneficial results. This factor is also considered if the total insulin dose exceeds 1.2 U/kg/day.

   (3) In spite of apparently poor control, these patients usually gain weight, are rarely ketoacidotic, and handle infections reasonably well. Hepatomegaly (from glycogen deposition) may develop, however. To stabilize the situation, a reduction in insulin dosage is necessary.

e. Insulin resistance is a rare event in the treatment of diabetes mellitus. In the adult, it is defined as an insulin requirement in excess of 200 U/day in the absence of acidosis. A change from beef to pork insulin may be effective in reducing the requirement.

D. Oral hypoglycemic agents The two types commonly used in the treatment of adult-onset diabetes, sulfonylurea compounds and the biguanides, have no place in the treatment of juvenile diabetes and are probably not even required in the management of young patients with adult-type diabetes. Dietary regulation, with emphasis on the maintenance of normal weight, will suffice in the latter case.

E. Guidelines for the diabetic diet

   1. The aim of the diabetic diet is to permit the patient to lead a comfortable, asymptomatic life and to attain normal growth and development. The nutritional needs of diabetic children are essentially no different from those of nondiabetic children. The diabetic diet is thus a normal, well-balanced diet with concentrated carbohydrates eliminated. Dietary manipulation is sometimes used as an adjunct to the insulin adjustment in the regulation of urinary sugar.

   The emphasis in the diabetic diet is on the regularity of meals and snacks and the consistency of quantity of foods eaten, rather than on a strictly controlled regimen. It is not recommended that foods be weighed, but rather that the food exchange and diabetic food lists be followed. The simplicity of this approach seems to aid acceptance of the disease by patient and family.

   2. Planning the diabetic diet A normal, well-balanced diet should contain representative proportions of each of the following four basic food groups:

a. **Skim milk,** three or more glasses/day for children (small glasses for those under age 6) and four or more glasses for teenagers.

b. **Meat,** two or more servings.

c. **Vegetables and fruit,** four or more servings.

d. **Bread and cereals,** four or more servings.

e. These foods should be taken in sufficient amounts to provide the following:

   (1) **Calories** It is desirable to keep the diabetic patient's weight in an ideal range for height and body build. The rule of thumb in caloric estimation is by age: 1000 calories daily at 1 year, plus 100 for each additional year up to 18 years for males, 15 years for females.

   (2) **Protein** Because of fat restriction in the diabetic patient, protein intake is usually increased to approximately 20 percent of the calories.

   (3) **Carbohydrates** are maintained at about 45–50 percent of the calories, largely by avoiding sweets and foods containing concentrated sugars.

   (4) **Fat** The fat allowance is moderately restricted, to about 30–35 percent of the dietary calories, to make up the balance of daily caloric needs.

f. **Snacks** The daily diet is usually planned to include three meals and two or three snacks.

   (1) The main purpose of snacks in a diabetic diet is to provide additional carbohydrate coverage at the peak of the insulin reaction and to aid in the prevention of possible nighttime hypoglycemia.

   (2) Snacks are usually scheduled at 3:00 P.M. and at bedtime, with an additional mid-morning snack for young children.

V. EDUCATION Patients and parents are taught the fundamentals of the pathophysiology and management of diabetes. Insulin preparation, injection technique, and a program for the management of acute illness are introduced. They are also made aware of the symptoms of hypoglycemia, its oral treatment, and the use of glucagon. Qualitative tests for sugar with Clinitest (the two-drop method) and acetone are taught. Patients are encouraged to participate in activities normal for their age. The importance of understanding of the dietary instructions, exchange lists, and food preparation guidelines should be pointed out. All patients are advised to carry a diabetic card and Medic Alert bracelet or necklace.

VI. SPECIAL PROBLEMS OF DIABETES MELLITUS

A. **Physical growth and maturation** In general, diabetic children follow the normal growth pattern. However, there may be a diminished growth rate in those whose diabetes is poorly controlled.

B. **Problems in emotional adjustment** Diabetic patients often become overly dependent and demonstrate anxiety and hostility. Understanding, patience, education of both patient and family, and, occasionally, psychiatric counseling are necessary in these cases. Heavy responsibilities (e.g., the administration of insulin) should not be levied on a diabetic child who is not mature enough to accept them.

C. Infection

1. The incidence of urinary tract infections, subcutaneous abscesses, candidal vulvitis, and cystitis is higher in teenage girls with diabetes than in nondiabetic female adolescents.

2. Pyelonephritis is more common in diabetic patients than in the nondiabetic.

3. If infection occurs, adequate doses of appropriate antibiotics and antifungal agents should be administered promptly, and the establishment of good diabetic control should be emphasized.

4. Diabetic children should receive pneumococcal vaccine.

15

Antibiotics and Infectious Diseases

I. **PRINCIPLES OF ANTIMICROBIAL THERAPY** Whenever possible, a single antimicrobial agent should be used, and the antimicrobial spectrum should be kept as narrow as possible. The use of multiple antimicrobials is associated with an increased likelihood of colonization and superinfection by drug-resistant organisms. However, severely ill patients or those whose defenses are impaired should be given broad-spectrum therapy pending the definitive results of cultures.

A. **Identification of the infecting pathogen** The most probable infecting pathogen(s) can frequently be determined from the site of infection, the results of rapid diagnostic procedures, the patient's underlying illness, and local epidemiologic factors. Specific considerations include

1. **Host factors**

   a. **Age** In the neonatal period the most common pathogens are *Escherichia coli*, other gram-negative enteric bacilli, group B streptococci, and *Staphylococcus aureus*. *H. influenzae* type B, pneumococci, and meningococci are common and serious pathogens between the ages of 3 months–5 years.

   b. **Granulocyte defects** The most common defect is granulocytopenia. As the granulocyte count falls below 1000/mm³, the risk of bacterial infection increases. The most common pathogens are gram-negative enteric bacilli (especially *Pseudomonas*) and *S. aureus*.
   Functional defects of granulocytes are also associated with an increased incidence of similar infections.

   c. **Defects of humoral immunity** See also Chap 18. Patients with congenital or acquired hypogammaglobulinemia or defects of certain components of complement, particularly C3, have an increased incidence of infections with encapsulated pyogenic organisms such as pneumococcus, meningococcus, and *H. influenzae*.
   Isolated deficiencies of C6, C7, and C8 have been specifically associated with infections due to meningococcus and gonococcus.

   d. **Defects in cellular immunity** The T lymphocytes and their effector cells are probably important in the defense against intracellular bacteria, fungi, certain viruses, and certain protozoa.

   e. **Miscellaneous defects**

      (1) Patients with splenic hypofunction are at increased risk of fulminant infections, most commonly due to the pneumococcus, meningococcus, and *H. influenzae* type B.

      (2) Patients with severe *hepatic dysfunction* have an increased frequency of bacteremias with *E. coli*, other enteric gram-negative bacilli, and occasionally the pneumococcus.

      (3) Patients with nephrotic syndrome have an increased incidence of infections caused by pneumococci and gram-negative bacilli.

(4) Primary peritonitis occurs almost exclusively in patients with ascites associated with cirrhosis or nephrosis.

2. **Site of infection** Table 15-1 lists the bacterial and fungal pathogens that cause acute infections at various sites. The common pathogens are those responsible for the majority of infections at a given site. The uncommon pathogens are rare or associated only with specific clinical situations, which are indicated. The list is not exhaustive.

Further discussion of specific sites of infection is found in **4**, p. 336.

3. **Rapid diagnostic procedures**

   a. A **Gram stain** should be performed on all body fluids and exudates from suspected sites of infection. Two common pitfalls are

      (1) Underdecolorization This problem is recognized by the blue staining of cell nuclei and can be avoided by repeating the decolorization step of the Gram stain.

      (2) Gram-stained artifacts most commonly resemble "sheets of gram-positive cocci." This problem is avoided by the use of fresh stains and gentle heat fixing.

   b. **Methylene blue** stains all bacteria dark blue and can be helpful in detecting small numbers of pleomorphic gram-negative bacteria that have been phagocytosed or are associated with gram-negative debris.

   c. **Microbial antigen detection** Rapid immunologic techniques for the detection of microbial antigens in serum, cerebrospinal fluid (CSF), and other body fluids may allow early etiologic diagnosis of hepatitis type B, cryptococcal meningitis, and infections with *H. influenzae* type B, meningococci, pneumococci, the K-1 capsular type of *E. coli*, group B streptococci, and other organisms.

   d. **Serology** In general, serologic procedures are unreliable in the diagnosis of *acute* infections. However, two helpful serologic tests are

      (1) Tests for **heterophil antibody,** which become positive during the second week of infectious mononucleosis.

      (2) Cold agglutinins, which are found in 75 percent of patients with *Mycoplasma* pneumonia during the second week of illness. A simple bedside test will detect a significant titer ($\geq 1:64$): add 2 or 3 drops of whole blood to an oxalate tube (blue top), place on ice for 2 min, and observe for agglutination by tilting the tube against the light.

   e. All microbiologic specimens should be plated on appropriate media as promptly as possible. Urine cultures may, however, be refrigerated overnight, if necessary.

      (1) Specimens containing cold-labile organisms, such as the meningococcus or gonococcus, should be aspirated into a syringe, sealed, and taken promptly to the laboratory. Many organisms, especially anaerobes, **will not survive on swabs that are allowed to dry.** On the other hand, group A β-hemolytic streptococci will survive at least 24 hours on a dry swab. If this organism is specifically sought, the swab need not be placed in liquid medium. Thus, irrelevant organisms may not survive, permitting better yield of streptococci.

      (2) *Shigella* and many *Salmonella* species do not survive cooling and storage of stool specimens. Therefore the stool must be cultured promptly, or a buffered transport medium should be used. *Salmonella* (but not *Shigella*) survive drying on rectal swabs.

Table 15-1 Bacterial Etiology of Acute Infections in Various Sites

Site	Common Organisms	Less Common Organisms	Comments
Skin (primary)	Group A streptococcus S. aureus	H. influenzae type B Gram-negative enteric bacilli Candida	Face, periorbital Impaired host Paronychia, intertriginous skin, diaper dermatitis
Skin (trauma)	S. aureus	Group A streptococcus P. aeruginosa Anaerobes	Burns and surgical wounds, early Burns, late, puncture wounds of foot Severe trauma and abdominal wounds
		Clostridium spp.	Severe trauma and abdominal wounds
		Gram-negative enteric bacilli	Severe trauma and abdominal wounds
		Erysipelothrix Pasteurella multocida	Animal products Animal bites
Conjunctiva	Pneumococcus H. influenzae	Gonococcus Trachoma inclusion conjunctivitis (TRIC) organism	Neonate, sexual history Neonate
	S. aureus	P. aeruginosa	Trauma, contact lens
Middle ear	Pneumococcus H. influenzae (nontypable) Group A streptococcus	Gram-negative enteric bacilli M. tuberculosis	Septic neonates Chronic drainage
Sinuses	H. influenzae (nontypable) Pneumococcus Oral anaerobes S. aureus	Gram-negative bacilli Group A streptococcus Aspergillus Phycomycetes	Cystic fibrosis Impaired hosts Impaired hosts
Cervical adenitis	Group A streptococcus S. aureus Oral anaerobes	Toxoplasma Atypical mycobacteria M. tuberculosis	Cats Children <4 years Contact history, abnormal chest x-ray

Table 15-1 (Continued)

Site	Common Organisms	Less Common Organisms	Comments
Mouth and pharynx	Group A streptococcus	Gonococcus *Candida* Oral anaerobes *Corynebacterium diphtheriae*	Sexual history Antibiotic therapy, impaired host Vincent's infection Gray pseudomembrane
Epiglottis	*H. influenzae* type B	*Corynebacterium diphtheriae* Group A streptococcus	Gray pseudomembrane
Lower respiratory tract	Pneumococcus *Mycoplasma pneumoniae*	*H. influenzae* *S. aureus* Group A streptococcus Group B streptococcus *Klebsiella* and other gram-negative bacilli Oral anaerobes *Bordetella pertussis* *M. tuberculosis* *Chlamydia*	Children < 4 years Influenza, impaired host, neonate Pharyngitis, large bilateral pleural effusions Respiratory distress in neonate Impaired hosts Aspiration, lung abscess Characteristic cough Exposure history Infants
Endocardium	Viridans streptococci *S. aureus* Enterococcus	*Staphylococcus epidermidis,* diphtheroids, etc. *P. aeruginosa* *Candida* and other fungi	Prosthetic valves Addicts Large emboli
GI tract	*Shigella* *Salmonella*	*Yersinia enterocolitica* *Vibrio parahaemolyticus* *Campylobacter* *Vibrio cholerae* *E. coli* *Entamoeba histolytica* *Giardia lamblia* *Clostridium difficile*	Symptoms of appendicitis Shellfish ingestion Foreign travel Foreign travel Foreign travel Foreign travel Antibiotic therapy

Site	Common organisms	Other organisms	Associated conditions
Urinary tract	*E. coli* and other enteric gram-negative bacilli	Enterococcus	Chronic recurrent infections
		P. aeruginosa	Chronic recurrent infections
		Staphylococcus epidermidis	Instrumentation
		S. aureus	Bacteremia, kidney abscess
Bone	*S. aureus*	*Salmonella*	Sickle cell disease
		Pseudomonas	Foot puncture
		Streptococcus	
		M. tuberculosis	
Joints	*S. aureus*	Gram-negative bacilli	Neonates
	H. influenzae type B	Gonococcus	Neonates, sexually active adults
	Streptococcus	Pneumococcus	
		Staphylococcus epidermidis	Prostheses
		M. tuberculosis	
Meninges	*H. influenzae* type B	Enteric gram-negative bacilli	Neonates, surgery
	Meningococcus	Group B streptococcus	Neonates
	Pneumococcus	*S. aureus*	Surgery and shunts
		Staphylococcus epidermidis	Shunts
		Listeria monocytogenes	Impaired host
		Cryptococcus	Impaired host
		M. tuberculosis	

B. Choice and dosage of antimicrobial agents

1. **Antibiotic susceptibility**   The recommended choice and dosage of antimicrobials for specific pathogens are outlined in Tables 15-2 and 15-3.

    a. Frequently, the likely pathogen(s) is (are) susceptible to several antimicrobials. A rational choice is then based on drug toxicity, pharmacologic factors relating to the patient (age, renal and hepatic function), and pharmacologic factors relating to the infection (antimicrobial penetration and activity at the site of infection).

    b. *Agents with potentially serious side effects should be used only when they offer a definite advantage over less toxic agents.*

2. **Combinations of antimicrobial agents**   Although a single antimicrobial agent should provide adequate therapy for the majority of infections, combination therapy is recommended for specific organisms or certain clinical situations. These include **endocarditis** (see p. 382) caused by enterococci or by viridans streptococci relatively resistant to penicillin, **severe *Pseudomonas* infection** (an aminoglycoside [gentamicin or tobramycin] and a penicillin [carbenicillin or ticarcillin]), **active tuberculosis** (see p. 385), **cryptococcal** meningitis and disseminated infections caused by other yeasts (amphotericin B and 5-fluorocytosine, *provided* the organism is sensitive to 5-fluorocytosine), and **empiric antibiotic therapy** for severely ill patients. Two widely used regimens are carbenicillin plus gentamicin and carbenicillin plus cephalothin. The latter regimen is particularly useful in patients with renal dysfunction.

3. **Monitoring antimicrobial dosage**   Treatment with antibiotics with a narrow toxic-therapeutic ratio should be monitored by measuring serum peak and trough levels. Table 15-4 gives the recommended therapeutic levels of such antimicrobials.

    a. **Peak levels** should be measured 1 hr after an IM dose or ½ hr after the end of a ½-hr IV infusion. **Trough levels** should be measured just before a dose. Peak and trough levels should be checked shortly after the initiation of and at least once per week during therapy. More frequent monitoring is recommended in neonates and in patients who are seriously ill or who have renal or hepatic dysfunction.

    b. In **endocarditis** and other serious infections such as osteomyelitis, **bactericidal** rather than bacteriostatic antibiotics are used, and the effectiveness of the patient's serum in killing the pathogen is monitored during therapy. The peak bactericidal level should be at least 1:8 and the trough at least 1:2.

4. **Antimicrobial activity at site of infection**   The levels of most antimicrobial agents in well-perfused tissues and serous spaces are adequate for treating infections at these sites. On the other hand, subtherapeutic levels are attained in sequestered sites such as abscess cavities and in the obstructed urinary or biliary tract. Hence surgery is vital in the management of these infections.

    a. **Antimicrobial penetration into the CNS**   Table 15-5 summarizes the ability of various antimicrobials to penetrate into the CSF in the presence of normal and inflamed meninges. These data are based on fragmentary and sometimes conflicting results.

        (1) Chloramphenicol, the sulfonamides, and most antituberculous agents penetrate normal meninges well.

        (2) The penicillins penetrate effectively, but only in the presence of

inflamed meninges. Large doses must be given **parenterally and maintained throughout therapy.**

(3) Cephalothin does not penetrate in therapeutic amounts. Meningitis due to sensitive organisms may develop during parenteral cephalothin therapy.

(4) The levels of aminoglycoside antibiotics in the CSF after parenteral therapy are unpredictable and are often inadequate for the therapy of gram-negative meningitis. Therefore these antibiotics should be given intrathecally. Intrathecal doses of aminoglycosides and other antimicrobials are summarized in Table 15-6.

(5) **Adjustment of intrathecal dosage for children** may be based on the relative CSF volume at various ages: neonates, 25 ml; 5 years, 50 ml; adults, 140 ml. If the dose is given by the lumbar route it should be given slowly in a large volume of saline (10 percent of the CSF volume) after prior removal of an equal volume of CSF.

(6) The **frequency of intrathecal dosage** is best monitored by measuring the antimicrobial activity in the CSF 24 hr after the first dose. Usually, injections are required q24–48h to maintain therapeutic levels.

b. Antimicrobial activity in the urinary tract (see p. 378) In patients with normal renal function, many antimicrobials reach much higher concentrations in the urine than in serum. As a result, routine sensitivity tests based on achievable serum concentrations are not always reliable predictors of antibiotic efficacy. **Therefore a report of antibiotic resistance should prompt a repeat urine culture** rather than a change in regimen, unless the patient's symptoms have failed to respond. An effective regimen should sterilize the urine within 12–24 hr.

(1) **Acidification** enhances the activity of the tetracyclines, nitrofurantoin, and the penicillins and cephalosporins. **Alkalinization** markedly enhances the activity of the aminoglycosides and erythromycin and extends the spectrum of the latter to include many gram-negative rods.

(2) Because of ionic partitioning into acid secretions, **trimethoprim** may be particularly useful in treating recurrent urinary tract infections in females (anterior urethra) and prostatitis in males.

5. Failure of therapy There is variation in the rate of resolution of infections. Causes for failure of treatment should be considered when fever and signs of infection are prolonged. These include inadequate antibiotic therapy, complication of original infection, and complications of treatment.

6. Pharmacologic considerations

a. Use of antimicrobial agents in infants and young children

(1) In **neonates,** antibiotic dosage must be individualized, and serum levels should be monitored, particularly when using toxic drugs. Guidelines for initial antibiotic dosage in neonates may be found in Chap. 5, Appendix Table 5-1.

(2) In general, dosage intervals are **longer** in younger infants than in older infants. Drug half-lives in premature infants are longer than in full-term infants. Similarly, decreases in renal function are as-

Table 15-2 Choice of Antimicrobial Agents for Specific Pathogens[a]

Organism	Infection	Drug of Choice	Pediatric Dose[a]
A. *Gram-positive cocci*			
1. Group A streptococcus	Pharyngitis,[b] impetigo	Penicillin G	25,000 U/kg/d PO *or* IM
	Cellulitis	(Alt.: erythromycin,	50,000–100,000 U/kg/d PO, IM *or* IV
	Pneumonia, empyema, bacteremia	cephalosporin, clindamycin)	100,000 U/kg/d IV *or* IM
	Meningitis		300,000 U/kg/d IV
2. Viridans streptococcus	Subacute bacterial endocarditis	Penicillin G (Alt.: cephalothin, vancomycin)	250,000 U/kg/d IV
3. Enterococcus	Urinary tract	Ampicillin (Alt.: Furadantin)	50–100 mg/kg/d PO
	Subacute bacterial endocarditis	Ampicillin or penicillin G plus gentamicin (Alt.: vancomycin and gentamicin)	300 mg/kg/d (ampicillin) 250,000 U/kg/d (penicillin G) 180 mg/M² *or* 3–7.5 mg/kg/d (gentamicin)
4. Pneumococcus	Pneumonia	Penicillin G (Alt.: See 1)	25,000–50,000 U/kg/d (penicillin G) PO, IM, *or* IV
	Meningitis, complications (empyema)		300,000 U/kg/d IV
5. *S. aureus* (penicillin-sensitive)	Soft tissue abscess Endocarditis, pneumonia	Penicillin G (Alt.: See 6)	50,000 U/kg/d PO, IM *or* IV 300,000 U/kg/d IV
6. *S. aureus* (penicillin-resistant)[c]	Mild infection Systemic infection	Semisynthetic penicillin (Alt.: cephalothin, erythromycin, clindamycin, vancomycin)	50–100 mg/kg/d PO *or* IV 300 mg/kg/d IV
7. *S. epidermidis*[d]	Endocarditis	Semisynthetic penicillin (Alt.: cephalothin, vancomycin)	300 mg/kg/d IV
B. *Gram-positive bacilli*			
8. *Clostridium perfringens*	Gas gangrene	Penicillin G (Alt.: chloramphenicol)	300,000 U/kg/d

Organism	Disease	Drug	Dosage
	Meningitis	(Alt.: tetracycline, cephalosporin) Human antitoxin (see Table 15-10)	300 mg/kg/d
10. *Listeria monocytogenes*	Meningitis	Ampicillin ± gentamicin (Alt.: erythromycin, tetracycline, chloramphenicol)	
11. *Corynebacterium diphtheriae*	Diphtheria	Penicillin G (Alt.: erythromycin) Horse antitoxin (see Table 15-10)	25–100,000 U/kg/d PO *or* IM
C. *Gram-negative cocci*			
12. Meningococcus	Meningitis Meningococcemia	Penicillin G (Alt.: chloramphenicol, ampicillin, erythromycin)	300,000 U/kg/d IV 150,000 U/kg/d IV
13. Gonococcus (see Table 15-13)	Gonorrhea	Penicillin G-plus probenecid	4.8 million U aqueous procaine penicillin G IM ½ hr after 1 gm probenecid
		(Alt.: spectinomycin, tetracycline, ampicillin or amoxicillin plus probenecid)	2 gm spectinomycin (4 gm in females) IM
			2 gm tetracycline daily for 5 days PO
			3.5 gm ampicillin IM *or* PO ½ hr after 1 gm probenecid PO
D. *Gram-negative bacilli*[t]			
14. *E. coli*	Urinary tract	Sulfisoxazole (Alt.: ampicillin, trimethoprim-sulfamethoxazole, cephalexin)	100 mg/kg/d PO
	Surgical wound, pneumonia, sepsis	Gentamicin (Alt.: ampicillin, cephalosporins, chloramphenicol, amikacin)	180 mg/M² *or* 4.5–7.5 mg/kg/d IV
	Meningitis	Chloramphenicol (Alt.: ampicillin, gentamicin, amikacin)	100 mg/kg/d IV

339

Table 15-2 (Continued)

Organism	Infection	Drug of Choice	Pediatric Dose[a]
15. Klebsiella	Urinary tract	Trimethoprim-sulfamethoxazole (Alt.: cephalexin, tetracycline, chloramphenicol)	8 mg/kg/d trimethoprim 40 mg/kg/d sulfamethoxazole
	Pneumonia, sepsis	Gentamicin (Alt.: cephalosporin, amikacin)	180 mg/M² or 4.5–7.5 mg/kg/d
16. Proteus mirabilis	Urinary tract	Ampicillin (Alt.: cephalexin, trimethoprim-sulfamethoxazole, chloramphenicol)	50–100 mg/kg/d PO
	Systemic	Gentamicin (Alt.: ampicillin, cephalosporins, amikacin, chloramphenicol)	180 mg/M² or 4.5–7.5 mg/kg/d
17. Proteus, indole-positive	Urinary tract	Trimethoprim-sulfamethoxazole (Alt.: chloramphenicol, carbenicillin, tetracycline)	8 mg/kg/d trimethoprim 40 mg/kg/d sulfamethoxazole
	Systemic	Gentamicin (Alt.: carbenicillin[e], cefamandole, cefoxitin, amikacin)	180 mg/M² or 4.5–7.5 mg/kg/d
18. Pseudomonas aeruginosa	Urinary tract	Carbenicillin (indanyl) (Alt.: tetracycline with acidification)	50–65 mg/kg/d
	Systemic	Gentamicin or tobramycin and carbenicillin[e]	4.5–7.5 mg/kg/d 400–600 mg/kg/d

	Systemic		
19. Salmonella		Chloramphenicol (Alt.: ampicillin, trimethoprim-sulfamethoxazole)	50–100 mg/kg PO, IM
20. Serratia		Gentamicin (Alt.: cefoxitin, chloramphenicol, carbenicillin,[e] amikacin)	180 mg/M² or 4.5–7.5 mg/kg/d IM or IV
21. Shigella		Ampicillin (Alt.: chloramphenicol, tetracycline)	50–100 mg/kg/d PO, IM, or IV
22. Bacteroides	Respiratory infections Abdominal abscess, bacteremia	Penicillin G Clindamycin (Alt.: chloramphenicol, cefoxitin, carbenicillin[e])	300,000 U/kg/d IV 25 mg/kg/d IV 50–100 mg/kg/d IV
23. Pasteurella multocida		Penicillin G (Alt.: tetracycline)	50,000 U/kg/d PO
24. H. influenzae	Otitis media	Ampicillin (Alt.: penicillin plus sulfonamide, erythromycin plus sulfonamide, trimethoprim-sulfamethoxazole)	50–100 mg/kg/d PO or IM
	Bacteremia Epiglottitis Pneumonia Meningitis	Chloramphenicol (Alt.: ampicillin, cefamandole, except for meningitis)	100 mg/kg/d IV

[a] See Table 15-3 for maximum doses and Chap. 5, Appendix Table 5-1 for doses in neonates.
[b] Always treat for 10 days to prevent postinfection sequelae.
[c] In life-threatening staphylococcal infections gentamicin may be added for initial therapy.
[d] May be resistant to semisynthetic penicillins. Usually sensitive to vancomycin, aminoglycosides, and rifampin.
[e] Ticarcillin may be used interchangeably with carbenicillin at two-thirds the dosage.
[f] Since sensitivity patterns vary, antibiotic choice should be based on specific sensitivity determination whenever possible.

Table 15-3 Doses of Antimicrobial Agents[a]

Antimicrobial	Daily Dose	Frequency	Route	Usual Maximum Adult Dose
A. Penicillins				
1. Oral penicillin G[b,c]	50,000–100,000 U/kg	q6h	PO	6.4 MU
Phenoxymethyl penicillin (V)[c]			PO	6.4 MU
2. Parenteral				
a. Aqueous penicillin G[a]	25,000–400,000 U/kg	q2–4h	IV	24 MU
b. Procaine penicillin G[a]	25,000–50,000 U/kg	q12–24h	IM	4.8 MU
c. Benthazine penicillin G[c]	600,000–1,200,000 U	single dose	IM	1.2 MU
3. Penicillinase-resistant				
a. Methicillin,[a] oxacillin,[a] nafcillin[a]	100–300 mg/kg	q4h	IM or IV	12 gm
b. Cloxacillin,[c] dicloxacillin[c]	25–100 mg/kg	q6h	PO	4 gm
4. Broad spectrum				
a. Ampicillin[a]	50–100 mg/kg	q6h	PO	4 gm
	50–400 mg/kg	q4h	IM or IV	12 gm
Amoxicillin	20–40 mg/kg	q8h	PO	3 gm
b. Carbenicillin[a]	50–65 mg/kg	q6h	PO	40 gm
	400–600 mg/kg	q2–4h	IM or IV	
c. Ticarcillin	200–300 mg/kg	q4h	IM or IV	30 gm
B. Cephalosporins				
1. Cephalothin[a]	60–150 mg/kg	q4h	IV	12 gm
2. Cephaloridine[c]	100 mg/kg	q6h	IM	4 gm
3. Cefazolin[c]	25–100 mg/kg	q4h	IM or IV	6 gm
4. Cephalexin[c]	25–50 mg/kg	q6h	PO	4 gm
5. Cefamandole	50–150 mg/kg	q4h	IM or IV	12 gm
6. Cefoxitin	50–150 mg/kg	q4h	IM or IV	12 gm
C. Erythromycins[c]	30–50 mg/kg	q6h	PO	4 gm
	50 mg/kg	q6h	IV[d]	4 gm

D. Lincomycins[c]	30–60 mg/kg	PO	q6h	5 gm
	20–100 mg/kg	IM or IV	q6h	5 gm
Clindamycin[c]	10–25 mg/kg	PO	q6h	5 gm
	10–40 mg/kg	IM or IV	q6h	5 gm
E. Sulfonamides[c]	150 mg/kg	PO	q6h	8 gm
	100 mg/kg	IV	q6h	
Trimethoprim-sulfamethoxazole	8–20 mg TMP/kg	PO	q12h	960 mg TMP
	40–100 mg SMZ/kg			4.8 gm SMZ
F. Aminoglycosides				
1. Neomycin	50–100 mg/kg	PO	q4–6h	0
2. Streptomycin[c]	20–30 mg/kg	IM	q12h	2 gm
3. Kanamycin	600 mg/M² or	IM	q8h	1.5 gm
	15 mg/kg			
4. Gentamicin[a]	180 mg/M² or	IM or IV	q8h	5 mg/kg
	4.5–7.5 mg/kg			
5. Tobramycin	150 mg/M² or	IM or IV	q8h	
	3–5 mg/kg	IM or IV	q8h	
6. Amikacin	600 mg/M² or	IM or IV	q8h	
	15 mg/kg			
G. Nitrofurantoin[c]	5–7 mg/kg	PO	q6h	400 mg
H. Chloramphenicol[a]	50–100 mg/kg	PO or IV	q6h	4 gm
I. Tetracycline,[c] Chlortetracycline,[c]	20–40 mg/kg	PO	q6h	2 gm
Oxytetracycline[c]	10–20 mg/kg	IV or IM	q12h	2 gm
1. Doxycycline[c]	2–4 mg/kg	PO	q12h	4 mg/kg/d
2. Minocycline[c]	4 mg/kg	PO	q12h	4 mg/kg/d

[a] For newborn doses see Appendix Table 5-1, p. 147.
[b] 1 mg = 1600 units.
[c] Not recommended for newborns.
[d] May be given in continuous drip.

Table 15-4 Therapeutic and Toxic Serum Levels of Antimicrobials with a Narrow Toxic-Therapeutic Ratio

Antimicrobial	Therapeutic Peak Levels (μg/ml)	Probably Toxic Peak Levels (μg/ml)	Probably Toxic Trough Levels (μg/ml)
Streptomycin	15–25	>30	>3 (24 hr)
Kanamycin	15–25	>30	
Amikacin	15–25 (?)	>30 (?)	
Gentamicin	4–8	>12	>2 (8 hr)
Tobramycin	4–8 (?)	>12 (?)	
Chloramphenicol (free)	10–25	>25[a] >50[b]	
Vancomycin	10–20	>25	
5-Fluorocytosine	40–100	>100	
Trimethoprim	5–10	>10	

[a]Reversible marrow suppression.
[b]Gray syndrome.

Table 15-5 Penetration of Antimicrobials into CSF

Antimicrobial	Normal Meninges (% of serum level)	Inflamed Meninges (% of serum level)
Antibacterial agents		
Penicillin, ampicillin, methicillin	5	10–30
Cephalothin	<1	<1
Cephaloridine	3	25–50
Streptomycin, kanamycin, gentamicin	<5	5–25 (unpredictable)
Chloramphenicol	33–100	33–100
Erythromycin, clindamycin	<5	10–40
Tetracycline	<10	15–25
Trimethoprim	60	
Sulfonamides	50	
Metronidazole	100	
Antituberculous agents		
Isoniazid	25	40–100
Para-aminosalicylic acid	low	30–50
Ethambutol	low	25–40
Rifampin	<5	10–20
Antifungal agents		
Amphotericin B	<1	5–25
5-Fluorocytosine		50

Table 15-6 Intrathecal Dosage of Antimicrobial Agents

Agent	Adults	Neonates
Streptomycin, kanamycin, amikacin	25–50 mg	5–10 mg
Gentamicin, tobramycin	5–10 mg	1–2 mg
Polymyxin	5–10 mg	0.5 mg (5000 U)
Amphotericin B	0.5 mg every 2–3 days	

sociated with long half-lives of aminoglycoside antibiotics. Therefore, doses and intervals near the lower limits of the ranges given in Chap. 5 should be chosen in these groups.

(3) To achieve a given blood level, older infants and children less than 10 years of age also require higher doses of antimicrobials (based on weight) than older children and adults require.

(4) Dosage of toxic antibiotics should be adjusted according to the age of the patient. For **gentamicin** the usually recommended dosage is 2.5 mg/kg q8h in children less than 5 years of age; 2.0 mg/kg in children 5–10 years; and 1.5 mg/kg in children over 10. However, these recommendations rarely produce levels above the therapeutic range, and levels may be subtherapeutic, particularly in cachectic patients. A single gentamicin dosage of 60 mg/M^2 q8h produces reproducible peak levels in all age groups regardless of body habitus.

b. Use of antimicrobial agents in renal failure The routes of metabolism and excretion of antimicrobials are summarized in Table 15-7.

(1) Antimicrobials handled mainly by the kidneys

(a) Antibiotics excreted primarily by renal mechanisms (group I) are best avoided in patients with severe renal failure. If they must be used, the dosage should be modified according to the following guidelines, and serum antibiotic levels should be monitored to ensure therapeutic levels (see Table 15-7).

(b) Adjustment of dosage is based on estimates of renal function.

i. The standard dose of the antibiotic is given. The dosage interval is prolonged in direct proportion with the increase in serum creatinine concentration.

Analogous calculations may be used for other aminoglycoside antibiotics and other group I drugs (Table 15-8). **The serum creatinine is unreliable in acute or unstable kidney disease in severe uremia and in intermittent dialysis.**

ii. All rules for the adjustment of dosage in renal failure provide only a rough estimate of what will happen in an individual patient. Such rules should therefore be used only to guide initial therapy. If therapy is continued, **serum antibiotic levels should be measured directly** in order to verify that they are in the therapeutic range.

(2) Antimicrobials handled by both the kidney and extrarenal mechanisms (group II, Table 15-7) may be used in standard doses in

Table 15-7 Metabolism and Excretion of Commonly Used Antimicrobial Agents

Mainly Renal	Renal and Nonrenal	Nonrenal
Antibacterial Agents—Systemic		
Aminoglycosides	Penicillins	Chloramphenicol
Streptomycin Kanamycin Gentamicin Tobramycin	Cephalosporins	
Amikacin	Lincomycin Clindamycin	Erythromycin[a]
Vancomycin	Tetracycline[b]	Doxycycline Minocycline
Polymyxins Polymyxin B Colistin		
Antibacterial Agents—Urinary Tract		
Methenamine[b]	Nitrofurantoin[a,b] Sulfonamides[b] Trimethoprim	Nalidixic acid[b]
Antituberculous Agents		
Ethambutol	PAS[a,b]	Rifampin INH
Antifungal Agent		
5-Fluorocytosine		Amphotericin B

[a] Should be avoided in severe hepatic failure.
[b] Should be avoided in severe renal failure.

patients with mild or moderate renal failure (creatinine clearance > 30 ml/1.74 M² or serum creatinine < 3 mg/100 ml). The dosage interval should be increased, as outlined in Table 15-9, if renal failure is moderate or severe. **Nitrofurantoin and all tetracyclines except doxycycline are contraindicated in severe renal failure.** In addition, sulfonamides and para-aminosalicylic acid (PAS) should be avoided in severe renal failure.

(3) Antimicrobials handled by nonrenal mechanisms When these agents are used in patients with renal failure, the dosage does not need to be adjusted. When possible, amphotericin B should be avoided in such patients, but if indicated, full doses should be given.

c. Use of antimicrobials in hepatic failure Among antimicrobials metabolized by the liver (see Table 15-7), metabolic and excretory pathways differ. Specific guidelines for dosage modifications in liver failure therefore cannot be formulated. Antimicrobials with a narrow toxic-therapeutic ratio **(nitrofurantoin)** or with a high risk of

Table 15-8 Adjustment of Dosage for Antimicrobials Excreted Mainly by the Kidney (Group I)

Antibiotic	Standard Dose	Normal Renal Function Half-Life (hr)	Normal Renal Function Dosage Interval (hr)	Moderate to Severe Impairment in Renal Function	Anuria[a] Half-Life (days)	Anuria[a] Dosage Interval (days)
Streptomycin	10–15 mg/kg/dose; maximum, 500 mg/dose	1–3	8–12	Increase dosage interval or decrease dose according to text	2–4	6
Kanamycin[b]	10 mg/kg/dose; maximum, 500 mg/dose	1–3	8	Same as above	2–4	6
Gentamicin[c]	2.5 mg/kg if < 5 years 2.0 mg/kg if 5–10 years 1.5 mg/kg if > 10 years or 60 mg/M² all ages	1–3	8	Same as above	2–4	6
Vancomycin	20 mg/kg/dose; maximum, 1 gm/dose	6	12		9	7–14
5-Fluorocytosine	40 mg/kg/dose	6	6			

[a] The half-life in anuria depends on the rate of extrarenal clearance of the antibiotic. Individual variation is great, and antibiotic levels must be measured.
[b] Amikacin closely resembles kanamycin in its pharmacology.
[c] Tobramycin closely resembles gentamicin in its pharmacology.

347

Table 15-9 Adjustment of Dosage for Antibiotics Excreted Renal and Other Routes (Group II) When Given in High Dosage

Antibiotic	Standard Dose	Renal Function (% of Normal)					
		Normal (50–100%)		Moderate Impairment* (10–30%)		Anuria* (0%)	
		Half-Life (hr)	Standard Dose Interval (hr)	Half-Life (hr)	Dose Interval (hr)	Half-Life (hr)	Dose Interval (hr)
Penicillin G	60,000 U/kg/dose	0.5	4	2	6	4	12–24
Ampicillin	50 mg/kg/dose	1	4	No modification		8	12
Carbenicillin	100 mg/kg/dose	1	4	3–6	6–12	16	24
Methicillin	50 mg/kg/dose	0.5	4	No modification		12	12
Oxacillin, nafcillin	50 mg/kg/dose	0.5	4	No modification		1–2	8
Cephalothin	25 mg/kg/dose	0.5	4	2	6	6	12
Cefazolin	25 mg/kg/dose	2.0	6	6–12	12–24	36	
Cephalexin	10 mg/kg/dose	1.0	6	4	12	24	48
Lincomycin	20 mg/kg/dose	4	6	No modification		12	24
Clindamycin	10 mg/kg/dose	4	6	No modification		12	24
Trimethoprim-sulfamethoxazole	10 mg trimethoprim/kg/dose; 50 mg sulfamethoxazole/kg/dose maximum dose, 480 mg trimethoprim/dose, 2.4 gm sulfamethoxazole/dose	12	12	24–36	24	Use not recommended	

* Further prolongation of the half-life occurs when hepatic failure is present concurrently.

hepatotoxicity (**erythromycin estolate, PAS**) are **contraindicated** in severe liver failure. When possible, **clindamycin, lincomycin, erythromycin, chloramphenicol, tetracyclines, INH**, and **rifampin** should be avoided in patients with severe liver failure. If used, serum levels should be monitored.

II. OTHER ASPECTS OF THERAPY AND PREVENTION

A. Treatment of fever See Chap. 1.

B. Surgery The need for adequate drainage of loculated pus, removal of necrotic tissue, relief of obstruction, and removal of foreign bodies should always be considered.

C. Immune serum globulin Passive immunization with human or animal immunoglobulins is useful in the prevention and treatment of certain viral and toxin-mediated infections (Table 15-10).

D. Isolation procedures Guidelines for hospital precautions and periods of contagiousness of common communicable diseases of childhood can be found in *Pediatrics* 53:663, 1974.

E. Antimicrobial prophylaxis Indications for antimicrobial prophylaxis are summarized in Table 15-11.

III. SPECIFIC ANTIMICROBIAL AGENTS Table 15-2 summarizes the drugs of choice and dosages for specific bacterial pathogens. Modification of drug dosage for neonates is discussed on p. 337 and in Chap. 5, and modifications in renal failure on p. 338. Penetration of antimicrobial agents in the tissues and CSF is discussed on p. 336. The antituberculous agents are summarized in Table 15-12 (p. 354). Antifungal agents are discussed on p. 363 and antiviral therapy and agents on p. 392.

A. Antimicrobial agents

1. The penicillins inhibit cell wall synthesis and kill growing bacteria by lysis.

a. Penicillin

(1) Spectrum and indications Penicillin is the drug of choice for infections due to pneumococci, streptococci, nonpenicillinase-producing *S. aureus*, **clostridia**, **Neisseria**, oral anaerobes, and spirochetes. It is also used in anthrax, diphtheria, actinomycosis, leptospirosis, and rat-bite fever. Penicillin G is more active than penicillin V.

(2) Pharmacology

(a) Oral preparations are penicillin G and penicillin V (phenoxymethyl penicillin). Because it is acid labile, the absorption of penicillin G is **variable.** Penicillin V is well absorbed, especially when given 1 hr before meals.

(b) Parenteral preparations differ in their peak serum level and half-life.

i. Aqueous penicillin G results in rapid attainment of high blood levels after IM or IV administration. Its rapid excretion in patients (except newborns) with normal renal function requires that it be administered frequently (usually

Table 15-10 Gamma Globulin Prophylaxis and Therapy

Disorder	Value	Purpose	Dose (IM)	Comment
		Standard Human Immune Serum Globulins		
Measles	Proved	Modification	0.05 ml/kg	Rarely indicated
		Prevention	0.25 ml/kg	Given immediately after exposure to unvaccinated children
			0.50 ml/kg (maximum, 0.15 ml)	For immunosuppressed patients
Viral hepatitis type A (HAV)	Proved	Prevention: Single exposure	0.02–0.04 ml/kg	Given as soon as possible after exposure
		Continuous exposure	0.06 ml/kg. Repeat in 5–6 months	Travel to endemic area
Viral hepatitis type B (HBV)	Proved	Prevention	0.12 ml/kg to maximum of 5 ml for adult. Repeat after 1 month. *Neonates*: 2.0 ml	Use when hepatitis B immune serum globulin is not available. See indications for use below
Varicella[a]	Limited	Modification	0.6–1.2 ml/kg	Give immediately after exposure if VZIG or zoster immune plasma is not available. Indicated only in serious underlying illness without history of previous chickenpox[a]
Rubella	Limited	Prevention	20 ml	For pregnant women in the first trimester who will not consider abortion
		Special Human Immune Serum Globulins[b]		
Tetanus (TIG)	Proved	Prevention	250–500 U	See p. 366 for indications
		Treatment	3000–6000 U	

Hepatitis B (HBIG)	Proved	Prevention	0.06 ml/kg to maximum of 5 ml for an adult. *Infants*: 0.5 ml. Repeat after 1 month.	Indications are: (1) needle puncture with contaminated needle; (2) infective blood (or blood products) splashed onto cuts or mucous membranes or ingested; (3) in infants of mothers with hepatitis B during pregnancy or carrying hepatitis B
Varicella-zoster (VZIG)		Prevention		
Pertussis	Unproved	Prevention (exposed infants) Treatment	1.5 ml IM, repeat after 1 week 3–6 ml IM	Protection not reliable. See Table 15-12 for antimicrobial prophylaxis
Mumps	Unproved	Prevention		No evidence that orchitis is prevented

Special Animal Immune Serums[b]

Botulism (trivalent ABE)	Proved	Treatment		As soon as possible after testing for sensitivity to serum
Diphtheria	Proved	Treatment	20,000–120,000 U	As soon as clinical diagnosis is made; higher doses for more extensive disease
Gas gangrene (polyvalent clostridial antitoxin)	Unproved	Treatment		No longer commercially available

[a] Zoster immune plasma (ZIP) from patients convalescing from herpes zoster may also modify illness, but carries the risk of hepatitis. The dose is 10 ml/kg IV.

[b] Detailed information about indications, source of supply, and dosage can be obtained from the Center for Disease Control (404) 633-3311 (8:00 A.M.–5:00 P.M. weekdays) and (404) 633-2176 or 633-8673 (off-duty hours).

Table 15-11 Antimicrobial Prophylaxis

Disease	Indication	Antimicrobial and Dosage
A. Preexposure		
1. Rheumatic fever	History of acute rheumatic fever; lifetime for patients with heart disease; to age 21 in patients without heart disease	Benzathine penicillin G, 1.2 million U IM monthly Sulfadiazine, single daily dose of 1.0 gm Penicillin V, 250 mg bid PO (children < 60 lb should receive ½ the above doses)
2. Endocarditis a. Viridans streptococcus	Patients with congenital or valvular heart disease undergoing dental procedures, including cleaning, or oral surgery, including tonsillectomy	*Parenteral (high-risk patients, e.g., with prosthetic valves)* 1.2 million U aqueous procaine penicillin G and 1 gm streptomycin IM 1 hr before procedure, followed by penicillin V, 500 mg PO q6h for 4–8 doses *Penicillin-allergic patients* 1 gm vancomycin IV 1 hr before procedure, followed by erythromycin 500 mg PO q6h for 4–8 doses *Oral* 2 gm penicillin V PO 1 hr before procedure, followed by 500 mg PO q6h for 4–8 doses *Penicillin-allergic patients* 1 gm erythromycin PO 2 hr before procedure, followed by 500 mg PO q6h for 4–8 doses
b. Enterococcus	Patients with valvular heart disease undergoing urinary tract, genital tract, or GI tract manipulation or surgery	2 million U aqueous crystalline penicillin G IV or IM and gentamicin, 60 mg/M² IV or IM at time of procedure, followed by 4 similar doses of penicillin q4h and 2 similar doses gentamicin q8h *Penicillin-allergic patients* 1 gm vancomycin IV and gentamicin, 60 mg/M² IV or IM, at

Table 15-11 (*Continued*)

Disease	Indication	Antimicrobial and Dosage
		time of procedure, followed by same dose of vancomycin 12 hr later and 2 doses of gentamicin at 8-hr intervals
B. Postexposure		
1. Tuberculosis	Recent tuberculin conversion or tuberculin-positive children	Isoniazid 10 mg/kg/day up to 300 mg/day for 1 year
	Household exposure to active disease[a]	
	Tuberculin test and chest x-ray positive	
2. Meningococcal disease[b]	Persons in intimate contact with index case (family members, and nursery school playmates, hospital personnel)	Rifampin, 10 mg/kg/dose, to maximum of 600 mg given bid for 4 doses
		If strain is sensitive to sulfonamides, sulfadiazine, 1 gm q8h for 3 days, may be used
3. Pertussis	Contacts not previously immunized	Erythromycin 30 mg/kg/day for 10 days if contact is broken, or for duration of cough in the infected contact
4. Gonorrhea	Neonatal ophthalmia	1% silver nitrate solution
	Contact of known case	4.8 million U aqueous procaine penicillin IM plus 1 gm probenecid PO
5. Syphilis	Contact of known case	2.4 million U benzathine penicillin G IM

[a] A PPD test should be performed after 3 months; if negative, prophylaxis may be discontinued if no further contact takes place.
[b] If serogroup A or C, immunization with meningococcal A or C vaccine may be helpful, since half the secondary cases occur more than 5 days after the index case.

q4h) for optimal therapy. It is prepared as a potassium or sodium salt (1.7 mEq/10^6 U).

ii. Procaine penicillin G is absorbed slowly from IM injections and so produces relatively low but prolonged serum concentrations. It should thus be used only in infections due to highly susceptible organisms or in large dosage.

iii. Benzathine penicillin G produces even lower blood levels, which last for as long as 3–4 weeks. It is used primarily against group A streptococci and *T. pallidum*, prophylactically in patients with rheumatic heart disease, and

Table 15-12 Drug Therapy in Tuberculosis

Drugs	Daily Dose/Kg Body Weight[a]	Route and Mode of Administration of Daily Dose	Major Adverse Reactions
Isoniazid	10–20 mg, max. 600 mg	PO, IM, or IV in 1 or 2 divided doses	Hepatotoxicity,[b] peripheral neuropathy[b]; GI irritation, skin rashes, fever less common
Streptomycin	20–40 mg, max. 1 gm	IM in 1 or 2 divided doses	8th cranial nerve toxicity (primarily vestibular); skin rashes, nephrotoxicity
Para-aminosalicylic acid	0.2–0.3 gm, max. 12 gm	PO in 3 divided doses	Gastrointestinal irritation (10%); liver damage, fever, skin rashes less common
Ethambutol	15–25 mg	PO in 1 dose	Retrobulbar optic neuritis (especially with higher doses—ophthalmologic monitoring recommended); skin rashes
Rifampin	10–20 mg	PO in 1 dose	Hepatotoxicity; GI disturbance; rarely, thrombocytopenia

[a] High dose is recommended for critically ill patients; low dose for prophylaxis and long-term therapy after improvement.
[b] Hepatotoxicity is rare in children. Therapy should not be stopped because of mild abnormalities in liver function tests unless the patient has clinical symptoms.

therapeutically when adherence to a program of oral penicillin is questionable.

b. Penicillinase-resistant penicillins

(1) Spectrum and indications These agents are resistant to hydrolysis by the β-lactamase produced by staphylococci and are therefore the drugs of choice for penicillin-resistant staphylococcal infections. They are approximately 10 times *less* active than penicillin G against penicillin-sensitive organisms.

(2) Pharmacology The only clinically significant difference between preparations is in their routes of administration. Because **methicillin, oxacillin,** and **nafcillin** are not well absorbed after oral administration they are used only parenterally. **Cloxacillin** and **dicloxacillin** are well absorbed orally.

c. Ampicillin and amoxicillin

(1) Spectrum and indications

(a) Ampicillin has the gram-positive spectrum of penicillin and is more active against enterococci and *Listeria*. Like penicillin, **it is inactive against penicillinase-producing staphylococci.** It is also active against many gram-negative organisms, including most *H. influenzae* strains, *Shigella, Salmonella, Proteus mirabilis,* and some *E. coli.* Ampicillin acts synergistically with sulfonamides or erythromycin against *Nocardia*.

(b) The spectrum of **amoxicillin** is similar to that of ampicillin, except that it is less effective against *Shigella* infections.

(2) Pharmacology The major difference between ampicillin and amoxicillin is that the latter is better absorbed after oral administration, even when given with meals. Amoxicillin is therefore given in lower dosage and may produce fewer GI side effects and a lower incidence of maculopapular rash than ampicillin.

d. Carbenicillin and ticarcillin

(1) Spectrum and indications These agents extend the spectrum of ampicillin to include *P. aeruginosa* and some *Proteus* species. Some strains of *Enterobacter* and *Serratia* may also be sensitive. Carbenicillin may also be effective against *Bacteroides fragilis*. Ticarcillin is more potent than carbenicillin against *P. aeruginosa* and is therefore used in lower dosage. **Carbenicillin (and other penicillins and cephalosporins) should not be mixed with aminoglycosides for simultaneous administration because they react at high concentrations to form an inactive complex.**

(2) Pharmacology Oral indanyl carbenicillin attains therapeutic levels only in urine and is indicated only for urinary tract infections caused by gram-negative organisms resistant to ampicillin and other oral agents.

e. Side effects of the penicillins

(1) Immediate allergic reactions include anaphylaxis, angioneurotic edema, and urticaria. **A previous maculopapular rash due to ampicillin does not signify an increased risk of immediate reactions.** Because penicillins share the same chemical structure, patients allergic to one preparation may react to others and occasionally may react to the cephalosporins.

(a) **Patients suspected of having a penicillin allergy** may be skin tested with two types of materials: penicilloyl-polylysine (PPL, available commercially as Pre-Pen) and a "minor determinant" mixture (not commercially available, but aqueous penicillin G may be substituted). Patients with a positive reaction to PPL are likely to have an allergic reaction to therapeutic doses of penicillin. Patients with a positive reaction to minor determinants are likely to have an immediate reaction such as anaphylaxis.

(b) **Intradermal skin testing with aqueous penicillin G** may cause severe reactions in the highly allergic patient. Therefore a scratch test with a dilute solution (5 U/ml in saline) should first be performed (together with a saline control). If no local reaction occurs within 20 min, a second scratch test is performed with a more concentrated solution (10,000 U/ml). If this is negative, a small skin bleb is raised by intradermal injection of the concentrated solution. A negative intradermal test suggests that an anaphylactic reaction to therapeutic penicillin G is unlikely **but does not absolutely exclude this possibility. Appropriate drugs and equipment for respiratory and circulatory assistance should be at the bedside during the skin-testing procedure and the first doses of penicillin.**

(2) **Aqueous procaine penicillin G** may produce a **nonallergic immediate reaction** simulating anaphylaxis, especially when mistakenly injected into the intravascular space.

(3) **Delayed reactions** include fever, eosinophilia, hemolytic anemia, serum sickness, and urticaria. Interstitial nephritis may occur with all penicillins but has been most often described with methicillin. Neutropenia and anicteric hepatitis occur rarely. The most common delayed reactions are maculopapular rashes, which occur during 8 percent of all treatment courses with ampicillin (100 percent in the presence of infectious mononucleosis); they are less common with other penicillins. When indications are clear, antibiotic therapy can be continued because the rash usually disappears. Very rarely, it may progress to erythroderma and exfoliative dermatitis.

(4) Dose-related effects include CNS toxicity, hypokalemia, and coagulation disorders, The last of these is most typical with carbenicillin, but may also occur with penicillin, especially in patients with renal failure. Diarrhea from oral preparations may also be dose related. The sodium or potassium contained in aqueous penicillin preparations can produce congestive heart failure or hyperkalemia.

2. **Cephalosporins**   Their mechanism of action is similar to that of the penicillins.

a. **Cephalothin and its analogues**

(1) **Spectrum and indications**   **Cephalothin** and its analogue **cephaloridine, cefazolin, cephalexin, cephapirin, cephacetrile,** and **cephradine** have a similar antimicrobial spectrum. They are active against gram-positive cocci, including penicillinase-producing *S. aureus*, many strains of *E. coli*, *Klebsiella*, and *P. mirabilis*. Generally, they have poor activity against enterococci, and, despite disk sensitivity tests indicating activity against

methicillin-resistant staphylococci, the cephalosporins are usually ineffective against these organisms. Cephalothin is more resistant to staphylococcal penicillinase than other cephalosporins and cephamycins, including the new agents listed in **a** and **b** and is therefore the cephalosporin of choice for serious staphylococcal infections.

(2) Pharmacology Cephalothin and its analogues differ in their pharmacologic properties, especially with respect to the routes of administration. Cephalothin, cephaloridine, cefazolin, cephapirin, and cephacetrile are available only for IM or IV administration. Cephalothin is painful when administered IM and should be given IV. Cephradine may be given parenterally or PO; cephalexin is given PO only. The half-life in blood of most of the agents is very short (30–60 min), and parenteral therapy should therefore be given at 4-hr intervals. Cefazolin has a half-life of 1.5–2.0 hr and may be given at 6-hr intervals. **All the cephalosporins (except cephaloridine) penetrate poorly into the CNS and should therefore not be used when meningitis is suspected.**

   (a) Cefamandole extends the spectrum of the older cephalosporins to resistant *E. coli, Enterobacter,* indole-positive *Proteus, Providencia,* and *H. influenzae* type B (including ampicillin-resistant strains).

   (b) Cefoxitin is a new semisynthetic cephamycin antibiotic. It extends the antimicrobial spectrum of the older cephalosporins to resistant *E. coli, Klebsiella,* indole-positive *Proteus, Providencia,* some *Serratia marcescens* and, most important, *B. fragilis.* Limited clinical experience suggests that cefoxitin may be an effective alternative antibiotic for anaerobic and mixed anaerobic-aerobic infections.

b. Side effects of the cephalosporins

   (1) Include allergic reactions, nephrotoxicity, thrombocytopenia, granulocytopenia, dose-related encephalopathy, and anicteric hepatitis.

   (2) Local irritation after IM injections and phlebitis from IV administration are common, particularly with cephalothin. Severe irritation may occur when cephalothin is added to wound irrigation fluids.

3. Aminoglycosides inhibit protein synthesis at the ribosome.

a. Spectrum and indications The aminoglycosides are bactericidal against a broad range of enteric gram-negative bacilli and *S. aureus,* but the various analogues differ in their antimicrobial spectrum.

   (1) They are not effective against streptococci and pneumococci, anaerobes, and spirochetes.

   (2) Many gram-negative bacilli, especially in hospitals, have become resistant to **streptomycin** and **kanamycin.** In addition, neither agent is active against *P. aeruginosa.*

   (3) Streptomycin is now used mainly as an antituberculosis agent.

   (4) Kanamycin may be used for the initial treatment of non-life-threatening, community-acquired gram-negative infections, or after sensitivity has been established.

   (5) Gentamicin is active against most gram-negative rods, including

P. aeruginosa, and is the aminoglycoside of choice for the empiric treatment of suspected gram-negative infections.

(6) Tobramycin is more active than gentamicin against *P. aeruginosa* (including isolates resistant to gentamicin).

(7) Amikacin is active against many enteric gram-negative bacilli that are resistant to gentamicin. Unless such organisms are common, this agent should be reserved for infections proved resistant to the other aminoglycosides.

b. Pharmacology

(1) The aminoglycosides are poorly absorbed from the GI tract. However, they may reach toxic levels after oral administration in patients with a damaged gut or with renal failure.

(2) Because the aminoglycosides have a narrow toxic-therapeutic ratio, dosage must be carefully adjusted to obtain safe, effective serum levels (see p. 336).

(3) Aminoglycosides are excreted almost entirely by the kidneys. The dosage must be adjusted even with a minor degree of renal impairment (see p. 337).

c. Side effects

(1) Nephrotoxicity due to renal tubular damage is enhanced by the concurrent use of cephalosporins, and diuretics (especially when sodium depletion occurs) and by preexisting renal disease. It is usually reversible. **The serum creatinine should be monitored in all patients on aminoglycoside therapy.**

(2) Ototoxicity (both vestibular and auditory) is enhanced by preexisting ear disease (e.g., otitis media), concurrent administration of diuretics, and preexisting renal disease. **It may be irreversible** unless recognized early. Patients should be examined daily for symptoms of "fullness" in the ears, tinnitus, or vertigo. Ability to hear a watch tick provides a simple bedside screening test for the high-tone hearing loss characteristic of aminoglycoside toxicity. Head shaking elicits symptoms of vertigo in patients confined to bed.

(3) Neuromuscular blockade with respiratory paralysis has been described, usually after peritoneal irrigation with high concentrations of aminoglycoside.

4. Erythromycin inhibits bacterial protein synthesis by binding to ribosomes.

a. Spectrum and indications Erythromycin is bacteriostatic at low concentrations against *M. pneumoniae,* spirochetes, and most gram-positive organisms. It is commonly used as an alternative drug in penicillin-allergic patients with β-streptococcal and pneumococcal infections. Some staphylococci may be resistant de novo, or resistance may emerge during therapy. It is moderately active against *H. influenzae.* Erythromycin is the drug of choice for Legionnaire's disease, mycoplasma pneumonia, pertussis, and diphtheria carrier state.

b. Pharmacology Erythromycin base is acid labile and poorly absorbed. Erythromycin estolate is well absorbed, even in the presence of food, but must be hydrolyzed to the active base by the liver. A variety of parenteral preparations are also available. Active erythromycin is excreted in low concentrations in urine and in higher concentrations in bile.

   c. **Side effects** include nausea, vomiting, and diarrhea. Erythromycin estolate occasionally causes a cholestatic jaundice, probably on a hypersensitivity basis.

5. Lincomycin and **clindamycin** inhibit bacterial protein synthesis.

   a. **Spectrum and indications**

      (1) Both drugs have a similar spectrum, but clindamycin is generally more active. Their antibacterial spectrum resembles erythromycin except that they are inactive against enterococci, some *Clostridium*, *M. pneumoniae*, *N. gonorrhoeae*, *N. meningitidis*, and *H. influenzae*. On the other hand, they are more active against *S. aureus* (but resistance may emerge) and against anaerobic organisms including *B. fragilis*.

      (2) Clindamycin is the drug of choice for serious anaerobic infections due to *B. fragilis*. These agents are alternatives to erythromycin for β-streptococcal and pneumococcal infections and alternatives to penicillinase-resistant penicillins for staphylococcal infections. However, staphylococcal endocarditis may relapse after clindamycin treatment.

   b. **Pharmacology** Both drugs are well absorbed. Most are metabolized by the liver.

   c. **Side effects**

      (1) **GI side effects** (nausea, vomiting, abdominal cramps, diarrhea) are common. Both drugs can produce **pseudomembranous colitis,** which may be severe if treatment is continued. Assays for the enterotoxin of *Clostridium difficile* in the stool may confirm the diagnosis.

      (2) Uncommon side effects include rashes, anaphylaxis, and hepatitis. *Rapid IV infusion may produce syncope or cardiopulmonary arrest.*

6. **Chloramphenicol** inhibits bacterial protein synthesis at the ribosomal level.

   a. **Spectrum and indications**

      (1) Chloramphenicol is active against most gram-positive organisms, most gram-negative bacilli (except *P. aeruginosa*), anaerobes, including *B. fragilis,* and *Rickettsia.* At low concentrations it is bacteriostatic for most organisms and bactericidal for highly sensitive organisms, such as *H. influenzae*; at high concentrations it is bactericidal for sensitive organisms.

      (2) It is the drug of choice for serious infections caused by *H. influenzae,* systemic *Salmonella* infections, including typhoid fever, and serious rickettsial infections, including Rocky Mountain spotted fever.

   b. **Pharmacology** Chloramphenicol is well absorbed from the GI tract and diffuses well into tissues and the CSF. Most of the drug is conjugated in the liver and excreted in the urine.

c. Side effects

(1) Aplastic anemia is a rare (1 in 50,000 courses of treatment) but serious side effect. It has been well documented only with the oral preparation.

(2) Dose-related bone marrow suppression is common and reversible, occurring regularly when plasma-free chloramphenicol levels exceed 25 μg/ml. Manifestations include increased serum iron, decreasing reticulocyte counts, and a falling hematocrit. Thrombocytopenia and leukopenia also occur. The bone marrow shows the characteristic vacuolation of erythroblasts. Free erythrocyte protoporphyrin may be elevated.

(3) In neonates in whom high serum levels of chloramphenicol (> 50 μg/ml) develop, a shocklike syndrome ("gray syndrome") may occur. Dosage should be reduced and serum levels monitored (see **d,** p. 145).

(4) Chloramphenicol may delay the metabolism of tolbutamide, dicumarol, and phenytoin sodium.

(5) Rare side effects include optic neuritis, peripheral neuritis with prolonged therapy, and allergic reactions.

7. The tetracyclines inhibit bacterial protein synthesis and are not used commonly in childhood because of their side effects.

a. Spectrum and indications

(1) The tetracyclines have broad-spectrum bacteriostatic activity against gram-positive organisms, enteric gram-negative bacilli, anaerobes, mycoplasmas, spirochetes, and rickettsiae. However, an increasing number of strains have become resistant. *Serratia, Proteus,* and *P. aeruginosa* are almost always resistant.

(2) Tetracyclines are the drugs of choice for brucellosis, cholera, Q fever, relapsing fever, tularemia, psittacosis, lymphogranuloma venereum, and nonspecific urethritis. They are second-line drugs for *Mycoplasma* pneumonia, gonorrhea, syphilis, and eradication of the meningococcal carrier state (minocycline).

b. Pharmacology
The absorption of tetracycline is impaired by concurrent food intake and the presence of divalent cations (calcium, iron). The serum half-life is relatively short (6 hr). Doxycycline and minocycline are absorbed more completely than tetracycline, and the half-life is long (14–20 hr). Most tetracyclines are excreted mainly by the kidney, but also reach high concentrations in bile. **Doxycycline,** which is eliminated mainly by nonrenal mechanisms, **is the only tetracycline that can be safely used in renal failure.**

c. Side effects

(1) Tetracyclines may produce **permanent yellow discoloration of the deciduous teeth** (when given during the second and third trimester of pregnancy and the first 3 months of life) and of permanent teeth (when given to children 3 months–6 years of age). Tetracyclines should therefore be avoided during these periods; if they must be used, oxytetracycline is the analogue associated with the least discoloration. Other side effects include upper and lower **GI symptoms,** candidal superinfection, and dose-related **hepatitis.**

(2) Preexisting renal dysfunction is exacerbated by all the tetracyclines except doxycycline.

(3) Rare side effects include allergy, photosensitivity (dimethyl chlortetracycline), benign intracranial hypertension, and reversible vestibular disturbance (minocycline).

8. Vancomycin inhibits bacterial cell wall synthesis.

    a. Spectrum and indications Vancomycin is bactericidal for most gram-positive organisms but only bacteriostatic for enterococci. It is active against staphylococci, β-hemolytic streptococci, viridans streptococci, pneumococci, *Corynebacterium*, and clostridia.

        (1) Vancomycin is useful in the treatment of serious infection caused by methicillin-resistant staphylococci.

        (2) Vancomycin and gentamicin combined are the treatment of choice for enterococcal endocarditis in penicillin-allergic patients.

        (3) Oral vancomycin is effective treatment for staphylococcal enterocolitis and antibiotic-induced colitis associated with enterotoxin-producing *Clostridium*.

    b. Pharmacology Vancomycin is not absorbed after oral administration. After parenteral administration it enters tissues well, but diffuses poorly across uninflamed meninges. It is excreted primarily by the kidneys, and dosage must be adjusted in renal failure (see p. 345). **It is not eliminated by hemodialysis.**

    c. Side effects include

        (1) Fever, phlebitis, and maculopapular and urticarial rashes. Anaphylaxis is rare.

        (2) Ototoxicity and **nephrotoxicity** may occur with high serum levels and may be enhanced when aminoglycosides are used concurrently. Renal and auditory function should be monitored with aminoglycosides (see **3.c**, p. 358).

9. The sulfonamides block the synthesis of dihydrofolic acid from para-aminobenzoic acid in bacterial cells.

    a. Spectrum and indications

        (1) Sulfonamides have a broad bacteriostatic spectrum, including most gram-positive cocci (but not enterococci), gram-positive bacilli, most gram-negative organisms including *H. influenzae*, *Chlamydia*, *Actinomyces*, *Nocardia*, and protozoa (malaria, *Toxoplasma* and *Pneumocystis*). Unfortunately, sulfonamide resistance has become common with most of the bacterial groups mentioned.

        (2) The **major indications** for sulfonamides include uncomplicated urinary tract infection, *Nocardia* infections, and, together with other drugs, toxoplasmosis and *P. carinii* pneumonia.

        (3) Penicillin or erythromycin with a sulfonamide remains an effective regimen for otitis media.

        (4) Sulfonamides provide effective rheumatic fever prophylaxis but cannot be relied on for the treatment of group A streptococcal infections.

    b. Pharmacology (e.g., sulfisoxazole) Most sulfonamides are well absorbed orally. They are metabolized by the liver, and both active drug and metabolites are excreted primarily by the kidney. Products of tissue necrosis inhibit the action of sulfonamides. Therefore these agents should not be used for severe suppurative infections.

c. Side effects

(1) Allergic reactions include fever, rash (usually maculopapular, occasionally urticarial, rarely exfoliative or the rash of Stevens-Johnson syndrome), systemic vasculitis, myocarditis, and pulmonary eosinophilia.

(2) Rare **hematologic effects** include reversible agranulocytosis and fatal aplastic anemia. Acute hemolytic anemia may occur in patients with glucose 6-phosphate dehydrogenase deficiency.

(3) Sulfonamides compete with bilirubin for albumin-binding sites, thereby increasing the risk of **kernicterus** in neonates. *They are contraindicated in pregnancy near term and during the first 2 months of life.*

10. Co-trimoxazole (trimethoprim-sulfamethoxazole) Both drugs inhibit folic acid synthesis.

a. Spectrum and indications

(1) The antimicrobial spectrum includes most gram-positive cocci, enteric gram-negative bacilli, *H. influenzae*, and *P. carinii*.

(2) The **major indications** include treatment and prophylaxis of urinary tract infections, prostatitis, and *P. carinii* pneumonia. It is an alternate drug in the treatment of otitis media. Co-trimoxazole may also be useful in systemic infections with gram-negative organisms resistant to other drugs, including *Salmonella* infections.

b. Pharmacology Currently, only oral preparations are available. The dosage should be decreased in patients with severe renal dysfunction (see p. 345).

c. Side effects (Also see **9.c**).

(1) High doses may produce GI irritation and hematologic suppression due to weak inhibition of folic acid metabolism. The latter is reversible with folinic acid. **Co-trimoxazole should be used with caution in patients with preexisting hematologic disease and in patients receiving immunosuppressive therapy.**

(2) Reversible renal impairment may occur.

11. Nitrofurantoin may inhibit bacterial carbohydrate metabolism.

a. Spectrum and indications

(1) Nitrofurantoin is active against most gram-positive cocci (including enterococci) and gram-negative bacilli that cause urinary tract infections. Sensitive organisms usually do not become resistant.

(2) The **only indication** for nitrofurantoin is the treatment and prophylaxis of urinary tract infections.

b. Pharmacology The drug reaches therapeutically effective levels only in the urine, which is its major route of excretion.

c. Side effects

(1) GI side effects (nausea, vomiting, abdominal cramps) occur frequently and are dose related. They are less common with the macrocrystalline form, which is more slowly absorbed but equally effective. Serious systemic toxicity may occur in renal failure.

(2) Other adverse reactions include allergy (rashes, fever, eosinophilia, hepatitis, asthma, and acute pneumonitis), dose-related peripheral neuritis, pulmonary fibrosis, and hemolytic anemia in patients with G-6-PD deficiency.

B. Antifungal agents

1. Amphotericin B and nystatin Both bind to a sterol constituent in the fungal cell membrane, thereby increasing its permeability.

a. Spectrum and indications

(1) Both drugs are active against *Candida* species, *Cryptococcus neoformans, Sporotrichum schenckii, Blastomyces dermatitidis, Histoplasma capsulatum, Coccidioides immitis, Aspergillus* species, and *Phycomycetes.*

(2) These drugs are the antimicrobials of choice for fungal infections on the skin and mucosal surfaces (nystatin) (see Chap. 23) or disseminated to other organs (amphotericin B). Severe mucosal infections may require systemic amphotericin B.

b. Pharmacology Both drugs are poorly absorbed after oral administration.

(1) Nystatin is available only for topical use on the skin, mucosal surfaces, and in the GI tract. Amphotericin is given by slow (3–6 hr) IV infusion in 5% dextrose. Premedication with an antihistamine and the addition of 1000 U of heparin and 10–50 mg of hydrocortisone to the infusate may minimize local phlebitis and systemic reactions. Dosage should be increased gradually, beginning with a dose of 1 mg on the first day. Nonetheless, in serious systemic fungal infections, it is important to increase dosage quickly to full therapeutic levels.

(2) Amphotericin B has a half-life of approximately 20 hr and may therefore be given in increased dosage every other day when prolonged treatment is necessary, especially on an outpatient basis.

c. Side effects

(1) Immediate side effects during infusion of amphotericin B are very common and include fever, chills, headache, nausea, vomiting, and rarely, hypotension. Reversible **nephrotoxicity** and **normochromic normocytic anemia** also occur.

(2) Rare adverse reactions include allergic reactions, peripheral neuropathy (with intrathecal administration), and cardiotoxicity with rapid infusion.

2. 5-Fluorocytosine (5-FC) may be converted to the antimetabolite 5-fluorouracil within the fungal cell and thereby interfere with nucleic acid synthesis.

a. Spectrum and indications

(1) 5-FC is active against *C. neoformans*, most species of *C. albicans*, and *Torulopsis glabrata.* All these organisms may become resistant during therapy, particularly when 5-FC is used alone in low dosage. Sensitivity must be confirmed before this agent is used alone for *Candida* infections.

(2) The **major indications** for 5-FC is its use together with amphotericin B for cryptococcal meningitis. This combination may also be useful for severe disseminated infections with sensitive *Candida* species and possibly *Aspergillus*.

   b. **Pharmacology** 5-FC is well absorbed orally, is not metabolized significantly, and is excreted almost entirely by glomerular filtration. In patients with renal dysfunction, the dosage should be adjusted and serum levels monitored (see p. 345).

   c. **Side effects include** bone marrow suppression and, rarely, hepatitis, GI side effects, and skin rashes.

3. **Clotrimazole** interferes with synthesis of the fungal cell wall. It is active against dermatophytes, most species of *Candida, C. neoformans,* and most filamentous fungi.

   Only topical forms of clotrimazole are currently available as an effective alternative for cutaneous dermatophyte and candidal infections and for vaginal candidiasis.

IV. TREATMENT OF INFECTIOUS DISEASES

A. Impetigo See **VII,** p. 508.

B. Cellulitis (including erysipelas)

1. **Etiology** *S. aureus,* β-hemolytic streptococci, and, less commonly, *H. influenzae* type B.

2. **Evaluation**

   a. Needle aspiration of the advancing border of an active lesion should be carried out for Gram stain and culture.

   b. A blood culture should be done in patients with severe cellulitis, fever, generalized toxicity, or impaired host defenses.

   c. Sinus x-rays should be done in patients with periorbital cellulitis (see p. 532).

3. **Diagnosis** is usually established by the characteristic warm, erythematous, tender, edematous, and indurated skin.

   a. Streptococcal cellulitis (erysipelas) is suggested by advancing, well-demarcated, heaped-up borders; facial involvement may assume a butterfly distribution.

   b. *H. influenza* type B is suggested by a fever greater than 102°F, facial involvement, and the characteristic purple color (which occurs in about half the patients) in a child 6 months–2 years old.

4. **Therapy**

   a. Application of local heat, e.g., warm compresses, 10–20 min qid or more.

   b. If feasible, immobilization and elevation of the affected extremity.

   c. Incision and drainage of any primary suppurative focus.

   d. **Antibiotics**

      (1) Localized cellulitis without fever may be treated with oral antibiotics. However, if evidence of systemic toxicity is present, parenteral antibiotics should be given until sustained clinical improvement has occurred.

(2) Streptococcal disease or erysipelas usually responds to benzathine penicillin G, 0.6–1.2 million U IM in 1 dose, or oral penicillin V, 125–250 mg qid. More severely ill patients may initially require procaine penicillin G, 600,000–900,000 U IM q12h, or even IV penicillin, 100,000 U/kg/day q4h. Treatment should be continued for 7–10 days.

(3) Staphylococcal cellulitis is treated either with penicillin or a penicillinase-resistant penicillin, depending on the organisms' in vitro sensitivity; e.g., nafcillin or oxacillin (100–200 mg/kg/day IV q4h) for severe infections, or dicloxacillin, 25–50 mg/kg/day qid PO for milder infections.

(4) *H. influenzae* cellulitis, in view of the high incidence of positive blood cultures in this disease, is treated initially with chloramphenicol, 100 mg/kg/day q5h, pending ampicillin sensitivity testing.

(5) **Orbital cellulitis** Hospitalization and high doses of antibiotics given IV are indicated (pp. 532 ff.). The initial choice should include a penicillinase-resistant penicillin and, in children, an antimicrobial effective against *H. influenzae*.

C. Scalded skin syndrome (Ritter's disease or toxic epidermal necrolysis), bullous impetigo, and **staphylococcal scarlet fever** represent a spectrum of dermatologic manifestations of staphylococcal infection, resulting from release of soluble toxins by *S. aureus*.

1. Etiology The infecting organism is *S. aureus* (usually bacteriophage group II).

2. Evaluation

a. Cultures of the skin, nose, throat, and blood should be made (exceptions include children with only localized bullous impetigo and older children who are afebrile and nontoxic).

b. Gram stain of the denuded skin or bullous fluid, or both, will differentiate direct staphylococcal skin invasion from the more common toxin-mediated skin changes.

3. The diagnosis is established by the clinical picture in association with recovery of *S. aureus* from the patient. Nikolsky's sign (gentle rubbing of the skin results in sloughing of the epidermis) is usually indicative of the scalded skin syndrome; its absence does not exclude this diagnosis.

4. Therapy

a. A 7–10-day course of a penicillinase-resistant penicillin (or penicillin V if the *S. aureus* is sensitive) usually is sufficient. The antibiotic is usually given parenterally (e.g., oxacillin, 100–200 mg/kg/day q4h IV) (see Appendix Table 5-1 in Chap. 5 for dosages in infants under 4 weeks of age).

b. After a good clinical response has been achieved, therapy may be completed with oral dicloxacillin, 25–50 mg/kg/day qid.

c. Contact precautions are indicated until the lesions have resolved.

d. Corticosteroids have not been demonstrated to be beneficial.

e. In patients with extensive skin losses, hydration and maintenance of normal body temperature are important. Avoid unnecessary skin trauma (e.g., adhesive from tape).

D. Animal bites   Initial management is primarily prophylactic.

1. Potential bacterial complications

a. Etiology   Potential pathogens include anaerobic and microaerophilic streptococci, other anaerobic cocci, *Clostridium* species (including *C. tetani*), *Pasteurella multocida*, *Streptobacillus moniliformis*, and *Spirillum minus* (the latter two cause the two types of rat-bite fever).

b. Evaluation includes an assessment of the patient's immunity to tetanus as well as the extent of the wound.

c. The **diagnosis** of a bacterial complication of an animal bite is suggested by the finding of cellulitis (see **B.2**).

d. Therapy   Besides local antisepsis and surgical care of the bite, including irrigation and débridement if necessary, the following prophylactic measures should be considered:

(1) Tetanus immunization

(a) Tetanus toxoid, 0.5 ml IM, is indicated only if the patient has not received a booster in the previous 5 years or has not completed the basic series of three tetanus immunizations.

(b) In the absence of a history of two (documented) preceding tetanus immunizations, patients with other than clean, minor wounds should receive passive immunization with human tetanus immunoglobulin, 5 U/kg IM, up to 250 U. In such cases, tetanus toxoid is given, but in a separate syringe and site, with subsequent completion of the recommended series at monthly intervals.

(2) Antibiotics are indicated only for severe or penetrating bites (e.g. cat bites). Since most of the potential bacterial pathogens are sensitive to penicillin, low-dose penicillin V, 300,000–600,000 U bid for 3–5 days, is recommended.

2. Rabies prophylaxis   The recommendations are based on those of the Public Health Service Advisory Committee, 1976.

a. Evaluation

(1) Species of biting animal involved   Carnivorous animals (especially skunks, foxes, coyotes, raccoons, dogs, cats, and bats) are more likely to be infective than other animals. Bites of rodents seldom, if ever, require specific antirabies prophylaxis.

(2) Vaccination status of the biting animal   An adult animal immunized properly with one or more doses of rabies vaccine has only a minimal chance of having rabies and transmitting the virus.

(3) Circumstances of the biting incident   An unprovoked attack is more likely to indicate that the animal is rabid than is a provoked attack. Bites during attempts to feed or handle an apparently healthy animal should generally be regarded as provoked.

(4) Extent and location of bite wound   The likelihood that rabies will result from a bite varies with its extent and location, as follows:

(a) Severe   Multiple or deep puncture wounds and any bites on the head, face, neck, hands, or fingers.

(b) Mild   Scratches, lacerations, or single bites on areas of the body other than head, face, neck, hands, or fingers. Open wounds, such as abrasions, suspected of being contaminated with saliva, also belong in this category.

b. Postexposure prophylaxis If adequate laboratory and field records indicate that there is no rabies infection in a domestic species within a given region, local health officials may be justified in modifying general recommendations concerning antirabies treatment after a bite by that species.

E. Acute otitis media See Chap. 23, Sec. **I.D.4.**

F. Tonsillar infections

1. Vincent's angina

a. Etiology Mixed oral anaerobic bacteria are the causative organisms.

b. Evaluation Culture of the ulcerated lesion is necessary to rule out diphtheria and group A streptococcus.

c. Diagnosis Painful, deep, punched-out ulcerations in a red edematous base are present, covered by a poorly adherent gray pseudomembrane whose removal produces only scanty bleeding. Involvement may include the tonsillar fossa, soft palate, and pharynx; inflammatory neck nodes are present. Culture and microscopic examination may confirm the diagnosis.

d. Treatment

(1) **Antibiotics** Penicillin V, 50 mg/kg/24 hr in 4 divided doses is given for 10 days.

(2) **Local hygiene** 3% Hydrogen peroxide mouthwash and gargles q2h, with normal saline gargles at alternate hours. Cēpacol or Chloraseptic mouthwashes may be soothing.

(3) **Analgesics** are given as necessary: acetaminophen and/or codeine, viscous lidocaine, or diclonine HCl mouthwashes and gargles q2–3h.

2. Streptococcal pharyngitis (tonsillitis)

a. Etiology Group A β-hemolytic streptococci.

b. Evaluation must include a properly obtained throat culture (vigorous swabbing of both tonsillar areas and the posterior pharynx, which, if done properly, usually induces a gag reflex).

(1) The disease should be suspected in any patient with a sore throat and fever. In infants, streptococcal infection is more likely to present as persistent nasopharyngeal discharge, with fever and excoriation of the nares.

(2) Any history in the patient or his family of recent streptococcal pharyngitis, scarlet fever, rheumatic fever, or penicillin allergy should be noted.

c. Diagnosis is supported by a positive throat culture and confirmed by a rising ASO titer.

d. Therapy

(1) **Penicillin** Prevention of rheumatic fever requires either benzathine penicillin G given IM, or a 10-day course of oral penicillin (see Chap. 10). The parenteral route ensures treatment for a sufficient length of time, while oral therapy is dependent upon the

cooperation of the patient. Treatment schedules recommended by the American Heart Association are as follows:

    (a) Intramuscular penicillin (benzathine)   Children should be given a single injection of 600,000–1,200,000 U. The larger dose is probably preferable for children over 10 years of age.

    (b) Oral penicillin   Children and adults are given 125 or 250 mg* 3–4 times a day for a full 10 days. Therapy must be **continued for the entire 10 days,** even though the temperature returns to normal and the patient is asymptomatic.

  (2) For patients with documented penicillin allergy, oral erythromycin, 30–50 mg/kg/day in 3 or 4 divided doses, or clindamycin, 10–20 mg/kg/day in 3 or 4 divided doses for 10 days, is recommended. Sulfonamides, while effective in prophylaxis, are ineffective in the treatment of streptococcal infections.

  (3) Bed rest is not necessary. Children can return to school as soon as the symptoms subside.

  (4) Throat cultures are indicated for symptomatic family members but are not necessary for others unless recurrent streptococcal pharyngitis occurs in the family. Such recurrences may necessitate antibiotic treatment of the entire family.

G. Cervical adenitis   Lymph nodes often enlarge in response to localized or systemic infection. Marked enlargement (3 cm or more) associated with tenderness and erythema indicates progressive infection within the node.

  1. The **etiology** varies with the location of the infected neck glands:

    a. Tonsillar nodes (at the angle of the jaw) are likely to be infected by throat pathogens.

    b. Submandibular node infection follows oral or facial disease. Unilateral "cold" submandibular nodes, in the absence of orofacial infection, suggest infection with atypical mycobacteria.

    c. Posterior cervical node infection suggests adjacent skin infection.

    d. Bilateral cervical node enlargement of marked degree indicates infectious mononucleosis, acute toxoplasmosis, secondary syphilis, a phenytoin reaction, or infiltrative node disease.

    e. Recurrent episodes of adenitis should raise the suspicion of chronic granulomatous disease or immunoglobulin deficiency.

  2. Evaluation and diagnosis   The history, examination of the area drained by affected lymph nodes, and routine laboratory data may reveal the likely cause of adenitis.

    a. Needle aspiration of the node offers a simple, safe means of diagnosis. Gram stains of aspirates provide immediately helpful information in 50 percent of patients. Aspirates should be cultured aerobically, anaerobically, and for mycobacteria.

---

* Of the various oral forms available, buffered penicillin G is satisfactory and least expensive. Although higher blood levels may be achieved with a-phenoxymethyl penicillin (penicillin V) or a-phenoxyethyl penicillin (phenethicillin), especially when taken near mealtime, their superiority in the prevention of rheumatic fever has not been documented.

b. Although *M. tuberculosis* adenitis is now uncommon, tuberculin testing is prudent.

c. Surgical drainage or excision biopsy is appropriate for infected nodes that are fluctuant ("pointing") (usually due to *S. aureus*) or re- ' fractory to broad-spectrum antibiotic therapy.

3. Therapy

a. Streptococcal adenitis Penicillin G, either IM (procaine, 600,000–1.2 million U/day) or IV (aqueous, 100,000–250,000 U kg/day) in severe cases, is given until the fever and localized inflammation have subsided. This response should occur within 2–3 days, after which a 10-day course of oral penicillin can be completed. Hot compresses and aspirin also are prescribed.

b. Staphylococcal adenitis Since the organism is often penicillin-resistant, one of the penicillinase-resistant semisynthetic penicillins is given initially and continued if the offending pathogen is resistant to penicillin. Severity of the illness determines whether or not the IV route and hospitalization are necessary.

(1) Recommended preparations and IV doses are as follows: nafcillin, oxacillin, or methicillin, 100–200 mg/kg/day q4h.
PO: dicloxacillin, 50 mg/kg/day qid.
PO: penicillin, 300,000–600,000 U qid.

(2) The duration of treatment is determined by the patient's response, but a 10–14-day course is usually sufficient.

c. Tuberculous adenitis Antituberculous drugs are given (see Table 15-12).

d. Atypical mycobacterial adenitis Although the natural history of this disease is variable, the adenopathy will often resolve spontaneously. The atypical mycobacteria are not communicable from human to human, and the patient presents no danger to siblings or classmates.

(1) Since atypical strains are frequently resistant in vitro to the usual antituberculous drugs, observation is usually the preferred management.

(2) Successful treatment of some infections has been reported with rifampin, which should be used in conjunction with other agents (INH, ethambutol).

(3) When increasing adenopathy or related symptoms indicate more aggressive management, complete surgical excision of the involved nodes is recommended. Antituberculous therapy should be given postoperatively until culture reports demonstrate that *M. tuberculosis* is not present.

H. Infectious mononucleosis is a common, self-limited infectious illness.

1. Etiology Infection is due to Ebstein-Barr virus.

2. Evaluation Pharyngeal symptoms are usually predominant (sore throat, nodes) but 20 percent of patients have a "typhoidal" illness with fever predominating. Physical signs may include continuous fever, lasting 2–5 weeks; lymphadenopathy, with nodes slightly tender; splenomegaly in 50–75 percent, **hepatomegaly** in 15–25 percent, and jaundice in 5–11 percent; periorbital edema in 30 percent; and rash in 3–6 percent (may be macular, scarlatiniform, urticarial, or resemble erythema mul-

370 Ch. 15 Antibiotics and Infectious Diseases

tiforme). A palatal exanthem (red spots on the soft palate) is briefly pre
ent in one-third to one-half of the patients.

3. Diagnosis The classic laboratory findings are

   a. Lymphocytosis (> 50%) with 10 percent atypical lymphocytes.

   b. Monospot tests become positive in most patients during the secon
week of illness and remain so for over 12 months in most patients.

   c. Paul-Bunnel heterophil titers are 1:32.

   d. A heterophil response is rarely seen in children under 3 years of ag
but occurs in 50 percent of those 3–8 years old and in most childre
over 9 years of age.

   e. The peak antibody response occurs 6 weeks after onset.

4. Therapy The full-blown illness lasts 5–20 days, and convalescence
often prolonged.

   a. Supportive therapy includes fluids, rest, and analgesics.

   b. For patients severely toxic or with marked splenomegaly wit
threatened rupture, prednisone, 1–2 mg/kg/day for 5–7 days, may t
beneficial.

   c. Ampicillin should be avoided.

   **d. To avoid splenic rupture, strenuous activity should be prohibited whil
splenomegaly persists.**

I. Epiglottitis is a rapidly progressive bacterial cellulitis of the supraglott
tissues resulting in narrowing of the airway inlet, with risk of total airwa
obstruction. **It is a medical emergency.**

1. Etiology The causative organism is *H. influenzae* type B in 95 percent (
cases. Rare causes are group A streptococci, pneumococci, diphtheri
and tuberculosis.

2. Evaluation and diagnosis To prevent death, skillful handling of patien
with a tentative diagnosis of epiglottitis is essential. The onset of resp
ratory difficulty is usually acute, with rapid progression, most often i
children 3–6 years old. Bacteremia is present in over 90 percent and
associated with fever and toxicity, dysphagia, drooling, inspirato
stridor, muffled voice, and extended neck.

   a. The swollen cherry-red tip of the epiglottis may be readily visible i
the throat of a cooperative child but examination must not be force
lest sudden, complete obstruction occur.

   b. Radiographs should be done only under controlled conditions wit
skilled personnel and equipment to evaluate the patient's ventilatic
and to secure the airway swiftly if necessary. Lateral radiographs
the neck delineate the epiglottis and aryepiglottic folds well and a
helpful in puzzling cases.

3. Therapy

   a. Conservative management of epiglottitis includes prophylactic nas
tracheal intubation to prevent sudden death. Skillful intubation ha
generally replaced the need for tracheostomy in patients with o
structed airways. Intubation is well tolerated and briefly require
(1–3 days).

   b. Antibiotic therapy directed against *H. influenzae* is begun immed ately (chloramphenicol, 100 mg/kg/day given IV). Later, treatment may be changed to ampicillin if the isolate is susceptible. Treatment is continued for 7–10 days.

    c. Early in convalescence, patients should be carefully evaluated for metastatic *Haemophilus* infection, such as pneumonia, pericarditis, meningitis, or septic arthritis.

J. Croup   Viral laryngotracheobronchitis is complicated by subglottic edema, resulting in a characteristic barking cough and a hoarse voice.

  1. Etiology   Parainfluenza, respiratory syncytial virus, adenovirus, and measles virus are the most common causes. Bacterial infection is rare.

  2. Evaluation

    a. History   A coryzal prodrome is common, with increasing cough and hoarseness, often at night and typically in a child under 3 years of age.

    b. Physical examination   High fever or toxicity is unusual. Examination is directed toward the extent of airway narrowing: inspiratory stridor at rest, tachypnea (40/min), retractions, and diminished breath sounds indicate critical narrowing. Restlessness, tachycardia, altered mental status, and pallor or cyanosis suggest hypoxia.

    c. Laboratory data   A CBC and arterial blood gas estimation are indicated if this can be done by skilled personnel. A lateral neck radiogram will clarify the clinical presentation.

  3. The **diagnosis** of croup is confirmed by neck radiographs showing subglottic narrowing.

  4. Therapy

    a. Hydration and **moisturized air**   Cool, moist air with O_2 is provided as necessary.

    b. Sedation   A quiet room where a parent may stay with the child and elimination of unnecessary procedures help to reduce the associated anxiety. In patients in whom excessive apprehension aggravates the respiratory distress, mild sedation (chloral hydrate, 10–15 mg/kg q6–8h) may be beneficial (see Chap. 1, p. 10).

    c. Steroids   A short course of high-dose corticosteroids (1–3 doses dexamethasone, 1 mg/kg q6h) in severe croup has become commonplace, although current studies have not yet shown a clear-cut benefit.

    d. Intubation is indicated for respiratory failure.

    e. Aerosolized racemic epinephrine therapy remains controversial; aerosolized saline appears equally beneficial.

    f. Home care   Most cases of croup are mild and can be managed at home. Therapeutic measures include a vaporizer, a steamed-up bathroom, and, occasionally, outdoor air. Parents should be instructed to call a physician if the child's respiratory distress increases.

K. Bronchiolitis is a syndrome of acute small airway obstruction in young infants, with the risk of respiratory failure.

  1. Etiology   Usually viral (most commonly, respiratory syncytial virus).

  2. Evaluation should include assessment of hydration and respiratory exchange.

3. The **diagnosis** is suggested by the onset of coryza, cough, and dyspnea i an infant and by prominent wheezing, hyperinflation of the lungs, an retractions. Fever may not be present.

4. **Therapy**

   a. **Humidified O$_2$** (40% or more) In severe cases, arterial blood gase should be monitored.

   b. **Adequate hydration** of the patient is important. Whether fluids ar administered PO or IV depends on the severity of the respirator distress. **In severe respiratory distress, administration of oral fluids ma induce vomiting and aspiration pneumonia and is contraindicated.**

   c. In severe cases, assisted ventilation may be required.

   d. Congestive heart failure can develop in severely ill patients, neces sitating digitalis (see Chap. 10, Sec. **D.1**).

   e. Antibiotics are not routinely given, but are indicated if associate otitis media or pneumonia are present.

   f. Glucocorticoids have *not* been shown to be beneficial.

   g. Bronchodilators given parenterally or by inhalation may be wort trying, but are not reliably effective (see Chap. 2, p. 46).

   h. Patients with bronchiolitis continue to excrete respiratory syncytia virus for several weeks and should be nursed in isolation to preven cross-infection of other infants.

L. Pneumonia See also Chaps. 5 and 20.

1. **Etiology**

   a. **Viruses** probably cause the majority of pediatric pneumonias. Resp ratory syncytial virus is a particularly prominent cause in infant Other common viral pathogens include the parainfluenza (1, 2, and 3 influenza A and B, and adenoviruses.

   b. *M. pneumoniae* is a common cause of pneumonia in school-age chi dren and adolescents.

   c. *S. pneumoniae* is the most frequent cause of bacterial pneumoni Lobar or segmental consolidation are most common, but pneumoco cal bronchopneumonia is not infrequent.

   d. **Staphylococcal pneumonia** is suggested by rapidly evolving respi ratory distress, empyema, and the characteristic radiologic feature of rapid progression, lobular ectasia, and pneumatoceles in an infan or child less than 3 years old. Even in an extremely ill child, however the initial x-ray film may demonstrate only faint focal mottling.

   e. Group B β-hemolytic streptococcal etiology is suggested by an inter stitial bronchopneumonia resembling a viral pneumonitis, sudde onset of symptoms, chills, leukocytosis, and often a preceding vira infection (e.g., measles). An early serosanguineous pleural effusion i characteristic (see Chap. 5).

   f. *H. influenzae* pneumonia can mimic any of the preceding types o pneumonia and should be suspected in a young child or infant who i toxic or fails to respond to adequate penicillin therapy.

   g. Other gram-negative organisms and *P. carinii*, fungi, and tuber culosis (see Sec. **T**) are rare causes of pneumonia in children, occurrin

primarily in neonates, leukemia patients, and others with immunologic deficiencies.

2. Evaluation may include the following:

a. Chest x-ray (posteroanterior and lateral).

b. Tuberculin skin test.

c. Sputum or deep tracheal aspirate for Gram stain and culture. Cultures from the nasopharynx should be interpreted with great caution.

d. Blood culture(s) in the patient who appears toxic.

e. If pleural fluid is present, a diagnostic thoracentesis should be done.

f. Cold agglutinin titer (see bedside method, p. 332).

g. ASO titer if group A streptococci are suspected.

h. Diagnostic lung puncture in critically ill children in whom a specific
etiologic diagnosis is of major importance to guide antimicrobial therapy (see *Pediatrics* 44:486, 1969).

i. Leukocyte and differential counts occasionally are helpful but, in
general, should not be relied on to distinguish bacterial from other
causes.

3. The **diagnosis** is usually established by the chest x-ray and physical signs
of consolidation. An etiologic diagnosis usually is made from the culture,
the clinical features described, and, in the case of *M. pneumoniae*, a cold
agglutinin titer > 1:64.

4. Therapy

a. Antibiotics

(1) Children who are mildly ill with features suggestive of viral disease can be managed without antibiotics, provided the patient can
be followed closely.

(2) Infants and hospitalized patients should receive antibiotics when
pneumonia is diagnosed.

(3) The choice of specific antibiotics is based on interpretation of
available gram-stained specimens, age of the patient, and other
suggestive clinical features.

(4) Specific recommendations

(a) The toxic, hospitalized patient age 2 months–5 years should be
treated with both a penicillinase-resistant penicillin (200 mg/
kg/day) and ampicillin (200 mg/kg/day) or chloramphenicol (75
mg/kg/day IV q6h).

(b) Infants less than 2 months old should receive a penicillinase-
resistant penicillin IV (200 mg/kg/day q4h for infants greater
than 4 weeks old–see Appendix Table 5-1, Chap. 5, for infants
less than 4 weeks old) and gentamicin IV, 5.0–7.5 mg/kg/day
q8–12h, or kanamycin IV, 30 mg/kg/day q8h.

(c) Nontoxic children with suspected pneumococcal pneumonia
should be treated with IM procaine penicillin G, 0.6–1.2 million
U/day for 1–3 days, by which time definite clinical improvement with uncomplicated pneumococcal pneumonia should
have occurred. Subsequently, a 7-day course can be completed

with oral penicillin V, 125–250 mg tid. Suspected *Mycoplasma* pneumonia is treated with oral erythromycin, 30–50 mg/kg day in 4 daily doses for 10 days.

(5) Identification of the pathogen or failure to respond to these regimens necessitates reevaluation of the choice of antibiotics.

(6) Duration of antimicrobial therapy is based on the individual patient's clinical response, but, in general, staphylococcal pneumonia requires 6 weeks of parenteral therapy, and *H. influenzae* and streptococcal pneumonia usually respond to 2–3 weeks of therapy.

(7) Recommended alternatives to the penicillins in the penicillin allergic patient are cephalosporins, erythromycin, and clindamycin.

b. Indications for hospitalization include the following: significant respiratory distress or toxicity, cyanosis, age under 6 months, empyema or pleural effusion, possible staphylococcal pneumonia, and inadequate home care.

c. In the case of empyema, drainage by repeated aspiration or insertion of a chest tube is necessary (Chap. 1, p. 5, Sec. **5**). (Loculated pleural fluid may explain persistent fever in the face of seemingly adequate antibiotic therapy.)

d. Symptomatic care should include O_2 if necessary, high humidity (such as the use of a vaporizer in the home), expectorants, bronchodilators if bronchospasm is present, and deep tracheal suction in patients with ineffectual cough.

e. Postural drainage and physiotherapy may be helpful, particularly with underlying bronchiectasis.

f. Initial follow-up of the ambulatory patient should be on a day-to-day basis until definite clinical improvement has occurred.

g. Although radiologic resolution may lag behind clinical improvement, persistence of radiologic abnormalities without improvement for more than 4–6 weeks should alert the physician to possible underlying pulmonary disease (e.g., tuberculosis, foreign body, cystic fibrosis).

M. For discussion of neonatal meningitis, see Chap. 5, Sec. **V.B.**

1. Etiology   Meningitis is a complication of bacteremia. *H. influenzae* type b (60–65 percent), meningococci, and pneumococci account for most cases of acute bacterial meningitis in children over 2 months of age. Infrequently involved organisms are β-hemolytic streptococci, *S. aureus*, and gram-negative enteric bacteria, except in neonatal meningitis.

2. Evaluation

a. In infants, the **presenting symptoms and signs** are nonspecific and include a high-pitched cry, irritability, anorexia, vomiting, lethargy, and/or a full fontanelle. Meningeal signs are uncommon, and fever is not invariably present. The closest attention must be paid to alterations in consciousness if an early diagnosis is to be made. Convulsions may be an early manifestation of meningitis. Thus convulsions associated with fever in infancy are generally an indication for CSF examination.

b. In older children, meningeal signs are more reliable. Brudzinski's sign (flexion of the neck eliciting pain in the lower back, and/or spas ticity of the quadriceps) can be helpful in determining the need for lumbar puncture (LP).

c. Patients with evidence of bacteremia should be carefully assessed for evidence of meningitis.

d. An **LP** should be performed as soon as the diagnosis is suspected (Chap. 1, p. 4). **Before** the LP is performed, a blood glucose should be obtained for comparison with the CSF glucose.

e. **Papilledema is a relative contraindication to LP,** and, if it is present, a neurosurgical consultation should be considered before proceeding. (Papilledema is rare in *acute* bacterial meningitis, and its presence may suggest other diagnostic possibilities, e.g., brain abscess.)

f. Other diagnostic procedures include blood culture, smears and cultures from any purpuric lesions, cultures of other body fluids (e.g., stool, urine, joint, abscess, middle ear), BUN, serum electrolytes, chest x-ray, and tuberculin test. In infants, transillumination should be performed and the head circumference carefully measured.

3. The **diagnosis** can be established only by the LP.

a. In bacterial meningitis, the CSF is characteristically cloudy and under increased pressure, with > 100 WBC/mm^3, predominantly neutrophils, elevated total protein, low glucose (less than one-half of the pre-LP blood glucose concentration), and organisms in the CSF gram-stained smear. However, some of these findings frequently may not be present, and any of these abnormalities must be viewed with suspicion, particularly the presence of *any* neutrophils. The CSF culture usually confirms the diagnosis.

b. Rapid etiologic diagnosis of bacterial meningitis may be possible by using methods to detect capsular polysaccharide antigens (see p. 332).

c. The limulus test for endotoxin in CSF is sensitive and reliable in detecting gram-negative bacterial meningitis.

4. Therapy Intravenous antibiotic therapy should be initiated immediately after bacteriologic specimens have been obtained. The initial choice of antibiotics usually is based on the CSF gram-stained smear and the patient's age.

a. **In children over 2 months of age** in whom there is no reason to suspect an unusual organism, chloramphenicol is the drug of choice (100 mg/kg/day IV in 4 divided doses), in combination with ampicillin (200–400 mg/kg/day given q4h) or penicillin. Since ampicillin-resistant *H. influenzae* type B has now been isolated in all areas of the United States, anticipatory use of chloramphenicol is advisable. If *H. influenzae* is recovered, and sensitivity is confirmed in vitro, ampicillin is used to complete therapy. If the culture discloses meningococci or pneumococci, penicillin G is the drug of choice.

b. **In infants less than two months old** (see Chap. 5, Sec. **V.B.1**).

c. The duration of therapy depends on the infant's clinical course, but antibiotics should be given for a minimum of 2 weeks.

d. **Other aspects of management**

(1) During treatment, frequent observations of **vital signs** should be made. All patients should be carefully evaluated for evidence of hypotension and abnormal bleeding.

(2) LP should be repeated after 24–48 hr of therapy in patients whose disease is severe or who respond poorly to treatment. Cultures and stains are usually negative after 48 hr if treatment is effective. LP is generally repeated at the end of treatment, by which time the CSF glucose is usually normal and the protein and cell count markedly improved. Criteria for the cure of meningitis based on these data are not precise; a few mononuclear cells at this time are not unusual. Glucose transport may remain impaired in the absence of infection. The persistence of neutrophils is worrisome, but seldom proves to be the result of persistent infection in patients who have responded well to therapy (see *Am. J. Dis. Child.* 131:46 1977).

(3) Persistence or recrudescence of fever during therapy most commonly results from phlebitis, drug, fever, nosocomial infection, subdural effusion, or coexisting viral infection. Nonetheless, localized infection in the subdural space, joints, pericardium, or pleura should be sought.

(4) Children should be observed for recurrence of fever for 24–48 hr after discontinuance of antibiotics and before discharge from the hospital.

N. Brain abscess Normal brain tissue is resistant to bacterial infection. However, ischemic brain injury (e.g., cyanotic heart disease), parameningeal infection (sinusitis, mastoiditis, skull osteomyelitis), and skull trauma increase the risk of brain abscess.

1. Etiology Causative bacteria are usually derived from the upper airway or mouth. Mixtures of aerobes (α-streptococci, *S. aureus*, diphtheroids, *Haemophilus*) and anaerobes (*Peptococcus*, *Bacteroides*) are common. Unusual agents are occasionally responsible, especially in immunocompromised patients.

2. Evaluation Brain abscess must be considered in patients with evidence of a rapidly progressive intracranial mass.

a. The **history** should focus on possible predisposing causes. Headache and seizures are common. Fever is seldom prominent.

b. In the **physical examination** attempts should be made to uncover extracranial infection and localize the neurologic lesion. An assessment should be made for elevated intracranial pressure.

c. Laboratory examination includes blood cultures, skull x-rays, emergency electroencephalography, and a CT scan. **CSF examination should be avoided in patients with increased intracranial pressure.** It seldom adds to the evaluation (CSF changes are not universally present nor pathognomonic for brain abscess). Leukocytosis may or may not be present.

3. The **diagnosis** is made by confirmation of an intracranial mass by CT scan. Even small abscesses can be localized in skilled hands and generally make an arteriogram unnecessary. When CT scan facilities are unavailable, other radiologic techniques are required.

4. Therapy

a. Surgical excision or drainage of the abscess is necessary for cure. Antibiotics may be started prior to operation **but will not cure (or halt the progression of) an established abscess.** Mortality and CNS sequelae are closely proportional to the depth of coma at the time of drainage.

b. Initial empiric antibiotic therapy usually includes chloramphenicol, 100 mg/kg/day IV in 4 divided doses, and penicillin IV (300,000 U/kg/ day q4h). This can be modified after bacteriologic evaluation of the abscess contents.

c. To reduce brain swelling, fluids should be restricted moderately to keep the patient "dry." Hyperosmotic agents such as mannitol are commonly used. Dexamethasone, 1 mg/kg/day IV, may also help to reduce cerebral edema (see Chap. 2, Sec. **V**, p. 43).

d. Follow-up radionuclide or CT scans are used to monitor resolution of the abscess and to determine the duration of antibiotic therapy.

e. Parameningeal foci of infection responsible for brain abscess may also require surgical drainage (sinus, mastoid).

O. Gastroenteritis (bacillary)   For other discussion, see Chap. 11, Sec. **II**.

  1. Etiology

  a. Bacterial agents cause diarrhea infrequently. The principal agents in the United States are *Salmonella* and *Shigella*. Enteropathogenic *E. coli* (EPEC), defined by demonstration of enterotoxin activity, is uncommon. It is, however, more common elsewhere. Other agents include *Yersinia enterocolitica* (noteworthy for its association with mesenteric adenitis), *Vibrio parahaemolyticus* (causing shellfish-related diarrhea), and *Campylobacter*, a newly appreciated invasive organism that may prove to be more common than *Salmonella*. *Clostridium difficile* may cause **pseudomembranous colitis** as it overgrows the residual flora of antibiotic-treated patients (i.e., clindamycin-associated colitis).

  b. Food poisoning can be caused by toxins from several bacteria, including staphylococci, *Clostridium perfringens*, and *Bacillus cereus*.

  2. Evaluation includes an epidemiologic history, assessment of the character and duration of the abnormal stools, and careful assessment of the patient's state of hydration.

  a. The demonstration of sheets of fecal leukocytes in diarrheal stools is well correlated with inflammatory (usually bacterial) disease.

  b. Indications for stool cultures are infancy, toxicity, severe diarrhea, chronic disease or impaired host, and epidemic diarrhea. (See Chap. 11, Sec. **I.B** for culture methods.)

  c. Hospitalized patients with fever and diarrhea should have one or more blood cultures.

  3. Diagnosis   The presence of bacterial gastroenteritis can be established only by the results of stool cultures. Routine stool cultures will identify only *Salmonella* and *Shigella*; EPEC are reliably identified only by special assays for enterotoxin and are usually recognized only in epidemics, e.g., nursery outbreaks. An invasive form of EPEC occurs rarely and is usually recognized only after the fact. A research assay is needed for confirmation of this entity. If *V. parahaemolyticus* or *Y. enterocolitica* are suspected, the laboratory should be alerted. The toxin of *C. difficile* can be identified directly in stool samples of patients with pseudomembranous colitis.

4. **Therapy** is directed primarily toward fluid and electrolyte management (see Chap. 8). Antibiotics are indicated in epidemic EPEC diarrhea, shigellosis, and in some cases of salmonellosis.

   a. *Shigella* Ampicillin, 50–100 mg/kg/day PO qid for 7 days.

   b. **EPEC** The choice of antibiotic depends on the antibiotic sensitivity of the organisms.

      (1) Antibiotics are given PO for a minimum of 7 days until negative stool cultures have been obtained on 3 consecutive days.

      (2) Agents that have been used include colistin PO (15 mg/kg/day tid), neomycin PO (50–100 mg/kg/day qid), and kanamycin IM (50–100 mg/kg/day qid). For newborns the lower doses are recommended.

      (3) Prophylactic antibiotics for travelers are not recommended.

   c. *Salmonella* Since antibiotics only prolong the carrier state, most patients with *Salmonella* in the stool are *not* treated.

      (1) **Indications for treatment** are infancy, impaired host defenses, sickle cell anemia, chronic inflammatory bowel disease, severe toxicity, and positive blood cultures.

      (2) *Salmonella* infections may be treated with ampicillin (200 mg/kg/day) or chloramphenicol (100 mg/kg/day) for 2 or 3 weeks. Trimethoprim-sulfamethoxazole may be effective for multiply resistant organisms.

P. Urinary tract infections Also see Chaps. 5 and 9.

1. **Etiology** First infections are most commonly caused by *E. coli*. Other pathogens include *Proteus, Klebsiella, Pseudomonas, Streptococcus faecalis, S. epidermidis*, and, rarely, *S. aureus*.

2. **Evaluation and diagnosis** Clinical manifestations of urinary tract infection (UTI) vary with age. UTI must be considered in any acutely ill or nonthriving infant.

   a. **Pyelonephritis** is suggested by high fever (>102°F), toxicity, and flank pain. It occurs in 10 percent of symptomatic infections and is commonly associated with ureteral dysfunction (reflux).

   b. At any age, UTI may be minimally symptomatic ("occult" bacteriuria). These children, often considered normal by their parents, frequently have enuresis, daytime wetting, and urgency beyond the expected ages for such behavior. In some children, UTI is symptomless. Occult UTI tends to persist without treatment but seldom becomes overtly symptomatic.

   c. **Physical examination** should include blood pressure, a search for congenital malformations and a careful review of the abdomen, genitalia, and perineum.

   d. **Laboratory studies**

      (1) **Urine microscopy** can provide an accurate provisional diagnosis of UTI if used to quantitate the concentration of bacteria in a fresh, clean sample: One or more bacteria per oil field in gram-stained, **uncentrifuged** urine = $\geqq 10^5$ colonies/ml. The presence of numerous bacteria per high-power field does not necessarily indicate infection.

      (2) Pyuria is not specific for infection. Proteinuria and hematuria are uncommon with UTI.

(3) Urine culture provides alternate proof of infection, but its value in young children is reduced by frequent sampling errors.

(a) Infected urine will contain $>10^5$ colonies/ml (except in some neonates, in whom $>10^4$ colonies may indicate infection). Negative cultures of voided samples are of value in ruling out infection.

(b) Repetition of cultures increases diagnostic precision in all age groups.

(c) Diagnostic precision is greatest with urine obtained by suprapubic bladder aspiration or sterile catheterization ($>10^3$ colonies/ml). In skilled hands, both procedures are safe. They are most appropriately used to resolve urgent or difficult diagnostic problems in younger children.

(d) Note that contamination of samples may provide $\geqq 10^5$ colonies/ml of a single species. More typically, contaminated cultures contain several species in concentrations $<10^5$ colonies/ml. Urine specimens should be refrigerated at 4°C and cultured promptly to avoid growth of contaminants.

(4) A **blood culture** should be obtained in patients with pyelonephritis and in neonates with UTI.

(5) Indications for an IVP and a voiding cystourethrogram are the following: age less than 2 years; toxicity or sepsis (suggestive of pyelonephritis); and first infection in a male and second infection in a female (unless the history, physical findings, and/or clinical response to the first infection suggests an early workup). In these circumstances, a serum BUN, creatinine, and creatinine clearance are also indicated.

(6) Contributing factors to recurrent infections include poor perineal hygiene, vulvovaginitis, pinworm infestations, constipation, and perhaps masturbation.

3. Therapy

a. Most initial and uncomplicated UTIs respond to oral sulfonamides, e.g., sulfisoxazole (Gantrisin), 150–200 mg/kg/day, administered qid. An effective alternative is ampicillin, 100 mg/kg/day PO qid, or nitrofurantoin, 5–7 mg/kg/day qid.

b. Children with **pyelonephritis** require parenteral antibiotics, hydration, and hospitalization. Ampicillin, 100–200 mg/kg/day q4h IV, is effective against many urinary tract pathogens, but a previous history of pyelonephritis or infection with a resistant organism indicates the need for a broad-spectrum antibiotic. Kanamycin, 15 mg/kg/day (up to 1 gm/day) q12h IM, is recommended in such cases; or, if *Pseudomonas* is suspected, gentamicin, 3.0–7.5 mg/kg/day q8–12h IM. The recommended duration of therapy is usually 10–14 days, but clinical improvement should be evident within 48–72 hr.

c. Infants, especially newborns, with UTI should have prompt urologic evaluation as well as aggressive antibiotic treatment.

d. Ongoing antimicrobial therapy is based on the clinical response of the patient and the results of subsequent urine cultures.

(1) A culture should be obtained 24–48 hr after therapy has been initiated, and at this time the urine should be sterile (or have $< 10^4$ bacteria/ml).

    (2) A Gram stain of the unspun specimen should not show organisms and the sediment should be significantly cleared of leukocyte 24–48 hr after therapy.

    (3) Adequate clinical responses may be seen despite in vitro resistance of the organism isolated, because of the high concentrations of certain antimicrobials in the urine (see **b,** p. 337).

    (4) Failure to respond should increase suspicion of an underlying anatomic abnormality.

  e. Adequate **hydration** of the patient is important.

  f. Continuous bladder drainage by an indwelling catheter should be done only when absolutely necessary and discontinued at the earliest possible time; a **closed drainage system is mandatory.** Bladder irrigation with a solution containing neomycin and polymyxin B in normal saline, or ¼% acetic acid, may reduce the incidence of catheter induced infection. In young adults, the use of a three-way catheter allowing continuous irrigation is possible and recommended. On removal of the catheter, a urine culture should be obtained.

4. Follow-up of a UTI should be carefully organized, since infection tends to recur (in more than 50 percent of patients), often in asymptomatic form. Recurrence is most likely during the first 6–12 months after an infection.

  a. After therapy is discontinued, urine cultures are indicated 1 week later, every 2 months during the subsequent 6 months, and less frequently thereafter. Yearly follow-up is appropriate for the remainder of the patient's childhood. There is increased risk of recurrence with marriage and pregnancy.

  b. Among patients with **significant reflux,** recurrent infection is prevented by prophylactic antibiotic therapy, which is continued until reflux resolves or is repaired.

  c. Some normal girls experience **multiple recurrences** of UTI. They should be carefully assessed for correctable contributing factors. When infections are frequent, socially distressing, or associated with renal scarring, prophylactic antibiotic therapy is often prescribed for 6–12 months. Sulfonamides, trimethoprim-sulfamethoxazole, or nitrofurantoin, are used in very small dosages.

  d. Home screening can improve the follow-up of UTI, using simple, inexpensive tests such as the nitrate chemical test for bacteriuria and agar-coated dip slides.

Q. Septic arthritis

1. Etiology Usually *S. aureus, H. influenzae,* or β-hemolytic streptococci. Penetrating injuries or skin infections are associated with *S. aureus* infections. Gram-negative enteric bacteria, *N. gonorrhoeae,* pneumococci, and *N. meningitidis* are less commonly involved. Tuberculous arthritis is uncommon.

2. Evaluation

  a. Careful **examination** of the patient for other foci of infection.

  b. **X-ray films** of the joint(s) and adjacent bones.

  c. Multiple **blood cultures.**

  d. **Arthrocentesis** To avoid introducing bacteria, joint aspiration is performed with full surgical asepsis. Analysis of the joint fluid includes gram-stain, culture (including plating on prewarmed chocolate agar if *H. influenzae* or *Neisseria* is suspected), WBC and differential, total protein, and joint-blood–glucose ratio.

   e. Joint infection may be overlooked in the toxic, prostrate patient with bacteremia. **Delayed diagnosis may result in extensive damage to growth cartilages.**

   f. Hip involvement is most common in children, and this joint is difficult to assess. **Repeated examinations of the hips and all other joints** is an important aspect of managing bacteremic patients.

3. The **diagnosis** can be established only by the presence of bacteria in the synovial fluid. Joint or blood cultures, or both, are positive in most patients with septic arthritis.

4. Therapy

   a. Drainage Prompt aspiration of the affected joint is both diagnostic and therapeutic, since adequate drainage is critical to the prevention of sequelae. Whether or not open surgical drainage or repeated needle aspiration is chosen depends on the *joint involved* (e.g., the hip and shoulder require surgical drainage); *age* (infants and young children usually require surgical drainage); *viscosity* of the synovial exudate; the offending *pathogen* (staphylococcal disease usually necessitates surgical drainage while meningococcal or gonococcal arthritis may require only needle aspiration); and the *response* of the patient to antibiotics.

   b. Antibiotics The initial choice of antibiotics is based on the gram-stained smear of the synovial fluid and the patient's age.

      (1) In the absence of a diagnostic Gram stain, the initial choice should include a penicillinase-resistant penicillin (e.g., oxacillin, 200 mg/kg/day q2–4h IV, up to 12 gm/day). For children 2 months–5 years of age, an agent effective against *H. influenzae* should be added (chloramphenicol 75 mg/kg/day q6h, IV).

      (2) Once the pathogen is identified, therapy may require modification, to provide the most effective drug with the least toxicity.

      (3) Because antibiotics diffuse well into synovial fluid, local instillation of antibiotics is not necessary.

      (4) Antibiotic therapy for 2–3 weeks is usually sufficient.

   c. Other therapeutic measures include early immobilization of the joint and physical therapy when the inflammation subsides.

R. Acute osteomyelitis

1. Etiology

   a. *S. aureus* is the organism responsible in 75–80 percent of cases.

   b. Other organisms include β-hemolytic streptococci, pneumococci, and *H. influenzae.* Special associations include *Salmonella* in sickle cell anemia, gram-negative enteric pathogens in neonates, and *P. aeruginosa* following penetrating injury of the foot.

2. Evaluation

   a. A careful search for metastatic infection in other bones and soft tissues is indicated.

   b. Multiple blood cultures, cultures of other sites, x-ray films, and radionuclide scans of suspected bony sites.

    c. In the presence of localized bony tenderness and a positive bone scan needle aspiration of the bone for Gram stain and culture is indicated

3. The **diagnosis** is based on the characteristic clinical picture and results of needle aspiration. Although radiologic evidence of disease does not appear until 10 or more days, deep soft tissue swelling **in conjunction with local bone tenderness,** is good evidence of osteomyelitis. Bone scans may provide early confirmation.

4. Therapy Prevention of chronic osteomyelitis and other sequelae depends on early diagnosis and treatment.

    a. Administration of a penicillinase-resistant penicillin (e.g., oxacillin 300 mg/kg/day q2–4h IV, up to 12 gm/day) is started as soon as the appropriate cultures have been obtained.

    b. A second antibiotic is chosen if an organism other than *S. aureus* is suspected.

    c. Patients with sickle cell anemia should also receive ampicillin, 200 mg/kg/day q2–4h IV; neonates should be given kanamycin, 30 mg/kg/day q8h IM, or gentamicin, 5.0–7.5 mg/kg/day q8–12h IM.

    d. *Pseudomonas* osteomyelitis usually requires surgical drainage as well as antibiotic therapy with gentamicin and carbenicillin.

    e. Surgical drainage should be considered for most long-bone infections unless the history prior to diagnosis is short and the response to antibiotic therapy is prompt.

    f. Antibiotic therapy is usually given for 3–6 weeks. In patients responding promptly, therapy may be completed with oral antibiotics provided the organism is known, compliance is certain (e.g., the child remains in the hospital), and serum inhibitory and bactericidal titers are monitored (see *J. Pediatr.* 92:485, 1978).

    g. Initial immobilization of the affected limb helps to relieve pain.

S. Bacterial endocarditis The incidence of infective endocarditis in children is increasing.

    1. Etiology Congenital heart disease is present in most cases. Predisposing lesions include tetralogy of Fallot, ventricular septal defect (VSD), patent ductus arteriosus (PDA), and aortic stenosis (AS) and coarctation Cyanotic children with shunts (Blalock, Waterston, Potts) are also at risk.

        a. A prior event leading to bacteriuria (e.g., dental manipulation, infection) is present in only 30 percent of cases.

        b. Viridans streptococci and *S. aureus* are most commonly involved.

        c. Other organisms include *S. epidermidis*, microaerophilic streptococci β-hemolytic streptococci, enterococci, *Haemophilus* species, *C. albicans*, and *S. pneumoniae*.

    2. Evaluation includes the following:

        a. A **history,** with special attention to fever (particularly its duration height, and time of onset), malaise, and symptoms of embolism (to the brain, kidneys, or spleen).

        b. **Physical examination,** with attention to cardiac auscultation, cutaneous manifestations such as petechiae, splinter hemorrhages, Osler's nodes, or Janeway lesions, and, if indicated, needle marks from illicit drug use.

    c. Laboratory studies should include a CBC, erythrocyte sedimentation rate (ESR), urinalysis (UA), and serum protein analysis (SPA). Three to six blood cultures should be obtained over a 48-hr period.

    d. Multiple urine cultures as well as cultures of possible noncardiac foci, multiple microscopic examinations of fresh urine sediment for red blood cells and red cell casts, a CBC, ESR, chest roentgenogram, serum complement, protein electrophoresis, and serum rheumatoid factor also are recommended.

    e. Once isolated, the causative organism should be saved. After appropriate antibiotics have been started, serum bactericidal levels should be determined (see Sec. **4.d**).

3. The **diagnosis** is established by positive blood cultures in association with a compatible clinical picture:

    a. Typically the bacteremia is low grade and continuous. Consequently, the majority (85–90 percent) of blood cultures are positive.

    b. Splenomegaly is common.

    c. The development of a new regurgitant murmur and extracardiac findings indicating systemic emboli or vasculitis are significant.

    d. **Laboratory abnormalities** include anemia (in 40 percent), leukocytosis with a shift to the left (in 50 percent), elevated ESR (in 80 percent), microscopic hematuria (in 50 percent), and hyperglobulinemia (in 50 percent).

    e. When the blood cultures are negative, a presumptive diagnosis is based on the typical clinical syndrome.

4. Therapy

    a. If the diagnosis is clinically evident, initiation of antibiotics is reasonable while the results of the blood cultures are still pending.

    b. In acute bacterial endocarditis, therapy with penicillinase-resistant penicillin and gentamicin **should be initiated within several hours of the patient's admission to the hospital.**

    c. Once the pathogen has been identified, recommended antibiotics are as follows (see Table 15-2):

        (1) Viridans streptococci, β-hemolytic streptococci, and microaerophilic streptococci: Give aqueous penicillin G, 250,000 U/kg/day q4h IV, up to 18 million U daily.

        (2) Enterococci: Give ampicillin, 300 mg/kg/day q2–4h IV, and gentamicin, 3.0–7.5 mg/kg/day q8h IM.

        (3) *S. aureus:* A penicillinase-resistant penicillin (e.g., nafcillin, 300 mg/kg/day q2–4h IV) should be given unless the organism is penicillin sensitive, in which case aqueous penicillin G, 300,000 U/kg/day q2–4h IV, should be used. In severely ill patients, gentamicin, 4.5–7.5 mg/kg/day q8h, may be added for the first 7–10 days.

    d. Drug therapy is individualized on the basis of the organism's in vitro sensitivities and the results of serum bactericidal tests. A serum bactericidal level of 1:8 or greater at the time of peak antibiotic concentration is desirable. Although subjective improvement (in appetite, for example) may be prompt, fever can remain elevated for several days to weeks after initiation of antibiotic therapy.

    e. In general, the duration of antibiotic therapy is 4 weeks.

    f. In addition to a daily physical examination, the erythrocyte sedimentation rate and urinalyses are useful parameters to follow.

    g. Recurrent manifestations attributed to embolization and associated vasculitis do not necessarily indicate failure of antibiotic therapy.

    h. Surgical replacement of the infected valve, when indicated, may be lifesaving. The indications for surgery in endocarditis are actively evolving but reflect either clinical deterioration or persistent infection.

5. Prevention of endocarditis Prophylactic antibiotic regimens are outlined in Table 15-11. The choice of regimen should be individualized according to the risk of the underlying heart disease and the risk of the procedure. The regimens requiring parenteral administration of potentially toxic antibiotics should be reserved for high-risk situations.

    a. Patients with prosthetic heart valves or grafts are at highest risk; patients with rheumatic heart disease are also at high risk; congenital heart diseases such as ventricular septal defect, atrial septal defect, patent ductus arteriosus, and the "click-murmur" syndrome are at lower risk.

    b. High-risk procedures are dental manipulations, especially surgery and tooth extractions in patients with poor oral hygiene, and manipulations of infected genitourinary tract, especially when enterococci are present. Procedures such as bronchoscopy, endoscopy, proctosigmoidoscopy, barium enemas, and liver biopsies may be associated with bacteremia but have a lower risk.

T. Tuberculosis (TB)

1. Etiology *M. tuberculosis* is the infecting organism.

2. Evaluation

    a. Clinical manifestations of childhood TB include

        (1) Persistent cough, pulmonary infiltrates, and pleural effusion or enlarged hilar nodes.

        (2) Chronic draining otitis media, cervical adenopathy.

        (3) Aseptic meningitis.

        (4) Occult fever, failure to thrive, weight loss, and anemia or hepatosplenomegaly.

        (5) Aseptic pyuria.

        (6) Monoarticular arthritis, dactylitis, back pain, or bony tenderness.

    b. Screening In the United States, approximately 0–2 percent of 5-year-old children and 0–7 percent of adolescents have been infected as determined by positive skin tests. Without treatment, overt disease will develop in 5–15 percent of infected children within 5 years. For screening, the tine test is adequate, but an intermediate strength PPD (5 TU) is indicated for patients whose tine tests are positive or who are suspected of having TB.

    c. When TB is suspected, a detailed inquiry into possible contacts with persons with active TB, an intermediate strength PPD (5 U) and a chest x-ray are essential.

    d. Atypical mycobacteria can cause cervical adenitis or (uncommonly) pulmonary infection. These strains are often resistant to conventional TB therapy. Specific skin test antigens are available. Atypical strains may cross-react with intermediate strength PPD, but the reaction is usually less than 10 mm unless infection is recent.

e. In the presence of a positive skin test and chest x-ray, the following should be done:

(1) Obtain and culture three **gastric** aspirates in the morning, immediately on the patient's awakening.

(2) Culture three **first-voided** morning urine collections.

(3) **Liver function tests** A liver biopsy, or bone marrow biopsy, may be necessary if miliary disease is suspected. A pleural biopsy should be performed in patients with pleural effusions.

f. In the presence of neurologic abnormalities, **CSF examination**, including culture and acid-fast stain, is necessary.

g. In proved cases of TB, **skin tests and chest x-rays of family members and contacts** are indicated.

3. **Diagnosis**

a. The demonstration of acid-fast bacilli in exudate or tissue is the most direct method of diagnosis. The judicious use of needle biopsy specimens of pleura, liver, or bone marrow often yields the diagnosis.

b. The culture may not become positive for 3–6 weeks, but a presumptive diagnosis of TB is often made on the basis of the clinical presentation, epidemiologic history, and skin test reactivity to tuberculin antigen. Induration greater than or equal to 10 mm from an intermediate strength PPD generally indicates prior infection with the tuberculosis bacillus (symptomatic or asymptomatic).

4. **Therapy** See also Table 15-12, p. 354.

a. **Asymptomatic converter** (positive skin test with a negative chest x-ray): oral isoniazid, 5–10 mg/kg (maximum of 300 mg) once daily for 1 year. Follow-up chest x-rays are obtained at 3–6 month intervals and again on completion of therapy.

b. **Primary nonprogressive pulmonary TB (including an effusion) and cervical adenitis:** oral isoniazid, 10 mg/kg once daily, and para-aminosalicylic acid (PAS), 0.2–0.3 gm/day, or rifampin (10–20 mg/kg/day). Ethambutol, 15 mg/kg/day, is given in place of PAS for patients over 13 years of age. The major side effect of ethambutol is optic neuritis (blurred vision, color blindness, visual field alteration), which is difficult to monitor in younger children.

c. Tuberculous meningitis, progressive pulmonary disease, miliary tuberculosis, and other forms of extrapulmonary tuberculosis. Isoniazid, 15 mg/kg/day, and, initially, streptomycin, 20–40 mg/kg/day, to 1 gm/day. After a satisfactory clinical response has occurred (minimum of 6–12 weeks), streptomycin is replaced by PAS or ethambutol. Therapy is continued for a minimum of 24 months. Initially, critically ill patients with meningitis should receive triple therapy (isoniazid, streptomycin, and rifampin).

d. If the isolated *M. tuberculosis* is resistant in vitro to isoniazid, rifampin, 10–20 mg/kg/day PO, given ½–1 hr before breakfast, is usually added to the regimen, and the dosage of isoniazid is increased to 20 mg/kg/day (up to 600 mg/day).

e. The infant of a tuberculous mother is given BCG vaccination and/or isoniazid. BCG is indicated when close medical supervision of the infant in the first year of life cannot be guaranteed. Isoniazid for 1 year is probably effective, but its potential neurotoxicity must be borne in mind.

f. Members of the household of a patient with active tuberculosis are given isoniazid, 5–10 mg once daily for 1 year, regardless of tuberculin status. Periodic tuberculin tests should be done and chest x-ray films taken in such cases.

g. Pyridoxine, 25–50 mg once daily, is indicated in children over 8 years of age and in children receiving high-dose isoniazid (more than 40 mg/kg/day).

h. Corticosteroids given in conjunction with antimicrobial therapy may lessen the inflammatory complications of tuberculous pericarditis, peritonitis, and possibly meningitis. They may also indicate when large hilar lymph nodes are obstructing the passage of air and when severe respiratory distress complicates diffuse pulmonary tuberculosis.

i. Isoniazid treatment commonly causes a transient asymptomatic elevation of liver enzymes during the first 3 months of therapy. The physician should be alert to signs and symptoms of overt hepatitis and discontinue the drug if they appear.

U. Venereal disease   See also Chap. 13.

1. Gonorrhea   The infecting organism is *N. gonorrhoeae*.

   a. Evaluation

     (1) In **males,** urethral specimens can be obtained by stripping the penis.

     (2) In **females,** pelvic examination allows the physician to evaluate cervical and adnexal tenderness as well as obtain culture material from the cervix.

     (3) The rectum and pharynx should be cultured in both males and females for *N. gonorrhoeae*.

     (4) *N. gonorrhoeae* is relatively fastidious, and specimens should be cultured promptly and placed in a high CO_2 atmosphere (e.g., candlejar). Transgrow medium is an excellent transport medium for *N. gonorrhoeae* and should be used when direct cultures are not practical.

     (5) A serologic test for syphilis should be performed in all patients with gonorrhea (see **2**).

     (6) The disease is seen with increasing frequency in children *under* 12 years.

   b. Diagnosis   *N. gonorrhoeae* is identified by demonstration of gram-negative diplococci on gram-stained smears of urethral discharge or by culture of appropriate specimens on Thayer-Martin media. Smears of cervical mucus are not reliable.

   c. Treatment   Treatment is outlined in Table 15-13. Case contact finding as well as sex education and counseling are as important as the drug therapy.

2. Syphilis   The infecting organism is *Treponema pallidum*.

a. Evaluation and diagnosis See also Chap. 5.

(1) Dark-field examination of skin lesions (chancre or rash). The material is infectious and should be handled with care.

(2) Serologic tests for syphilis are usually nonreactive when the chancre first appears, but become reactive during the following 1–4 weeks. Biologic false-positive test with nonspecific antigens (VDRL, RPRCT, Wasserman, Hinton, Kolmer) may be caused by a variety of other illnesses and should be confirmed by tests specific for *T. pallidum* (FTA-ABS, TPI).

b. Therapy for syphilis is outlined in Table 15-14. Case contact findings, as well as sex education and counseling, are as important as the drug therapy. Child abuse must be investigated in cases involving younger children.

V. Candidiasis

1. Etiology *C. albicans* is the most common pathogen, but other species, including *C. tropicalis, C. krusei, C. parapsilosis, C. guillermondii,* and *Torulopsis glabrata,* may also cause invasive disease.

2. Evaluation

a. Cultures of the blood, urine, oropharynx, and stool.

b. Gram stain of mucosal lesions.

c. If esophageal involvement is suspected, a barium swallow and esophagoscopy (with biopsy and culture of lesions) are most helpful.

d. If disseminated disease is suspected, the ocular fundi and skin should be carefully examined. Cardiac ultrasound and lumbar puncture may be indicated.

3. Diagnosis The demonstration of yeasts and pseudohyphae in scrapings of skin or mucosal lesions or tissue specimens is diagnostic. Repeated isolation of *Candida* from the blood suggests endocarditis, an infected intravascular device (e.g., hyperalimentation line), or disseminated candidiasis.

4. Treatment Duration of therapy depends on severity of disease and speed of response.

a. GI disease may respond to oral nystatin therapy, 500,000 U q1–4 h. For oral and esophageal lesions, use of the oral tablets or lozenges is superior to the suspension.

b. Disseminated infection, endocarditis, and **meningitis** should be treated with full doses of amphotericin B (1.0 mg/kg/day). Fluorocytosine 150 mg/kg/day may be added in seriously ill patients, but only if the organism is sensitive to this agent.

c. Candidal infection restricted to the bladder may respond to continuous irrigation with amphotericin B (maximum dose of 1 mg/kg/day in sterile **distilled water**). Infection restricted to the bladder or kidney may also be treated with 5-fluorocytosine alone.

W. Cryptococcosis

1. Etiology The causative organism is *C. neoformans.*

2. Evaluation

a. History Respiratory symptoms and subtle neurologic symptoms, including headache and diplopia.

Table 15-13 Recommended Treatment Schedules for Gonococcal Infections

Type	Drugs of Choice	Dosage	Alternatives
Anogenital and urethral	Tetracycline HCl *or*	500 mg oral qid × 5 days	Spectinomycin (2 grams IM once)
	Penicillin G procaine	4.8 million U IM divided into 2 sites at one visit	Cefoxitin (2 grams IM once)
	plus		*plus* probenecid (1 gram oral)
	probenecid, *or*	1 gram oral	
	Amoxicillin[a]	3 grams oral[b]	
	plus probenecid	1 gram oral	
Pharyngeal	Tetracycline HCl *or*	as for anogenital	
	Penicillin G procaine	as for anogenital	
	plus probenecid		
Pelvic inflammatory disease	Tetracycline HCl *or*	500 mg oral qid × 10 days	
	Penicillin G procaine	as for anogenital	
	plus probenecid		
	followed by amoxicillin[a] *or*	500 mg oral qid × 10 days	
	Amoxicillin[a]	3 grams oral[b]	
	plus probenecid	1 gram oral	
	followed by amoxicillin[a]	500 mg oral qid × 10 days	
Acute epididymitis	Tetracycline HCl *or*	500 mg oral qid × 10 days	
	Penicillin G procaine	as for anogenital	
	plus probenecid		
	followed by amoxicillin[a] *or*	500 mg oral qid × 10 days	
	Amoxicillin[a]	3 grams oral[b]	
	plus probenecid	1 gram oral	
	followed by amoxicillin[a]	500 mg oral qid × 10 days	
Bacteremia and arthritis	Penicillin G crystalline	10 million U IV daily × 3 days	Tetracycline (500 mg oral qid × 7 days)
	followed by amoxicillin[a]	500 mg oral qid for 4 additional days	Spectinomycin (2 grams IM bid × 3 days)
			Erythromycin (500 mg oral qid × 7 days)

Neonatal		
Ophthalmia	Penicillin G crystalline *plus* saline irrigation	50,000 U/kg/day IV in 2 doses × 7 days
Arthritis and septicemia	Penicillin G crystalline	75,000 to 100,000 U/kg/day IV in 2 or 3 doses × 7 days
Meningitis	Penicillin G crystalline	100,000 U/kg/day IV in 3 or 4 doses for at least 10 days
Children (under 45 kg)		
Anogenital, urethral, or pharyngitis	Amoxicillin *plus* probenecid, *or* Penicillin G procaine *plus* probenecid	50 mg/kg oral once 25 mg/kg (max. 1 gram) 100,000 U/kg IM once 25 mg/kg (max. 1 gram)	Spectinomycin (40 mg/kg IM once) Tetracycline (over 8 years old) (40 mg/kg/day oral in 4 divided doses × 5 days)
Ophthalmia	Penicillin G crystalline *plus* saline irrigation	100,000 U/kg/day IV × 7 days	
Arthritis	Penicillin G crystalline	100,000 U/kg/day IV × 7 days	Tetracycline (over 8 years old) (40 mg/kg/day oral in 4 divided doses × 7 days) Erythromycin (50 mg/kg oral in 4 divided doses × 7 days)
Meningitis	Penicillin G crystalline	250,000 U/kg/day IV in 6 divided doses for at least 10 days	Chloramphenicol (100 mg/kg IV/day for at least 10 days)

[a] Or ampicillin.
[b] Or 3.5 grams ampicillin.
Modified from *Med. Lett. Drugs Ther.* 21(16):68, 1979. Issue 537.

Table 15-14 Recommended Treatment Schedules for Syphilis*

Stage	Choice	Dosage	Alternatives
Early (primary, secondary, or latent less than one year)	Penicillin G benzathine *or* Penicillin G procaine	2.4 million U IM once 600,000 U IM/day × 8 days	Tetracycline HCl (500 mg oral qid for 15 days) Erythromycin (500 mg oral qid for 15 days)
Late (more than one year's duration, cardiovascular)	Penicillin G procaine *or* Penicillin G benzathine	600,000 U IM/day × 15 days 2.4 million U IM weekly for 3 doses	Tetracycline HCl (500 mg oral qid for 30 days) Erythromycin (500 mg oral qid for 30 days)
Neurosyphilis	Penicillin G crystalline *or* Penicillin G procaine *or* Penicillin G benzathine	2 to 4 million U IV q4h for 10 days 600,000 U IM/day × 15 days 2.4 million U IM weekly for 3 doses	Tetracycline HCl (500 mg oral qid for 30 days) Erythromycin (500 mg oral qid for 30 days)

Congenital
  CSF normal
  CSF abnormal
	Penicillin G benzathine
	Penicillin G crystalline *or* Penicillin G procaine
		50,000 U/kg IM once
		25,000 U/kg IM or IV bid for at least 10 days
		50,000 U/kg IM daily for at least 10 days	

* Modified from "Handbook of Antimicrobial Therapy." *The Medical Letter on Drugs and Therapeutics.* Revised Edition Supplement 19:26, 1978

b. CSF examination, including India ink preparation, culture for fungus, and cryptococcal antigen test. Culture yields are improved by culturing a large volume of CSF.

c. Sputum and urine culture for fungus.

d. Cryptococcal antigen test on the serum and urine.

e. Chest x-ray; occasionally, a lung biopsy is necessary.

3. Diagnosis The presence of cryptococcal antigen in CSF, serum, or urine or a "positive" India ink smear strongly suggests the diagnosis. The diagnosis is established by the growth of cryptococci from CSF or lung tissue.

4. Treatment

a. Cryptococcal meningitis may be treated with a combination of amphotericin B, 0.3 mg/kg/day, and 5-fluorocytosine, 150 mg/kg/day for 6 weeks. Patients with severe marrow impairment in whom further marrow suppression from 5-fluorocytosine may develop may be treated with amphotericin B alone (1 mg/kg/day) to a total dose of 2 or 3 gm.

b. Treatment should be monitored with weekly examination of the CSF by culture and India ink smear and for cryptococcal antigen concentration. Cultures should become sterile promptly. Microscopy should show a decrease in the number of organisms, and antigen testing should show at least a fourfold decrease in level during treatment.

c. After completion of treatment, the CSF should be examined q2–3 months for 1 year to detect relapses.

5. Cryptococcal pneumonia, in the absence of dissemination to the CNS, may not require therapy unless it is progressive.

X. Invasive aspergillosis

1. Etiology A variety of *Aspergillus* species are pathogenic in humans, the most common being *A. fumigatus.*

2. Evaluation

a. Careful examination for sinusitis, necrotic nasal lesions, pneumonia, pleuritic pain, and necrotizing skin lesions.

b. X-rays of the sinuses and chest.

c. Direct microscopic examination and **culture of sputum** and **biopsy specimens from suspected sites.** Early diagnosis is essential, and biopsies should be performed promptly.

3. Diagnosis

a. Demonstration of septate fungal mycelium 3–4 μ in diameter with acute angle branching in tissues is diagnostic of invasive aspergillosis.

b. A chest x-ray showing a ball within a cavity is suggestive of aspergilloma.

4. The **treatment** for invasive aspergillosis is amphotericin B, 1 mg/kg/day, and surgical débridement of cutaneous and sinus lesions. In severely ill patients, 5-fluorocytosine or rifampin may be added.

V. ANTIVIRAL THERAPY

A. Principles

1. Viruses are obligate intracellular parasites that depend on the host cell for growth and replication. Clinically useful antiviral agents must act at stages of infection or replication involving virus-specific metabolic activities. Relatively few of these activities are recognized, and there are correspondingly few opportunities for selective chemotherapy (see **B.3**).

2. The **toxicity** of antiviral drugs is due to the same mechanism of action that produces the antiviral effect.

B. Antiviral agents in clinical use

1. **Amantidine** combines with plasma membrane and inhibits penetration and uncoating of virus.

   a. **Antiviral spectrum** Active against influenza A strains H_2N_2 (Asian) and H_3N_2 (Hong Kong) as well as the newer H_1N_1 (Russian) strains but not against influenza B.

   b. **Pharmacology** Complete absorption from the GI tract, with peak blood levels at 1–4 hr after an oral dose. Amantadine is excreted unmetabolized in the urine and has a half-life of 12–24 hr.

   c. **Adverse effects** Amantadine is well tolerated in children but may cause CNS symptoms. Adverse reactions are more likely in patients receiving concomitant anticholinergics or antihistamines or having impaired renal function.

2. **Idoxuridine (IUdR) (Stoxil)** slows DNA synthesis by inhibition of DNA polymerase and of enzymes necessary for thymidine synthesis. In addition, DNA replication is abnormal.

   a. **Antiviral spectrum** IUdR is active in **herpetic** keratitis, although there is *no* antiviral effect in **adenoviral** keratoconjunctivitis.

   b. **Pharmacology** It is *not* effective when administered parenterally because of rapid degradation (half-life 30 min). There is no absorption of the topical preparation.

   c. **Adverse effects** Topical use in the treatment of herpetic keratitis can result in corneal ulcers, local allergic reactions, and emergence of drug-resistant viruses.

3. **Adenosine arabinoside** (vidarabine, ara-A) (Vira-A) inhibits virus-specific DNA polymerase.

   a. **Antiviral spectrum** Ara-A has in vitro activity against many of the herpesviruses, vaccinia, and certain other viruses (e.g., hepatitis B virus). The drug is licensed only for the treatment of **herpetic keratitis** and **herpes simplex encephalitis.**

   b. **Pharmacology** Ara-A is poorly soluble (0.5 mg/ml) in aqueous solution and, when administered parenterally, must be given in a large volume of fluid. It is rapidly deaminated, and is then excreted in the urine. The 3% ophthalmic preparation is not absorbed into the anterior chamber unless there is severe corneal ulceration.

   c. **Adverse effects** Parenteral administration can produce nausea and vomiting, weight loss, megaloblastosis, thrombocytopenia, and leukopenia. Encephalopathy with tremors, confusion, and abnormal electroencephalographic findings can occur.

C. Treatment of viral disease

1. Herpes simplex virus encephalitis

a. Etiology Usually, herpes simplex virus (HSV type 1; rarely, HSV type II).

b. Evaluation

(1) The **history** often includes olfactory hallucinations, headache, and confusion.

(2) **Physical examination** may reveal focal neurologic signs.

(3) A brain scan, EEG, and computerized axial tomography will usually reveal a focal defect, most often in the temporal lobe(s).

(4) An **accurate** diagnosis requires isolation of virus from a **brain biopsy specimen.**

(5) **Immunofluorescence assays** for HSV antigen on frozen brain sections are less sensitive than viral cultures, but can result in an earlier diagnosis.

(6) Although helpful, clinical signs, orofacial HSV infection, or even rising antibody titers are *not* diagnostic.

c. Therapy

(1) Careful attention to the management of increased intracranial pressure and to the treatment of the comatose patient is essential (see Chap. 2, p. 43). Dexamethasone or other adrenocorticotropic hormones **should not be used** unless other therapeutic agents fail.

(2) **Adenine arabinoside**

(a) The **dosage** is 15 mg/kg/day, given by slow IV infusion over 12 hr for 10 days.

(b) A brain biopsy specimen must be obtained for virus culture **prior to initiation of therapy.** Therapy should be discontinued if the culture is negative after 5 days.

(c) The low solubility of the drug in aqueous solution requires suspension of each milligram in at least 2 ml of 5% D/W or a salt solution. Fluid overload should be avoided.

(d) The white cell, platelet, and reticulocyte counts should be followed.

2. Herpes simplex keratoconjunctivitis   See p. 545.

3. Mucocutaneous and orofacial herpes simplex   See p. 534.

4. Herpes zoster, disseminated zoster, and disseminated varicella

a. Etiology Herpes zoster and varicella (chickenpox) are caused by varicella zoster virus (VZV). The reactivation of VZV months or years after chickenpox occurs in a dorsal spinal or cranial nerve ganglion, with spread to the appropriate cutaneous dermatome and occasionally to distant sites. Spread of infection to visceral organs (disseminated zoster or chickenpox) is usually due to underlying immunodeficiency.

b. Evaluation and diagnosis

(1) In zoster patients, the **history** should exclude other causes of localized vesicular disease.

(2) Physical examination should include careful inspection for the number and character of vesicles and for evidence of complications such as bacterial superinfection, cutaneous dissemination, tenderness in the abdomen or liver, and paresis of the muscles in the involved area (e.g., urinary retention). When cranial nerve V is involved, vesicles on the top of the nose (innervated by the nasociliary branch) suggest the possibility of keratoconjunctivitis and/or uveitis.

(3) A Tzanck preparation is done to look for the presence of multinucleated giant cells. Without a viral culture, the diagnosis of herpes zoster is not completely reliable, since herpes simplex virus can also cause dermatomal involvement.

(4) In immunosuppressed persons, the tempo of disease and extent of viral spread should be determined by periodic pox counts, serial chest x-rays, serum liver enzyme analyses, and CNS examinations.

c. Treatment

(1) Wet-to-dry soaks are applied to involved dermatomes tid using Burow's solution to facilitate débridement. Superinfection is treated with a semisynthetic oral penicillin and topical antibiotics.

(2) Pain symptoms are treated appropriately (see Chap. 1, p. 6). Since postherpetic neuralgia is not a problem in children, there is *no indication* for systemic corticosteroids.

(3) When **cranial nerve V** is involved, referral to an ophthalmologist is indicated.

(4) Scopolamine eyedrops (0.3%) are used to produce **mydriasis** and **cycloplegia.** Corticosteroid drops are indicated when **interstitial keratitis** or **uveitis** is present (in the absence of dendritic keratitis).

(5) Disseminated skin vesicles of previously healthy persons can occur in 10 percent. This does not indicate adverse prognosis and need not be treated.

(6) In the immunosuppressed person, the presence of fever, rapidly increasing numbers of new vesicles, failure of vesicle maturation, elevation of serum liver pancreatic enzymes, and onset of respiratory or CNS symptoms are indications for experimental treatment with adenine arabinoside (10 mg/kg/day) or with the newer antizoster drugs. **There is no indication for the use of zoster immunoglobulin or plasma.**

(7) Broad-spectrum antibiotics are indicated in the febrile neutropenic patient (see **b,** p. 331 and **2,** p. 336).

(8) Hospital contacts of patients with zoster or chickenpox who have no history of prior chickenpox or whose VZV immunofluorescent antibody tests are negative must be isolated in the hospital, discharged, or kept away from work from the eighth to twenty-first day after exposure.

(9) Immunosuppressed children who have not had chickenpox should receive varicella-zoster immunoglobulin (see Table 15-10) or zoster immune plasma (10 ml/kg) following close exposure to zoster or chickenpox.

5. Hepatitis See Chap. 11 discussion of hepatic failure.

a. **Etiology** Hepatitis is due to a wide range of viruses. In addition to hepatitis A (infectious hepatitis), hepatitis B (serum hepatitis), and antibody, *Toxoplasma* antibody.

  (1) Congenital infection (see also **A**, p. 136): TORCH series.

  (2) Exposure to small animals: *Leptospira* culture (blood, urine, and/or antibody), *Toxoplasma* antibody.

b. **Treatment**

  (1) There is no specific therapy for viral hepatitis.

  (2) Prophylactic immune serum globulin should be given to household contacts of patients with **hepatitis A,** and hepatitis B immunoglobulin should be given to needle-stick contacts of **hepatitis B** patients (see Table 15-11).

  (3) The patient with hepatitis should be monitored initially at weekly intervals and later at monthly intervals for evidence of resolution of the disease. If liver enzymes remain markedly elevated after 3 months, the patient should be evaluated by liver biopsy for evidence of chronic disease. In hepatitis B, a small proportion of patients will remain HBsAg positive after 3 months. These patients should be followed closely for evidence of chronic hepatitis.

16

Parasitic Infections

Infections with protozoa and helminths are subject to rational principles of diagnosis and therapy. Most parasitic infections occur in temperate as well as tropical environments. Their incidence varies with climate, sanitation, and socioeconomic conditions. The frequency with which the clinician in temperate areas encounters parasitic infections is increasing, both as a result of intercontinental travel and the use of immunosuppressive agents.

I. **PRINCIPLES OF DIAGNOSIS** The diagnostic features of common parasitic infections are summarized in Table 16-1.

A. **General**

1. **The diagnosis of parasitic infection can rarely be made on clinical grounds alone.** The clinical picture in many parasitic infections may be identical, and different clinical presentations may be produced by a single parasite. In addition, parasitic infections are often asymptomatic or produce only mild symptoms. Commonly, a diagnosis of parasitic infection is suspected only because of an abnormal, unexpected laboratory finding.

2. **The diagnosis of most helminthic or protozoal infections requires the demonstration of the parasite in body excreta, fluids, or tissue.**

3. Many parasites have an intricate route of migration through the human host and affect several organs successively or simultaneously. The choice of appropriate diagnostic techniques and materials thus rests on some understanding of the life cycles of the possible infecting agents.

4. Knowledge of the **geographic distribution** of parasitic infections and their **mode of acquisition** and **means of spread** often aids diagnosis and therapy. Detailed information is available from standard parasitology texts.

5. **Patients commonly harbor several parasites.** A complete evaluation must be made to avoid overlooking the most important infecting species in each clinical setting.

B. **Hematologic changes in parasitic infections**

1. **Erythrocytes** Anemia is an inconstant and nonspecific finding in most parasitic infections. It reflects the general nutritional status of the patient rather than any direct effect of the infecting parasite. Iron deficiency anemia in hookworm disease and hemolytic anemia in malaria are exceptions.

2. **Eosinophils**

a. Eosinophilia is often the first clue to the presence of a **helminth** infection. **Protozoa,** conversely, do *not* evoke an eosinophilia. The finding of eosinophilia in amebiasis, malaria, toxoplasmosis, or giardiasis suggests an additional helminth infection.

Table 16-1 Diagnostic Features of Commonly Encountered Parasitic Infections

Disease	Mode of Spread	Location in Man	Clinical Features	Laboratory Diagnosis	Eosino-philia*	Remarks
Roundworms (nematodes)						
Ascariasis	Fecal-oral	Adult: small intestine; Larvae: lung	Vague abdominal distress; cough and pneumonia during lung migration	Eggs in feces	Usually mild; moderate to marked during migration	Aberrant wanderings may cause clinical disease
Hookworm	Larvae in soil, skin penetration	Small intestine	Vague abdominal distress; anemia in severe infections	Eggs in feces	Mild to moderate	Distinguish infection from disease
Whipworm	Fecal-oral	Large intestine	Rarely symptomatic	Eggs in feces	Absent to mild	
Strongyloidiasis	Larvae in soil; skin penetration	Upper small intestine	Duodenitis; hyperinfection syndrome rarely	Larvae in *fresh stool*; duodenal aspirate	Moderate to marked	
Pinworm	Fecal-oral	Large intestine, perianal area	Perianal pruritis	Scotch-tape swab for eggs; gross examination of area for worms	Absent	Very common; usually asymptomatic
Creeping eruption (cutaneous larva migrans)	Larvae in soil; skin penetration (larvae from dog, cat feces)	Skin	Intensely pruritic, serpiginous skin lesions	Physical examination	Variable	
Visceral larva migrans	Fecal-oral, via pica (eggs from	Liver, lung, muscle	Fever, hepatosplenomegaly	Clinical diagnosis	Marked	

	Mode of infection	Site	Symptoms	Diagnosis	Eosinophilia	Geographic distribution
Trichinosis	Ingestion of undercooked pork	Striated muscle	Fever, diarrhea, periorbital edema, muscle pain	Biopsy of muscle, skin; serologic tests	Marked	
Tapeworms (cestodes)						
Beef tapeworm	Ingestion of undercooked beef	Small intestine	Asymptomatic	Proglottid segments passed with feces	Absent	
Pork tapeworm	Ingestion of undercooked pork	Small intestine	Asymptomatic; rare autoinfection with CNS symptoms (cysticercosis)	Proglottid segments passed with feces	Absent	
Hydatid disease	Fecal-oral (eggs from carnivore feces)	Liver, lung, bone, brain	Usually asymptomatic; occasionally, pressure symptoms in affected organ	Removal of cyst; skin and serologic tests	Variable	
Flukes (trematodes)						
Schistosoma mansoni	Cercarial in streams; skin penetration	Venules of large intestine	Fever, colitis, hepatomegaly, portal hypertension	Eggs in feces; rectal biopsy	Moderate to marked	Africa, S. America; common in Puerto Ricans
Schistosoma haematobium	Same	Venules of urinary bladder	Fever, malaise, hematuria	Eggs in urine; bladder or rectal biopsy	Moderate to marked	Africa
Schistosoma japonicum	Same	Venules of small intestine	Fever, malaise, abdominal pain, diarrhea, hepatomegaly	Eggs in feces; rectal biopsy	Moderate to marked	S.E. Asia
Protozoa						
Intestinal amebiasis	Fecal-oral	Lumen and wall of large intestine	Bloody diarrhea, fever, abdomi...	Trophozoites in fresh stool or...	Absent	

Table 16-1 (Continued)

Disease	Mode of Spread	Location in Man	Clinical Features	Laboratory Diagnosis	Eosinophilia*	Remarks
			nal pain; mild, intermittent GI symptoms	proctoscopic material, cysts in stool		
Extraintestinal amebiasis	Fecal-oral	Liver, lung	Hepatomegaly, fever	Trophozoites from abscess or sputum; serologic tests	Absent	
Giardiasis	Fecal-oral	Upper small intestine	Diarrhea, abdominal pain, malabsorption	Cysts and trophozoites in *fresh stool*; duodenal aspirate	Absent	
Toxoplasmosis	Congenital, raw meat, cat feces (?)	All organs, blood, reticuloendothelial system	Congenital, acute mononucleosis-like illness, asymptomatic	Biopsy; serologic tests	Absent	
Malaria	Bite of infected *Anopheles* mosquito; transfusion rarely	Erythrocytes, reticuloendothelial system	Fever, splenomegaly, anemia, collapse, encephalopathy with *P. falciparum*	Repeated blood smears	Absent	Important to distinguish *P. falciparum* from relapsing malarias
Pneumocystosis	Unknown	Lungs	Fever, cough, dyspnea, lung infiltrates in compromised host	Sputum; bronchial brushings; lung biopsy	Absent	Compromised host

*W[...]

b. The level of eosinophilia is of diagnostic aid. In general, tissue-living helminths evoke a profound eosinophilia, and those that exist within the lumen of the bowel evoke a mild eosinophilia or none at all (Table 16-1).

C. Direct identification of parasites Many techniques are available to identify parasites in excreta, fluids, and tissue. Examination of specimens is usually done by hospital, public health, or private laboratories. However, there are several simple procedures, requiring little equipment, that the physician can perform when the patient is seen. It is helpful to have charts of diagnostic stages of helminths and protozoa available for accurate interpretation. If more sophisticated procedures are needed, standard texts of parasitology can be consulted.

1. Blood

a. The **thin dry smear** is useful in detecting malarial parasites. The technique is identical to routine blood smears used for hematologic studies. Wright's or Giemsa stain is used in the usual fashion, and parasites are seen within red blood cells. Species differentiation is of therapeutic importance once malaria parasites have been identified.

b. The **thick dry smear** for the detection of malaria parasites yields a much higher concentration of parasites than the thin smear and thus is useful when the parasites are few and thin smears are negative. However, the thick smear is harder to interpret, since the erythrocytes are lysed, and the parasites are seen on a background of stained proteinaceous debris. The technique is as follows:

(1) Spread a drop of blood on a clean microscope slide, using an applicator or corner of another slide. (The smear should be about the diameter of a dime and of a thickness sufficient to allow for transparency when the hemoglobin is removed.)

(2) Allow the smear to dry for 1–2 hr at 37°C.

(3) Cover the slide with distilled water until the color of the hemoglobin has disappeared.

(4) Dry the slide and cover it with Wright's stain as for routine blood smears, or with dilute Giemsa stain for 45 min.

(5) Examine for parasites under the oil immersion lens.

2. Stool Examine feces as soon after passage as possible and before barium or cathartics are given. Helminth ova and protozoal cysts can be identified in older specimens, but the identification of free-living, motile forms requires the examination of **freshly passed, warm stool.**

a. Direct examination of stool enables the rapid identification of intestinal parasites. Free-living, motile forms and ova and cysts can be identified, particularly if there is a heavy infestation. The procedure takes a few minutes and makes use of supplies found in all laboratories.

(1) Examine the specimen grossly for flecks of blood and mucus. If present, take a sample from these areas.

(2) Place a match-head-size sample on each of two microscope slides with a wooden applicator.

(3) Mix one sample with 2 drops of saline and cover with coverslip.

(4) Add 2 drops of dilute iodine solution to the other sample, mix, and cover similarly.

      (5) Observe for the presence of erythrocytes and leukocytes. **Erythro cytes** suggest amebic colitis, and **leukocytes,** bacterial infection o inflammatory bowel disease and *not* parasitic infection.

      (6) Examine the stained slide for the presence of helminth eggs unde low power and for protozoal cysts under high power and oil im mersion.

      (7) Examine the unstained slide under low and high power for th presence of motile organisms (ameba, trophozoites, larvae).

  b. Concentration A number of techniques are available for examinatio of larger quantities of feces for parasites. The formalin-ether tech nique will concentrate ova and cysts more than 20 times. It is pe formed as follows:

      (1) Emulsify 1–2 gm of feces in 10 ml of a 10% formalin-saline solutio

      (2) Strain through gauze into a tapered centrifuge tube.

      (3) Add 3 ml of ether and shake vigorously for 1 min.

      (4) Centrifuge at 2000 rpm for 3 min.

      (5) Four distinct layers will appear. Loosen and decant off the uppe three layers.

      (6) Examine the deposit for ova and cysts.

  c. Quantitation In certain helminthic infections, estimation of the wor burden by quantitation of egg excretion is of great importance. Th method of Stoll is commonly employed (D. L. Belding, *Textbook c Parasitology* [3rd ed.], New York, Appleton-Century-Crofts, 1965).

  d. Scotch-tape examination is a useful and simple technique for the dem onstration of pinworm eggs.

      (1) Evert a strip of Scotch tape, gummed side outward, on the edge a tongue blade.

      (2) Dab the perianal area first thing in the morning.

      (3) Place on a microscope slide, sticky side down, on a drop of toluene.

      (4) Examine under low power for characteristic eggs.

D. Serologic tests in parasitic diseases

  1. Immunodiagnostic tests are helpful in several parasitic infections. The are to be used and interpreted **in conjunction with** clinical and laborator evaluation and should not be solely relied on for diagnosis.

  2. The tests are specifically helpful in invasive amebiasis, trichinosi toxoplasmosis, and echinococcosis.

  3. The serologic tests referred to in Table 16-1 are performed at the Cente for Disease Control, Atlanta, Georgia, and by some local health depart ments.

II. PRINCIPLES OF TREATMENT See Table 16-2.

  A. Protozoal infections are always treated. The principles of treatment consi of the identification of the responsible parasite and the selection of a appropriate therapeutic agent, administered in appropriate dosage (se Tables 16-2 and 16-3). For the efficacy of therapeutic agents and their e pected side effects, see Tables 16-2 and 16-3.

B. **Helminthic infections are not always treated.** After identifying the causative parasite, the clinician must weigh several additional factors before initiating treatment. These include

   1. The number of worms harbored by the patient and the life span of the infecting worm(s)

   2. The likelihood and seriousness of personal and public health complications resulting from infection

   3. The availability and efficacy of therapeutic agents and their expected side effects and toxicity (Table 16-3)

C. Treatment must be individualized and arbitrary rules avoided.

D. **Follow-up clinical and laboratory assessment** is always indicated to determine if treatment has been efficacious. Stools should be examined several weeks after the treatment of intestinal parasites is completed, and re-treatment given if cure has not been achieved. In general, re-treatment with the same drug is more desirable than proceeding to an alternate agent that is more toxic, less efficacious, or both.

E. **Patient education** The physician should always combine treatment with patient education aimed at **prevention** of future parasitic infection. Attention should be given to the environmental circumstances that resulted in the child's acquisition of infection.

III. SPECIFIC PARASITES

A. **Roundworms (nematodes)**

   1. **Ascaris**

      a. **Etiology** Fecal-oral passage of infective ova of *Ascaris lumbricoides*. The human is the only susceptible host. The infection is worldwide in distribution.

      b. **Evaluation and diagnosis** Two distinct clinical phases occur:

         (1) **Transient blood-lung migration phase of the larvae** Pneumonia occurs, with cough, blood-tinged sputum, patchy pulmonary infiltrates, and fever. A marked peripheral eosinophilia is typical. Characteristic larvae may be found in the sputum.

         (2) **Prolonged intestinal phase of the adults** The patient is usually asymptomatic, although vague abdominal discomfort may occur. On rare occasions, more serious manifestations may occur, including intestinal obstruction, appendicitis, and regurgitation and aspiration of wandering adult worms.

         (3) The **diagnosis** is confirmed by:

            (a) Characteristic ova in feces by direct examination or concentration techniques

            (b) Regurgitation or stool passage of adult worms

            (c) Occasionally, demonstration of adult worms on abdominal x-ray films

      c. **Treatment** The occasional aberrant wanderings of individual worms and subsequent serious consequences require that **all** ascaris infections be treated. Tetrachlorethylene, used in the treatment of hookworm infection, may provoke ascaris wandering. Ascaris intestinal infections should thus be treated first if a combined infection is present and this agent is used.

Table 16-2 Treatment of Common Parasitic Infections

Disease	Parasite	Drug of Choice[a]	Alternate Drugs[a]
Roundworms (nematodes)			
Ascariasis	A. lumbricoides	Pyrantel pamoate	Piperazine citrate, mebendazole
Hookworm	A. duodenale	Mebendazole	Thiabendazole, pyrantel pamoate, bephenium
	N. americanus	Mebendazole	Thiabendazole, pyrantel pamoate
Whipworm	T. trichiuria	Mebendazole	
Strongyloidiasis	S. stercoralis	Thiabendazole	
Pinworm	E. vermicularis	Mebendazole	Pyrvinium pamoate, pyrantel pamoate, piperazine citrate
Creeping eruption	A. braziliense	Thiabendazole	
Visceral larva migrans	T. canis, T. cati	Thiabendazole and treatment with steroids for severe symptoms	
Tapeworms (cestodes)			
Beef tapeworm	T. saginata	Niclosamide	Quinacrine
Pork tapeworm	T. solium	Quinacrine	
Hydatid disease	E. granulosus	None	

Disease	Organism	Drug of Choice	Alternative Drugs
Schistosomiasis	*S. mansoni*	Stibophen	Antimony sodium dimercaptosuccinate Niridazole Lucanthone
	S. haematobium	Niridazole	Stibophen
	S. japonicum	Antimony potassium tartrate	Stibophen
Protozoa			
Intestinal amebiasis (see text)	*E. histolytica*	Metronidazole	Paromomycin, diiodohydroxyquin
Extraintestinal amebiasis	*E. histolytica*	Metronidazole	Above, plus dehydroemetine HCl, chloroquine phosphate
Giardiasis	*G. lamblia*	Quinacrine	Metronidazole, furazolidone
Toxoplasmosis	*T. gondii*	Pyrimethamine plus sulfadiazine	
Malaria (see text)	*P. falciparum*	Chloroquine phosphate	Quinine sulfate, pyrimethamine, sulfadiazine (all for resistant malaria)
	P. vivax, P. ovale, and *P. malariae*	Chloroquine phosphate plus primaquine phosphate	
Pneumocystis pneumonia	*P. carinii*	Trimethoprim-sulfamethoxazole	Pentamidine isethionate[b]

[a] See text for dosages.

[b] Available through Parasitic Drug Service, Parasitic Diseases Branch, Center for Disease Control, 1600 Clifton Road, NE, Atlanta, Ga. 30333.

Table 16-3 Adverse Effects of Antiparasitic Drugs

Drug	Frequent	Infrequent
Antimony potassium tartrate	Cough, vomiting, myalgia, ECG changes	Cardiovascular collapse, hepatic damage
Antimony sodium dimercaptosuccinate (Astiban)	Similar to but less frequent and severe than with antimony potassium tartrate	
Bephenium hydroxynaphthoate (Alcopar[a])	Anorexia, nausea, vomiting	
Chloroquine phosphate (Aralen Phosphate)	Anorexia, nausea, visual disturbances	Retinopathy—only with prolonged, high dosage
Dehydroemetine	Diarrhea, nausea, vomiting, myalgias, ECG changes	Hypotension
Furazolidone (Furoxone)		Anorexia, nausea, hypersensitivity reactions*
Lucanthone HCl (Miracil D)	Anorexia, nausea, vomiting	Convulsions, psychosis (in adults only)
Mebendazole (Vermox)		Diarrhea, abdominal pain
Metronidazole (Flagyl)	Anorexia, nausea, vomiting, metallic taste	Peripheral neuropathy, ataxia, neutropenia*
Niclosamide (Yomesan)		Nausea
Niridazole (Ambilhar)	Anorexia, nausea, vomiting	Convulsions, psychosis (in adults only)
Paromomycin (Humatin)	Anorexia, nausea, vomiting	Nephrotoxicity
Pentamidine isethionate	Dizziness, tachycardia, headache, vomiting, hypotension	Nephrotoxicity, hepatotoxicity
Piperazine citrate (Antepar)		Anorexia, rash, ataxia
Primaquine phosphate	Anorexia, nausea	Hemolytic anemia in G-6-PD deficiency, methemoglobinemia
Pyrantel pamoate (Antiminth)	Anorexia, nausea	
Pyrimethamine (Daraprim)		Folate-deficient macrocytic anemia
Pyrvinium pamoate (Povan)	Anorexia, nausea, red-colored stool	
Quinacrine HCl (Atabrine Hydrochloride)	Nausea, vomiting, dizziness	Psychoses, exfoliative dermatitis, hepatic necrosis, yellowing of skin
Quinine sulfate	Tinnitus, nausea, vomiting, vertigo	Hypotension, hemolytic anemia

Table 16-3   (*Continued*)

Drug	Frequent	Infrequent
Stibophen (Fuadin)	Similar to but less frequent and severe than with antimony potassium tartrate	
Thiabendazole (Mintezol)	Anorexia, nausea, vomiting, dizziness	Tinnitus, drowsiness
Trimethoprim-sulfamethoxazole (Bactrim, Septra)		Rash, hemolytic anemia

*Carcinogenic in rats and mutagenic in bacteria (see *Med. Lett. Drugs Ther.* 17:53, 1975). Significance for humans not known.

> **(1) Ascaris pneumonitis**   Symptomatic treatment.
>
> **(2) Intestinal ascariasis**   Pyrantel pamoate, 11 mg/kg in 1 dose
> Mebendazole, 100 mg bid for 3 days
> Piperazine citrate, 75 mg/kg/day for 2 days

d. Prevention   Sanitary disposal of feces.

2. Hookworm

a. Etiology

> **(1)** Human hookworms belong to two genera, *Necator* and *Ancylostoma*. The former are prevalent in the southern United States, South and Central America, Asia, and Africa. The latter are rarely seen in the United States.
>
> **(2)** Infections spread by skin penetration of soil-living larvae hatched from eggs passed in infected feces.

b. Evaluation and diagnosis   Three clinical phases of hookworm infection are recognized:

> **(1) Penetration of the skin by larvae**   A local papulovesicular dermatitis and a history of walking barefoot in feces-contaminated soil suggest the diagnosis.
>
> **(2) Transient blood-lung migration by larvae**   A mild pneumonitis with peripheral eosinophilia is suggestive. Hookworm larvae may be found in the sputum.
>
> **(3)** The **prolonged intestinal phase** results from the attachment of blood-feeding adult worms to the small intestinal mucosa of the host.
>
> > **(a)** In **hookworm infection** the number of infecting worms is small, and diarrhea and abdominal cramps may be the only clinical findings. Infection is confirmed by demonstrating hookworm ova in feces.
> >
> > **(b)** In **hookworm disease** large numbers of worms are present, and significant blood loss occurs. The disease is confirmed by
> >
> > > **i.** Signs and symptoms of anemia.
> > >
> > > **ii.** Documentation of iron deficiency.

iii. The finding of occult blood in the feces.

iv. The demonstration of large numbers of hookworm ova in the feces by the method of Stoll (see reference in Sec. **I.C.2.c** or other standard text for details).

c. Treatment

(1) Drugs

(a) *Ancylostoma*
Mebendazole, 100 mg bid for 3 days
Bephenium, 2.5 gm if < 20 kg in 1 dose
 5.0 gm if > 20 kg in 1 dose
Pyrantel pamoate, 11 mg/kg in 1 dose
Thiabendazole, 25 mg/kg bid for 2 days

(b) *Necator*
Mebendazole, 100 mg bid for 3 days
Pyrantel pamoate, 11 mg/kg in 1 dose
Thiabendazole, 25 mg/kg bid for 2 days

(2) Differentiation between *Necator* and *Ancylostoma* infections is difficult. Infections acquired in the Western Hemisphere should be assumed to be due to *Necator* and treated accordingly.

(3) Moderate to very heavy infections should always be treated with antihelminthics, as should hookworm disease. Light infections need not be specifically treated if the patient is adequately nourished.

(4) Iron supplementation should be given to patients with hookworm disease.

d. Prevention   Sanitary disposal of feces and wearing of shoes to prevent contact of bare feet with contaminated soil.

3. Whipworm

a. Etiology   Fecal-oral spread of *Trichuris trichiura*. The infection is worldwide, and the human is the natural reservoir and only susceptible host.

b. Evaluation and diagnosis

(1) Diarrhea and abdominal pain have been associated with trichuriasis, but the vast majority of infections are asymptomatic.

(2) The presence of typical ova in feces by direct fecal smear or concentration techniques is diagnostic.

(3) Eosinophilia is not associated with trichuriasis, and its presence should suggest another parasitic infection.

c. Treatment   Treatment is toxic and rarely indicated, since symptoms are so infrequent.

d. Prevention   Sanitary fecal disposal and wearing of shoes to prevent skin penetration by the larvae.

4. Pinworm

a. Etiology   Fecal-oral spread of *Enterobius vermicularis*, a 4-mm worm just visible to the naked eye and the most common helminth found in humans in the United States. The infection often affects entire households. Autoinfection is also common. Humans are the only known hosts.

b. Evaluation and diagnosis

(1) Perianal itching, vulvitis, and vaginitis in young children suggest the presence of pinworms. Symptoms may be intense enough to cause insomnia, restlessness, and hyperactivity.

(2) Adult worms may be seen in the perianal area and on the surface of freshly passed feces, particularly in the early morning.

(3) Characteristic ova are demonstrated by Scotch-tape swab (see Sec. **d**, p. 402). Examination should be made first thing in the morning and repeated on consecutive days if necessary. A single swabbing reveals only about 50 percent of infections; three swabbings will uncover 90 percent; and five examinations are required before the patient is considered free from infection. Scrapings from beneath the fingernails may show eggs in 30 percent of infected children.

(4) If diagnostic procedures fail to reveal pinworms, a therapeutic trial is reasonable in markedly symptomatic children.

c. Treatment
Mebendazole, 100 mg in a dose
Pyrvinium pamoate, 5 mg/kg in 1 dose
Piperazine citrate, 65 mg/kg daily for 7 days
Pyrantel pamoate, 11 mg/kg in 1 dose
If repeated symptomatic infections occur, it is reasonable to treat all members of a household simultaneously.

d. Prevention Boiling of sheets, undergarments, pajamas, and the like is of little or no value. Hand washing and fingernail cleanliness may reduce transmission and autoinfection.

5. Strongyloides

a. Etiology Skin penetration of *S. stercoralis* larvae passed in infected feces. Autoinfection may occur.

b. Evaluation and diagnosis Children may be asymptomatic or complain of upper gastrointestinal distress since the adult worms live within the duodenal submucosa. Larvae (not ova) are found in freshly passed feces or by aspiration of duodenal contents. Infections are associated with a moderate to marked eosinophilia. Fatal, overwhelming infection may occur in children who harbor this parasite and who are undergoing immunosuppression.

c. Treatment Thiabendazole, 25 mg/kg bid for 2 days

d. Prevention Sanitary disposal of feces and wearing of shoes.

6. Visceral larva migrans

a. Etiology Ingestion of the ova of dog and cat ascarids, *Toxocara canis* and *Toxocara cati*. Larvae emerge in the intestine and migrate extensively throughout the body.

b. Evaluation and diagnosis

(1) The presumptive diagnosis is based on clinical manifestations in a child known to ingest dirt. These include fever, cough, hepatosplenomegaly, and transient pneumonia.

(2) Hypergammaglobulinemia, marked eosinophilia, and leukocytosis are present.

    (3) The parasite is rarely demonstrated; stool examination and tissue biopsy are useless.

  c. Treatment

    (1) The disease is often mild and self-limited, lasting several weeks. Specific treatment is usually unnecessary.

    (2) In severe cases, antihelminthic therapy may be beneficial (thiabendazole, 25 mg/kg bid for 2 days).

    (3) Antiinflammatory therapy with corticosteroids or antihistamines, or both, may offer relief of severe symptoms.

  d. Prevention Avoidance of contamination of play and work areas by dog and cat feces.

7. Trichinosis

  a. Etiology Ingestion of raw meat containing encysted larvae of *Trichinella spiralis* (pork is the principal source of human infection). The infection is more common in temperate than in tropical environments.

  b. Evaluation and diagnosis

    (1) A history of ingestion of uncooked pork.

    (2) The clinical picture may suggest the diagnosis, but is often unclear until the second or third week of infection. At this time the full-blown picture of fever, facial and periorbital edema, headache, photophobia, conjunctivitis, and severe muscle pain and tenderness may develop. Signs of encephalitis, meningitis, and myocarditis may appear.

    (3) A muscle biopsy specimen showing the characteristic larvae. (Crush a thin slice of muscle between two slides and inspect it under the microscope to verify the presence of larvae.) Histologic examination of tissue for the presence of an inflammatory reaction is essential to confirm **recent** infection. A negative biopsy does not rule out the diagnosis.

    (4) Marked peripheral eosinophilia (in 20–80 percent) after the third week of infection, which may persist for months.

    (5) A positive intracutaneous skin test with *Trichinella* larval antigen (85–100 percent sensitivity). An immediate wheal and flare reaction occurs after injection of 0.1 ml of antigen. The test becomes positive about 3 weeks after infection and remains positive for 5–7 years.

    (6) Agglutination or flocculation reactions with rising titer demonstrated on paired samples (tests turn positive in the third week of infection and may remain positive for months to years).

  c. Treatment

    (1) The efficacy of specific antihelminthic therapy is in question. In severe cases, thiabendazole may be tried.

    (2) Corticosteroids may ameliorate severe symptoms, but they are not universally considered beneficial.

  d. Prevention Consumption of only well-cooked pork. Pork is *not* inspected for trichinosis in the United States.

B. Tapeworms (cestodes)

1. Beef tapeworm

a. Etiology The disease is transmitted by the ingestion of undercooked beef containing *Taenia saginata* larval cysts. The infection is worldwide in distribution; the human is the definitive host, and cattle are the intermediate host.

b. Evaluation and diagnosis Most patients are asymptomatic, and the infection is noted only when migrating proglottids pass through the anus. Observation of gravid proglottids is diagnostic.

c. Treatment

(1) Niclosamide achieves a 90 percent cure rate.

(a) No prior bowel preparation is required. Dosage is as follows:

< 10 years of age, 1 gm in 1 dose
> 10 years of age, 2 gm in 1 dose

(b) The worm will be macerated, and search for the scolex (head) is thus unprofitable.

(c) Re-treat if proglottids reappear in subsequent months.

(2) Quinacrine achieves a 75 percent cure rate. The total dose is 25 mg/kg. Treatment is as follows:

(a) Give a cathartic the evening before treatment and a cleansing enema (Fleet's) in morning.

(b) Quinacrine on an empty stomach is given in 4–5 divided doses q10 min until the total dose is given. Each dose is given with 250 mg sodium bicarbonate.

(c) Give a saline purge several hours later and follow by a stool examination for scolex for the next 24 hr.

(d) Re-treat if proglottids reappear in subsequent months.

d. Prevention Thorough cooking of beef.

2. Pork tapeworm

a. Etiology Ingestion of uncooked pork containing larval cysts of *Taenia solium*.

b. Evaluation and diagnosis Adult worms rarely produce symptoms. The passage of gravid motile proglottids through the anus raises the suspicion of infection. Confirmation is obtained by laboratory examination of the proglottid.

c. Treatment **Quinacrine** is the drug of choice [see **1.c.(2)**].

d. Prevention Thorough cooking of pork.

3. Hydatid disease

a. Etiology Humans acquire the infection by ingesting the eggs of *Echinococcus granulosus* passed in the feces of carnivores.

b. Evaluation and diagnosis

(1) A slowly growing, usually asymptomatic cyst in the proper epidemiologic setting suggests the diagnosis. Two-thirds occur in the liver; one-fourth in the lung; and the remainder are widely scattered.

    (2) The **x-ray** appearance is typical but not pathognomonic.

    (3) Casoni's intradermal skin test An immediate wheal and flare con stitute a positive test specific for *E. granulosus* and 75 percen sensitive.

    (4) Hemagglutination and bentonite flocculation tests are positive i the majority of cases.

    (5) Demonstration of the characteristic gross and histologic appear ance on removal of the cyst. **(Aspiration is dangerous and shoul not be done.)**

  c. Treatment Easily accessible cysts are removed surgically. Most cyst are asymptomatic and may, in fact, be left untreated. Freezing of th cyst and subsequent surgical removal have given favorable result (*N. Engl. J. Med.* 284:1346, 1971).

C. Trematodes (flukes): schistosomiasis

  1. Etiology Schistosomiasis is caused by one of three species of bloo flukes. Each species has a different geographic distribution and ana tomic localization in the infected host and produces different clinica manifestations. The human host acquires the infection through ski penetration in freshwater streams. The infection is spread through uri nation or defecation into streams.

    a. *Schistosoma mansoni* is found in Africa, South America, and th Caribbean area, including Puerto Rico (5–10 percent of Puerto Rican residing in the United States are infected). Its pathologic effects ar primarily in the GI tract.

    b. *S. japonicum* is found in the Far East and also primarily affects the G tract.

    c. *S. haematobium* is found in Africa and causes disease of the genitouri nary system.

  2. Evaluation and diagnosis

    a. Schistosome infections are not acquired or transmitted in the conti nental United States. A history of residence or travel in an endemi area is thus required if the diagnosis is suspected.

    b. The clinical manifestations of schistosomiasis are varied and reflec acute and chronic stages of infection.

      (1) In the acute stages, a **localized dermatitis** is produced at the site o skin penetration; this subsides in a few days. In some patients a **acute illness,** characterized by fever, chills, abdominal pain, urti carial eruptions, and marked eosinophilia may occur 2—4 week later.

      (2) The deposition of eggs begins 1–3 months after infection. Th symptoms reflect the sites of egg deposition. *S. japonicum* cause abscesses and ulceration of the ileum and cecum. *S. mansoni* in fections involve the sigmoid colon and rectum. Both result in ab dominal pain and bloody diarrhea. *S. haematobium* infections in volve the bladder, producing hematuria, dysuria, and suprapubi pain and tenderness.

      (3) The process may become chronic and result in granulomatous inflammation and fibrosis of the intestine, or bladder, or both Eggs carried to the liver via the portal circulation in *S. mansoni* and *S. japonicum* infections may produce periportal cirrhosis with portal hypertension, although liver function is usually not impaired. Eggs carried to the lungs may produce an obliterative, endarteritis with cough, hemoptysis, pulmonary hypertension, and cor pulmonale. Eggs carried to the CNS and skin may produce local lesions in these organs.

(4) A moderate eosinophilia is usually found.

(5) Demonstration of typical eggs is required for diagnosis.

  (a) The number of eggs in feces or urine is small, and **concentration techniques** are usually required and should be specifically requested if samples are examined by outside laboratories.

  (b) If the clinical picture is suggestive and eggs are not found, a **rectal or bladder biopsy is done.** The sample should be crushed between two slides and examined directly for eggs.

3. Treatment

  a. The serious potential consequences of schistosome infections and the long life span (20–40 years) of egg-laying adults usually mandate treatment of all schistosome infections. Treatment should not be undertaken lightly; the agents used have significant toxicity and treatment is prolonged.

  b. Specific therapy

   (1) *S. haematobium*
   Niridazole (age < 16), 25 mg/kg for 7 days
   Lucanthone (age > 16), 5 mg/kg tid for 7 days
   Stibophen, 1 ml IM, day 1; 2 ml IM, day 2; 3 ml IM, day 3; 4 ml IM every other day for 18 injections. (For age and weight modification see H. L. Barnett, *Pediatrics* [15th ed.], New York, Appleton-Century-Crofts, 1972, p. 815.)

   (2) *S. mansoni*
   Stibophen, as in **(1)**
   Antimony sodium dimercaptosuccinate, 8 mg/kg IM weekly for 5 weeks
   Niridazole (age < 16), 25 mg/kg for 7 days

   (3) *S. japonicum*
   Antimony potassium tartrate (see *Med. Lett. Drugs Ther.* 14(2), 1972)
   Stibophen, as in **(1)**
   Antimony sodium dimercaptosuccinate, as in **(2)**

  c. The patient should have **repeat stool or urine examinations** monthly for 6 months to ensure cure.

4. Prevention
Avoidance of infected water; proper disposal of human feces and urine.

D. Protozoa

1. Amebiasis

  a. Etiology Fecal-oral passage of cysts of *Entamoeba histolytica*. Amebiasis is worldwide in distribution, and the human is the only known host. Sporadic localized epidemics occur in the United States, and the disease is endemic in many institutionalized populations.

b. Evaluation and diagnosis

(1) Intestinal amebiasis

(a) Intestinal amebiasis varies in presentation from the asymptomatic carrier state (by far the most common) to fulminant colonic disease.

   i. **Mild colonic infection** is characterized by alternating diarrhea and constipation.

   ii. **Amebic dysentery** presents most frequently as subacute illness. Mild tenderness, bloody diarrhea, low-grade fever, weakness, and malaise are characteristic. The tempo of the illness may clinically distinguish it from more acute, bacillary dysentery. Abdominal tenderness is common, particularly over the sigmoid and cecal areas; appendicitis is sometimes erroneously diagnosed.

(b) Confirmation in acute cases is obtained by demonstrating motile amebic trophozoites in **fresh stool,** or cysts in the carrier state. Proctoscopy may be useful if multiple stool samples are negative.

(c) Erythrocytes are plentiful and leukocytes are minimal in the stool, which is helpful in distinguishing between amebic and bacillary dysentery.

(d) Eosinophilia is *not* found.

(2) Extraintestinal amebiasis most commonly affects the liver.

(a) Disease may occur without the signs or symptoms of intestinal infection. Fever, chills, an enlarged, tender liver, elevated right diaphragm, minimal liver function abnormalities, and the finding of a filling defect on liver scan are highly suggestive. Of all amebic abscesses, 95 percent are single and situated in the upper part of the right lobe of the liver.

(b) Serologic tests for invasive amebiasis (indirect hemagglutination, complement fixation) are extremely accurate.

(c) Percutaneous liver aspiration is recommended in large abscesses only. Aspirated material may show amebas. However, their absence does not rule out hepatic infection, since organisms tend to be located at the margins of the abscess.

(d) A therapeutic trial with metronidazole or dehydroemetine is an accepted diagnostic measure **in a severely ill patient.**

c. Treatment

(1) All stages of amebiasis are treated.

(a) **Asymptomatic carrier state**

Metronidazole, 7–10 mg/kg tid PO for 10 days

(b) **Intestinal infection**

Metronidazole, 7–10 mg/kg tid PO for 10 days
   or
Diiodohydroxyquin, 7–10 mg/kg tid PO for 3 weeks,
   and
Paromomycin, 25–30 mg/kg PO tid for 10 days,
   and, **if severe,**
Dehydroemetine HCl, 1.0–1.5 mg/kg IM for 10 days

(c) Hepatic infection

> Metronidazole, 7–10 mg/kg PO tid for 10 days
> *or*
> Chloroquine phosphate, 10 mg/kg PO qid for 10 days,
> *and*
> Dehydroemetine HCl, as in **(b)**,
> *and*
> Paromomycin, as in **(b)**,
> *and*
> Diiodohydroxyquin, 7–10 mg/kg tid PO for 3 weeks

(2) In addition to specific amebicidal therapy, **supportive care** is important in invasive amebiasis. Hospitalization, bed rest, and good nutritional intake may contribute to rapid recovery.

(3) Follow-up stool examinations should be done at 1 and 2 months to ensure that a cure has been achieved.

d. Prevention Sanitary disposal of feces and treatment of asymptomatic cyst passers.

2. Giardiasis

a. Etiology Fecal-oral spread of *Giardia lamblia.* Infection is worldwide and is common in institutionalized populations.

b. Evaluation and diagnosis

(1) There are often no symptoms. Abdominal pain, chronic and recurrent diarrhea, and weight loss may occur. The diarrhea is not bloody; stools may be bulky and offensive. Steatorrhea and malabsorption may occur.

(2) The diagnosis is confirmed by the demonstration of characteristic motile trophozoites in **fresh diarrheal stool** or **duodenal aspirate** by direct examination. Cysts may be seen in formed stools by direct or concentration methods.

c. Treatment

(1) Specific therapy is highly effective.
> Quinacrine, 2–3 mg/kg tid for 5 days
> Metronidazole, 3–5 mg/kg tid for 7 days
> Furazolidone, 1 month–1 year, ½–1 tsp qid for 10 days
>   1–4 years, 1–1½ tsp qid for 10 days
>   > 5 years, 1 tsp qid for 10 days

(2) Supportive measures and restoration of nutritional status are important in patients with malabsorption.

d. Prevention Sanitary disposal of feces.

3. Malaria

a. Etiology Malaria, among the most common worldwide infections of man, is transmitted by the bite of an *Anopheles* mosquito infected with *Plasmodium.* Four species of *Plasmodium* infect man: *P. falciparum, P. vivax, P. ovale,* and *P. malariae.* Transfusion-induced malaria occurs infrequently.

b. Evaluation and diagnosis

(1) The clinical manifestations of malaria infection are nonspecific. Fever, rigors, malaise, headaches, myalgias, and arthralgias commonly occur in acute infections. **Splenomegaly** is the most consistent physical finding.

Table 16-4   Differentiation of Malarial Parasites

Falciparum	Relapsing *(P. vivax, ovale, malariae)*
Small ring forms	Large ring forms
High parasite count (10% or more of RBCs)	Low parasite count (1–2% or less of RBC
Only ring forms	
Parasites at margins of RBCs	Intermediate forms
No Schüffner's stippling	Schüffner's stippling
Crescent-shaped gametocyte (pathognomic if present)	Schüffner's stippling

    (2) The fever pattern may become periodic after infection is well established: every 48 hr in *P. vivax* and *P. ovale* infections; every 72 hr in *P. malariae* infections; and every 36–48 hr in *P. falciparum* malaria. Typically, the patient appears well between fever paroxysms.

    (3) **It is exceedingly important to distinguish between relapsing malaria (*vivax, ovale,* and *malariae*) and falciparum malaria** (Table 16-4). The former group usually produces a self-limited illness that may relapse after months or years. The latter species can infect red blood cells of all ages, with resultant heavy parasitemia, serious complications, and possible fatal outcome. Also, *P. falciparum* may be resistant to antimalarial drugs.

    (4) The complications of *P. falciparum* infection include cerebral malaria (presenting as coma, delirium, and convulsions), massive hemolysis, disseminated intravascular coagulation, renal failure, pulmonary edema, and cardiovascular collapse.

    (5) A history of residence or travel in an endemic area is almost always elicited.

    (6) **The diagnosis rests on the demonstration of malaria parasites in the peripheral blood** (see **B,** p. 397 and **C,** p. 401).

        (a) Clinical sequelae reflect the level of parasitemia. In patients with serious complications, 10 percent or more of red cells are likely to be parasitized, and the infection is thus easily diagnosed by thin smear.

        (b) As previously noted, laboratory differentiation between falciparum malaria and the relapsing malarias is of great importance and will affect the choice of antimalarial agents (Table 16-4). Textbooks of parasitology should be consulted to aid in species differentiation.

  c. **Treatment**   The choice of antimalarial drugs depends on the infecting species and the geographic area of acquisition of infection.

    (1) **Falciparum infections** acquired in Southeast Asia and localized areas of Central and South America must be assumed to be resistant to chloroquine phosphate. Alternative drugs should be given, as outlined in **(4)(b).**

    (2) In **relapsing malaria,** therapy must be directed against both the erythrocytic and exoerythrocytic parasites to prevent relapse

There is no resistance to chloroquine, but relapse may occur if this agent is used alone.

(3) In addition to vigorous antimalarial therapy, the complications of falciparum malaria require intensive supportive measures. Transfusions with packed RBCs are given in severe hemolytic anemia. Corticosteroids, mannitol, or both have been used effectively in cerebral malaria. Mannitol may be used in renal failure, and dialysis may be necessary. Heparin may be useful in disseminated intravascular coagulation. Careful attention to fluid and electrolyte balance in each of these situations is essential.

(4) Recommended treatment regimens

(a) Relapsing malaria

Chloroquine phosphate, 10 mg/kg PO (or IM if necessary), followed by 5 mg/kg q12h for 3 doses

Primaquine, 0.3 mg/kg daily for 14 days. Patients deficient in glucose 6-phosphate dehydrogenase may demonstrate a hemolytic anemia with primaquine

(b) Falciparum malaria

i. Nonchloroquine-resistant area

Chloroquine phosphate, as in **(a)**

ii. Chloroquine-resistant area

Quinine HCl, 10 mg/kg PO q8h for 10 days (IV, if severely ill, with 10 mg/kg diluted to 0.5 mg/ml in saline, administered 1 ml/min, with ECG and blood pressure monitoring)

Pyrimethamine, 0.3 mg/kg PO tid for 3 days

Sulfadiazine, 10 mg/kg PO qid for 7 days

(5) Treatment with pyrimethamine requires folinic acid supplementation, since the drug is a folic acid antagonist.

(6) Response to therapy is followed by dramatic clinical improvement. Repeated blood smears show disappearance of parasitemia.

d. Prevention   Persons traveling through or residing in malarious areas should receive prophylactic suppressive therapy with chloroquine phosphate, 5 mg/kg weekly. To prevent relapsing malaria, a 14-day course of primaquine should be taken after leaving an endemic area.

4. Toxoplasmosis

a. Etiology   *Toxoplasma gondii*, an obligate intracellular parasite, is responsible for this infection. Congenital transmission has been clearly established. The mode of acquisition of postnatally acquired infection remains obscure. Transmission by meat ingestion and spread by cat feces are strong possibilities.

b. Evaluation and diagnosis

(1) Infection is largely asymptomatic. Serologic evidence of prior infection is demonstrated in 25–40 percent of the population of the United States. Several symptomatic forms are recognized:

(a) Congenital infection is usually the result of asymptomatic acute infection in the mother. Prematurity or spontaneous abortion may occur. Newborns with toxoplasmosis are asymptomatic at birth, and most remain so. In a small number, chorioretinitis, microcephaly, hydrocephaly, mental retardation, cerebral calcification, or seizure disorders develop.

   (b) Acquired infection shows clinical variations ranging from a mild viral-like illness with lymphadenopathy to fatal pneumonia and encephalitis (seen in compromised hosts).

(2) Demonstration of **rising antibody titers** by complement-fixation (CF), hemagglutination (HA), indirect fluorescent antibody tests (IFA), and the Sabin-Feldman dye test establishes the diagnosis. Newborn infections can be diagnosed by demonstration of IgM *Toxoplasma* antibodies or the persistence of high titers of CF, HA, or IFA beyond 4 months of age.

(3) Rarely, in special circumstances, the diagnosis may be established by the demonstration of organisms in tissue sections or smears of body fluids. Intraperitoneal mouse inoculation is required for isolation. To determine if an infection is recent, however, rising serologic titers are still required.

c. Treatment

(1) There have been no controlled clinical trials to establish the efficacy of drug therapy.

(2) Infants with active disease should be treated in the hope of preventing further destruction of tissue.

(3) Treatment of acquired toxoplasmosis depends on the clinical severity of the illness. Patients with underlying severe illness and immunoincompetence should be strongly considered for treatment if infection is clinically apparent.

(4) Specific therapy
      Pyrimethamine, 0.5 mg/kg daily for 1 month
                          and
      Sulfadiazine, 0.15 mg/kg qid for 1 month

(5) With pyrimethamine treatment, supplemental folinic acid should be given. **Pyrimethamine is contraindicated in pregnancy.**

d. Prevention   Since the mode of spread of infection remains unknown, preventive measures are speculative. Avoidance of ingestion of raw meat and areas of cat feces contamination, particularly during pregnancy, may be of benefit.

5. Pneumocystis pneumonia

a. Etiology   *Pneumocystis carinii*, an organism of uncertain classification, is the etiologic agent. Little is known of the route of infection or the pathogenesis of disease, but the pulmonary focus suggests a respiratory portal of entry.

b. Evaluation and diagnosis

(1) *P. carinii* produces a bilateral diffuse interstitial pneumonia in immunologically compromised hosts. The pneumonia is perihilar in distribution, and symptoms are usually insidious in onset. The diagnosis must be considered when pneumonia develops in patients with leukemia, lymphoma, hypogammaglobulinemia, and those receiving immunosuppressive therapy. Bacterial pathogens should be ruled out by appropriate sputum studies.

(2) Diagnosis requires the demonstration of the parasite by methenamine silver stains in tissue sections obtained at lung biopsy. Rarely, sputum and bronchial brushings may show organisms.

c. Treatment

(1) *Pneumocystis carinii* pneumonia is usually present as a terminal event in patients with severe underlying illness. Spontaneous recovery has been documented; the effect of therapy is thus difficult to assess.

(2) Recovery from or remission of the underlying illness or withdrawal of immunosuppressive therapy may have a beneficial effect on *P. carinii* infection.

(3) Oxygen and other respiratory supportive measures are of great importance.·

(4) Trimethoprim-sulfamethoxazole, 20 mg trimethoprim and 100 mg sulfamethoxazole/kg/day in 4 divided doses PO, has become the drug of choice for therapy of *P. carinii* pneumonia. Vigorous attempts should be made to confirm the diagnosis before instituting therapy. In a desperately ill patient in whom this is impossible, the drug may be started when the disease is suspected.

(5) Pentamidine isethionate, 4 mg/kg IM daily in 1 dose for 12–15 days, is a more toxic alternative. Its IV use is associated with significant side effects, including hypotension, vomiting, facial flushing, and transitory hallucinations. It is rarely justified to give pentamidine empirically. The side effects and toxicity of the drug and the possibility of misdiagnosis strongly favor proof of infection by lung biopsy before institution of therapy.

(6) The use of trimethoprim and sulfamethoxazole (Bactrim) for prophylaxis, 5 mg trimethoprim and 20 mg sulfamethoxazole/kg/day in 2 divided doses, has been successful in preventing *P. carinii* pneumonia in immunocompromised patients when the disease is strongly suspected. Experience is too limited at this point to make general recommendations, however.

17

Blood Disorders

I. MICROCYTIC HYPOCHROMIC ANEMIAS

A. Iron deficiency

1. Etiology

a. Inadequate stores provided at birth (prematurity, fetal-maternal bleeding, severely iron-deficient mother).

b. Failure of dietary iron intake to keep up with increasing requirements of an expanding blood volume as the child grows (usually seen in the first few years of life in children with inordinately high milk intake [> 1 quart/day], and again in menstruating adolescents because of a combination of inadequate iron intake and increased iron loss).

c. Iron loss (hemorrhage).

2. Evaluation and diagnosis See Table 17-1.

a. Microcytic hypochromic smear, decreased serum iron, and increased iron-binding capacity; the iron-binding protein (transferrin) is less than 15 percent saturated. A quick and usually reliable bedside test is to look at the patient's serum in a spun hematocrit tube; in iron deficiency it is strikingly pale.

b. Hemoglobin electrophoresis shows a low hemoglobin A_2 level, but otherwise normal findings.

c. Bone marrow examination shows absent stainable iron.

3. Therapy The goal of therapy is to replenish marrow iron stores as well as to achieve a normal hemoglobin value. Therefore treatment should be continued at least 6 months after a normal hemoglobin level has been reached. Since dietary iron rarely provides sufficient replacement, a supplement is required. Oral therapy is preferred unless the patient is unable to tolerate it, or the family is not considered sufficiently dependable to administer the dose regularly.

a. Oral therapy The recommended therapeutic dose is 4–6 mg/kg/day of elemental iron given in 3 daily doses. Ferrous sulfate is probably the most effective and least expensive iron-containing drug. Since it consists of 20 percent elemental iron by weight, the usual daily dose is 30 mg/kg.

b. Parenteral therapy

(1) The calculated total dose should aim at raising the hemoglobin concentration to 12.5 gm/100 ml and to provide 20 percent of total blood iron to replenish depleted body stores. The dose is calculated by using the formula

Table 17-1   Findings in Iron Deficiency Anemia and Thalassemia Trait

Iron Deficiency	Thalassemia Trait
Decreased serum iron	Normal or increased serum iron
Increased iron-binding capacity	Normal or increased iron binding capacity
Clear plasma	Yellowish plasma
Increased free erythrocyte protoporphyrin	Normal free erythrocyte protoporphyrin
Decreased serum ferritin	Increased serum ferritin
MCV/RBC × 10^{-6} > 13	MCV/RBC × 10^{-6} < 12
Decreased A₂ on hemoglobin electrophoresis	Increased A₂ and/or F on hemoglobin electrophoresis (in β-thalassemia)
Can occur in any ethnic group	Seen predominantly in groups of Mediterranean (β-thalassemia), black or Oriental (α-thalassemia) origin
Responds to iron	No response to iron
Iron replacement and maintenance therapy usually necessary	No therapy indicated or necessary; genetic counseling may be appropriate

mg iron

$$= \frac{(\text{blood volume}) \times [12.5 - \text{observed hemoglobin}] \times (3.4) \times (1.2)}{100}$$

where blood volume = 75 ml/kg and 3.4 = iron content in mg/gm hemoglobin.

   (2) Imferon, an iron-dextran complex containing 50 mg elemental iron per milliliter is used for deep IM injection in the buttock. Since this dark brown solution tends to stain superficial tissues, separate needles should be used for withdrawing it from vial and injection, and the Z-tract injection technique should be used. Adverse reactions include local pain, headaches, vomiting, fever, urticaria, angioneurotic edema, arthralgias, and anaphylaxis. **The total dosage should be spaced over 2–3 weeks and should not exceed 0.1 ml/kg/ dose.**

B. Lead poisoning   See Chap. 3, Sec. III for a detailed description.

C. The thalassemias   The thalassemias are hereditary defects in globin chain synthesis transmitted as autosomal recessive traits.

   1. β-Thalassemia (homozygous condition)   Inadequate production of beta chains in β-thalassemia leads to unbalanced production of alpha chains and the excess alpha chains precipitate as intracellular inclusions. This leads to destruction of RBCs in the bone marrow (ineffective erythropoiesis) and marked shortening of the RBC life span. The RBCs that manage to reach the peripheral blood contain reduced hemoglobin levels and are therefore hypochromic.

   a. Evaluation and diagnosis

      (1) Clinical manifestations vary with the age of the patient and the severity of the anemia. It is clinically undetectable in the early months of life, due to the relatively large amount of fetal hemoglobin present. However, as gamma chain synthesis recedes, normal beta chain production does not occur, and anemia and hepatosplenomegaly develop. The characteristic facies is apparent by 1 year of age.

(2) The combination of increased oral iron absorption and transfusion therapy leads to increased iron overload, resulting in hemosiderosis of vital organs and a bronzed complexion.

(3) Congestive heart failure due to myocardial hemosiderosis is an important source of morbidity and mortality in these patients.

b. Treatment

(1) Transfusion with packed RBCs (10–20 ml/kg) should be given at sufficiently frequent intervals to maintain a hemoglobin level of 10–12 gm/100 ml to allow for normal growth and development and to decrease the erythropoietic activity of the bone marrow. The long-term effects of a hypertransfusion regimen started early in life are not yet clear.

(2) Iron chelating agents (e.g., deferoxamine and ascorbic acid) have been utilized with varied results in an attempt to mobilize the increased iron stores. At present this is an experimental procedure that should be conducted only under a research protocol.

(3) Splenectomy The indications for this procedure are generally considered to be

  (a) Hypersplenism as manifested by increasing transfusion requirements.

  (b) Symptoms (e.g., "small stomach syndrome") resulting from marked splenic enlargement.

  (c) Hypermetabolism by spleen, with generalized wasting.

  (d) After splenectomy, thalassemic patients have a significant increase in the risk of **septicemia**, especially if they are under 4 years old. The procedure should be deferred, if possible, until the child is over 4 because of this increased risk. Patients should receive pneumococcal vaccination prior to splenectomy. Some advocate antibiotic prophylaxis after splenectomy (see Tables 15-2 and 15-11, pp. 338 and 352).

(4) Folic acid (1 mg/day) is useful in preventing megaloblastic crises induced by the rapid turnover of erythropoietic cells.

(5) These patients should not be treated with iron preparations because they already have increased tissue iron deposition.

2. β-Thalassemia trait (heterozygous condition) The major significance of this condition is that its presentation as a mild microcytic hypochromic anemia frequently causes it to be confused with iron deficiency and mistakenly treated with iron. The major differential points are a normal or increased serum iron level and an increased hemoglobin A_2 on hemoglobin electrophoresis in thalassemia trait (see Table 17-1). **Iron therapy is contraindicated** in this condition unless there is concomitant iron deficiency.

3. α-Thalassemia (heterozygous condition) Patients with this problem may have a hypochromic anemia similar to, but usually milder than, β-thalassemia trait. Anemia is rare.

4. α-Thalassemia (hemoglobin H disease) In this form of α-thalassemia, the abnormal gene from one parent is combined with a so-called silent carrier gene from the other parent.

   a. Affected patients have a moderately severe anemia (8–12 gm/100 ml) and an abnormal band on hemoglobin electrophoresis. The band corresponds to hemoglobin H (beta tetramer) and may total 12–40 per cent of the total hemoglobin.

   b. The need for transfusion therapy will depend on the severity of the anemia.

II. MACROCYTIC ANEMIAS The most common causes are vitamin B_{12}, folate deficiency, and drugs that interfere with folic acid metabolism such as phenytoin sodium and certain antimetabolites (methotrexate, trimethoprim, pyrimethamine). Less common causes are hereditary orotic aciduria, liver disease, thiamine deficiency, sideroachrestic anemia, and Di Guglielmo syndrome. Establishment of a correct etiologic diagnosis is of primary importance, since incorrect treatment of B_{12} deficiency with folate may result in hematologic improvement but progressive neurologic damage.

A. Vitamin B_{12} deficiency

   1. Etiology The causes may be intrinsic factor deficiency (congenital or acquired), congenital transcobalamin deficiencies, generalized intestinal malabsorption, selective B_{12} malabsorption, or resection of the distal ileum.

   2. Evaluation and diagnosis

   a. Physical examination may demonstrate the neurologic signs associated with subacute combined degeneration of the spinal cord.

   b. Peripheral smear shows macro-ovalocytes, marked variation in RBC size and shape, and a high mean corpuscular volume (MCV) (> 110). Although nucleated RBCs may be present, there is a reticulocytopenia. Neutropenia and thrombocytopenia may also be present as well as hypersegmentation of the neutrophils.

   c. Bone marrow examination shows megaloblastic erythroid maturation and giant metamyelocytes and may also show dysplastic erythroid cells.

   d. Nonspecific laboratory findings may include a positive Coombs test, hyperbilirubinemia, and elevated lactic dehydrogenase (LDH). The most specific findings are low serum B_{12} (except in transcobalamin II deficiency), abnormal Schilling test results, and a successful response to a therapeutic trial of vitamin B_{12}.

   3. Treatment

   a. Therapeutic trial Give 1–3 μg **vitamin B_{12}** daily (IM) for 10 days. If the patient is B_{12}-deficient, the response will be as follows: within 24–48 hr the marrow will convert from megaloblastic to normoblastic morphology. Reticulocytosis should appear within 3 days and peak around the fifth day. Hemoglobin should return to normal levels within 4–weeks. (Although folate-deficient patients may respond to very high doses of B_{12}, they will not respond to this very low dose.)

   b. Subsequently, 100 μg/day IM for 2 weeks should be given to replenish body stores; then 100–1000 μg IM once monthly for the rest of the patient's life or until the underlying disorder is cured.

c. Life-threatening hypokalemia may occur during early treatment, and serum K+ values should be carefully monitored.

d. A rise in serum uric acid frequently accompanies the reticulocytosis, usually reaching its peak at about the fourth day after the start of treatment. This may be prevented by allopurinol.

B. In **folic acid deficiency,** body stores of folate are relatively small. Deficiency may be manifested within 1 month of folate deprivation, and full-blown megaloblastic anemia is seen within 3–4 months.

1. Etiology   Causes include dietary inadequacy, congenital and acquired malabsorption syndrome, antimetabolite therapy, and conditions that create a high folate demand because of increased hematopoiesis (chronic hemolysis, pregnancy, leukemia).

2. Evaluation   This condition is often seen in infants with a history of poor growth, serious infection, chronic diarrhea, and goat's milk feeding. The neurologic signs associated with B_{12} deficiency are absent.

3. Diagnosis   Hematologic findings are similar to those associated with B_{12} deficiency. The major differences noted in laboratory studies are a normal B_{12} level, low folate level, and normal Schilling test results. Folic acid deficiency can coexist with iron deficiency anemia, in which case macrocytosis will not be seen. (Folic acid levels should be checked in all patients with iron deficiency believed to be on a nutritional basis.)

4. Treatment

a. A therapeutic trial of **folate** consists of 20–200 μg folic acid IM daily for 10 days. If malabsorption does not appear to be a problem, this dose can be given PO. B_{12}-Deficient patients do not usually respond to this small dose of folate.

b. A dose of 1–5 mg PO daily for 4–5 weeks is usually adequate to replenish body stores even in patients with malabsorption. Patients with simple dietary deficiency can usually stop therapy at this point if they are on a proper diet, while patients with malabsorption or increased need for folate may require therapy indefinitely.

III. HEMOLYTIC ANEMIAS

A. Congenital hemolytic anemias

1. Hereditary spherocytosis

a. Etiology   This condition results from autosomal dominant inheritance. Erythrocytes are unusually susceptible to splenic sequestration and destruction, and the patient has a chronic hemolytic anemia that may manifest itself as early as the first day of life (neonatal jaundice) or be sufficiently mild to be noticed only on a routine examination.

b. Evaluation

(1) A peripheral smear shows small, round RBCs that lack the normal areas of central pallor.

(2) There is increased osmotic fragility and high mean corpuscular hemoglobin concentration (MCHC > 36).

c. Treatment

   (1) In general, the anemia is rarely severe enough to require transfu
   sion, but, following viral infection, there may be a temporar
   slowdown of erythropoiesis, causing a sudden drop in hematocrit
   Such aplastic crises are associated with an increase in pallor,
   drop in bilirubin level and reticulocyte count, and, if sever
   enough, cardiac decompensation. The process is usually sel
   limited, but the patient must be observed closely until the retur:
   of reticulocytosis.

   (2) Secondary folate deficiency may lead to a megaloblastic crisis un
   less prevented by a prophylactic administration of folate (1 m
   daily).

   (3) **Splenectomy** is the treatment of choice. It results in a decrease i
   bilirubin and reticulocyte count and a rise in hematocrit, despit
   persistence of spherocytes and abnormal osmotic fragility. If pos
   sible, splenectomy should be deferred until the patient is over 4 t
   lessen the risk of sepsis. Antibiotic prophylaxis should be consid
   ered after splenectomy (see Table 15-2) and pneumococcal vaccina
   tion should be given prior to splenectomy.

2. Congenital nonspherocytic hemolytic anemias

   a. Etiology   This is a heterogenous group of hereditary RBC enzym
   defects.

   (1) **Type of defect**   In some patients the Embden-Meyerhof pathwa
   (e.g., pyruvate kinase [PK], triose phosphate isomerase) may b
   involved. In others, involvement is in the hexose monophosphat
   shunt (e.g., glucose 6-phosphate dehydrogenase [G-6-PD], gluta
   thione reductase).

   (2) **Pattern of inheritance**   This varies with each enzymopathy. P
   deficiency has an autosomal recessive pattern, while G-6-PD defi
   ciency follows an X-linked recessive pattern. The latter is mos
   commonly seen in males of Mediterranean origin and black males.

   b. Evaluation   These conditions may present with hemolytic jaundice i
   the neonatal period, hemolytic anemia at any age, or gallstones
   Acute hemolytic episodes following infection or exposure to oxidan
   drugs is characteristic of hexose monophosphate shunt defects (Tabl
   17-2).

   c. Diagnosis   PK deficiency may be associated with burr cells, whil
   hexose monophosphate shunt defects may be associated with Hein
   bodies in the RBCs (brilliant cresyl blue staining). The precise diag
   nosis can only be made by assay for the specific enzyme defect.

   d. Treatment

   (1) **Splenectomy** may be useful in increasing the hemoglobin level i
   patients with Embden-Meyerhof defects. It is best deferred **be
   yond the age of 4 years** to reduce the risk of overwhelming sepsis
   No treatment is needed in mild cases.

   (2) In hexose monophosphate shunt defects, therapy consists mainl
   of avoidance of the large number of oxidant drugs that precipitate
   hemolysis.

   (3) Occasionally, during a severe infection or after exposure to ar
   oxidant drug, anemias may be sufficiently severe to warran

Table 17-2   Drugs Provoking Hemolysis in G-6-PD–Deficient Red Cells

Acetanilid	Pamaquine
Acetophenetidin (phenacetin)	Para-aminosalicylic acid
Acetylsalicylic acid (aspirin)	Phenacetin
N^2-acetylsulfanilamide	Phenylhydrazine
Antipyrine	Primaquine
Colamine	Probenecid
Fava bean	Pyramidon
Furazolidone	Salicylazosulfapyridine
Isoniazid	Sulfamethoxypyridazine (Kynex)
Naphthalene (mothballs)	Sulfacetamide
Naphthoate	Sulfisoxazole (Gantrisin)
Nitrofurantoin (Furadantin)	Sulfoxone
	Synthetic vitamin K compounds
	Thiazolsulfone

transfusion of packed RBCs. More commonly, adequate treatment of infection or discontinuation of the offending drug is sufficient.

3. Sickle cell anemia

  a. Etiology   The RBCs contain hemoglobin S, which consists of two normal alpha chains and two abnormal beta chains (α_2^A, β_2^S). Hemoglobin S forms a linear polymer on deoxygenation that produces a sickle-shaped cell. These cells cannot pass through capillaries, which leads to thrombosis and infarction. Sickle cell anemia is a hereditary disorder, affecting mainly blacks. (Approximately 10 percent of black Americans carry the trait, while 0.2 percent have the homozygous form of the disease.)

  b. Evaluation

    (1) There are usually no clinical manifestations of the disease until a high proportion of the RBCs contain hemoglobin S (at about 6 months of age). An exception to this is the increased risk of infection in infants with sickle cell anemia before other manifestations of the disease are apparent.

    (2) The earliest clinical presentation is often painful swelling of the dorsum of the hand or foot due to ischemic necrosis of the metacarpal or metatarsal bones.

    (3) Other manifestations are hepatosplenomegaly, pallor, cardiomegaly, icterus, and isosthenuria. Progressive episodes of infarction and scarring in the spleen cause it to shrink in size as the patient becomes older, and it is usually no longer palpable by adolescence. The patient may, however, be functionally asplenic even before that time, as demonstrated by the absence of a spleen on a technetium scan and the presence of Howell-Jolly bodies on a peripheral smear.

    (4) Laboratory findings   These include severe anemia (hemoglobin 5–9 gm/100 ml), associated with bizarre RBC shapes (0.5– > 20% are in the sickled form), reticulocytosis (usually 10–20%), and variable hyperbilirubinemia. Exposure of the blood to a reducing agent (e.g., sodium metabisulfite) produces the characteristic sickling change. Hemoglobin electrophoresis demonstrates the abnormal band corresponding to hemoglobin S; no hemoglobin A is seen, and there are variable amounts of hemoglobin F. The degree of hemolysis is related to the number of irreversibly sickled cells. **But the number and severity of the crises are more often related to the amount of hemoglobin F present.**

c. **Treatment** is palliative and revolves about the various "crises" that afflict these patients.

(1) **Painful (thrombotic crises)** are produced by vaso-occlusive episodes due to plugging of vessels with sickled cells. The signs and symptoms depend on which organ's microvasculature is involved (e.g., bone, liver, spleen, GI tract). Among the precipitating causes are infections, dehydration, acidosis, and hypoxia. Treatment consists of reversing these factors and providing analgesia.

(a) **Adequate hydration** is the mainstay of therapy. These patients, even when dehydrated, are frequently unable to concentrate their urine, so urine specific gravity should not be used as a guide to fluid therapy.

(b) Parenteral therapy is preferred if pain or dehydration is severe. Use ½ NS containing 5% dextrose infused at 1½–2 times maintenance. Sodium bicarbonate may be added to the IV fluid in sufficient quantity to raise the urine pH to 6.5–7.0. Extra care must be taken with older patients who have cardiac decompensation, to guard against fluid overload.

(c) Oxygen should be considered in severe crises, especially if there is concomitant pulmonary infection.

(d) In severe vaso-occlusive episodes (especially if the CNS is involved), dilution of the sickle cells with normal RBCs has been found to be beneficial. This can be achieved by transfusions of packed RBCs (10 ml/kg), with or without concurrent phlebotomies, q12h until the hemoglobin is increased to 12–13 mg/100 ml, or by performing a partial exchange transfusion with packed RBCs. The risks are circulatory overload, isoimmunization, hepatitis, and increasing blood viscosity. If the sickle crisis has not terminated, the latter problem can lead to increased severity.

(e) Long-term transfusion therapy (to turn off production of hemoglobin S) should be seriously considered in children with neurologic foci of thrombotic crises, recurrent severe, painful crises, or recurrent priapism. This is usually done for a period of 1–2 years to try to break the cycles of recurrent crises. Long-term therapy involves the additional risk of sensitization and iron overload. Therefore **any patient with sickle cell anemia should have a complete blood typing,** and, unless it is an emergency, the patient should be transfused with blood as closely matched as possible, and should be monitored for signs of iron overload.

(2) **Aplastic crises**   Infections can sometimes result in complete cessation of RBC production for 7–14 days, with disappearance of reticulocytes, a rapid drop in hemoglobin level, and a decrease in serum bilirubin.

(a) These episodes are usually self-limited. However, when anemia is severe or when symptoms of congestive heart failure are present, the patient should be slowly transfused with relatively fresh packed RBCs at a rate of 2–3 ml/kg q8h until the hemoglobin level reaches 7–8 gm/100 ml and the cardiac status stabilizes.

(b) Oxygen should be given to dyspneic patients, but digitalization is usually not necessary.

(c) In severe congestive heart failure, transfusion should be monitored by frequent central venous pressure readings.

(3) Sequestration crises   Sudden pooling of large amounts of blood in the spleen or liver may result in significant hypovolemia and marked organomegaly. Treatment must be prompt and directed toward correction of hypovolemia with plasma expanders or whole blood transfusion while monitoring the patient's central venous pressure.

(4) Hyperhemolytic crises are probably not frequent, but may occur when the patient is coincidentally G-6-PD–deficient and has an infection or is exposed to an oxidant drug. Treatment consists of appropriate antibiotic therapy if a bacterial infection is present, removal of an offending oxidant drug, and correction of dehydration and acidosis. If severe anemia is present, packed RBCs should be given slowly.

(5) Megaloblastic crises are due to the increased folate requirements of rapid erythropoiesis. Treatment with **folic acid,** 1 mg/day, is preventive.

(6) Miscellaneous problems

(a) Infection   Patients with sickle cell disease have increased susceptibility to bacterial infections, notably *Streptococcus (Diplococcus) pneumoniae, Salmonella,* and *Haemophilus influenzae* in the young patient. This should be borne in mind when unexplained fever is present. Young patients with sickle cell anemia should be treated as if they were asplenic and should be placed on prophylactic penicillin. All patients above the age of 2 should be given pneumococcal vaccination.

(b) Gallstones are common in sickle cell patients after the age of 10. Surgical intervention must be carefully considered in patients with obstructive jaundice, fever, and abdominal pain because this constellation can also be produced by intrahepatic cholestasis secondary to sickling.

(c) In operations on patients with sickle cell disease, general anesthesia must be approached with caution and with scrupulous avoidance of hypoventilation, hypoxia, acidosis, and dehydration. It is generally a good idea to increase O_2-carrying capacity and dilute hemoglobin S (to < 40 percent) by slowly transfusing the patient preoperatively with packed RBCs (10 ml/kg). A sickle screen should be performed on all black patients prior to general anesthesia.

(d) Interactions with other hemoglobins   Sickle hemoglobin may interact with other hemoglobins (SC) or thalassemias (S-thal) to produce a hemolytic anemia with milder symptoms. The incidence of crisis is less in these conditions, but sequestration crises of the spleen do occur. Retinopathy should be carefully watched for in older children with hemoglobin SC, as in patients with homozygous hemoglobin S disease.

4. Other hemoglobinopathies

a. Hemoglobin C

(1) Evaluation Homozygous hemoglobin C disease is a mild disord℮ characterized by hemolytic anemia and splenomegaly. Among th symptoms seen are fleeting abdominal pain and cholelithiasis.

(2) Diagnosis Laboratory findings include mild normocytic norm℮ chromic anemia, with many target cells present and a mild r℮ ticulocytosis (1–7 percent). A very slow-moving band is seen ne℮ the origin on hemoglobin electrophoresis.

(3) Treatment is symptomatic. Splenectomy does not appear t influence the clinical course.

b. Unstable hemoglobins These patients have a congenital hemolyt℮ anemia associated with Heinz bodies in the RBCs and abnorm℮ findings on a hemoglobin heat stability test. In general, these p℮ tients have a mild, compensated hemolytic anemia; patients with h℮ moglobin Zurich can exhibit a marked increase in the hemolytic rat℮ when challenged by an infection or an oxidant drug (see Table 17-2℮ Splenectomy is useful on some occasions.

B. Acquired hemolytic anemias

1. Autoimmune Patients with this condition produce antibodies directe℮ against their own erythrocytes that are demonstrable either in the RBCs or in the plasma. This condition may occur secondary to collage℮ diseases, lymphoma, infections, drug therapy (e.g., penicillin, methy℮ dopa, quinine), or any of a miscellaneous group of diseases. It is usuall℮ idiopathic in children.

a. Evaluation and diagnosis

(1) Routine hematologic studies show anemia associated with r℮ ticulocytosis. The sine qua non for diagnosis is the Coombs, ℮ antiglobulin, reaction. A positive direct Coombs test indicate℮ antibody coating the erythrocytes; a positive indirect Coomb℮ test indicates antibody in the patient's plasma.

(2) If the reaction is maximal at about 37°C, a "warm" antibody i℮ present, which is usually of the 7-S globulin variety and require℮ addition of albumin to the RBC suspension in order to caus℮ agglutination.

(3) "Cold" antibodies are of the 19-S variety, react best at low temper℮ ature, fix complement, and agglutinate RBCs in saline suspension℮

(4) This differentiation is important for therapy, since patients wit℮ cold antibodies respond poorly to corticosteroid therapy ℮ splenectomy and should avoid exposure to low temperature.

b. Therapy

(1) If the condition is secondary to a known disease or drug, therap℮ should be directed at this process.

(2) In addition, **corticosteroid therapy** is frequently useful in hemolyti℮ anemia associated with *warm* antibodies. Prednisone, 2–4 mg/k℮ day (up to 60–100 mg/day), may be used. Several weeks may elaps℮ before a favorable response is noted, at which time prednison℮ dosage should be reduced to the minimal amount necessary t℮ keep the hemoglobin and reticulocyte count within an acceptabl℮ range.

(3) If the patient fails to respond to prednisone or requires an unacceptably high dose, **splenectomy** should be considered. If corticosteroid and splenectomy fail to control the process, immunosuppressive drugs should be considered.

(4) Blood transfusion is hazardous in these patients and should be used only in conjunction with corticosteroid therapy if life-threatening anemia develops, because the patient's anti–RBC globulin usually will cross-react with antigens on the donor RBCs and cause a hemolytic transfusion reaction. If the blood bank can identify a specific antigen against which the antibody is directed, blood may be given from a donor whose erythrocytes are negative for this factor. Otherwise, the unit of blood that is **least** reactive with the patient's plasma should be used and should be infused extremely slowly, with close monitoring of the patient for evidence of transfusion reaction.

2. Nonautoimmune

a. Etiology This condition has multiple causes, including mechanical trauma from prosthetic heart valves, chemical agents and drugs, severe burns, and infections (malaria, *Clostridium perfringens*).

b. Diagnosis The Coombs test is negative. The smear usually contains many fragmented RBCs and spherocytes.

c. Therapy consists of treatment of the primary disease, as well as transfusion with packed RBCs when anemia is severe.

IV. ANEMIAS ASSOCIATED WITH PRIMARY BONE MARROW DISEASE

A. Aplastic anemia (pancytopenia) There are two general types of aplastic anemia: constitutional and acquired.

1. Constitutional aplastic anemia, or Fanconi's anemia, is commonly associated with skeletal, renal, and pigmentary anomalies and chromosome breaks in lymphocyte culture. Some patients may have the chromosomal anomalies without the phenotypic ones; thus chromosome studies are mandatory in all patients with aplastic anemia. Although this is an autosomal recessive hereditary condition, the patients commonly do not show signs of hematologic disorder until after infancy. The most common presenting age for boys is 4–7 years and for girls, 6–10 years.

a. Diagnosis Pancytopenia, reticulocytopenia, and hypoplastic marrow associated with skeletal anomalies and chromosome breaks are diagnostic. Decreased sister chromatid exchange in cultured lymphocytes is found only in this disease.

b. Therapy

(1) In addition to supportive care with RBCs and platelets when necessary, combined administration of **an androgen and a corticosteroid** has been successful in most cases. The usual plan of therapy is to give up to 5 mg/kg/day of oxymetholone and 1 mg/kg/day of prednisone until the hemoglobin is normal.

(2) These medications are then slowly tapered until the hemoglobin falls below 12 mg/100 ml, at which point they are maintained indefinitely. These patients require continued therapy in order to maintain hematologic stability.

(3) Liver function should be monitored in patients on oral androgen therapy.

c. Prognosis Despite marked improvement in survival with the use of androgens, leukemia and other malignancies develop in many of these patients. In addition, some become refractory to therapy.

2. Acquired aplastic anemia

a. Etiology This condition may be secondary to hepatitis, radiation toxicity, drugs (e.g., chloramphenicol), or chemicals (e.g., benzene), or it may be idiopathic.

b. Evaluation and diagnosis Pancytopenia, reticulocytopenia, and marrow findings that may show varying degrees of hypoplasia or aplasia are characteristic. However, there is generally no family history of anemia nor phenotypic or chromosome anomalies. Fetal hemoglobin is usually elevated.

c. Therapy

(1) Supportive therapy with RBCs and platelets, preferably HLA matched single donor units.

(2) Androgens and corticosteroids are also used as in constitutional aplastic anemia, but the response rate in acquired disease is much lower. However, when a response is obtained, it is often possible to taper and then discontinue drugs completely.

(3) **Early bone marrow transplantation** should be considered in severe cases (i.e., reticulocyte count < 1 percent, platelet count < 20,000 mm³, and a bone marrow that is hypocellular with > 70 percent lymphoid elements). This procedure is feasible only if an appropriate HLA-matched donor is available and should be performed only in a medical center that has the necessary personnel and equipment. **If transplantation is even remotely considered, non-RBC transfusions should be limited, related donors avoided, and washed, frozen RBCs used when RBCs are required.**

B. Hypoplastic anemia (pure red cell anemia, Diamond-Blackfan syndrome)

1. Etiology The familial incidence suggests hereditary involvement, but no definite inheritance pattern has been established.

2. Diagnosis Anemia is associated with normal leukocyte and platelet counts. The reticulocyte count is low. Red cell indexes may show slight macrocytosis. Bone marrow examination is diagnostic (an aspirate of normal cellularity containing normal myeloid elements and megakaryocytes, but with a striking paucity of erythroid cells).

3. Therapy

a. Corticosteroid therapy has been very effective in some cases, especially if begun early in the disease.

(1) The starting dose is 1–2 mg/day of prednisone. A response is usually seen within 2–4 weeks if the regimen is going to be successful.

(2) This dose should be maintained until the hemoglobin concentration attains normal or near-normal levels, at which time gradual tapering of the dosage should be attempted. Growth retardation may be ameliorated to some extent by giving the prednisone on alternate days once remission has been attained.

b. Patients who do not respond to prednisone can be supported with **periodic transfusion of packed red cells,** although this may lead to hemochromatosis or hepatitis.

V. ACUTE LYMPHOBLASTIC LEUKEMIA (ALL) is the most common malignant disease of childhood, occurring in approximately 4 children/100,000. Acute lymphoblastic leukemia accounts for 70–80 percent of childhood leukemias.

A. Etiology Although there are many theories involving viruses and immune surveillance, there is no known cause.

B. Evaluation and diagnosis The manifestations of ALL are protean, but most of the clinical presentations are related to the lack of normal hematopoietic elements (i.e., pallor of anemia, purpura or bleeding of thrombocytopenia, prolonged or unusual infection of neutropenia). In addition, invasion of organs by leukemic cells can also lead to symptomatology (bone pain, meningeal irritation, respiratory distress due to mediastinal involvement, etc.). The disease is usually suspected when the peripheral blood smear shows unexplained leukoerythroblastic changes such as nucleated red blood cells in the absence of reticulocytosis, tear-drop shaped RBCs, myeloblasts, and other early myeloid elements, without an increase in bands. Whether or not these abnormalities are present, a bone marrow aspiration and often a biopsy must be performed whenever leukemia is suspected; and, if necessary, special stains should be used to determine the nature of the blasts.

C. Treatment The goal of all forms of therapy for leukemia is to destroy the leukemic cells while allowing normal cells to grow. Because of the complexity of this task, treatment approaches are guided by protocols in referral centers.

D. Prognosis The prognosis for childhood ALL is constantly improving. Protocols used at various cancer centers are projecting a 5-year disease-free survival of 60–80 percent. Certain prognostic features are associated with a less favorable initial response and final response to therapy. These include (1) an anterior mediastinal mass, (2) a white cell count less than 50,000/mm^3, (3) massive hepatosplenomegaly, (4) CNS involvement at presentation, (5) T-cell markers on lymphoblasts, (6) a more undifferentiated leukemia, and (7) an age of onset less than 2 years or over 12 years.

VI. ACUTE NONLYMPHOBLASTIC LEUKEMIAS These disorders include acute myeloblastic leukemia, acute promyelocytic leukemia, acute monomyelocytic leukemia, erythroleukemia, and acute stem cell leukemia. They account for about 25 percent of all childhood leukemias.

A. Therapy for these disorders has not had the same success as that for ALL. With most aggressive types of chemotherapy, 50–75 percent of patients with these forms of leukemia will go into remission. However, the remissions are of short duration (< 12 months), and death usually rapidly follows relapse. The same chemotherapeutic agents are employed, but the doses and scheduling vary. Prophylaxis is controversial, since in most of the patients the initial relapse is in the bone marrow.

B. Bone marrow transplantation has been performed in patients with acute myeloblastic leukemia (AML) in relapse and has had limited success. Even when there was successful engraftment, however, most patients have succumbed to a recurrence of the disease. Investigation is under way in the use of bone marrow transplantation in patients with AML who are in remission and who have an HLA-identical sibling.

C. Immunotherapy with bacillus Calmette Guérin (BCG) and autologous tumor cells has been shown to lengthen remissions, and its use in childhood nonlymphoblastic leukemia is currently being studied.

VII. DISORDERS OF COAGULATION
Bleeding secondary to abnormalities in the coagulation mechanism may be due to a deficiency or abnormality in either clotting factors or platelets. The deficiency may be secondary to decreased production or increased consumption.

A. Deficiency of clotting factors

1. Hemorrhagic disease of the newborn

a. Etiology Hemorrhage in the first few days of life occurs due to a relative deficiency of factors II, VII, IX, and X (the vitamin K-dependent factors). This follows from the patient's not receiving or being able to utilize vitamin K. ↑ *capillary fragility*

exchange
2vol −
↓ PLT by
90%

b. Evaluation

(1) Check the history for vitamin K administration.

(2) Evaluate the patient's gestational age.

(3) Determine the source and extent of bleeding.

(4) Prothrombin time (PT), partial thromboplastin time (PTT), platelet count.

(5) Specific factor assays.

c. Diagnosis

(1) The diagnosis is strongly supported by lack of vitamin K administration.

(2) The condition is more common in prematures than in full-term infants.

(3) Bleeding may occur from any site and with any degree of severity.

(4) The platelet count and fibrinogen are normal; PT and PTT are prolonged.

(5) Factors II, VII, IX, and X are decreased.

d. Treatment

(1) Prophylaxis

(a) Administer 0.5–1.0 mg natural vitamin K_1 IM (Aqua MEPHYTON) or vitamin K_1 oxide (Konakion) to all newborn at birth.

(b) The synthetic form of vitamin K_1, menadiol, is felt to have less of a margin of safety than natural vitamin K_1.

(2) Corrective treatment

(a) Give 1–2 mg of aqueous colloidal suspension of vitamin K slowly IV. A rise in clotting factors will be noted in 2–4 hr approaching normal in 24 hr.

(b) For severe bleeding, transfuse with **fresh frozen plasma** (FFP) 10 ml/kg, and packed red blood cells to correct the anemia.

2. Liver disease

a. Etiology Patients with mild destructive liver disease may have bleeding secondary to vitamin K deficiencies in factors I, II, V, VII, IX, and X due to decreased protein synthesis. In addition, they may have decreased factor VIII due to consumption of clotting factors.

b. Evaluation

(1) Liver function tests.

(2) PT, PTT, platelet count, fibrinogen, fibrin split products, and factors V and VIII.

c. The **diagnosis** is confirmed by a prolonged PT and PTT. Consumption should be suspected if the platelet count is low, factor VIII is low, and there is marked increase in fibrin split products (these may be slightly elevated in liver disease in the absence of consumption).

d. Treatment **Vitamin K** (1–5 mg) is given slowly IV and the PT and PTT are repeated in 2–4 hr. If there is no response and if bleeding is severe, fresh frozen plasma, 10 ml/kg, should be administered to correct the clotting abnormality. The prophylactic use of FFP is not recommended because of the short half-life of factors V and VII.

3. Hemophilia (hemophilia A; factor VIII deficiency)

a. Etiology X-linked recessive deficiency of factor VIII.

b. Evaluation

(1) Personal and family history.

(2) Physical examination.

(3) Activated partial thromboplastin time (APTT) and PT.

(4) Factor assay.

(5) Bleeding time.

(6) Platelet adhesiveness.

c. Diagnosis

(1) History and physical examination

(a) In most mild-to-moderate cases there is positive *family* history, but no *personal* history or stigmata, unless the patient has been exposed to trauma or surgery.

(b) In many severe cases there is no positive family history (de novo mutations), but the patient has a personal bleeding history dating from about 1 year of age or earlier.

(c) Most patients with mild to moderate disease and some with the severe form show no bleeding tendency during the neonatal period and early infancy.

(d) The older patient with severe hemophilia may show chronic joint deformities and contractures secondary to bleeding into joints and muscles.

(2) Laboratory studies

(a) The bleeding time is normal.

(b) The platelet count and platelet adhesiveness are normal.

(c) The PT is normal.

(d) The APTT is prolonged.

(3) Assay for factor VIII

(a) Mild deficiency: 5–30 percent of normal.

(b) Moderate deficiency: 1–5 percent of normal.

(c) Severe deficiency: < 3 percent of normal.

d. Therapy

(1) Factor VIII-containing materials For each U/kg of factor VIII a[d]ministered, plasma levels will rise by 2 percent. Adequacy of the[r]apy should be monitored with APTT. This becomes prolonge[d] when factor VIII levels fall below 40 percent of normal.

(a) Fresh frozen plasma (must be type-specific or compatible)

i. The amount to be used is limited by volume consideration[s]. Sufficient factor VIII levels to stop closed soft tissue blee[d]ing (10–20% factor VIII) may be obtained, but not enough [to] stop surface bleeding.

ii. **Dose** 15 ml/kg initially and then 10 ml/kg q12h.

(b) Cryoprecipitate This plasma fraction is obtained by slo[w] thawing of rapidly frozen plasma and dissolving in 10–20 [ml] supernatant plasma. It contains factor VIII concentrated a[p]proximately 20 times. Factor VIII content (expressed as unit[s]) in different containers of cryoprecipitate varies, depending [on] donor and manufacturer.

(c) Lyophilized factor VIII preparations Concentrations of fact[or] VIII vary from 20- to 100-fold. Preparation from pooled plasm[a] involves a greater risk of hepatitis when compared with cry[o]precipitate, which is produced from single units of plasma.

e. Treatment of bleeding

(1) Bleeding into joints

(a) For minor bleeding (incipient hemarthrosis not requiring joi[nt] aspiration) a single dose of factor VIII concentrate (20 U/k[g]) will suffice. Immobilization with plaster splints is not usual[ly] necessary. If used, early mobilization is essential.

(b) For hemarthrosis with a swollen painful joint, administer [?] U/kg of factor VIII concentrate followed by ½ this dose q1[2h] for about 2 days. **Aspiration** of the joint should be considere[d] after the first dose of factor VIII. Immobilization for sever[al] days with splints may be necessary to prevent contracture[.] The joint should be slowly rehabilitated with physical therap[y,] serial splinting to gain full extension, and eventual weig[ht] bearing.

(2) Other soft tissue bleeding

(a) Localized or early bleeding into skin or muscle responds to [a] single dose of factor VIII concentrate (20 U/kg). Ice packs m[ay] also be helpful.

(b) Bleeding into more vital areas such as the mediastinum, flo[or] of the mouth, and retroperitoneum may require addition[al] maintenance doses q12h for up to 48 hr.

(c) The use of traction or splinting must be considered in [in]tramuscular hemorrhage to prevent contracture.

(3) Bleeding in surgery   Plasma alone is inadequate to increase factor VIII levels to a range safe for operation.

 (a) Administer **factor VIII concentrate** in a loading dose of 50 U/kg, followed by 25–30 U/kg q12h. Factor VIII must be administered for 7–10 days (the duration of wound healing). The dose may be decreased by ⅓ during the second week. Higher doses are used in brain surgery or in the presence of infection.

 (b) Epsilon-aminocaproic acid (EACA), in an initial dose of 3 gm/M^2 PO, is helpful in dental procedures, as is topical thrombin.

 (c) Therapy should be monitored with APTT determinations.

(4) Bleeding from surface wounds

 (a) Small skin wounds and minor epistaxis may respond to ice packs and pressure.

 (b) The patient with severe lacerations should be treated like the patient with surgical wounds [see **(3)**].

 (c) GI bleeding not involving the mesentery or retroperitoneum usually responds to 3 or 4 doses of factor VIII concentrate in amounts used for enclosed soft tissue bleeding. However, consider the need for a diagnostic workup to determine the cause of GI bleeding.

 (d) Hematuria, if mild, may stop spontaneously over a few days. Severe or persistent hematuria requires replacement therapy for 1–2 days with high doses of factor VIII sufficient to attain levels 50 percent of normal. **EACA is contraindicated in renal bleeding** because of the risk of calyceal and ureteral clotting. Prednisone has been advocated for renal bleeding, but its efficacy is unproved.

 (e) Bed rest is indicated.

f. Complications

 (1) Patients with hemophilia should avoid salicylates, antihistamines, and other drugs that interfere with platelet function.

 (2) Inhibitors   Antibodies against factor VIII develop in about 8–16 percent of patients receiving factor VIII transfusions.

 (a) *Inhibitors rarely develop in patients who have had more than 100 days of replacement therapy without their development.*

 (b) The presence of inhibitors is suggested by failure of apparently adequate therapy and is documented by demonstrating inhibition of coagulation of normal plasma by the patient's plasma.

 (c) Patients with inhibitors should not receive factor VIII. For mild bleeding, **local measures** and **rest** are the best treatment. For serious bleeding problems and surgery, **activated factors** have recently been employed.

 (3) Preparations of Proplex and Konȳne have activated factors that bypass factor VIII and allow coagulation to proceed. The concentration of activated factors in these preparations is variable. The initial dosage is usually 50–100 factor IX U/kg. The adequacy of therapy is measured by hemostasis and a shortening of the APTT tȯ about 40 sec. This therapy has been associated with complications such as disseminated intravascular coagulation (DIC), and thus the patients should be carefully observed. Preparations of activated factors are now being made so that a more uniform dose may be given.

4. Factor IX deficiency (Christmas disease, hemophilia B) is one-fifth as common as factor VIII deficiency. Clinically, the two diseases are very similar. Plasma levels can be raised from 0.5–1.5 percent with 1 U/kg of factor IX. Therapy should be monitored with APTT. This disease is also transmitted as an X-linked recessive disorder.

   a. Plasma   Regular bank plasma or fresh frozen plasma may be used but it is adequate only for treatment of enclosed soft tissue bleeding. The dose is 15 ml/kg loading with 10 ml/kg q12h.

   b. Lyophilized factor IX concentrates

   (1) These are made from pooled plasma and thus increase the risk that hepatitis will develop.

   (2) For surgery, administer a loading dose of 40 U/kg, followed by 15 U q12h.

5. von Willebrand's disease (vascular hemophilia)   Patients with this autosomal dominant inherited disorder have a mild, lifelong bleeding tendency but may have prolonged epistaxis, gingival and GI bleeding, and easy bruising. Females may be troubled by menorrhagia.

   Although there are many forms of the disease and a wide spectrum of severity, most patients with von Willebrand's disease have decreased factor VIII activity, prolonged bleeding time, and a normal platelet count.

   a. The **diagnosis** is suspected when the patient has a prolonged PTT and a normal PT in addition to a prolonged bleeding time and a normal platelet count. The diagnosis is established by a demonstrated decrease in factor VIII (both activity and antigen) and an abnormal ristocetin-induced platelet aggregation.

   b. Treatment is with fresh plasma or cryoprecipitate. Both contain the factor deficient in von Willebrand's disease, and a dose of 10 units of FFP/kg will correct the factor VIII level and the bleeding time for 24–48 hr to over 50 percent of the normal level.

B. Disseminated intravascular coagulation

   1. Etiology

   a. There is abnormal consumption of clotting elements, leading to their decrease and to thrombosis and bleeding.

   b. Consumption may be initiated by any pathologic state that triggers the cascade of clotting elements at some point in its course.

   2. Evaluation

   a. In the setting of any conditions known to produce DIC, **unexplained bleeding** requires laboratory investigation with the tests listed in Table 17-3.

   b. Physical examination should reveal evidence of bleeding, peripheral thrombosis, or both.

   3. Diagnosis   See Table 17-3.

Table 17-3 Laboratory Evidence of Disseminated Intravascular Coagulation

Platelets decreased
Prothrombin time prolonged
Partial thromboplastin time prolonged
Fibrinogen decreased
Thrombin time prolonged
Fibrin split products: elevated titers
Microangiopathic changes on blood smear
Factor VIII decreased, *[handwritten: Vↆ Hemolytic anemia]*

*[handwritten margin notes:
1) Hypoxia - acidosis
2) Infections + TORCH
3) OB complications
4) Rh incompat.]*

4. Therapy

a. Treat the cause of the consumption, e.g., sepsis, acidosis, hypoxia.

b. Most patients who succumb to DIC die because of bleeding, not clotting. FFP, 10 ml/kg, should be administered, together with platelet transfusions, to control bleeding.

c. Heparin has not been shown to alter the mortality from this disorder and is not recommended for DIC crises. Thrombosis rather than bleeding is the major clinical problem. If heparin is given, it is best done as a continuous infusion of 12–25 U/kg/hr IV. The response to therapy is best monitored by following fibrinogen levels. Platelet levels can also be followed, but their return toward normal is usually slower than that of fibrinogen.

C. Deficiency in platelets Most platelet deficiencies are secondary to increased destruction with the exception of drug-induced aplasia and some congenital thrombocytopenias. *[handwritten: Overall, ↓ PLT function in neonatal]*

1. Hypersplenism

a. Thrombocytopenia due to hypersplenism is usually mild and does not cause bleeding. The platelet count does not normally fall below 25,000/mm³. There is often accompanying anemia and neutropenia.

b. If hypersplenism occurs in severe liver disease with depression of clotting factors, abnormal bleeding may be more of a problem.

c. Therapy Splenectomy is curative but is usually done for symptoms of hypersplenism other than platelet deficiency, such as an increasing transfusion requirement or recurrent infections.

2. Drug-induced thrombocytopenia

a. Etiology This condition may result from bone marrow depression or increased peripheral destruction due to drug-induced **antibody production.** Drugs most commonly associated with a toxic insult to the bone marrow are diuretics such as the thiazides and furosemide, trimethoprim, tolbutamide, and thioridazine. Drugs that produce thrombocytopenia by an immunologic mechanism include quinidine, phenylbutazone, sulfonamides, penicillins, digitalis, and tricyclic antidepressants. *[handwritten: Dilantin,]*

b. Therapy

(1) The primary treatment for drug-induced thrombocytopenia is to **withdraw the drug.** In addition, drugs that adversely affect platelet

[handwritten: Also. phototherapy.]

function (e.g., aspirin) should be avoided. Cerebral hemorrhage is the major cause of death in drug-related thrombocytopenia, and bed rest is advisable if bleeding is more than mild. Coughing, straining, and other activities that cause increased intracranial pressure should be avoided.

(2) Steroids acutely increase vascular stability and may prevent immunologic destruction of platelets. Prednisone, 1–2 mg/kg/day for 1–2 weeks, is helpful if bleeding is a problem.

use maternal
PLT, if
possible

(3) Platelet transfusion is helpful in stopping the bleeding from thrombocytopenia secondary to bone marrow suppression. If the platelet count is less than 20,000/mm³ on the basis of decreased production, significant bleeding is likely, and platelet concentrations (6 U/M²) should be used. In some cases of severe thrombocytopenia on an immune basis, massive platelet transfusions with high-dose steroids may be indicated.

3. **Immune thrombocytopenic purpura** (ITP) is an autoimmune thrombocytopenia that in 60 percent of reported cases follows a viral infection with about 15 percent following common exanthemas.

   a. **Etiology** The cause is unknown but the pathogenesis may be related to immunologic stimulation by a virus. *TORCH*

   b. **Evaluation**

      (1) Petechiae and purpura are almost invariably present, and 30 percent of patients have epistaxis. While hemoglobin, hematocrit, and white blood count may be normal (atypical lymphocytes may be present), the platelet count is less than 50,000/mm³, and there is a preponderance of large platelets on the peripheral smear.

Maternal
IgG

      (2) Antiplatelet antibodies are found in 60 percent of children with ITP and if facilities for the test are available, it should be performed.

      (3) A **Coombs test** should be done to rule out autoimmune hemolytic anemia. But in childhood, acute ITP is not associated with other autoimmune disorders. *Like Rh incompatib:*

   c. The **diagnosis** of immune thrombocytopenia is made by doing a bone marrow aspiration to document the adequacy of megakaryocytes. Often eosinophilia is present in the marrow. If the clinical history is suggestive and the thrombocytopenia is mild, observations of serial platelet counts to document recovery may be used in place of bone marrow examination. If, however, therapeutic intervention is considered, bone marrow aspiration should be performed to rule out infiltrative diseases.

   d. **Therapy** Most children with ITP do very well without therapy. In about 70 percent, platelet counts return to normal within 4 months. Another 10 percent of cases resolve in the next 8 months; 20 percent go on to have chronic ITP. Postpubertal children do not do as well with only 20–30 percent resolving spontaneously. Mortality in childhood ITP is less than 1 percent. Death, when it occurs, is due to intracranial, pulmonary, or gastrointestinal hemorrhage. Of children who die, 90 percent do so within the first few days of the onset of their disease. Although the risk of significant bleeding is greatest early in the disease, some deaths have been reported among children with chronic ITP.

      (1) Drugs that interfere with platelet function **should be avoided.**

EtoH, NSAID, maternal ASA ↓ 1in 10 days
of delivery

(2) Corticosteroids usually have not increased the number of children achieving a normal platelet count, although they probably affect the **rate** of rise in platelet count. Acutely, however, steroids have been shown to enhance the rate at which bleeding disappears in ITP, which is probably related to their effect on vascular stability. **Prednisone,** 2 mg/kg/day, should be given to patients with ITP who have a platelet count of $< 10,000/mm^3$ or who show evidence of mucosal bleeding. The drug is given for 2 weeks and then tapered over the next week **regardless of the platelet count.** The use of steroids is to protect against early severe bleeding. Some authorities advocate an additional trial of prednisone for 2–4 weeks for patients who have not spontaneously recovered after 4 months.

(3) Splenectomy Of the 20 percent of patients in whom chronic ITP develops, only one-tenth will recover spontaneously. Of patients with chronic ITP who undergo splenectomy, 60–70 percent are cured, probably because the spleen, in addition to being the organ of platelet destruction, is a site for production of antiplatelet antibodies.

(a) Before splenectomy, patients should receive **prednisone** or **hydrocortisone,** and, although postoperative bleeding is rare, **platelets** should be available for administration.

(b) The platelet count peaks about 4 days after splenectomy and then reaches a plateau at 2–4 weeks.

(c) Splenectomy is to be avoided in children under 5.

(d) **Most children who undergo splenectomy are placed on prophylactic penicillin (400,000 units bid) for at least 2 years** or are given pneumococcal vaccine preoperatively. There are no data, however, to suggest that this affects the risk of sepsis.

(e) About 2–3 percent of patients will continue to have thrombocytopenia after splenectomy. Some may respond to intermittent steroids. Others require immunosuppressive agents, such as vincristine, azathioprine, or cyclophosphamide. The risk of these drugs should be weighed against risk of bleeding from the thrombocytopenia, which in children is low.

18

Inflammatory and Immunodeficiency Disorders

I. INFLAMMATORY DISORDERS

A. **Juvenile rheumatoid arthritis (JRA)** is a generalized systemic inflammatory disease involving the joints, connective tissue, and viscera. The disease may occur at any age, but the peak incidence is at 1–4 years and at puberty.

1. **Evaluation** There are three distinct modes of onset: acute febrile or systemic, polyarticular, and pauciarticular. Each may be confused with other diagnoses.

   a. **Acute febrile or systemic** This group of children has prominent systemic symptoms with various manifestations of fever, rash, lymphadenopathy, hepatosplenomegaly, abdominal pain, pericarditis, myocarditis, or pleuritis. Joint symptoms may be absent or minimal at presentation. The characteristic fever has one to two daily spikes to 103°F or higher and subsequent rapid return to normal or subnormal levels. Arthritis will eventually develop in most of these patients.

   b. **Polyarticular** The arthritis may begin in the large joints, but the small joints of the hands and feet, the cervical spine, and the temporomandibular joint are often involved. The affected joints are swollen, warm, and tender, with limitation of movement and morning stiffness. Low-grade fever, anorexia, and malaise are common.

   c. **Pauciarticular** The arthritis is limited to four or fewer joints and usually involves large joints, namely, the knees, ankles, elbows, or hips. The small joints are usually spared. Iridocyclitis occurs in over 25 percent of the patients with this type of presentation and may precede the joint symptoms.

2. **Diagnosis** There is no single laboratory test that confirms the diagnosis. Assessment is based on the clinical presentation, laboratory abnormalities, and exclusion of other diseases.

   a. There are no uniformly agreed-on diagnostic criteria. However, the following criteria are useful:

      (1) **Polyarticular or monoarticular arthritis persisting for 6 weeks** is sufficient for diagnosis if other diseases are excluded. **Arthritis** is defined as swelling of a joint or limitation of motion with heat, pain, or tenderness. The latter two symptoms alone are not sufficient for the diagnosis. Temporomandibular joint involvement, cervical spine involvement, small joint involvement, a nonmigratory pattern, and morning stiffness are suggestive of the diagnosis. The joint involvement may be symmetrical and associated with subcutaneous nodules. The only early x-ray abnormalities are soft tissue swelling and osteoporosis without erosive joint changes. Painless contractions without swelling may occur.

      (2) **The acute systemic form will be associated with fever and a characteristic rash** consisting of recurrent, evanescent, pale red macules,

often with central clearing and found predominantly on the chest axilla, thighs, and upper arms.

b. Although there are no diagnostic tests, certain **laboratory findings** may be abnormal in some patients. These include the following:

    (1) An elevated white blood count, anemia, elevated erythrocyte sedimentation rate (ESR), thrombocytosis, and an increase in acute phase reactants.

    (2) The assay for anti–gamma globulin (rheumatoid factor) as commonly performed is usually persistently positive in 5–20 percent of all patients with JRA. Positive tests are more frequent in older children with polyarticular onset disease. Its presence correlates with a chronic destructive arthritis.

    (3) Antinuclear antibody (ANA) may be found in 10–40 percent of patients with oligoarticular or polyarticular onset disease. An increased percentage of children with chronic iridocyclitis have a positive ANA.

    (4) Aspirated joint fluid in JRA is yellow to greenish, cloudy, with low viscosity, and has a poor mucin clot. The white count is 10,000 to 50,000 mm^3, with approximately 75 percent polymorphonuclears Inclusion-bearing cells may be seen.

    (5) There is an increased incidence of the histocompatibility antigen HLA–B27 in ankylosing spondylitis, Reiter syndrome, spondylitis with inflamed bowel disease, and arthritis following *Yersinia* or *Salmonella* infection. Laboratory studies to exclude other diseases will often be required.

3. Therapy   The goal of therapy is to relieve acute symptoms, control the inflammatory process, preserve functional capacity, prevent deformities and care for the psychological and social needs of patient and family There is no curative drug. With adequate care, at least 75 percent of children will be left with no significant disability. The worst prognosis is for patients with polyarticular involvement, especially those who have a positive rheumatoid factor.

    a. Relief of symptoms and control of inflammation   No drug has been specifically approved by the Food and Drug Administration for the treatment of JRA, but aspirin is universally used. The Pediatric Rheumatology Collaborative Study group is currently conducting controlled trials of other antiinflammatory agents (meclofenamic acid, fenoprofen, ibuprofen).

        (1) Aspirin is the drug of choice for relief of acute symptoms and fever.

            (a) The dose is 70–100 mg/kg/day in 4–6 divided doses to attain a blood level of 20–25 mg/100 ml 2 hr after a dose.

            (b) In the younger child (< 25 kg) the lower doses should be used and a dose of 4 gm should not be exceeded without checking levels. Occasionally, in patients with high intermittent fever to relieve symptoms, the dosage will need to be increased (to up to 120 mg/kg and a level close to 30 mg/100 ml).

            (c) Because of the wide individual differences in the level obtained, resulting from differences in absorption, metabolism and excretion, **blood levels should be checked in all patients about 1 week into therapy.** A small increase in the dose of patients on long-term therapy may have a dramatic effect on the level.

(d) Side effects

i. Patients and parents should be warned about **symptoms of intoxication,** which include lethargy, hyperventilation, dizziness, sweating, headache, vomiting, and tinnitus.

ii. Aspirin should not be taken on an empty stomach, and if gastric irritation is a problem, antacids may be helpful. However, antacids may lower the salicylate level. **Enteric-coated aspirin** may also be helpful, but levels should be checked after ingestion to confirm absorption.

iii. **Hepatotoxicity,** with elevation of serum transaminases, occurs in some patients with JRA on aspirin therapy. It is said to occur more commonly with levels over 25 mg/100 ml, but can occur with lower levels. Liver enzymes should be checked about 7–10 days into therapy and any time that nausea, vomiting, or abdominal discomfort occurs.

iv. Aspirin should be discontinued if prothrombin time is grossly prolonged, enzymes are very high, or clinical evidence of bleeding or liver dysfunction occurs.

(e) The patient should receive a trial of at least 6 weeks of aspirin at therapeutic levels before it is discontinued. If the patient responds to aspirin, it should be continued for several months after the patient is asymptomatic.

(2) Tolmetin sodium, a nonsteroidal antiinflammatory agent, has been recently investigated and recommended by the Pediatric Rheumatology Collaborative Study group for the treatment of JRA.

(a) It should be used for patients in whom allergy or intolerance precludes the use of aspirin, whose liver enzyme function is of concern, or in whom aspirin produces an unsatisfactory therapeutic effect.

(b) The **initial dose** is 15 mg/kg/day, with increases at 5 mg/kg/day at weekly intervals until efficacy is noted, adverse reactions appear, or a dose of 30 mg/kg/day or 1,800 mg is reached.

(c) **Side effects** include gastric intolerance and a slight decrease in hemoglobin.

(3) Other drugs Patients unresponsive to an adequate trial (3–6 months) of aspirin or tolmetin sodium and to good physical management with disease progression will require another drug. The choice of this drug will vary at different institutions; controlled trials with these drugs have not been conducted in children. None of the drugs is as benign as aspirin. The choice of drugs includes

(a) Gold compounds If the patient has progressive joint disease despite aspirin administration and can return for regular injections and follow-up, gold may be indicated. Gold can control symptoms and prevent further joint damage, but has little effect on systemic manifestations and will not improve joints deformed from damaged cartilage. This potentially toxic drug is given as a weekly injection over a long period and a response will not be seen for 3–4 months.

i. The dose is 1 mg/kg (up to 50 mg) IM of gold sodium thiomalate (Myochrysine) as a weekly injection into a buttock. A test dose of 2.5 to 5 mg is given, to detect any idiosyncratic reaction.

ii. If there is no intolerance, ¼ of the weekly dose is given followed by 2 weekly injections of ½ and ¾ of the full dose until the full dose is instituted once a week for 6 months. This is followed by a reduction to every other week for months, then to every third week for four injections, and then to a monthly injection indefinitely if the patient has shown a response.

iii. Toxicity can affect the skin, kidney, bone marrow, and liver. Before initiation of therapy, liver function tests, BUN, creatinine, the CBC, platelet count, and urinalyses should be checked. Before each injection a history of rash, pruritis, and stomatitis should be elicited. In addition, a urinalysis for proteinuria or hematuria, hemoglobin, white blood cell count, differential, and platelet count should be obtained.

iv. Gold therapy should be discontinued if rash, albuminuria, hematuria, leukopenia, thrombocytopenia, or eosinophilia occurs. It is sometimes possible to reinstitute therapy at a lower dose in spite of a mild dermatitis.

(b) Hydroxychloroquine (Plaquenil) has been used in some patients unresponsive to aspirin who have progressive joint disease. It has also been used to decrease the dose of steroids a patient is taking.

i. The dose used is 5–7 mg/kg, up to 250 mg/day. A therapeutic response will not be seen for 1–3 months.

ii. Some rheumatologists do not use the drug because of its potentially serious **side effects**. A **retinitis** with irreversible macular degeneration may occur. **Patients should be warned to report difficulty with vision, accommodation, photophobia or field defects and should wear sunglasses in bright light.** Every 3 months an ophthalmologic examination should be done to check for corneal deposits, visual-field changes, and scotomata. The drug should be reserved for children who can cooperate with this type of examination.

iii. Accidental ingestion of the drug is potentially fatal.

iv. The duration of treatment should not exceed 1 year.

(c) Indomethacin, when added to salicylate, has helped certain patients. Some centers use this drug for patients with high fever that is unresponsive to aspirin or to help decrease a steroid dose. Others feel that it is contraindicated in small children (at this time the FDA does not sanction its use in children 14 and under).

i. The **dosage** is 1–2 mg/kg/day up to 100 mg, divided into 2–3 doses, given after meals. Before starting the full dose, a test dose of ¼ of the total daily dose should be given for 2 days followed by ½ of the daily total for 2 days.

ii. Side effects include GI intolerance, headache, and bone marrow depression. The hemoglobin, white blood count, and urinalyses should be followed.

iii. Usually, if a response is going to occur, it will be seen in 2–3 weeks.

(d) Corticosteroids are not indicated for routine long-term treatment, since they do not alter the long-term course or prevent permanent joint damage.

  i. The **indications** for their use are severe pericarditis and myocarditis, iridocyclitis unresponsive to topical steroids, and severe incapacitating systemic symptoms with high fever that are unresponsive to other medication.

  ii. The **dosage** should be the minimum necessary to control the symptoms, and the drug should be discontinued as soon as possible. Steroids do not prevent progression of joint destruction, and, once started, they may be difficult to discontinue without causing a flare of activity. They may also increase the excretion of aspirin. When treating **cardiac complications,** aggressive treatment with prednisone, 1–2 mg/kg/day, should be started and maintained for a week; if there is improvement the level may be slowly decreased. Other indications can often be treated with lower doses (prednisone, 0.2–0.4 mg/kg/day) or with steroids every other day.

  iii. Intrasynovial steroid injections may be helpful if one or two joints are refractory to treatment.

b. Exercise, physical therapy, and rest An active program of daily physical therapy is essential to preserve range of motion, maintain muscle strength, and prevent deformities. The most valuable form of therapy is exercise, as long as it does not traumatize an inflamed joint.

(1) Even before aspirin has had its full effect, **passive range of motion and mild muscle stretching and strengthening exercises** should be started. The prior application of heat will allow for better results. Passive range of motion therapy should be replaced by active assistive and then active exercises. Moist heat (tub baths and hot packs) will relieve morning stiffness and pain.

(2) Adequate rest is important, and a firm mattress should be used.

c. Psychological adjustment Attention to the parents' and child's reaction to JRA is important in interpreting symptoms and judging compliance with the therapeutic regimen. The parents should not be overprotective, and the child should resume an active life with attendance at school as soon as possible.

d. Orthopedic measures Early in the disease, acutely painful joints may require intermittent resting splints to prevent flexion contractures and preserve functional alignment. Later, serial splinting may be required to correct contractures. Work splints, skin traction, braces, corrective devices, and intraarticular steroids may be indicated.

e. Eyes All patients should be checked by an ophthalmologist with a slit lamp examination to detect **iridocyclitis** when JRA is diagnosed and should be rechecked at least twice a year.

(1) Patients with pauciarticular disease, especially with a high ANA titer, are at an increased risk of the development of eye complications, and their eyes should be examined at least every 3 months. Patients in whom iridocyclitis develops usually do not have severe joint disease. The onset is insidious and often independent of joint activity.

(2) Patients should be warned to report a red eye, eye pain, photophobia, or visual difficulties. Topical steroids, mydriatics, and, at times, systemic steroids will be required. A close follow-up is mandatory.

B. Systemic lupus erythematosus (SLE)

1. The **etiology** of this multisystemic inflammatory disorder is unknown, but an interaction of genetic, viral, and immunologic factors has been invoked. Persons with SLE produce autoantibodies, and the deposition of the immune complex of DNA and anti-DNA in the kidney results in nephritis. Immune complexes may involve other antigens, and it is probable that the type of antibody, its avidity, and the size of the complex determine the symptoms. Autoantibodies to clotting factors and cells account for the circulating anticoagulant, thrombocytopenia, and positive Coombs tests seen. The majority of patients (88 percent) are females in whom the peak onset is during adolescence; in males, a more uniform age distribution is seen.

In occasional patients the disease can be provoked or exacerbated by sun exposure. In others, SLE or a mild reversible form of the disease can be precipitated by drugs (Table 18-1). Complement deficiency (C1, C2, C4, C5, and C8) may predispose to SLE.

2. Evaluation and diagnosis

a. Clinical

(1) The disease may be highly variable in its manifestations and course, but the most common presenting symptoms are rash (facial butterfly, erythematous blush), fever, malaise, and arthralgia or arthritis. On the initial presentation, only one of these symptoms may be present, or the symptoms may reflect involvement of one organ, such as the kidney.

(2) The American Rheumatism Association has designated preliminary criteria for the classification of SLE (Table 18-2). A diagnosis of SLE can be established if four or more of those symptoms are present. Hepatomegaly and lymphadenopathy may be especially prominent in childhood SLE.

b. Laboratory studies will be necessary to confirm the clinical impression.

(1) Almost all patients with SLE have an **ANA** that is usually directed to native double-stranded DNA. This type of antibody displays a peripheral immunofluorescence pattern of stained nuclei. An ANA may be found in other collagen disorders or chronic inflammatory states, but the titer usually is not as high and the specificity is not usually directed to double-stranded DNA. The titer of anti-DNA

Table 18-1   Drugs Precipitating Systemic Lupus Erythematosus

Hydralazine	Sulfonamides
Procainamide	Phenylbutazone
Trimethadione	Para-aminosalicylic acid
Phenytoin sodium	Isoniazid
Penicillin	

Table 18-2 American Rheumatism Association Classification Criteria for SLE

Facial erythema
Discoid lupus
Raynaud's phenomenon
Alopecia
Photosensitivity
Oral or nasopharyngeal ulceration
Arthritis without deformity
LE cells
Chronic false-positive serologic test for syphilis (STS)
Profuse proteinuria
Cellular casts
Pleuritis, or pericarditis, or both
Psychosis, or convulsions, or both
Hemolytic anemia, leukopenia, or thrombocytopenia

Modified from American Rheumatism Association.

antibody may correlate with the presence of clinical symptoms. A rising titer should suggest impending clinical activity.

(2) The level of **C3 and C4** may be decreased during active disease secondary to deposition of immune complexes. Circulating immune complexes may be detected, and their levels may also correlate with symptoms.

(3) Anemia, a positive Coombs test, leukopenia, abnormal clotting, an elevated ESR, hematuria, and proteinuria may be found.

(4) A **renal biopsy** is indicated if renal function is abnormal or urinary abnormalities are present. The biopsy will determine the type of nephritis, which may dictate therapy and the prognosis. Severe (diffuse) proliferate glomerulonephritis is more commonly associated with heavy proteinuria, hypertension, and renal insufficiency and has a worse prognosis than mild (focal) proliferative or minimal (mesangial) lupus nephritis. Membranous lupus nephritis may also present clinically with the nephrotic syndrome and hematuria, but azotemia is less common at onset, and the progression to renal insufficiency is slow when compared with that in diffuse proliferative glomerulonephritis.

3. The goals of **therapy** are prevention of progressive tissue damage, relief of incapacitating symptoms, prevention of death from treatment or the disease itself, and restoration of a normal daily routine.

a. General measures

(1) **Adequate rest** and **emotional support** are important. Emotional upsets can trigger an exacerbation.

(2) **All unnecessary medications should be discontinued** because of the possibility of drug-induced disease. If sunlight exacerbates the disease, exposure should be limited and a sunscreen containing 10% para-aminobenzoic acid prescribed.

(3) Cold should be avoided if the patient suffers from Raynaud's phe nomenon.

b. Drugs

(1) Aspirin is prescribed to control arthralgia and fever. To attain a blood level of about 20 mg/100 ml, give 30–60 mg/kg/day.

(2) Corticosteroids are indicated for patients with active renal hematologic, or CNS disease. They may also be required for severe skin disease and for fever and arthralgia unresponsive to aspirin or hydroxychloroquine.

(a) Prednisone, 1–2 mg/kg/day, is given PO in divided doses until the disease is brought under control, which may take 3–6 weeks (although fever, malaise, and arthralgia may improve after a few days). An increase in the complement level and a decrease in the ANA titer or DNA binding, ESR, and level of circulating immune complexes should occur, and some symptoms should be ameliorated. If the serologic abnormalities are not brought under control, the dosage may have to be increased.

(b) With remission or a plateau in improvement, the steroid dose should be **gradually** tapered to 5 mg or less (10 percent of the total daily dose) of prednisone per week to the minimum dose at which the disease is quiescent. **Rapid tapering can precipitate a flare-up.**

(c) An increase in DNA binding, a fall in complement, or a deterioration of renal function indicates the need for an increased steroid dose.

(d) Side effects and complications of steroids should be anticipated and treated.

(e) Topical steroids can be used on skin lesions in patients not requiring systemic steroids.

(3) Hydroxychloroquine, used with prednisone, may allow a reduction in the dose and duration of administration of steroids. Hydroxychloroquine may also be used in patients with skin and joint symptoms unresponsive to aspirin and topical steroids. Skin manifestations may improve quickly, but joint symptoms may continue for 1–2 months. The duration of therapy should not exceed 1 year (see **b**, p. 446, for toxicity and dose).

(4) Immunosuppressive agents The role of these agents in the treatment of childhood SLE has not been clearly defined. Azathioprine, cyclophosphamide, and chlorambucil in conjunction with steroids have been prescribed in patients in whom complications develop with high-dose steroids or who are unresponsive to high doses. They have been used for patients with diffuse proliferative glomerulonephritis and with CNS lupus, in which their effectiveness is under investigation. Abrupt cessation of these agents may precipitate an exacerbation of symptoms. They have potentially serious side effects that should be considered before they are used.

c. Other measures

(1) Infections SLE patients on steroids or immunosuppressants are highly susceptible to serious infection. Cultures should be done and the patient should be treated at the first sign of infection.

(2) **Hemodialysis** and **renal transplantation** should be considered in patients with terminal renal failure.

C. Dermatomyositis

1. Etiology The childhood form is a systemic disease with diffuse angiitis involving skeletal muscle, skin, fat, the GI tract, and parts of the CNS. The cause is unknown, but patients have been shown to have lymphocyte sensitization to muscle and deposition of immunoglobulin and complement in skeletal muscle blood vessels.

2. Evaluation and Diagnosis The characteristic clinical picture of muscle weakness with some pain occurring with constitutional symptoms and the characteristic rash should suggest the diagnosis. The diagnosis will be confirmed by elevated levels of muscle enzymes, an electromyogram, and a muscle biopsy. Myositis may also occur in SLE, JRA, scleroderma, and arteritis, as well as in virus infections.

3. Therapy

a. General measures Active physiotherapy, positioning, and splinting will be necessary to rebuild muscle strength and prevent contractures. Children should sleep in the prone position to prevent hip contractures.

b. Drugs Early diagnosis and early initiation of treatment are necessary to prevent further muscle damage and atrophy.

(1) Corticosteroids

(a) High-dose prednisone, $1-2$ mg/kg or 50 to 75 mg/m^2/day up to a dose of 80 mg/day, should be prescribed for 4–6 weeks or until clinical improvement of constitutional symptoms and skin manifestations and an increase in muscle strength occur. Muscle enzyme levels will usually decrease with clinical improvement.

(b) The steroid dose should be tapered gradually over 2–3 months and the patient maintained on 0.25 mg/kg/day or 5–10 mg/day or the lowest possible dose that keeps the disease quiescent and nonprogressive.

(c) Maintenance therapy should continue for 1–3 years. During this period, patients are susceptible to periods of relapse, with exacerbation of symptoms. If this occurs, high-dose steroids must be reinstituted. Rarely, exacerbations may occur several years later.

(2) Immunosuppressants In a limited number of cases, IV methotrexate and other immunosuppressants have been prescribed to control the disease in patients unresponsive to or requiring continuous high-dose steroids.

c. Involvement of the palatal-respiratory muscles, as clinically evidenced by dysphagia, regurgitation, or a change in the voice, demands close attention to **suctioning, postural drainage,** and **respiratory function.**

d. Long-term follow-up is mandatory to treat chronic contractures and atrophy and to attend to the psychological and social needs of the patient.

D. Vasculitis: Polyarteritis nodosa, mucocutaneous lymph node syndrome **Schönlein-Henoch purpura.** (For serum sickness and urticaria, see Chap. 19.)

1. Etiology Usually, the etiology is unknown. However, it is believed that in many cases the vessel inflammation is secondary to the deposition of immune complexes or antibody or cells directed to antigen existing in the vessel wall. The inciting antigen may be drugs (e.g., amphetamines, sulfonamides), infectious agents (e.g., hepatitis B [HBsAg]), streptococcal antigens, or autologous immunoglobulins (cryoglobulinemia).

2. Evaluation

   a. The **clinical symptoms** reflect the protean manifestations of multisystemic involvement. The symptoms may include the following:

   (1) Fever

   (2) Symptoms of **skin and mucosa involvement** (purpura, livedo reticularis, pyoderma gangrenosum, subcutaneous nodules, conjunctivitis, and enanthemata)

   (3) Kidney involvement (hematuria, proteinuria, renal insufficiency)

   (4) Heart involvement (congestive heart failure, myocardial infarction)

   (5) GI tract involvement (abdominal pain, melena, pancreatitis, hepatitis, cholecystitis)

   (6) Lung involvement (cough, wheezing)

   (7) CNS involvement

   (8) Myositis

   (9) Hypertension

   b. Laboratory investigations

   (1) All **tests for dysfunction of various organ systems,** especially the kidney, GI tract, lungs, and heart, should be performed.

   (2) Studies of cryoglobulins, anti–gamma globulins, circulating immune complexes, levels of C3 and CH50, ANA, and hepatitis B surface antigen should be made.

   (3) Arteriography may demonstrate microaneurysms or irregularities of the vessel wall.

   (4) Biopsies of the skin, muscle, kidney, or testis may be necessary.

3. Diagnosis

   a. Polyarteritis nodosa may present in an infantile form in children under 1 year of age or in older children and adolescents.

   (1) Clinical symptoms of the **infantile form** include an intermittent or prolonged fever, fleeting erythematous rash, conjunctivitis, cough, cardiomegaly, hypertension, or congestive heart failure, abdominal pain, and abnormal findings on urinalysis.

   (2) The **childhood form** is more variable. Arteriography of the coronary arteries may show microaneurysms, and a biopsy may show necrotizing vasculitis of small- and medium-sized arteries with fibrinoid necroses and aneurysm formation. Eosinophilia and an elevated IgE level are often found.

b. **Mucocutaneous lymph node syndrome** (MCLS, Kawasaki disease)

(1) **Clinical symptoms**

(a) Typically, there is fever lasting over 5 days, which does not respond to antibiotics, and reddening and indurative edema of the palms and soles, with membranous desquamation from the fingertips during convalescence, polymorphous exanthem of the trunk, bilateral conjunctivitis, reddening and fissuring of the lips with a strawberry tongue, reddening of the naso-pharyngeal mucosa, and swelling of the cervical lymph nodes.

(b) Other symptoms include tachycardia, gallop rhythm, heart murmurs, abdominal pain and diarrhea, and, rarely, arthralgia, aseptic meningitis, and mild jaundice.

(c) A mortality of 1 to 2 percent is secondary to **myocardial infarction** due to coronary thromboarteritis.

(2) **Laboratory findings** include leukocytosis, thrombocytoses, abnormal acute-phase reactants, elevated IgE level, and ECG abnormalities.

(3) **Coronary angiography** may reveal aneurysms, dilatation, stenosis, and irregularities in a large percentage of patients. Other vessels may be involved. Such vessel involvement should be sought, since it may dictate the type of treatment and the prognosis. The relationship between this syndrome and infantile polyarteritis is under investigation.

c. **Anaphylactoid purpura (Schönlein-Henoch purpura)**

(1) **Clinical symptoms** The typical clinical picture of involvement of the skin, joints, GI tract, and kidneys secondary to a vasculitis of capillaries and precapillary and postcapillary vessels makes the diagnosis evident.

(a) The **characteristic skin lesions** occur especially on the buttocks and lower extremities, appearing initially as urticarial, with rapid evolution into pink maculopapules that become either small and discrete or enlarged, blotchy, and confluent. The initial red color becomes brownish, and ecchymotic areas may appear. Petechial lesions may be seen.

(b) The **joints,** especially the ankles and knees, **are swollen in the periarticular spaces** and are often painful.

(c) **GI symptoms** include abdominal pain, melena, vomiting, and hematemesis.

(d) **Renal involvement** occurs in 20–70 percent of patients. The spectrum varies from microscopic hematuria to acute, rapidly progressive nephritis or nephrotic syndrome. The renal manifestations usually appear within a month of the other manifestations, but occasionally may present later and sometimes before the skin lesions.

(e) **Recurrent attacks** of the syndrome are not uncommon.

(2) **Laboratory investigations** may reveal an abnormal urinalysis, elevated serum IgA level, and a normal C3 level and antistreptolysin O titer. Bleeding times and platelet counts are normal.

4. Therapy

a. Any unnecessary drugs should be discontinued and a **careful histor**
taken to determine exposure to infectious agents, insect stings
foreign proteins, and medications. Before any drug is used a history o
previous adverse reactions should be elicited. To prevent serum sick
ness, **human hyperimmune globulin** should be used in place of foreign
serum proteins. If heterologous serum proteins must be used, the
patient should have a **skin test.**

b. Rigorous symptomatic treatment of various symptoms, including con
gestive heart failure, myocardial insufficiency, renal insufficiency
and hypertension, should be undertaken because the clinical course
may be self-limited.

c. Specific therapy

(1) Polyarteritis nodosa High-dose corticosteroids (prednisone,
mg/kg/day) should be started promptly. The clinical condition, in
cluding heart involvement, and the laboratory findings should be
followed to assess the response. Patients unresponsive to predni
sone may require a higher dose, and immunosuppressants should
be considered.

(2) Patients with the **mucocutaneous lymph node syndrome** should be
treated symptomatically. Coronary artery involvement should be
looked for, and, if found, should be treated with high-dose predni
sone (2 mg/kg/day) although its effectiveness has not been proved.

(3) Anaphylactoid purpura

(a) Patients with **severe arthralgia** may be helped with aspirin
initially at 60 mg/kg, which may have to be increased to higher
levels for relief (see **A.3,** p. 444).

(b) Acute renal failure should be treated vigorously because there
is a considerable spontaneous cure rate.

(c) Patients with **GI involvement** should be watched carefully for
the complications of severe hemorrhage, intussusception, and
perforation. If melena occurs, patients should be prophylacti
cally crossmatched.

(d) There has been no controlled study of the use of **corticosteroids**
in anaphylactoid purpura. They do not affect the total duration
of the illness, the frequency of recurrences, or the renal dis
ease. However, some physicians have used them for patients
with severe colicky abdominal pain and melena to provide a
more rapid relief of symptoms and prevent intussusception. I
abdominal pain does not respond to corticosteroids, a fixed le
sion of the GI tract should be suspected. The drug is given
either parenterally (IV hydrocortisone, 4 mg/kg/day) or PO
(prednisone, 1–2 mg/kg/day for 48–72 hr).

II. IMMUNODEFICIENCY DISORDERS   Defects of the immune system (Table 18-3)
may involve antibody-mediated immunity, T cell–mediated immunity, the
phagocytic system (which includes circulating neutrophils and monocytes and
tissue-fixed macrophages), or the complement system.

A. Etiology and evaluation

1. An immunodeficiency should be suspected if a child has an increased fre
quency of infection or infections of unusual severity, prolonged duration

Table 18-3   Evaluation of Defects of the Immune System

Antibody Deficiency	Cellular Deficiency
History of pyogenic infections after age 6 months	History of fungal and viral infection anytime after birth
Quantitation of IgG, IgA, IgM	Absolute lymphocyte number
Specific antibody production	X-ray for thymus shadow
Isohemagglutinins	Skin tests
Schick test	*Candida*, streptokinase-streptodornase, PPD, *Trichophytin*, mumps
Antibody titer to previous bacterial and viral immunizations	
Anamnestic response to boost of tetanus toxoid or killed antigen	Quantitation of T cells
Quantitation of B cells	Evaluation of T cell function
Evaluation of in vitro B-cell function	Responses to mitogens (PHA, *Concanavallin A*), allogeneic cells, and antigens
Immunoglobulin and specific antibody production	Lymphokine production
Other	Other
Lateral neck film	Enzyme levels of adenosine deaminase, nucleoside phosphorylase
Lymph node biopsy after local antigen injection	
IgG subclasses	
IgE level, IgD level	
Secretory IgA, immunoglobulin survival	

or with unusual complications. Unusual or opportunistic organisms may cause the infections. Although the normal child may have up to six respiratory infections in a year, the child with an immunodeficiency will have more prolonged infections and may not recover completely between infections. Chronic candidiasis or bronchiectasis, chronically draining ears, or chronic diarrhea may be the presenting symptom.

2. Abnormal humoral immunity will predispose to recurrent pyogenic infections such as otitis, sinusitis, pneumonia, and meningitis caused by *Pneumococcus, Haemophilus influenzae, Staphylococcus,* or *Streptococcus* spp. Antibody is necessary for opsonization for phagocytosis of these organisms. Maternal IgG protects the infant for the first 3–4 months, so that the child with isolated antibody deficiency will be asymptomatic for the first 6 months of life (Fig. 18-1).

3. Immunity to many fungal and viral infections resides in cellular or T cell–mediated processes. The infant with a T-cell deficiency has no maternal protection, so that symptoms begin during the first 3 months. Chronic candidiasis resistant to treatment in an infant, or a complication after viral infection or immunization, may reflect such a deficiency.

4. Complement is necessary for opsonization and immune adherence, and circulating white cells and fixed macrophages phagocytize and kill ingested organisms. Deficiency of any of these components results in pyogenic infections, recurrent abscesses, or recurrent stomatitis.

5. An immunodeficiency may be primary (congenital or acquired) or secondary to another disease or to treatment.

   a. **Congenital immunodeficiencies** with known inheritance include X-linked disorders (congenital hypogammaglobulinemia, severe com-

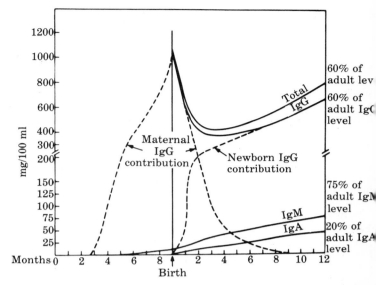

Figure 18-1 Immunoglobulin (IgG, IgM, and IgA) levels in the fetus an
infant in the first year of life. The IgG of the fetus and newborn infant
solely of maternal origin. The maternal IgG disappears by the age of nir
months, by which time the endogenous synthesis of IgG by the infant
well established. The IgM and IgA of the neonate are entirely endoge
nously synthesized, since maternal IgM and IgA do *not* cross the placent
(From E. R. Stiehm and V. A. Fulginiti, *Immunologic Disorders in In
fants and Children*, Philadelphia, Saunders, 1973. Reproduced by permi
sion.)

bined immunodeficiency, Wiskott-Aldrich syndrome, chronic gran
lomatous disease) and those inherited in an autosomal manne
(combined immunodeficiency, with or without absence of the enzyn
adenosine deaminase, and ataxia-telangiectasia).

b. Acquired immunodeficiencies may be associated with congenit
rubella, Epstein-Barr virus infection, malnutrition, malignancy, im
munosuppression, protein-losing diseases, transcobalamin II def
ciency, and use of phenytoin.

6. **Physical examination** should involve a search for the presence of lym
phoid tissues (tonsils, lymph nodes, spleen), signs of infection, and in
capacitation from chronic infection (hearing loss, failure to thrive, ev
dence of malabsorption). Skin involvement with eczema, candidiasi
telangiectasia, or petechiae should be noted.

7. The **laboratory evaluation** should be used to confirm a clinical suspicio
based on the type of infection, the age of onset, family history, and phys
cal examination.

a. Antibody deficiency and combined deficiency are more common tha
isolated T-cell deficiency or phagocytic and complement disorders. I
an immunodeficiency is suspected, **certain diagnostic and therapeuti
procedures are contraindicated.**

(1) Injection of live attenuated virus may cause a chronic viral disease.

(2) A **transfusion of blood products** may induce the **lethal** complication of graft-versus-host disease from transfused viable allogeneic lymphocytes. Irradiation of whole blood, packed red cells, frozen washed red cells, platelets, or frozen or fresh plasma with 5000 rads will prevent this complication.

b. The laboratory evaluation should proceed from the simpler to the more complicated tests. Results should be interpreted in relation to age-matched controls. The levels of immunoglobulins vary at different ages, and there is a wide normal range (see Fig. 18-1).

B. Diagnosis and therapy of specific disorders

1. Antibody deficiency

a. Diagnosis

(1) Congenital X-linked hypogammaglobulinemia This disorder of males is associated with absence of antibody responses, total immunoglobulin levels less than 200 mg/100 ml, and IgG less than 100 mg/100 ml. Circulating B cells are not usually present, although a few rare exceptions have been described. There is scanty tonsillar and adenoidal tissue on a lateral neck film. A lymph node biopsy shows abnormal architecture and absence of plasma cells.

Hypogammaglobulinemia with increased IgM can be an X-linked disorder or an acquired trait. IgG and IgA are decreased. Lymphadenopathy and large tonsils may occur. Neutropenia, thrombocytopenia, and hemolytic anemia are common.

(2) Transient hypogammaglobulinemia of infancy In some infants there is a delay in immunoglobulin synthesis, so that the nadir of IgG seen at 3–4 months (approximately 300 mg/100 ml) is prolonged and continues to decrease (see Fig. 18-1). IgG levels remain low (often less than 200 mg/100 ml), and IgM and IgA may be normal or low. Some specific antibody responses can be seen, and B cells are present. Plasma cells are present in the lymph nodes and in the GI tract. Wheezing, respiratory infections, and diarrhea may be the clinical symptoms.

(3) Common variable hypogammaglobulinemia This heterogeneous group of disorders occurs at any age. The type of defects described include absence of B cells, B cells that do not differentiate to produce immunoglobulin, B cells that synthesize but do not secrete immunoglobulin, circulating plasma inhibitors, and abnormal suppressor T lymphocytes. Pyogenic infections, chronic diarrhea with malabsorption, and *Giardia* infestation of the gut are frequently seen.

(4) In **IgA deficiency,** an IgA level less than 5 mg/100 ml is found, with normal levels of IgG and IgM and normal antibody responses. The lack of serum IgA is accompanied by absence of secretory IgA, and it is the latter that accounts for the sinopulmonary infections, diarrhea, or malabsorption seen. Circulating B cells with IgA are usually present.

(5) Selective immunoglobulin deficiency is associated with sepsis, meningitis, malignancies, and GI disorders. Usually, the IgM level is less than 20 mg/100 ml. Rarely, patients have borderline decreased levels of total IgG with deficiency of an IgG subclass and

associated with recurrent *H. influenzae* infections. Levels of su
classes are age dependent so that a critical interpretation of va
ues is imperative.

b. Therapy

(1) Patients who have clinical disease and low levels of IgG or la
specific antibody responses will benefit from **IgG replaceme**
Commercial gamma globulin is a 16% (160 mg/ml) solution of p
marily IgG, with only trace amounts of IgM and IgA.

(a) The usual dose is 0.6 ml (100 mg/kg) as a monthly IM injectio
The initial loading dose is 1.8 ml (300 mg/kg) in 3 doses of (
ml/kg over 1 week. The serum level of IgG is raised by 1
mg/100 ml with an injection of 100 mg/kg (the normal half-life
about 25–30 days). The IM injection should be divided betwee
sites if a large volume is given.

(b) If infections are not controlled, the interval between injectio
should be shortened.

(c) Rarely, systemic reactions occur after an injection of gamm
globulin. Treatment should include epinephrine, antih
tamines, and general support.

(2) IV administration of **frozen plasma** has been used in some patien
not responding to gamma globulin. The IgM and IgA are increas
only for a short time because of their short half-life. High titers
a specific antibody can be administered this way by prior immu
zation of the donor, and larger amounts of total gamma globul
can be given. Donors must be screened for hepatitis. Preferabl
the same donor should be used for repeated infusions. The dose
10–20 ml/kg every 3–4 weeks. An initial loading dose of two
three times the maintenance dose should be given over the first
weeks.

(3) **IgA deficiency will not be helped by commercial gamma globuli**
which may also sensitize the patient, so that anti-IgA antibodi
that may cause anaphylactic reactions after plasma or blo
transfusions may develop. If an IgA-deficient patient requires
transfusion, washed packed red cells should be used.

(4) Aggressive and immediate **antibiotic treatment** should be institut
for infection. Bronchiectasis should be managed with physic
therapy, postural drainage, and antibiotics. Hearing loss should
prevented. Malabsorption and diarrhea should be treated with
etary restriction, and if *Giardia* infestation is demonstrated
duodenal aspirate, the patient should be treated with m
tronidazole.

(5) Family members should be screened for immunodeficiencies.

2. Cell-mediated immunodeficiency

a. Diagnosis

(1) Congenital thymic aplasia (DiGeorge syndrome) This develo
mental abnormality of the 3rd and 4th pharyngeal pouch results
absence of the thymus and parathyroid glands, cardiac defects, and
characteristic facies. Neonatal tetany, candidiasis, heart murmur
and absence of a thymic shadow should suggest the diagnosi
Decreased T cells and poor in vitro lymphocyte responses will
seen. An incomplete form of the disease occurs.

(2) Chronic mucocutaneous candidiasis is characterized by chronic *Candida* infection of the nails, skin, and mucous membranes. Absence of delayed hypersensitivity skin tests to *Candida* will be found. Endocrinopathies, especially hypoparathyroidism and Addison's disease, are frequent occurrences.

(3) Miscellaneous disorders Absence of the enzyme nucleoside phosphorylase, malnutrition, drug immunosuppression, and lymphocyte loss will cause T-cell dysfunction.

b. Therapy

(1) DiGeorge syndrome Transplantation of a fetal thymus corrects the immune defect. Children with a partial defect may gradually acquire T-cell function without treatment. Irradiate all transfusions (see **A.7**).

(2) Mucocutaneous candidiasis has been treated with intravenous amphotericin B, oral and topical nystatin, and transfer factor prepared from a *Candida*-reactive person. Responses are variable. Experimental trials of miconazole, an antimycotic agent, suggest that it may be a useful alternative to amphotericin (see p. 363).

(3) Associated endocrinopathies should be treated.

3. Combined (antibody and cellular) immunodeficiency

a. Diagnosis

(1) Severe combined immunodeficiency may be inherited as an X-linked or autosomal recessive disorder, and the latter may be associated with absence of the enzyme adenosine deaminase.

(a) The diagnosis is confirmed by low immunoglobulin levels, absent antibody responses, and low numbers of circulating T cells with abnormal in vitro responses. Adenosine deaminase should be assayed in red cells.

(b) Bony abnormalities may be seen on x-rays of the rib cage, pelvis, and spine in ADA deficiency.

(c) If the child has inadvertently been given a nonirradiated transfusion or had a maternal-fetal transfusion, a graft-versus-host reaction may complicate the clinical picture with skin rash, diarrhea, hepatosplenomegaly, and failure to thrive.

(2) Wiskott-Aldrich syndrome is diagnosed by the clinical picture of eczema, thrombocytopenia, and recurrent infections in a male with absent isohemagglutinins and often with low IgM and abnormal T-cell function.

(3) Ataxia-telangiectasia is diagnosed by the occurrence of ataxia, choreoathetosis, dysarthric speech, telangiectasis, sinopulmonary infection, and the frequently found IgA deficiency and abnormal T cell function. Alpha-fetoprotein is often elevated.

b. Therapy

(1) In severe combined immunodeficiency, transplantation of histocompatible bone marrow can restore immunocompetence. A donor is selected on the basis of HLA and MLC typing. Some degree of graft-versus-host (GVH) disease may occur. The effectiveness of decontamination and laminar flow isolation in ameliorating GVH and preventing infections is being investigated. Infections from bacteria, viruses, and *Pneumocystis* may occur.

(2) The use of cultured thymus epithelium transplants, fetal live transplants, fetal thymus transplants, thymosin, transfer factor and correction of the defect in adenosine deaminase deficiency with packed red cell transfusions are at an experimental stage of evaluation.

(3) Blood products should be irradiated prior to transfusion [see **A.7.a.(2)**, p. 457].

(4) Aggressive treatment with antibiotics is necessary. Multiple organisms may be responsible for clinical disease. Lung infiltrates may be secondary to *Pneumocystis*, which is treated with pentamidine or trimethoprim-sulfamethoxazole (see Chap. 15). **Gamma globulin prophylaxis** is indicated for viral exposures.

(5) Siblings of affected children should be isolated at birth and screened for severe combined immunodeficiency with E rosetting, phytohemagglutinin (PHA) responses, and a chest x-ray for the presence of a thymus. Prenatal diagnosis of adenosine deaminase deficiency is possible with amniocentesis.

4. Phagocytic and complement disorders

   a. Diagnosis

   (1) Phagocytic disorders include chronic granulomatous disease, neutropenia, lazy leukocyte syndrome, myeloperoxidase deficiency, Chédiak-Higashi syndrome, Job syndrome, and splenic dysfunction or asplenia. These disorders are diagnosed by studying white cell number, morphology, and function (Table 18-4).

   (2) Complement abnormalities

   (a) Deficiency of C1 associated with a lupuslike syndrome and susceptibility to bacterial infection.

   (b) C2 deficiency associated with anaphylactoid purpura and SLE.

   (c) C3 deficiency and C3b inactivator deficiency associated with history of recurrent pyogenic infections that mimics hypogammaglobulinemia.

   (d) C4 deficiency with SLE.

   (e) C5 deficiency associated with recurrent infection and SLE.

   (f) C5 dysfunction with seborrhea, sepsis, and diarrhea.

   (g) C7 deficiency with Raynaud's phenomenon.

Table 18-4   Laboratory Investigations of Phagocytic, Opsonic, and Complement Deficiency

1. White blood cell count, differential, and morphology
   Examination of Howell-Jolly bodies, sickle preparation, and myeloperoxidase stain
2. Rebuck skin window
3. Nitroblue tetrazolium dye test; chemotactic, phagocytic, and bacterial killing assays
4. Spleen scan
5. Total hemolytic complement; individual complement component levels and function

(h) C6 and C8 deficiencies associated with recurrent *Neisseria* infections.

b. Therapy

(1) Antibiotics are indicated for infections. Because of the risk of overwhelming sepsis in patients with splenic absence or dysfunction, IV antibiotic administration should be instituted while awaiting cultures. Prophylactic antibiotics have been used in some of the white blood cell disorders.

(2) C5 dysfunction has been treated with fresh plasma infusions. Cellular immunodeficiency must be excluded.

(3) Prevention of infections There is no generally accepted practice for the prevention of infections in patients with splenic dysfunction.

(a) For patients at increased risk, some centers advocate prophylactic oral penicillin, 200,000 units bid, or ampicillin, 125 mg bid and 250 mg bid (for younger and older children respectively).

(b) It is important to educate parents about the risk of sepsis and the need to seek immediate medical attention at the first sign of infection. If prompt attention cannot be sought, some advise that the parents should be supplied with oral penicillin, 25,000 units/kg/6 hr, or ampicillin, 25 mg/kg/6 hr, which can be instituted at the first sign of infection.

(c) Controlled trials are being conducted to evaluate the effectiveness of immunization with pneumococci, *H. influenzae*, and meningococcal polysaccharides in preventing infections. Currently, patients over 2 years of age who have splenic absence or dysfunction **should be immunized with polyvalent pneumococcal-polysaccharide vaccine.**

5. Hereditary angioneurotic edema This autosomal dominant disorder of dysfunction or deficiency of the inhibitor of the activated first component of complement results in unopposed C1 activation, consumption of C4 and C2, and release of a vasoactive peptide that causes attacks of subcutaneous and submucosal edema by altering the postcapillary venule permeability. Intermittent episodes of nonpruritic edema of the skin of the extremities and face occur after minor trauma, emotional stress, or without a precipitating cause. The swelling may involve the mucous membranes of the hypopharynx and the larynx, causing **laryngeal obstruction and asphyxiation.** Abdominal pain with vomiting or diarrhea secondary to edema of the intestinal wall may occur without skin manifestations, but urticaria does not occur.

a. Diagnosis

In the majority of patients the level of C1 esterase inhibitor is decreased, but about 15 percent of persons with the disease have a normal level of nonfunctional protein. In both groups, C4 levels are low and fall during attacks.

b. Therapy

(1) The major complication of acute attacks is laryngeal obstruction, and thus patients or parents should be instructed to seek medical attention without delay if hoarseness, voice changes, or difficulty in breathing or swallowing occurs. A tracheotomy will be necessary for laryngeal obstruction. Epinephrine and hydrocortisone are of benefit in controlling swelling in only a rare patient, which

contrasts with the relief of urticaria and laryngeal obstructio
they afford in anaphylaxis and serum sickness (see Chap. 19).

(2) Fresh frozen plasma has been advocated for acute attacks to pr
vide C1 esterase inhibitor. However, fresh plasma has more sub
strate for C1 than C1 inhibitor, so that administration may exac
erbate symptoms.

(3) Prophylaxis has been attempted with the fibrinolytic inhibitor
epsilon-aminocaproic acid (EACA) and its analogue, tranexami
acid. Their usefulness is limited by the side effects of myopathy
predisposition to thromboses, phlebitis, nasal congestion, an
hypotension. But tranexamic acid has been used for short period
prior to surgery requiring dental extractions or tracheal intuba
tion with successful results.

19

Allergic Disorders

I. DIAGNOSTIC PROCEDURES

A. Skin tests Good correlations between the results of skin tests for pollens and inhalants and other in vitro or in vivo tests for immediate hypersensitivity are obtained when **appropriate controls** and **purified allergens** are used.

A small quantity of a suspected allergen is introduced (by scratch, prick, or intradermal method) into the skin. A *wheal and flare reaction* that occurs within 15–20 min and is larger than a control site where the diluent has been injected is interpreted as a positive reaction. A positive **histamine control** should be employed to be certain that the skin can respond properly, especially when all allergen sites are negative. Similarly, a **diluent control site** is important to document dermatographia in a patient who has all positive reactions. Skin testing for foods or drugs is in general less reliable, and the validity of the results must be individualized for each allergen.

B. The **radioallergosorbent test (RAST)** is a semiquantitative assay for allergen-specific IgE. The advantage of this test is that it can be performed in vitro, thus avoiding patient exposure to the allergen.

The RAST is recommended for patients who have skin conditions precluding accurate skin testing (e.g., urticaria pigmentosa, dermatographia) for patients who must remain on chronic antihistamines; for infants, in whom skin tests are generally unreliable; and for antigens that may be toxic or may sensitize the subject being tested.

C. IgE levels Total serum IgE levels are useful in evaluating infants under 12 months of age. In this group, levels greater than 100 IU/ml are strongly associated with asthma or rhinitis in which standard skin tests are negative. The finding of a significantly elevated level should stimulate further investigation for the source of allergen.

D. Challenge In rare cases it may be necessary to challenge a patient with a suspected allergen either orally (see Chap. 11) or by inhalation to confirm a relationship between exposure and symptomatology. This should be undertaken only with appropriate precautions to treat any undue reactions that may be precipitated.

II. SPECIFIC ENTITIES

A. Asthma See Chap. 2, Sec. **VII** and Chap. 20, Sec. **V.**

B. Anaphylaxis

1. Etiology Systemic anaphylaxis may be a life-threatening allergic reaction. It is caused by the IgE-triggered release of the mediators of immediate hypersensitivity from mast cells. Activated complement components ($C3_a$ and $C3_b$) may also be involved. "Anaphylactoid reactions" clinically resemble anaphylaxis but are caused by direct activation of the

Table 19-1 Major Causes of Anaphylaxis

Antibiotics
  Penicillin, cephalosporin, tetracycline, streptomycin, and others
Biologicals
  Insect venoms, allergen extracts, gamma globulin, blood transfusion, antitoxin
    antilymphocyte globulin, hormones, asparaginase, and others
Diagnostic agents
  Iodinated contrast media, BSP dye
Other drugs
  Aspirin, local anesthetics, dextran plasma expanders
Foods
  Especially eggs, milk, fish, shellfish, peanuts, nuts, chocolate

mast cell. The most common cause in children are antibiotics, allergen extracts, foods, and stinging-insect hypersensitivity (see Table 19-1).

2. Evaluation and diagnosis

  a. Anaphylactic reactions generally occur within minutes of exposure to the precipitating agent. When reactions are delayed, a carefully obtained **history** may suggest potential offenders.

  b. Laboratory evaluation

   (1) When available, RASTs are useful. A CBC may reveal eosinophilia.

   (2) Skin testing In the case of penicillin, foods, insect venoms, and other protein antigens, skin tests for immediate hypersensitivity may be diagnostic.

  c. Penicillin test Penicillin is the major drug implicated in anaphylactic reactions. **Appropriate skin testing** can identify patients at risk for serious reactions. The skin test procedure is, however, complex and should be undertaken only by experienced individuals. Penicillin testing should be performed only if the history suggests a previous hypersensitivity reaction in an individual who has an acute illness or chronic disease and makes future use of penicillin therapy likely (e.g. congenital heart disease, cystic fibrosis). (See also, **e**, p. 355.)

   (1) Following administration, penicillin is rapidly degraded into several breakdown products. Since any one of these products could produce an allergic reaction, several different preparations must be used in the skin test procedure. Furthermore, **dilute** solutions must be used initially to avoid systemic reactions.

   (2) The *penicilloyl* moiety is the major degradation product, and a skin test preparation (Penicilloyl-Polylysine, Kremers Urban Pharmaceutical Company) is available commercially. Reactions to this material are most frequently associated with late onset **urticaria** or **serum sickness.**

   (3) The multiple degradation products present in smaller amounts and referred to collectively as **minor determinants** are most important in **acute** anaphylactic reactions.

   (4) Minor determinant preparations for skin testing are not available

Table 19-2 Penicillin Skin Test Procedure

	Fresh Penicillin	Aged Penicillin	Penicilloyl-Polylysine[a]
Scratch[b]	500,000 U/ml	500,000 U/ml	6×10^{-5} M
Intradermal	500 U/ml	500 U/ml	6×10^{-5} M
Intradermal	5000 U/ml	5000 U/ml	—
Intradermal	50,000 U/ml	50,000 U/ml	—

[a] Pre-Pen, Kremers Urban Pharmaceutical.
[b] Always include a negative diluent and positive histamine (2.75 mg/ml) control with the initial scratch test.

commercially, but use of *both* fresh and aged penicillin (a solution that has been kept at room temperature for 1–2 weeks), which are presumed to contain minor determinants, are usually employed as a substitute.

(5) The breakdown products of the **semisynthetic penicillins** may differ from those in benzyl penicillin and, when possible, the specific penicillin product implicated should be incorporated into the test procedure.

(6) A RAST test for the major determinant is presently in use and could be obtained as an adjunct to skin testing. Positive reactions to the major determinant (either RAST or skin test) is the most consistent response with late or delayed sensitivity.

(7) Test procedure Table 19-2 outlines the sequential skin test procedure.

(a) Initially, a **scratch** test is performed followed by **intradermal** testing using 0.02 ml of increasing concentrations of fresh and aged penicillin. Test sites are read at 15–20 min. A negative diluent and positive histamine control should always be included. A positive reaction with any of these allergens must be viewed as evidence of sensitization.

(b) Entirely negative skin testing when all the solutions are employed suggests that sensitization is unlikely. As discussed in **(4)**, however, since a well-standardized minor determinant mixture is not available, negative skin tests in the presence of a strongly suggestive history must be interpreted with due consideration.

(c) "Desensitization" in a sensitized individual should **never** be attempted, **except** when penicillin therapy is an absolute indication in a life-threatening illness, and then only by an **experienced physician** who has appropriate resuscitative equipment available.

d. Anaphylactic symptoms vary in severity. Clinically, one or all of the following may be recognized in an anaphylactic reaction:

(1) Cutaneous Diffuse flushing may occur as the initial symptom, followed by urticaria, angioedema, or both.

(2) Respiratory Edema of the larynx and upper airway may result in stridor or even complete respiratory obstruction; or bronchospasm may predominate.

(3) **Cardiovascular**   Hypotension, tachycardia, or shock may occur.

(4) **Gastrointestinal**   Ingested allergens may cause nausea, abdominal pain, vomiting, and diarrhea.

(5) The diagnosis is made primarily on the basis of the clinical syndrome and a history consistent with exposure to an agent that may be responsible.

3. **Therapy** (see **d,** p. 40)   It is imperative that therapy be instituted **immediately** on recognition of the process. If the responsible agent is still being administered (e.g., IVP dye, blood products), **it must be discontinued promptly.**

   a. **General** measures include **epinephrine, fluid therapy, corticosteroids,** and **tourniquets.**

   b. For treatment of **bronchospasms, laryngeal edema, urticaria,** and **angioedema** (see **d,** p. 40).

   c. **Prophylaxis**   To prevent recurrence, cautious avoidance of reexposure to the specific allergen implicated in the original episode is mandatory.

      (1) **Stinging-insect allergy**   Injection therapy with venoms, when these become available, should provide significant protection.

      (2) Ready availability of an **anaphylaxis kit** that contains epinephrine should be emphasized for all persons who have had food or stinging-insect anaphylaxis. In addition, they should wear a Medic Alert necklace or bracelet engraved with the appropriate information.

C. Serum sickness

1. **Etiology**   Serum sickness is a condition resulting from the presence of circulating antigen-antibody complexes with resultant complement activation. Tissue-fixed IgE antibodies also participate. At the present time, drugs (e.g., penicillin, streptomycin, phenytoin), antilymphocyte globulin, and stinging-insect venoms are most frequently implicated. The syndrome also occurs in the preicteric phase of viral hepatitis, and possibly in other viral infections.

2. **Evaluation and diagnosis   Symptoms** most frequently begin 7–14 days after injection of the offending agent and may persist for weeks. Less frequently, an accelerated reaction may occur, with the onset of symptoms only hours or days after exposure. Fever, adenopathy, urticaria, angioedema, and arthralgias or arthritis, or both, are the most frequent presenting signs and symptoms. Less frequently, vasculitis occurs in other systems, including the gastrointestinal, pulmonary, and cardiovascular system and the CNS.

3. **Laboratory findings**

   a. **CBC**   The **differential diagnosis** may reveal a leukocytosis with a shift to the left, leukopenia, or eosinophilia. The finding of circulating plasma cells is very suggestive, since few conditions elicit plasmacytosis. The erythrocyte sedimentation rate is usually elevated.

   b. **Serum proteins**   With serosal, pleural, or pericardial involvement, there may be a reduction in both total and individual serum protein components. Gamma globulins are generally increased and serum complement is decreased.

c. Urinalysis   Rarely, proteinuria or hyaline casts are seen.

d. Other C_{1g} precipitins are positive, as is a non-gamma globulin Coombs test secondary to activation of complement (C3 and/or factor B activation products).

4. Treatment

a. Antihistamines   Therapeutic doses of antihistamines should be used throughout the symptomatic period to relieve pruritus. In addition, antihistamines may prevent deposition of immune complexes by partially diminishing the increased vascular permeability.

b. Corticosteroids   Since serum sickness is usually a benign, self-limited condition, systemic steroid therapy should be reserved for patients with the most severe symptoms who show evidence of organ involvement with vasculitis. If indicated, treatment should be initiated with 1–2 mg/kg/day of prednisone or methylprednisolone in divided doses, with tapering after clinical improvement and discontinuation after a total course of 10–14 days.

c. Aspirin may be used as an antipyretic and for generalized symptoms.

d. Epinephrine, 0.01 ml/kg (maximum dose 0.4 ml) will decrease acute urticaria and angioedema, but the effects are transient.

D. Allergic rhinoconjunctivitis   See also Chaps. 23 and 24.

1. Etiology

a. Release of the mediators of hypersensitivity in the conjunctiva and nasal membranes initiated by an allergen-IgE interaction is responsible for the edema, increased secretions, and pruritus associated with this symptom complex.

b. Among the **nonallergic causes** for perennial rhinitis or nasal congestion are hypothyroidism, pregnancy, and certain drugs (e.g., reserpine, birth control pills). The major causes are vasomotor rhinitis and perennial nonallergic rhinitis.

2. Evaluation and diagnosis

a. A careful **history** may suggest either seasonal variations in symptoms or possible offending perennial allergens.

b. Eosinophilia, both in a peripheral blood count and nasal smear is consistent with allergic rhinitis, but may be found also in perennial nonallergic rhinitis.

c. Skin tests are useful in confirming the significance of pollen or mold allergens in seasonal rhinitis. They are most important, however, in suggesting an allergic basis for perennial symptoms where the cause is not obviously allergic in origin.

d. Serum IgE levels are often elevated in allergic rhinitis.

e. Physical examination of the nasal mucosa in allergic rhinitis may reveal the following:

(1) Often, a bossy, pale edema of the turbinates with a clear, watery discharge.

(2) Nasal polyps may be seen in association with rhinitis. **(Whenever**

polyps are found in children a sweat test must be obtained to rule o
the possible diagnosis of cystic fibrosis.)

(3) Conjunctival inflammation is frequently seen in association wit
seasonal rhinitis. **Periorbital edema** and **infraorbital swelling** ("a
lergic shiners," or black eyes) are also frequently observed. Th
upper lids should be everted, to examine for the presence o
"cobblestoning," a hallmark of **vernal** conjunctivitis.

3. Treatment

a. Pharmacologic

(1) Therapy should be initiated either with a **pure antihistamine**, e.g
diphenhydramine (Benadryl), 5 mg/day, or chlorpheniramin
(Chlor-Trimeton), 0.35 mg/kg/day, or a **decongestant-antihistamin**
combination (e.g., Dimetapp, Actifed, Demazine). In general, mo:
effective control is obtained with maintenance therapy throug
out a symptomatic season than by intermittent symptomatic i
tervention. However, since tachyphylaxis may develop in respon:
to antihistamines after prolonged use, it may be necessary
change preparations during one course of treatment.

(2) Intranasal therapy (e.g., phenylephrine hydrochloride, Afrin) **shou**
be used with caution, since rebound rhinitis (*rhinitis medicame*
tosa) frequently occurs with prolonged use. Intermittent trea
ment is often very effective.

(3) Systemic corticosteroids are rarely necessary. However, **intranas**
dexamethasone (Decadron Phosphate Turbinaire), used for limit
periods (e.g., 2–4 weeks), is very effective. This steroid is partial
absorbed, and **prolonged administration should be avoided** becau
of the potential for suppression of the pituitary-adrenal axis.

(4) Treatment of **allergic conjunctivitis** should be initiated, with fr
quent instillation of a methylcellulose preparation. Intraocul
antihistamines (Vasocon A, Albalon A) can cause rebound co
junctivitis, as with intranasal antihistamines, and they should I
used only intermittently for this reason. Because of the pote
tial intraocular complications of steroids (e.g., glaucoma, herpe
they should be used only following consultation with an ophtha
mologist.

b. Specific allergies When a specific allergy or allergies is identifie
attempts should be made to remove it from the patient's immedia
environment. When this is not possible, a course of immunothera
may be considered. This mode of treatment is most effective f
pollen-induced rhinitis. Considerations for initiation of this treatme
are as previously discussed.

E. Urticaria Approximately 20 percent of the population experiences at lea
one acute episode of urticaria or angioedema. Of these cases, only a sm:
percentage progress to the chronic form, defined as recurrence of lesio
over a period of 6 weeks. The incidence of **acute urticaria** is slightly higher
an atopic than in a nonatopic population, but the incidence of **chronic ▪**
ticaria is unaffected by hereditary background.

The **clinical recognition** of urticaria or angioedema rarely presents
problem. On the other hand, in the chronic form, identification of the pr
cipitating factor or factors is often a perplexing, if not impossible, task.

Urticaria and angioedema frequently coexist. Attacks may last fro
hours to days. However, it is not unusual for patients with chronic urticar

Table 19-3 Etiology of Urticaria and Angioedema

Allergic
  Atopic (inhaled allergens)
  Anaphylaxis:
    Ingested allergens (foods, drugs)
    Injected allergenic drugs (e.g., penicillin, biologicals)
Physical
  Dermatographia
  Pressure
  Vibration
  Cold
  Heat
  Solar
  Aquagenic
  Cholinergic
Infections
Agents affecting prostaglandin synthesis
  Nonsteroidal antiinflammatory agents (aspirin)
  Azodyes and preservatives
Necrotizing vasculitis
Hereditary angioedema
Drugs (serum products and mast cell–releasing agent)
Neoplasms
Endocrine related
Psychogenic
Idiopathic

Table 19-4 Urticaria and Angioedema: Laboratory Evaluation

Suspected Cause	Procedures
(General screening)	(CBC, urinalysis, chemical profile)
Vasculitis or complement related	Sedimentation rate, immunoglobulin analysis, antinuclear factor, quantitative complement (C3, C4, $C\bar{1}$-inhibition, CH50), skin biopsy
Cold urticaria	Cryoglobulins, cryofibrinogens, VDRL
Infections	Culture, x-ray, stool for ova and parasites, hepatitis-associated antigen
Atopic	Eosinophil count, IgE, skin testing and/or RAST for suspected allergen
Physical	
Cholinergic	Mecholyl test/stress induced
Dermatographism	Firm stroking of skin
Cold	Ice-cube application
Solar	Light exposure
Heat	Warm-water immersion
Hereditary angioedema and acquired angioedema with lymphoma and other neoplasms	$C\bar{1}$-inhibition, $C1_a$, CH50, C4, C2

with angioedema to have recurrent episodes for years. Both because of th
long-term morbidity suffered by those whose attacks recur over a pro
longed period, as well as the occasional association with a significant un
derlying disorder (Table 19-3), complete evaluation of patients with chroni
urticaria should be undertaken (Table 19-4).

1. **Etiology**

   a. **Mechanism** Although caused by a number of mechanisms, a fina
   common pathway for urticaria or angioedema is release of chemica
   mediators of immediate hypersensitivity.

   b. **Specific agents** It is difficult to estimate the frequency with whic'
   the cause of acute urticaria is identified, since many persons witł
   mild acute episodes may not seek medical assistance. Of those evalu
   ated for chronic forms of the disease, however, it has been estimate
   that a cause is determined in less than 20 percent of cases. Because c
   the diversity of causes and mechanisms involved in this symptor
   complex, a rational classification is difficult to make. The classifica
   tion in Table 19-3 merely lists the known causes without attention t
   mechanism.

2. **Evaluation and therapy** If the urticaria or angioedema is associate
   with a specific ingested or inhaled substance, avoidance is obviously th
   preferred approach. Similarly, with physical urticaria, avoidance of th
   precipitating factor, such as cold or sunlight, is advisable. Sunscreen
   have been beneficial in solar urticaria.

   a. **Antihistamines** Urticaria, whether acute or chronic, is best cor
   trolled by antihistamine therapy. In general, antihistamine dosage
   should be increased slowly, either to tolerance or until symptoms ar
   controlled. There is no good evidence that any one antihistamine i
   more beneficial than another.

   b. **Steroids** There is no role for topical steroid therapy is this conditior
   and only rarely should systemic corticosteroid treatment be consic
   ered.

   c. In **hereditary angioedema,** androgen therapy, using oxymetholone,
   mg, has clearly prevented life-threatening attacks. Of major concer
   in this entity has been the treatment of acute episodes. Recent stud
   ies suggest that the use of the purified Cl inhibitor protein would b
   lifesaving. A more practical approach is the utilization of 5 gm c
   epsilon-aminocaproic acid (EACA), administered q6h in conjunctio
   with oxymetholone, 10 mg q6h, until the reaction is controlled.

   d. If a more serious underlying entity has been ruled out, reassurance '
   often the best therapy.

20

Pulmonary Disorders

I. GENERAL PRINCIPLES OF THERAPEUTICS

A. Smoking If possible, one should convince the patient and those in the immediate environment to break the habit. This approach applies to **all** pulmonary diseases (and to good health in general).

B. Environmental control

1. Control should be most vigorous in the child's bedroom. Feather-containing products should be avoided. Airtight plastic covers should be put on bedding not already stuffed with a polyester fiber. It is best to keep furry pets out of the immediate environment. The furniture should be easily cleanable. Hot-air heating should be avoided, as should chronic moisture that usually encourages mold growth.

2. In extreme situations, the physician may be forced to recommend a change in geographic location for the patient, although this is not always beneficial.

3. The preceding suggestions should be applied judiciously. When a child has mild or only questionable atopic disease, it is not helpful to disrupt the home environment with expensive and difficult changes.

C. Chest physical therapy Postural drainage.

1. **Indications** Chest physical therapy is useful in any clinical situation when excess fluid is not removed by the normal cough or ciliary action of the airways. It is sometimes recommended prophylactically for conditions in which future difficulties are anticipated.

2. The **frequency** depends on the severity of the illness. It is usually possible to have postural drainage performed at least once and usually twice daily without any great change in the family routine.

3. The best method of **learning the technique** is for the parents and the child to be taught by a qualified physical therapist.

D. Aerosol therapy Particles 5μ in diameter are best, since they are most likely to enter the small airways when inhaled through the mouth. Aerosol therapy should be given just **prior** to chest physical therapy, particularly in patients who have difficulty raising sputum.

E. Antibiotics See Chap. 15, Sec. III, p. 349.

F. Psychiatric support (see also Chap. 7) The severe and demanding nature of many childhood chronic respiratory diseases virtually requires that the physician, often with the help of the social worker, psychiatrist, or both, give added support to the family.

II. PHARMACOLOGIC AGENTS USED IN CHRONIC RESPIRATORY DISEASES

A. Adrenergic drugs

All the drugs discussed have both beta-1 (cardiovascular) and beta-2 (pulmonary muscular) effects. The beta-2 stimulators have greater beta-2 than beta-1 effects.

1. Epinephrine

  a. Action Epinephrine increases cyclic adenosine monophosphate (AMP). This produces a relaxation of bronchial smooth muscle and a decrease in bronchial hypersecretion. There is a concomitant increase in heart rate, cardiac output, and O_2 utilization.

  b. Side effects include cardiac arrhythmias, especially in hypoxemic patients, drying of secretions, anxiety, restlessness, headache, dizziness, pallor, and vomiting.

  c. Administration and dosage Epinephrine is most useful during acute episodes of bronchospasm. If 1:1000 aqueous epinephrine is used, give 0.01 ml/kg/dose SQ or IM (not more than 0.4 ml in a single dose). Repeat at intervals of 15–30 min. If using 1:200 epinephrine aqueous suspension (Sus-Phrine), the dosage is 0.005 ml/kg/dose, with a maximum dose of 0.3 ml in children. Do not repeat before 4 hr, since this is a long-acting preparation.

2. Ephedrine sulfate

  a. The **action** is similar to that of epinephrine.

  b. Side effects are CNS stimulation and palpitations.

  c. Administration and dosage 0.5–1.0 mg/kg/dose q4h PO.

3. Isoproterenol (Isuprel)

  a. The **action** is similar to that of epinephrine.

  b. The **side effects** are similar to those of epinephrine. Isoproterenol has been shown to cause a fall of 5–10 mm Hg in PO_2. It thus may be dangerous to have the patient use hand-held precharge nebulizers during a severe attack, especially if O_2 is not being administered. Also in an occasional patient, bronchospasm actually increases following the administration of isoproterenol by aerosol. This is rare, but may be detected using pulmonary function tests before and after administration.

  c. Administration and dosage Isoproterenol for aerosol use is supplied in a 1:200 solution; 0.25–0.5 ml of which is combined with 0.5 ml–4.0 ml saline for use in either a hand spray or O_2-driven nebulizer.

4. Beta-2 stimulants

  a. Action This class of drugs is said to have the advantage of causing bronchodilation without significant cardiovascular effects. Recent studies have called this assumption into question. It appears that these agents do have more beta-2 than beta-1 effects, but the beta-1 (cardiovascular) effects cannot be ignored.

  b. Preparations Metaproterenol, salbutamol, terbutaline, fenoterol, ritodrine, isoetharine, quinterenol, and soterenol are selective beta-2 preparations. Salbutamol is under study in the United States and has not yet been released for general use.

  c. Side effects Nervousness, weakness, drowsiness, and tremor are the most frequent problems.

d. Administration and dosage The usual dosage of **metaproterenol** is 20 mg PO qid for children over 9 years of age or weight over 60 lb. For children ages 6 to 9 years, or weights under 60 lb, give 10 mg tid or qid. The usual dosage of **terbutaline** for children is 2.5 mg tid. If side effects occur, the dosage can be reduced to 2.5 mg bid.

B. Xanthines: aminophylline The xanthines are phosphodiesterase inhibitors, which result in an increase in cyclic AMP.

1. Action Aminophylline stimulates CNS and cardiac muscle and relaxes smooth muscle. When used in combination with beta stimulators, aminophylline potentiates their action.

2. Side effects Nausea, vomiting, hypotension, arrhythmias.

3. Administration and dosage

a. IV aminophylline (5–7 mg/kg/dose) is more effective if given over 10–15 min rather than over 1 hr, but the patient must be observed more closely if this method is used. Theophylline levels must be monitored. Levels should be $15-20$ μg/ml. Occasional patients require and can tolerate blood levels as high as 30 μg/ml, but they must be monitored closely for adverse side effects.

b. A constant infusion of aminophylline can be used in critically ill children but must be undertaken **with great caution. Cardiac monitoring and measurement of theophylline levels are mandatory.** Rectal aminophylline is not recommended because of its irregular and unreliable absorption.

C. Corticosteroids See Table 20-1.

1. Action Antiinflammatory. Corticosteroids activate the release of cyclic AMP.

2. Side effects include the Cushing syndrome, osteoporosis, immunosuppression (in high doses), ulcers, and growth retardation. Corticosteroids have less toxicity if given on an alternate-morning dose program.

3. Route and dosage For acute attacks, IV hydrocortisone, 4 mg/kg q4–6h, is given. By the oral route, 1–2 mg/kg/24 hr prednisone is given initially in a single A.M. dose. As soon as the patient's condition permits, he or she may be switched to an alternate-morning dose program. A child with chronic asthma may be aided by minute amounts on this basis.

D. Expectorants

1. Iodides are not presently recommended.

2. Glyceryl guaiacolate is of questionable value. The dose is 5 ml q4–6h.

E. Mucolytic agents

1. Acetylcysteine (Mucomyst) is perhaps the most effective of the mucolytic agents.

a. Action Its mucolytic action is due to breakage of disulfide bonds in the mucoid secretions. It **may cause bronchospasm**, however, especially in patients with asthma.

b. Administration Acetylcysteine loses activity rapidly if in a solution of less than 10% concentration or if in contact with rubber or metal, and it inactivates many antibiotics given by aerosol. Properly administered, it often results in a great outpouring of secretions, which may require mechanical suctioning if the patient has an inadequate

Table 20-1   Equivalent Glucocorticoid
Effects of Various Corticosteroids

Cortisone	100 mg
Hydrocortisone	80 mg
Prednisone	20 mg
Prednisolone	16 mg
Triamcinolone	8 mg
9α-Fluorocortisol	5 mg
Dexamethasone	2 mg

cough, or inadequate ciliary action, or both. Many children object t
the taste and odor. If often works best if given with a bronchodilator

   c. The **dose** is 3–5 ml of a 20% solution q4–6h by aerosol.

2. **Saline** given directly as an ultrasonic aerosol may liquefy secretions. I
   has been reported to cause bronchospasm on occasion. It is of questiona
   ble value when delivered by a mist tent. Particle size is critical (best a
   2–5 μ) and studies question the amount of the aerosol delivered to th
   terminal bronchi. The use of mist tents is no longer recommended excep
   to deliver humidified oxygen when other methods are not possible. A
   though still occasionally recommended by others, they are not used b
   our patients with cystic fibrosis.

F. **Fixed combinations**   About 150 bronchodilators, either alone or in fixe
   combinations, are listed in the 1979 *Physicians' Desk Reference*. If, despit
   the increased cost, fixed combinations are prescribed, **the dosage calcu**
   lated should be based on that of the bronchodilator agent. The newer high
   dose theophylline regimen, with monitoring of serum levels, allows for indi
   vidualization of the therapeutic response. The combination products mak
   this approach difficult because of the undesirable side effects of the othe
   agents when dosage is based on the theophylline component. For thes
   reasons, combination products are rarely useful.

G. **Newer drug**   See **9**, p. 478.

III. VENTILATORS

A. General principles

1. **Assisted ventilation**   The ventilator will respond to an inspiratory effor
   initiated by the patient (a sudden reduction in the airway pressure). The
   method of ventilation will usually improve alveolar ventilation an
   oxygenation, but does not completely relieve the work of breathing
   especially when the "sensitivity control," which regulates the pressure
   needed to initiate flow, is set at high pressure.

2. In **controlled ventilation** a triggering device regulates the operation dur
   ing **all** phases of the respiratory cycle.

3. **Intermittent mandatory ventilation** (IMV) allows for a selected number o
   breaths per minute and for the patient to breathe in between these se
   numbers of breaths. It is helpful for guaranteeing adequate ventilatio
   while weaning patients from the respirator.

B. **Types of ventilators**

    1. **Pressure-cycled ventilators** The Bird (Mark VIII) ventilator is gas powered (either by compressed air or O_2). In this machine the inspiration ends when the pressure in the system (and thus in the airway) rises to a preselected value.

    2. **Volume-cycled ventilators** The tidal volume is delivered to the patient irrespective of the patient's airway resistance or compliance.

    3. **Negative-pressure ventilators** are tank and chest respirators of various configurations in which pressure and inspiration-expiration time are the determinants of tidal volume and respiratory rate. These respirators may be considered for patients who have relatively normal lungs and airways and who have a defect in the neuromuscular component of respiration.

C. **Continuous positive airway pressure (CPAP)** (see also Chap. 5, pp. 116 ff.) This technique has proved useful in improving the oxygenation of patients who fail to maintain an adequate arterial PO_2 on IPPB despite high concentrations of inspired oxygen. Recruitment of gas exchange units and prevention of terminal airway closure appear to be the physiologic reasons for the beneficial effects. This is especially useful in patients with RDS, after partial drowning, and in other conditions involving alveolar collapse. The risks of elevated $PaCO_2$ is real, and therefore arterial blood gases must be followed closely.

D. Although **IPPB** is widely used in many centers, it probably is rarely useful. Patients who can take a deep breath would probably benefit from medication delivered by aerosol, which delivers the drug more effectively and with less mechanical complications.

E. **Complications of mechanical ventilation**

    1. Infection.

    2. Pneumothorax, pneumomediastinum, and subcutaneous emphysema.

    3. Overcorrection of hypercapnia, with sudden changes in pH, cardiac arrhythmias, tetany, and so on.

    4. Interference with venous return and a drop in cardiac output and blood pressure (sometimes as a consequence of a previously borderline hypervolemic condition), especially worrisome in patients on CPAP.

    5. Positive fluid balance.

    6. Inappropriate antidiuretic hormone (ADH) secretion.

    7. "Stiff" lung.

    8. Accidental kinking or accidental displacement of the endotracheal tube into the right main bronchus.

    9. Tracheal inflammation, erosion, granuloma formation, and, later, stenosis.

    10. Oxygen toxicity: impairment of the defense mechanisms of the lung.

    11. Retention of secretions above the "cuff" (orotracheal suction before deflating the cuff essential to prevent aspiration).

    12. Gastrointestinal: dilatation, or bleeding, or both.

    13. Psychological: dependence on mechanical respiration, for example.

    14. Exhaustion: lack of sleep due to constant "intensive" care.

IV. RESPIRATORY FAILURE   See Chap. 2, Sec. **VII.**

V. MANAGEMENT OF CHRONIC CHILDHOOD ASTHMA   For management of acut asthma, see p. 49.

A. Tľ.e etiology is unknown.   There is an increase in the responsiveness of th bronchi of the asthmatic patient to histamine and acetylcholine and a de creased responsiveness of beta receptors. Precipitating factors include ir fection, environmental allergens, emotional upset, exercise, exposure t cold, and drugs (notably aspirin).

B. Evaluation and diagnosis   In the acute situation, the dyspnea of asthma i generally obvious. Evaluation of the "subclinical" case is often more com plex and includes the following:

1. **History**   Asthmatic children often have had repeated episodes of bron chitis or pneumonia as infants. Coughing in asthmatic children usuall continues longer after upper respiratory infections than in other chi dren. The child wheezes after exercise, colds, or while asleep. Symptom tend to be seasonal and occasionally date from changes in geographi area, the acquisition of a pet, or some other environmental factor. Ofte there is a family history of atopic disease.

2. **Physical examination**   It is often possible to induce a wheeze or an in crease in the expiratory phase by having the patient take a deep breatl and forcefully expire through a wide-open mouth. An increase in th anteroposterior (A-P) diameter of the chest and clubbing should b looked for. In the case of the latter, other entities must be considered since **clubbing is extremely rare in simple asthma.**

3. **Laboratory studies**

   a. **Chest x-ray studies** should be done.

   b. **Pulmonary function test**   In most cases there is a decrease in the pea flow rate, forced expiratory volume in 1 sec (FEV_1), and vital capacit (VC), along with an increase in the residual volume and total lun capacity. However, maximal midexpiratory flow rate (MMFR) an flow volume curves may be required to demonstrate abnormalities ir mild cases. Inhalation of isoproterenol will generally increase th vital capacity and FEV_1 more than 20 percent in the asthmatic pa tient. Occasionally, a patient will demonstrate bronchospasm onl after exercise.

   c. **Skin testing** is occasionally helpful (see Chap. 19, Sec. **I.A**).

   d. **Examination of sputum**   Eosinophilia may be seen on Wright's stain

   e. A **peripheral eosinophil count** of over 500/mm^3 is suggestive of atopic o parasitic disease, or both (see Chap. 16, Sec. **I.B.2**).

C. Treatment   A spectrum of therapeutic maneuvers is available to the physi cian, but they must be organized in a manner that avoids enslavement o the child and family to the disease process. The goal is normal school atten dance and unlimited activity, with few, if any, hospitalizations (see Tabl 20-2).

1. **Environmental control**   See Sec. **I.B.**

2. **Bronchodilators**   See Secs. **II.A** and **II.B** for pharmacology and dosages.

   a. If the patient has moderate to severe disease, bronchodilators shoul

Table 20-2 Outpatient Management of Acute Asthmatic Episode

Current Pharmacologic Regimen	Suggested Revision of Current Program	Duration of Therapy
1. None	Institute therapy with theophylline tablets or syrup,[a] 5–6 mg/kg q6h	5–7 days after symptoms have abated. Maintenance dose if indicated on follow-up
2. Theophylline (± cromolyn)[b]	Optimize theophylline dosage on basis of calculated total daily dose or available blood levels. Consider addition of oral beta-adrenergic agent, e.g., metaproterenol, 5–20 mg tid–qid, or terbutaline, 2.5–5.0 mg tid Discontinue cromolyn[b]	As above
3. Theophylline and beta-adrenergic agent	Add oral prednisone, 1–2 mg/kg/day in divided doses (bid–tid) for 3–4 days. Then taper to a qA.M. dose by decreasing the P.M. dose by 2.5–5.0 mg/day. **Physician visit within 7–10 days is mandatory**	Decision to use qd regimen of inhaled steroids or taper prednisone should be made on basis of clinical status
4. As in 2 or 3, plus steroids qd	If patient recently on high-dose suppressive regimen or in presence of significant obstruction, give IV hydrocortisone. Discharge on daily prednisone and arrange follow-up visit as above	Appropriate adjustments made at follow-up visit
5. As in 2 or 3, plus inhaled steroids	Unless the hypothalamic-pituitary-adrenal axis is known to be intact (rare), systemic steroids should be administered, except in very mild attacks. During acute episode, convert to oral prednisone as outlined in 3	As above
6. As in 2 or 3, plus daily steroids	Hospital admission likely if steroid dose is adequate and compliance good. Do not delay with prolonged emergency room therapeutic trial before decision to admit is made	

[a] When using episodic bronchodilator therapy, give rapidly absorbed (syrup or tablet and not timed-release) preparations to achieve therapeutic blood levels rapidly.
[b] In general, cromolyn should be discontinued during acute asthmatic attacks.
Courtesy of Dr. Frank Twarog.

be used on a long-term basis, although they may be required only during particular seasons. Occasionally, a bedtime dose is sufficient.

   b. In the mildly ill patient who has no difficulty with recurrent atelectasis and whose pulmonary function tests are normal or near normal, there is little need for continual administration of these agents. However, oral bronchodilators may be kept at home, to be started by the parents at the first sign of a cold, cough, or wheezing. By early administration of effective agents, a visit to the emergency room or even hospitalization may sometimes be avoided. Time must be set aside to educate the family about the potential side effects and toxicity of bronchodilators.

3. Corticosteroids (Only outpatient, long-term administration will be discussed here; for dosage, administration, and side effects, see p. 473.)

   a. In general, corticosteroids should be used only after **vigorous treatment** with the more benign program fails to keep the child well and relatively active.

   b. Once there appears to be no choice, corticosteroids should be titrated to the **minimum effective dose** on an alternate-day A.M. schedule. Beclomethasone inhalers used on the off-steroid day may allow alternate-day steroid usage by alleviating the need for daily steroid medication by mouth.

   c. It is better to maintain a child on low dosages of prednisone and leading a full life than to have him or her missing school or in the hospital, frequently because such medication is withheld.

4. Chest physical therapy See Sec. I.C.

5. Expectorants may aid some chronic asthmatic patients (see Sec. II.D).

6. Desensitization seems to help occasional asthmatic patients when relatively few specific antigens can be identified.

7. Aerosols (see Sec. I.D) The use of **isoproterenol** aerosols has been associated with **overdosages and fatal cardiac arrhythmias,** particularly in the presence of hypoxemia. If these devices are prescribed in the pediatric age group, **it is best to have the specific dosage administered by a parent.**

8. Psychotherapy (see F, p. 471) Generally, the pediatrician or social worker who develops an ongoing relationship with the patient can give the needed support. Occasionally, the psychiatrist will be useful in coping with more severe behavior problems. It is also important to remember that some of the behavioral changes seen are induced by the drugs used in the treatment of asthma.

9. Disodium cromoglycate (Aarane, Intal), which presumably acts as a mast cell stabilizer, has been licensed in the United States. The patient is instructed to inhale a 20-mg capsule qid as a prophylactic measure, using a device supplied by the company. Thus far, about 25–50 percent of severely asthmatic patients are afforded some relief using this drug. The major disadvantage is its cost, which is about $1.00/day.

VI. CYSTIC FIBROSIS See also Chap. 11, Sec. II.A.1.

   A. Evaluation The findings vary according to the time at which the diagnosis is made. In the **neonate,** meconium ileus, rectal prolapse, and prolonged jaundice can be seen. In the **infant,** tachypnea, retractions, and a prominent tympanitic abdomen are typical. Often, the infant presents with the picture of bronchiolitis. Later in **childhood** or **adolescence,** isolated pulmonary disease may be the only manifestation. Diffuse rhonchi and rales and clubbing of the extremities may be found. Nasal polyps and sinusitis are associated findings.

B. Diagnosis   See also Chap. 11, Sec. **VI.A.**

1. The **chest x-ray picture** may vary from normal to that of extreme "fibrosis," hyperinflation, and hilar adenopathy. Occasionally, the changes tend to be confined to one or two areas of the lung.

2. **Pulmonary function tests results** vary from normal to the pattern of obstructive disease with overinflation, as demonstrated by an increase in the residual volume (RV), in RV/TLC (total lung capacity), and a decrease in vital capacity (VC). Expiratory flow rates are decreased. Blood gases also vary from normal to the extremes of hypoxemia and, finally, hypercapnia.

3. **Sputum analysis**   The sputum is typically thick and viscous. *Pseudomonas aeruginosa* and *Staphylococcus aureus* are frequently isolated from sputum cultures.

C. Treatment of pulmonary disorder

1. Adequate hydration is of primary importance, and mobilization and loosening of secretions are essential.

2. Mist tents are no longer used in many institutions. Studies demonstrating lack of particle deposition in the small airways and worsening pulmonary function tests (PFT) in some patients when tents were used support this practice.

3. **Aerosol drugs**   Any generator properly suited to deliver medications can be used. Most of the preparations include normal saline as the base solution.

4. **Acetylcysteine**   See Sec. **II.E.1.**

5. **Bronchodilators**   See Secs. **II.A.3** and **II.B.**

6. **Expectorants**   See Sec. **II.D.**

7. **Chest physiotherapy** can be carried out by the patient, by a therapist, or by an electric vibrator.

8. **Antimicrobial agents** (see **d,** p. 355, and **5,** p. 357)   Hospitalized patients receive IV therapy (carbenicillin, gentamicin).

   a. **Electrolyte abnormalities** (hypochloremic alkalosis) are seen more frequently in patients receiving large doses of carbenicillin, and hypocalcemia and hypomagnesemia are occasionally seen in association with gentamicin.

   b. **Prognosis**   The average life expectancy is now in excess of 18 years, and an optimistic outlook must be maintained.

VII. PNEUMOTHORAX

A. Etiology   Spontaneous pneumothorax may be an idiopathic occurrence in a previously healthy person, or it may be a complication of underlying pulmonary disease.

B. Evaluation and diagnosis

1. **History**   A high index of suspicion is present whenever a patient with

known lung disease experiences the **acute onset** of severe respirator
distress.

2. **Physical examination** Decreased fremitus, decreased breath sound
and hyperresonance are present on the affected side. Percussion over th
clavicles on opposite sides reveals minor differences in percussion tone
In the infant and in patients with severe cystic fibrosis lung disease, th
physical findings may be minimal, even in the face of extensive collapse

3. **Chest roentgenogram** Sometimes, an expired posteroanterior view wi
aid diagnosis when the pneumothorax is small.

4. **Classification** Generally, a pneumothorax is well tolerated after an in
tial period of distress because of an adjustment of perfusion to ventila
tion. (**Pneumothorax can enlarge during reduced in-flight cabin pressure**
which can be a problem when transporting sick infants.)

   a. **Minor to moderate** Less than 30 percent collapse.

   b. **Major** 30–70 percent collapse.

   c. If **complete collapse** occurs, the possibility of tension pneumothorax
   should be suspected.

C. **Treatment** (For infants, see Chap. 5, Sec. **IV.B.4.**) The following point
should be observed:

1. **If the clinical condition is critical, immediate lifesaving maneuvers become
more important than diagnostic procedures.**

2. If the leak is in visceral pleura, **positive-pressure breathing** can aggravat
the situation. If there is a leak in the **parietal pleura** (flail chest), on th
other hand, positive pressure may be lifesaving.

3. **Simple observation** will suffice if the patient can be watched, the clinica
condition is stable, there is no evidence of an "open" leak, and th
radiologic diagnosis is "minor."

4. **Cough suppression** If necessary, dextromethorphan, codeine, or mor
phine should be used to suppress coughing. The use of respiratory de
pressants is dangerous and necessitates frequent arterial blood ga
measurements.

5. **Thoracentesis** Needle aspiration of air at the 2nd anterior intercosta
space, midclavicular line (see Chap. 1, Sec. **II.B.5**) may be lifesavin
whenever tension pneumothorax is present. Later, a closed thoracos
tomy drainage system will be in order.

6. **Thoracostomy** **Tube thoracostomy** is indicated when the pneumothora
is likely to reaccumulate. The term *closed thoracostomy* is used to desig
nate a thoracostomy tube connected to a water-seal bottle. With th
water seal (which can be improvised by placing the end of the tube unde
the surface of some sterile normal saline contained in anything with a
air vent), air (and also fluid) drain from the chest, but air cannot reente
the submerged tube tip **if the end of the tube and water seal are below th
level of the patient's chest**. It is customary to place the "bottle" on th
floor. If the system is functioning well, the fluid will be lifted a few cen
timeters up the tube as the patient breathes and produces negativ
(subatmospheric) inspiratory pressure. Later, when the visceral an
parietal pleura are adherent, this will not be seen.

7. Recurrent pneumothoraces require parietal pleural stripping when pos
sible or quinacrine instillation if an operation is precluded by the sever
ity of the underlying lung disease.

21

Disorders of the Nervous System

I. PAROXYSMAL DISORDERS

A. Convulsive disorders—epilepsy   See also III, p. 40.

1. Classification

a. **Grand mal convulsions** are the most common convulsive disorders, except in infancy. An aura may precede tonic-clonic movements of the extremities and a sudden loss of consciousness. The ictal event usually lasts for 2–4 min, after which the child may be somnolent, confused, and fatigued and may complain of headache.

   (1) **Etiology**   Lead intoxication, birth trauma, cryptogenic.

   (2) **Evaluation**   History, x-rays, measurement of blood glucose, calcium, phosphorus, and electrolytes, and an electroencephalogram (EEG) are required.

   (3) **Diagnosis**   Spike discharges may be seen on the EEG.

   (4) **Treatment**   See Table 21-1.

b. **Psychomotor (temporal lobe) seizures** are seen throughout childhood and early adolescence. The patient may exhibit a variety of automatic behavior, including lip-smacking, staring, grimaces, hand posturing, laughing, and grasping motions. Some patients experience an aura of bewilderment and act irrationally. Episodes of such behavior last longer than grand mal seizures and may be followed by a convulsion. The patient is often aware of his initial symptoms and aura, but is unable to terminate the automatisms.

   (1) **Etiology**   Trauma, cryptogenic, or (rarely) due to a mass lesion.

   (2) **Evaluation**   The same procedures should be done as for grand mal convulsions. The EEG should include sleep tracing.

   (3) **Diagnosis**   Characteristic history and EEG abnormality.

   (4) **Treatment**   See Table 21-1.

c. **Focal motor seizures** and hemiconvulsions are usually related to structural damage of the motor cortex and may not be associated with loss of consciousness.

   (1) **Evaluation** is the same as for grand mal convulsions. Tomography (CAT scan) should be performed to rule out a surgically remediable lesion. Cerebral angiography may also be necessary.

   (2) **Diagnosis** requires a reliable witness and, commonly, a focal spike discharge on the EEG.

   (3) **Treatment**   See Table 21-1.

d. **Myoclonic seizures** are sudden, brief jerking movements of the arms and legs and may occur singly. They are frequent just before rising. The patient does not lose consciousness.

(1) Etiology   Cryptogenic; early subacute sclerosing panencephalitis (SSPE).

(2) Evaluation is the same as for grand mal convulsions.

(3) Diagnosis   By history; the EEG may be normal.

(4) Treatment usually requires trial of and combinations of anticonvulsants (see Table 21-1).

e. **Petit mal, or centrencephalic, epilepsy** is a term restricted to certain EEG abnormalities of synchronous spike and wave discharges that accompany a clinical picture of staring, loss of consciousness, and blinking or lip-smacking and rarely last more than 10–15 sec. Onset is usually at about age 5–8 years.

(1) Etiology   Cryptogenic. The family history may be positive.

(2) Evaluation   Hyperventilation for 1–2 min may produce a spell.

(3) Diagnosis is made by a history of brief lapses of consciousness and the characteristic EEG findings.

(4) Treatment   See Table 21-1.

(a) Treatment is successful when appropriate "anti-spike-wave" medications (e.g., ethosuximide [Zarontin], valproic acid [Depakene], or trimethadione [Tridione]) are employed. Children with petit mal should also receive maintenance doses of phenobarbital or phenytoin (Dilantin) because convulsions develop in many of these children.

(b) A ketogenic diet may be necessary.

f. **Akinetic and absence spells** are variants of centrencephalic epilepsy characterized by frequent bouts of staring, head nods, and a blank facial expression for 5–10 sec. Some patients are propelled to the ground with the ictus.

(1) Etiology   Cryptogenic.

(2) Evaluation   By EEG.

(3) Diagnosis   The EEG shows atypical spike and wave discharges, many of which transiently disappear when diazepam (Valium) is injected IV.

(4) Treatment   See e.(4).

g. **Infantile spasms (massive myoclonic seizures)** represent a syndrome of severe, diffuse CNS malfunction during the first 6 months of life. The spells are massive attacks of flexion of the head and extension of the arms, legs, or both in salaam fashion and occur in series or as isolated events. The frequency may approach 100 times per day. Tactile stimuli may precipitate the spells. They have been mistaken for colic.

(1) The **etiology** is nonspecific.

(2) Evaluation usually reveals a significant neurologic abnormality (microcephaly, developmental retardation). A search for metabolic etiology and examination with a Wood's light for early cutaneous signs of tuberous sclerosis should be performed.

(3) Diagnosis   By history and classic hypsarrhythmia on EEG.

(4) Treatment Untreated, the prognosis is grave, and more than 90 percent of those surviving to 3 years of age are severely retarded.

(a) ACTH gel (150 U/M² IM/day) should be administered. Blood pressure, hematocrit, and electrolytes should be measured and stool guaiac tests done while the patient is receiving ACTH. Antacids should be administered with feedings.

(b) Initial treatment should continue for 10–14 days, with follow-up EEGs each week. If the clinical response is favorable, and the EEG abnormalities are no longer seen, treatment can be terminated after 6 weeks of ACTH.

(c) Oral therapy with **hydrocortisone cypionate** (liquid Cortef, 10 mg/5 ml) should be continued for 3–4 months. Babies should receive 20 mg PO tid.

(d) When no favorable response (as measured by an EEG and clinical evaluation) is evident after 2–3 weeks of ACTH therapy, tne drug should be stopped and trials of **anticonvulsants** begun. Diazepam, in doses up to 30 mg PO/day, has been a useful adjunct to other anticonvulsants for some children who did not respond to ACTH.

h. Breathholding spells are periods of apnea followed by transient unconsciousness, are usually precipitated by emotion or minor injury, and have their onset in children 4–18 months old. The apnea always **follows expiration.**

(1) Two types of breathholding spells are described:

(a) The **pallid breathholding spell** follows a frustrating stimulus in response to which the child becomes apneic and pale and may experience a brief tonic seizure with prompt spontaneous recovery. The EEG may be abnormal during ocular compression, producing bradycardia and > 2 sec of asystole.

(b) In **cyanotic breathholding spells,** violent crying is followed by apnea, cyanosis, and flaccidity. Prompt resolution with return of consciousness is seen, and the child appears normal. Spells of this type are rarely seen after 2–3 years of age. The EEG is normal during ocular compression.

(2) Treatment with anticonvulsants is not indicated. Infants with unprovoked periods of apnea should be evaluated for epilepsy.

i. Febrile convulsions are brief (2–5 min), generalized tonic-clonic seizures with loss of consciousness in an otherwise healthy, febrile child, age 5 months–3 years.

(1) Etiology A rapid increase in body temperature has been postulated as triggering the convulsion.

(2) Evaluation [See **1.a.(2),** p. 481 when no site of infection is evident.] There is little evidence that a lumbar puncture is indicated in a child older than 16–18 months when an extracranial source of fever has been satisfactorily identified **and** no meningeal signs are present.

(3) Diagnosis The child who has any of the following is **excluded** from the classification of simple febrile convulsion and must be evaluated for a cause other than fever:

(a) First seizure when under 6 months or over 3 years old

  (b) Evidence of head trauma

  (c) Abnormal cerebrospinal fluid (CSF) suggestive of infection « hemorrhage

  (d) Prolonged convulsive activity (> 6 min)

  (e) Persistently abnormal EEG

(4) Treatment See also **E**, p. 42.

  (a) There is a limited role for **anticonvulsants** in the managemer of a **single** febrile convulsion because of the brevity of the spe and the rapid return to normal activity. Any child experiencin a **second** febrile seizure should receive daily anticonvulsar therapy for a minimum of 2–3 years.

  (b) Administration of anticonvulsants during subsequent febri illnesses has little proved value in preventing recurrent simp febrile convulsions.

  (c) Should the patient have a recurrence of seizures when afebril(or after age 4 years, or both, anticonvulsant therapy should b given for 2–3 years. **Phenobarbital** is the drug of choice (se Table 21-1).

j. Hysterical fits (psychogenic epilepsy) These spells are occasionall seen as conversion symptoms in children and adolescents with bon fide epilepsy, as well as in previously healthy patients. The spell rarely occur when the patient is alone and lack the true tonic-cloni rhythmic jerking of a grand mal convulsion.

  (1) Etiology Overwhelming conversion symptom complex.

  (2) Evaluation should include an EEG during a "spell." If tempora lobe seizures are considered, a complete workup should be in tiated.

  (3) The **diagnosis** is confirmed when one witnesses opisthotonic post uring, flailing, beating movements of the arms, tightly close eyelids, and spitting and crying out with hyperventilation unac companied by urinary incontinence or tongue biting.

  (4) Treatment Initially, one should be very supportive and under standing. The ultimate therapy is psychiatric.

2. Approach to therapy of convulsive disorders

a. General measures

  (1) Treatment is aimed at preventing further seizures and allowin the patient to lead a normal life. This will be the case in th majority of children with seizures.

  (2) Treatment of the child with **one** seizure should be individualize(depending on the severity of the seizure, the child's age, an understanding of the parents. When there is reasonable doubt a to the authenticity of the seizure, it may be wise to await a secon spell and seek out witnesses before initiating treatment.

  (3) Every child who has had a seizure should have an EEG to establish baseline of reference to define focal abnormalities. This is mos useful if obtained at least 5–7 days after the seizure, sinc nonspecific postictal electric changes will be minimized. If child *appears* postictal but there are no witnesses to a convulsior an EEG may be helpful in defining the episode closer to the event. There is no reason to withhold therapy until after the EEG.

(4) The pediatrician should consider the impact of both the disease and its management on the developing child and adolescent. This is especially important in evaluating management failures.

b. Anticonvulsant therapy

(1) General principles

(a) The general principle of using the **single drug** that is most effective and least toxic is stressed when patients fail to respond to recommended therapy. It is advisable to obtain **blood levels** of the anticonvulsant in question.

(b) When a single drug is used, if seizure control is not optimal initially, the drug should be increased to near-toxic levels before being abandoned. This usually requires 4–6 weeks per drug.

(c) Always continue a medication, **decreasing it gradually,** when a second or replacement preparation is introduced. This lessens the chances of status epilepticus from drug withdrawal.

(d) Medications should be prescribed in capsule or tablet form whenever possible. Tablets may be crushed for infants and disguised with sweets for toddlers. This assures a uniform dose, prevents error in dispensing medication of more than a single concentration (and short shelf life), and is easily transported in a unit dose.

(2) Anticonvulsant drugs

Table 21-1 lists the most commonly used, safest anticonvulsants for each general class of seizure disorder. It is not intended to be exhaustive. The medications are listed in the order of efficacy (balancing anticonvulsant properties with sedative effects and toxic side reactions).

(a) **Phenobarbital** is one of the most effective anticonvulsants. It is well tolerated.

 i. **Side effects** include hyperkinesis, drowsiness, and ataxia.

 ii. **Therapeutic blood levels** are 0.5–1.5 mg/100 ml.

(b) **Mephobarbital (Mebaral)** may be used as a substitute for phenobarbital and causes hyperkinesis infrequently. Side effects are uncommon.

(c) **Phenytoin** (Dilantin) is presently the most effective of all anticonvulsants and has a relatively low incidence of serious side effects. Dosage must be individualized, and blood level determinations in refractory cases are helpful.

 i. The **therapeutic blood level** is 15–25 μg/100 ml. Lateral gaze nystagmus is seen when this level is reached.

 ii. **Common side effects** include (a) gingival hyperplasia, which is not entirely treatable by good oral hygiene and has required gingivectomy; (b) hypertrichosis of the face, arms, and trunk; (c) megaloblastic anemia, responsive to folic acid therapy; and (d) asymptomatic depression of normal values of T_4 and RT_3.

 iii. **Toxic effects** are infrequent and include agranulocytosis,

Table 21-1   Maintenance Therapy of Seizure Disorders

Seizure Disorder	Medication	Daily Dose (mg/kg, bid–tid)
Grand mal, focal motor, or psychomotor seizures	*Group A*	
	Phenobarbital	3–5
	Mephobarbital	3–10
	Phenytoin sodium[a]	5–8
	Primidone	5–25
	Carbamazepine[b]	
Centrencephalic (petit mal), akinetic, or myoclonic seizures	One medication from group A[b] plus one from group B	
	Group B	
	Ethosuximide	5–25
	Valproic acid	15–30
	Clonazepam	0.1–0.2 mg/kg/d
	Methylphenyl-succinimide	20–40
	Methsuximide	5–20
	Diazepam	0.5–2
	Trimethadione	15–40
	Paramethadione	15–40
	Acetazolamide	5–25

[a] Phenytoin may aggravate petit mal seizures.
[b] Carbamazepine dosage varies. In children 6–12 years of age, the total daily dose should not exceed 1 gm; in those 12–15 years old, it should not exceed 1.2 gm; and in those 15 or more years old, it should not exceed 1.6 gm.

ataxia, diplopia, dysarthria, eosinophilia, eliptocytosis, exfoliative dermatitis, hematuria, hepatitis, leukopenia, lymph adenopathy, macrocytosis, peripheral neuropathy, skin rashes, Stevens-Johnson syndrome, and thrombocytopenic purpura.

iv. Usage in pregnancy   About 11 percent of infants exposed to phenytoin in utero develop the fetal hydantoin syndrome (*Pediatrics* 63:331, 1979).

(d) Primidone (Mysoline) is used in the treatment of psychomotor and grand mal epilepsy. Its action is believed similar to that of barbiturates.

i. Frequent side effects are noted when the medication is instituted in full dosage. For this reason, it is recommended that treatment be started with ⅕ to ⅒ of the full dose and increasing the dosage every 4 days until the maximum dosage is reached. Behavior changes, irritability, drowsiness, vomiting, and ataxia may cause the patient to discontinue this medication if the dose is not increased gradually.

ii. Toxic effects from long-term therapy are infrequent. Megaloblastic anemia responsive to folic acid has been reported.

(e) Carbamazepine (Tegretol) is chemically unrelated to other anticonvulsants. It is indicated alone or in combination with other anticonvulsants for the treatment of partial seizures (focal motor, psychomotor), grand mal seizures, and absence seizures and petit mal. It is not a first-line anticonvulsant and **may cause serious and sometimes fatal hematologic complications** (aplastic anemia, agranulocytosis, thrombocytopenia). A pretreatment CBC and platelet count should be obtained, with weekly CBCs during the first 3 months of therapy and monthly thereafter. Carbamazepine must be started gradually (100 mg bid) and slowly increased to a therapeutic dose over 10–20 days. Serum levels can be measured.

(f) Ethosuximide is useful for petit mal epilepsy in combination with other drugs. However, it is available only in gelatinous 250-mg capsules, which challenges parental ingenuity in administering it. The medication must usually be removed from the capsules for young children, or the capsule may be frozen and cut into small bits.

    i. The **minimal effective dose** for a toddler may be 125 mg tid.

    ii. Toxic effects Agranulocytosis is the most serious toxic effect, and an initial CBC and periodic checks should be done. It is less toxic than trimethadione and usually is effective in less than 24 hr after therapy starts. Hiccups are seen as an idiosyncratic reaction.

(g) Valproic acid (Depakene) is also unrelated to other anticonvulsants and is indicated for the control of petit mal or absence seizures. It may be used in combination with other anticonvulsants, but is contraindicated in combination with clonazepam, since it may cause absence status. Dosage should be initiated at 15 mg/kg/day and increased weekly by 5–10 mg/kg/day until good seizure control or a dosage of 30 mg/kg/day is reached. Its **toxic effects** are related to liver damage, and serial tests of liver function should be monitored.

(h) Clonazepam (Clonopin) is a benzodiazepine type of anticonvulsant useful for adjunctive treatment of petit mal, absence or akinetic seizures, and myoclonic seizures. The **side effects** are predominantly those of CNS depression. There is a wide range of dosage, but the maximum recommended daily dose for adults is 20 mg.

(i) Trimethadione (Tridione) and **paramethadione (Paradione),** because of their serious toxic effects, should **not** be used before ethosuximide is tried and is unsuccessful.

    i. Toxic effects include "yellow vision," leukopenia, and agranulocytosis.

    ii. Side effects are vomiting, hiccups, rashes, photophobia, and alopecia.

    iii. The **minimal effective dose** is probably 150 mg tid.

    iv. Initial and weekly CBCs are mandatory. Thereafter they may be performed monthly.

(j) Methylphenylsuccinimide (Milontin) and **methsuximide (Celontin)** are not often used, but may be if ethosuximide fails. Toxic effects on bone narrow have been observed. **Side effects** of GI disturbance and drowsiness are seen.

(k) Acetazolamide (Diamox) is a carbonic anhydrase inhibitor, useful in conjunction with another anticonvulsant for ce trencephalic seizures.

   i. There is no minimal effective dosage, and children ha been given more than 2 gm/day to control seizures.

   ii. Side effects are probably dose related and include anorex polyuria, paresthesias, and hyperpnea when an acido state occurs.

   (l) Diazepam (Valium) has been shown to be an effective oral a ticonvulsant. For the poorly controlled centrencephalic seizu disorder, it is a useful drug in combination therapy.

   i. The dose should be increased slowly and withheld wh toxic symptoms appear. There is a wide safety margin, a children have taken up to 30–40 mg daily with cessation seizures and minimal side effects.

   ii. Drowsiness, amnesia, nystagmus, ataxia, and dysarth are commonly seen and are dose related. Amphetamin have successfully counteracted the somnolence.

B. Neonatal seizures   (See also p. 40, Sec. III.) Convulsive disorders during t first 2–3 weeks of life are a relatively common problem in any special ca nursery. Etiology, evaluation, and treatment of seizures in the neonate a unique. Seizures frequently are unrecognized in newborns because of the atypical form.

   1. Etiology   The most common causes are metabolic disturbance, birth i jury, and infection (see Table 21-2).

   2. Evaluation and diagnosis

      a. Convulsions as such are almost never seen. Instead, the seizure di charges are manifested clinically by apnea, twitching of the eyelids of one extremity, abnormal crying, deviation of the eyes, or cyanos The lack of organization and myelination of the neonatal nervo system is responsible for the poorly differentiated spells.

      b. Laboratory studies

         (1) Each infant must have appropriate **blood chemistry studies** i cluding glucose, calcium, magnesium, electrolytes, protein, phc phate, and BUN.

         (2) A lumbar puncture, skull x-ray, EEG, evaluation for sepsis, he circumference measurements, transillumination of the skull, a subdural taps when indicated are also required. A **CAT** scan ma be helpful in confirming a subdural hematoma or the source of subarachnoid hemorrhage.

         (3) Urinalysis should include amino acid screening, ferric chlorid dinitrophenylhydrazine, a test for reducing substance with gl cose oxidase dipstick, and Benedict's test to rule out galactosemi

      c. Hypocalcemia is a leading cause of seizures in neonates and is mo likely to appear between the fourth and eighth days of life. It is mo common in prematures and after a difficult delivery. Classic signs tetany are absent, although Erb's sign is usually present. *Ioniz* serum calcium is usually < 7.5 mg/100 ml and phosphate, > 7.5 mg/1 ml. Focal seizures are common, with EEG abnormalities most str ing during the ictus. The cause is usually speculative.

Table 21-2 Etiology of Neonatal Seizures Grouped According to Response to Therapy

---

I. Perinatal hypoxia-ischemia
II. Metabolic disorders
    Hypocalcemia
    Hypoglycemia
    Hyponatremia, hypernatremia
    Pyridoxine dependency
    Withdrawal
      Barbiturates
      Narcotics
III. Infections
    Meningitis (bacterial)
    Sepsis
    Viral meningoencephalitis
IV. Trauma
    Intracerebral hemorrhage
    Subarachnoid hemorrhage
    Skull fracture
    Subdural hematoma
    Cortical vein thrombosis
V. Postmaturity
VI. Congenital cerebral defects

---

d. Hypoglycemia (blood sugar < 30 mg/100 ml) is usually noted in the first 72 hr of life and may be seen with sepsis, in intracranial hemorrhage, and in infants of diabetic mothers. It is an infrequent cause of neonatal seizures.

e. Hypomagnesemia (serum magnesium < 1.2 mg/100 ml) is uncommon and may present with symptoms identical to hypoglycemia.

f. Pyridoxine dependency is not accompanied by clinical abnormalities except seizures, and the diagnosis is made by prompt response to pyridoxine given IV (see Table 21-3). If this diagnosis is made, treatment must be continued indefinitely to prevent recurrence.

g. Pyridoxine deficiency is seen after the neonatal period and is caused by a lack of exogenous vitamin B_6.

h. Hyponatremia and **hypernatremia** are rare causes of neonatal seizures and may be noted after therapy has been instituted for seizures due to another metabolic etiology. Prognosis is favorable when the electrolyte imbalance is not associated with sepsis.

i. Meningitis and **sepsis** account for a significant number of seizures in neonates.

j. Birth injury often causes seizures, and these occur on the second to fifth day of life.

3. Treatment

a. General

(1) Support ventilation, BP, pH.

(2) Use a reliable IV.

(3) Maintain the blood sugar even if it is not the primary cause seizures.

b. Treatment of metabolic deficiency with EEG   Therapeutic trials to cor rect metabolic deficiency should not be postponed until the results blood chemistry studies are available. Trials should be done while a EEG is being recorded (Table 21-3). One should wait 10–15 minute between IV trial infusions for therapeutic effect (begin with th treatment least likely to cause an effect).

c. Anticonvulsant drugs   If hypoglycemia and other metabolic problem have been ruled out, administer anticonvulsant medications (se **b.(2).(b)**, p. 485).

(1) **Phenobarbital**   Give 3–10 mg/kg IV over several minutes. If se zures continue, repeat one-half of the initial dose in 30 min.

    (a) **Maintenance**   5–8 mg/kg/day divided in q12h doses.

    (b) If the infant is not currently experiencing a seizure, admini ter 10–15 mg/kg/day IM or IV in two divided doses over th first day, followed by maintenance doses, to provide adequat blood levels (optimum levels, 15–30 μg/ml).

(2) **Phenytoin**   After 5–10 min, if there is no response to phenobar tal, give 5–10 mg/kg phenytoin IV initially; the dose can be r peated in 5–10 min.

    (a) If phenytoin was necessary for acute treatment, a mainte nance dose of 4–7 mg/kg/day divided in q12h doses can b given IV or PO **(not IM; IM administration fails to provid adequate blood levels).**

    (b) Phenytoin interferes with binding of bilirubin by albumi and bilirubin displaces phenytoin from albumin, causing i creased levels of unbound or active phenytoin. Thus phen toin should be used with caution in jaundiced infants. Opt mum levels are 5–15 μg/ml.

(3) **Diazepam (Valium)**   The vehicle for IV diazepam contains sodiu benzoate, which interferes with bilirubin binding. In additio when used with barbiturates, there is a risk of circulatory collap and respiratory failure.

    (a) The therapeutic dose is very variable.

    (b) It has a short duration of action.

    (c) Give 0.5–2 mg *slowly* IV until the seizure stops.

    (d) Diazepam is not reliable for maintenance. Phenobarbital phenytoin should be used instead.

(4) With resistant seizures, give diluted **paraldehyde,** 0.2 ml/kg p rectum; otherwise give IV or IM.

(5) At discharge, try to discontinue all medications except phenoba bital.

Substance	Amount	Note
Glucose, 50% (dilute to 25%)	0.5–1.0 gm/kg over 3 min to max. of 0.5 gm/kg/hr	Check Dextrostix frequently Maintain BS with 0.25–0.5 gm/kg/hr (10% D/W at 100 ml/kg/q4h = 0.25 gm/kg/hr)
Pyridoxine	50 mg	Cessation of seizures with normalization of EEG in minutes if this is the cause Maintenance: Dependency 10–100 mg PO/day Deficiency 5 mg PO/day
Calcium gluconate, 10%	2 ml/kg + equal volume sterile water, IV over 3 min with ECG	1. ECG; rapid infusion causes bradycardia 2. Do not mix with NaHCO$_3$ 3. Do not use UV line unless in IVC 4. Observe peripheral vein directly to avoid extravasation and tissue necrosis
Magnesium sulfate, 50% (MgSO$_4$)	0.2 ml/kg IM q12h	1. 50% of hypocalcemic infants also have hypomagnesemia. Failure to give Mg will aggravate hypocalcemia 2. Excessive Mg can cause weakness and hypotonia due to neuromuscular blockade

Table 21-4 Prognosis of Neonatal Seizures in Relation to Neurologic Disease

Neurologic Disease[a]	Normal Development (%[b]
Hypoxic-ischemic encephalopathy	10–20
Primary subarachnoid hemorrhage	90
Intraventricular hemorrhage	5
Hypocalcemia[c]	
Early onset	50
Late onset	80–100
Hypoglycemia	50
Bacterial meningitis	20[d]–50[e]
Developmental defect	0

[a] Includes cases accompanied by seizures.
[b] In general, periods of follow-up do not extend to school age.
[c] Prognosis is worse if due to asphyxia than if due to metabolic causes.
[d] Term infants with group B streptococcal meningitis.
[e] Premature infants with gram-negative meningitis.
Source: Adapted from J. J. Volpe, Neonatal seizures, *Clin. Perinatol.* 4:43, 1977.

    4. Prognosis of neonatal seizures is primarily related to the cause (Tab 21-4).

      a. The type of seizure is helpful in predicting the prognosis.

        (1) Tonic, multifocal clonic indicates a poor prognosis.

        (2) Focal clonic indicates a good prognosis.

      b. A markedly abnormal interictal EEG may indicate a poor prognosi Interpretation should be withheld until a follow-up EEG 4–7 day after the first one shows similar abnormalities.

   C. Headache The child with persistent or recurrent headache presents challenging diagnostic problem. When the headache is not due to acu infection, systemic illness, or trauma, the physician must consider n **graine.** The incidence of migraine is about 3 percent in the general popul tion of children. Most are 6–12 years of age when initial symptoms begi Girls frequently experience their initial attack with menarche.

    1. Evaluation Skull x-rays, blood pressure recordings, and an EEG wi strobe stimulation should be done.

    2. Diagnosis The diagnosis is made by history. Sometimes, an excessi response to strobe light stimulation is seen on the EEG.

      a. Common migraine is the most frequent type of headache seen, ar there is usually no prodrome. The pain is a steady, severe ache, whi may become throbbing, and lasts 4–6 hr. It is usually unilateral (b not always on the same side).

      b. Classic migraine often consists of an aura for 20–30 min prior to th pain. Visual symptoms (scotomas, flashing lights, blurred visio fortification spectra) are followed by a severe unilateral frontal pai that becomes throbbing, and the patient may then vomit. He or sh prefers to sleep in a cool, dark place, and this may terminate th episode. Variants include mild hemiparesis, ophthalmoplegia, and severe abdominal cramps. During an attack of migraine, children may present with an acute confusional state.

    c. Cluster headaches (histamine or Horton's headaches) are characterized by severe unilateral neuralgialike pain in the retroorbital region and are very rarely seen in childhood.

  3. Treatment Prophylaxis is the best therapy. Maintenance barbiturates in anticonvulsant dosage are beneficial to children with migraine, and ergot preparations are generally not needed until adolescence (Table 21-5).

D. Abdominal epilepsy is a syndrome of paroxysmal pain, altered state of consciousness, and postictal symptoms. It may occur alone or in association with other convulsive disorders. Psychomotor seizures are frequent accompaniments. Cyclic vomiting may occur.

  1. Etiology Cryptogenic.

  2. Evaluation Systemic causes of abdominal pain should be ruled out, particularly porphyria and plumbism.

  3. Diagnosis Abnormal EEG.

  4. Treatment Anticonvulsants (as for grand mal; see Table 21-1).

II. ALTERATIONS IN THE STATE OF CONSCIOUSNESS

A. Nontraumatic alterations An outline of management is given on page 43 (Chap. 2).

B. Traumatic alterations

  1. Evaluation

    a. If the child did not lose consciousness following head trauma and is alert and normally responsive, a careful general evaluation and neurologic examination may be done following the accident and superficial injuries treated.

    b. Evaluation for focal neurologic deficit such as hemiparesis and pupillary abnormalities must be made, and signs of increased intracranial pressure should be sought.

    c. Skull roentgenograms must be done and a search made for basal skull fractures. A **CAT scan** may be indicated after discussion with a neurosurgical consultant.

    d. CNS rhinorrhea may be a clue to a basal fracture, as are "raccoon eyes." Glucose in the nasal secretions (detected by a Dextrostix) is diagnostic of CSF rhinorrhea. Blood behind the tympanic membrane is another finding pathognomonic of basal skull fracture.

    e. Neurosurgical consultation is necessary for further management. **Lumbar puncture should not be performed.**

    f. Regardless of age, any child with a vague or incomplete history of single or repeated bouts of head trauma should be admitted to the hospital and evaluated for signs of the battered child syndrome (see p. 57). Roentgenograms of the skull, chest, and long bones should be made, and subdural hematoma must be ruled out.

Table 21-5 Drugs Used for Treatment of Migraine

Medication	Daily Dose	Frequency
Aspirin	65 mg/year of age/dose PO or PR	q4–6h prn
Phenobarbital	3–5 mg/kg/day	Continuous treatment bid
Phenytoin	5–8 mg/kg/day	Continuous treatment bid
Fiorinal (butalbital, 50 mg; caffeine, 40 mg; aspirin, 200 mg; phenacetin, 130 mg)	Under age 5: ½ tablet Over age 5: 1 tablet	qid qid
Cafergot (ergotamine tartrate, 1.0 mg; caffeine, 100 mg)	1 or 2 tablets with initial symptoms, then 1 q30min prn up to a total of 4 tablets in 12 hr Suppository: ½ PR initially and ½ q45min prn up to a total of 3	
Ergotamine tartrate sublingual	2 mg q30min prn up to total of 5 tablets per day	
Propranolol (prophylaxis only)	10–30 mg tid–qid	
Methysergide (prophylaxis only)	2 mg bid–tid	Continuous treatment

2. Head trauma syndromes

a. Cerebral concussion

(1) **Retrograde amnesia,** which is loss of memory for events immediately preceding the trauma, often occurs.

(2) **Anterograde amnesia** (memory loss after the trauma) usually lasts longer than retrograde amnesia.

(3) The **physical examination** should include a detailed neurologic evaluation. The patient with a mild concussion is usually lethargic and diaphoretic, and vomiting and headache may be seen in the first 24–48 hr.

(4) **Treatment** Any scalp lacerations should be treated to prevent infection, and then evaluation should be continued. The patient whose evaluation is negative usually becomes increasingly alert and responsive. Many of these children can be discharged to the care of responsible parents. It is useful to give them a list of guidelines for care. A sample set of such guidelines may be obtained from Emergency Services Department, Children's Hospital Medical Center, Boston, 02115.

b. Subdural hematoma and effusions

(1) **Evaluation**

(a) A history of irritability, vomiting, poor feeding, apathy, failure to thrive, convulsions, delayed motor milestones, anemia, and an enlarged, "boxy" head should alert the physician.

(b) One should check for a tense, bulging fontanelle, retinal hemorrhages, decreased percussion note of the skull, positive transillumination, and increase of head size above normal percentiles. In long-standing hematomas the skull roentgenogram may show abnormally split cranial sutures. **Lumbar puncture is contraindicated.**

(c) This diagnosis in infants is excluded only after bilateral subdural taps have been performed, as 50 percent of affected children are found to have hematomas over *both* hemispheres. In older children with closed sutures the definitive study is a CAT scan, cerebral angiography, or both.

(2) **Treatment** is by removal of the subdural fluid (alternating hemispheres daily) and may be successful in "drying up" the effusion in 2–3 weeks. In unusually large subdural hematomas—or when signs referable to compression of underlying brain are evident— early consultation with a neurosurgical colleague in necessary.

C. Benign increased intracranial pressure (pseudotumor cerebri)

1. **Etiology** includes changes in hormone balance, termination of corticosteroid therapy, administration of fluorinated corticosteroids, and administration of tetracycline, penicillin, and vitamin A. Also, a small percentage of these patients are found to have a cerebral venous sinus thrombosis.

2. Evaluation

a. Affected children may present with the symptoms and signs of intracranial hypertension: headache, vomiting, cranial nerve palsy, and papilledema without an antecedent illness.

   b. Physical examination may show enlarging head size if sutures are i
   the process of closing. Papilledema is present and a VIth nerve pals
   is common.

   c. Cerebellar signs and meningeal irritation are not present; this shoul
   alert the physician to the possibility that a posterior fossa mass c
   basilar meningitis may be responsible for such signs. Skull roen
   genograms, EEG, and a technetium brain scan are necessary.

3. **Diagnosis**   A CAT scan may reveal swollen cerebral hemispheres wit
   slitlike ventricles. Cerebral angiography and venography may be neede
   to rule out a sinus thrombosis when focal neurologic signs are not othe
   wise explained.

4. **Treatment**   Many patients will show spontaneous recovery after lumba
   puncture. Careful follow-up examination is needed, and the patier
   should be checked for visual changes associated with papilledema. Thos
   who remain symptomatic may be treated as follows:

   a. Acetazolamide (Diamox), 25 mg/kg/day

   b. Dexamethasone (Decadron), 2–4 mg q8h initially for 3–4 days, the
   2–4 mg q12h for 10 days, with a tapering dose

III. MISCELLANEOUS DISORDERS

A. **Myasthenia gravis** may present as diffuse weakness at any age and is see
   in newborns. Three forms are known in childhood.

   Transient neonatal myasthenia gravis occurs at or shortly after birth. A
   infant of a myasthenic mother may be floppy and have ptosis and stridor, b
   a poor eater, and have diminished reflexes, which may last 3–4 week
   Immediate treatment with neostigmine may be lifesaving. The disorde
   does not recur after symptoms disappear at about age 1 month (Table 21-5).

   Persistent neonatal myasthenia gravis is seen in infants of health
   mothers who do not have myasthenia. Fetal movement may have de
   creased during the latter part of the pregnancy. Symptoms are similar t
   those in infants who have transient myasthenia gravis, but respirator
   distress is usually absent. External ophthalmoplegia is common in thi
   group. It is also seen at birth. Many children are refractory to therap
   (Table 21-5).

   Juvenile myasthenia gravis occurs after the first year of life and is seen i
   girls 5 times as often as in boys. Ptosis (unilateral or bilateral) may be th
   only presenting sign. Generalized weakness, bulbar muscle weakness, an
   a flat, expressionless face are seen later.

   1. **Diagnosis** is by a positive response to edrophonium (Tensilon) (see Tabl
      21-5), and an electromyogram (EMG) confirms this finding.

   2. **Treatment**   (See Table 21-6.) Anticholinesterase medications usuall
      produce a marked improvement in muscle strength, but long-term re
      sults of medical therapy alone are discouraging. A child who become
      unresponsive to medications should be considered for thymectomy, sinc
      this may produce a lasting remission. Treatment with ACTH and predni
      sone is controversial but frequently helpful, although not thoroughl
      studied in children.

   3. **Crises**   Cholinergic or myasthenic crisis (see **a, b, c**) in a myastheni
      child is a medical emergency and presents as acute respiratory failur
      (see p. 46).

Age Group	Diagnostic Dose of Edrophonium (Tensilon, 10 mg/ml)	Oral Maintenance Dose		
		Neostigmine (Prostigmin)	Pyridostigmine (Mestinon)	Ambenonium (Mytelase)
	IV response in 30 sec[a] IM response in 2–8 min	15 mg =	60 mg =	6 mg
Neonatal[b]				
Transient	1 mg IV or 2 mg IM	1–5 mg[c]	6 mg, then is increased	Not to be used for neonates (no blood-brain barrier exists, and convulsions occur with overdose)
Persistent	Same	Same	Same	
Juvenile				
> 2 yr old	< 30 kg, 1–5 mg IV or 2–10 mg IM	Initial dose, 3.75 mg	Initial dose, 15 mg	Initial dose, 2 mg
	> 30 kg, 5–10 mg IV or 10–20 mg IM	Increase these increments until desired effects are attained or side effects occur. Adjuvant drugs (ephedrine, 12.5–25.0 mg tid) may be used.		

[a] Atropine must be available for cholinergic side effects.

[b] Positive response = improved respirations, good cry, Moro reflex, increased tone.

[c] Oral dose is 30 times parenteral dose. Parenteral neostigmine is available as 0.25, 0.5, and 1.0 mg/ml.

a. **Myasthenic crisis** occurs when the patient becomes unresponsive to the regular dose of medication and can be seen with intercurrent infection.

b. **Cholinergic crisis** is due to an overdose of anticholinesterase medication. The symptoms of cholinergic crisis are pallor, bradycardia, increased blood pressure, increased secretions, miosis, fasciculations, severe abdominal cramps, and dysarthria.

c. **Treatment of crises** begins with supported respirations. Assisted pulmonary ventilation may be needed. The differentiation between myasthenic and cholinergic crises may be difficult, and IV edrophonium, 1 mg q60sec, up to a total of 4 mg, should be administered. If the symptoms decrease abruptly, one can assume that inadequate medications (myasthenic crisis) are the cause.

   (1) **Treatment of myasthenic crisis** should proceed with prostigmine IV as needed, not to exceed 2.5 mg/hr. Atropine sulfate should be administered (0.1–0.3 mg IV) to decrease the muscarinic effects of increased bronchial secretions and diarrhea. **Do not give any of the following to patients in myasthenic crisis:** sedatives; hypnotics; quinine (including tonic water); or antibiotics of the neomycin bacitracin, streptomycin, or kanamycin groups.

   (2) **Treatment of cholinergic crisis** Atropine sulfate is the drug of choice and should be given in a dose of 0.2–1.0 mg IV as needed to decrease production of copious secretions and prevent further respiratory embarrassment.

B. **Bell's palsy** usually refers to involvement of the VIIth cranial nerve at or near the stylomastoid foramen and presents with a sudden onset of ipsilateral weakness of the upper and lower portions of the face.

1. **Physical examination** reveals a characteristic deformity that is rarely mistaken. The child has a flat nasolabial fold, cannot close the eyelids, pucker the lips, or wrinkle the brow. Saliva may drool from the corner of the mouth. Speech is abnormal. The deficit is accentuated when the patient smiles.

   Almost all children with incomplete Bell's palsy recover in 3–6 weeks. Denervation occurs only when facial paralysis is clinically complete. Such patients should be evaluated for decompressive surgery after EMG has confirmed total denervation.

2. **Treatment** to prevent secondary deformity should begin at onset.

   a. **Massage** The facial muscle should be massaged upward by placing the thumb inside the mouth and index finger on the cheek.

   b. **Eyedrops** Instillation of methylcellulose eyedrops should be done qid, keeping the lids opposed with the use of an eye pad to prevent corneal injury. Older children should wear clear plastic glasses.

   c. **Corticosteroids** The use of corticosteroids for a short time is controversial, but has benefited some patients. (Children 8 years of age or older may be given prednisone, 40 mg/day in divided doses for 4 days, tapering to 5 mg/day, to end at 8 days; children under 8 should be given 20 mg/day for 4 days, tapering off to 5 mg, to end at 8 days.)

C. **Wilson's disease** In this condition there is hepatolenticular degeneration with abnormal deposits of copper in the brain, liver, cornea, and kidney.

1. **Etiology** This is a hereditary (autosomal recessive) disease. A major

defect is an almost total absence of ceruloplasmin in the plasma, with resultant decreased copper binding.

2. Evaluation and diagnosis

a. The onset is usually in the early teens and may begin as a tremor of the hands, ticlike movements under stress, and tremulous speech when the tones are sustained. Hypertonia, "winged-beating" tremors, mental changes, behavior changes, and dysarthria are later manifestations.

b. Hepatomegaly may be present, and a thorough evaluation of the corneal limbus for Kayser-Fleischer rings should be made. A presumptive laboratory diagnosis is made by finding < 25 mg/100 ml ceruloplasmin in a child over 6 months of age. Liver biopsy with findings greater than 250 μg copper dry weight is pathognomonic. Sibs of affected children should be screened, although treatment of a carrier is not indicated.

3. Treatment   D-penicillamine, 15–30 mg/kg/day in 3 oral doses, will increase urinary copper excretion. A **low-copper diet,** with avoidance of mushrooms, chocolate, liver, and shellfish, should be prescribed. For discussion of side effects of D-penicillamine, see **C.(5),** p. 88.

4. Prognosis   Patients with mild neurologic symptoms becomes functionally normal after 6–12 months of penicillamine treatments. Those who are severely affected may not improve. The natural history of the untreated illness is progressive disability, with liver failure and death in about 5 years.

22

Skin Disorders

I. ACNE

A. Etiology At puberty, increased blood levels of androgenic steroids stimulate activity of the pilosebaceous apparatus. Sebum becomes trapped, and bacterial (*Corynebacterium acnes*) enzymes hydrolyze sebaceous lipids to free fatty acids. The sebaceous ducts, distended by inspissated sebaceous material, rupture and release irritating free fatty acids into the dermis, where an inflammatory reaction occurs. *Diet is not thought to play a role in the pathophysiology of the disease.*

B. Evaluation Determine the social problem presented by the disease. Ask if flares of disease activity are associated with periods of emotional stress or with menstruation. Note what topical preparations are being used for treatment or cover-up; moisturizers, oil-based cleansing creams, and makeup may aggravate preexisting acne.

C. Diagnosis

1. Subjective findings Flares of activity may be associated with emotional stress or with menstrual periods.

2. Objective findings The skin is oily. Scattered over the face, chest, and back are comedones, inflammatory papules and pustules, and, in some cases, deep, interconnecting, fluctuant cysts. Scarring may be disfiguring.

D. Therapy

1. Soaps Drying and abrasive soaps promote superficial desquamation and opening of plugged follicular orifices. They should be used 2 or 3 times daily. Representative products are Pernox, Fostex, and Brasivol.

2. Comedolytic agents The most useful comedolytic products contain either benzolyl peroxide (Benoxyl, Desquam-X, PanOxyl, Vanoxide) or tretinoin (Retin-A). Because irritant reactions often occur with the use of 0.05% tretinoin liquid, begin therapy with the 0.05% or 0.1% cream or the 0.025% gel. These preparations are applied to affected areas nightly or every other night, as tolerated.

3. Ultraviolet light Either sunlight or artificial ultraviolet light (UVL) will promote faster and more complete control of the disease. Commercially available UV lamps must be used regularly (3 times weekly at least) with stepwise increases in exposure time.

4. Antibiotics *C. acnes* organisms are exquisitely sensitive to tetracycline. For inflammatory pustular and cystic acne, start **tetracycline,** 500 mg PO bid, until control is obtained. Then decrease the dosage to a maintenance level, which may be 250 mg bid. Tetracycline should be administered on an empty stomach. An alternative antibiotic is **erythromycin,** administered in the same dosage as tetracycline. The combination of **erythromycin and clindamycin** is effective when applied topically as 1–2% solutions.

These preparations are not available commercially and must be com
pounded by a pharmacist.

5. **Estrogens** Whereas the more androgenic oral contraceptive agent
(Norlestrin 2.5/50, Ortho-Novum 10 mg, Ovral) may provoke acne
anovulatory drugs with a high estrogen content (0.1 mg mestranol) ma
be helpful in girls with severe acne that has not responded to conven
tional therapy. A gynecologic consultation should be obtained befor
starting a patient on anovulatory drugs. (See also Chap. 13.)

II. ATOPIC DERMATITIS

A. **Etiology** Patients with atopic dermatitis tend to have elevated serur
levels of IgE and decreased cell-mediated immunity. However, the role
these abnormalities in the pathogenesis of the dermatitis is still unknowr

B. **Evaluation** Allergy testing with scratch or intradermal skin tests is unre
warding. A careful history to determine the precipitants (foods, pollens
dusts, dander) of pruritus or dermatitis is much more helpful.

C. **Diagnosis**

1. **Subjective findings**

   a. Atopic dermatitis evolves in three stages: (1) the infantile stage,
   months–3 years; (2) the childhood stage, 3 years–puberty; and (3) th
   adolescent stage, puberty–25 years. Pruritus is common to all.

   b. Extremes of heat or cold, soap and water, alkalis, chemical irritant
   infection, wool, inhalants (pollens, dust, dander), particular foods, an
   psychic stress worsen atopic dermatitis.

   c. The family history is positive for some feature of the atopic syndrom
   in over 70 percent of cases.

2. **Objective findings**

   a. **Infantile stage** Erythematous papules with microvesicles, oozing
   and crusting involve the scalp, face, neck, the extensor aspects of th
   arms, and the ankles. Scattered patches occur on the trunk. Ar
   tecubital and popliteal fossae are often spared.

   b. **Childhood stage** Erythematous papules with less vesiculation an
   crusting than in the infantile stage, but with more scaling an
   lichenification, occur commonly on the trunk and extremities. The
   is less facial involvement than in the earlier stage. Papules an
   lichenification may be present in the antecubital and popliteal fossae

   c. **Adolescent-adult stage** The face, neck, and upper chest are dry an
   scaly. Transverse, parallel lines of rugalike lichenification of the ar
   tecubital and popliteal fossae are the hallmarks of this stage.

D. **Treatment**

1. **Topical corticosteroids** (see XIV.A, p. 518) are the single most effectiv
   therapeutic agents. Applied 2–4 times daily, they rapidly suppres
   inflammation and pruritus.

2. **Emollients** (Eucerin, hydrated petrolatum) are applied as often a
   needed for control of cracking and fissuring of dry, lichenified area
   Emollients should always be applied **immediately** after bathing to mair
   tain the benefits of hydration.

3. Soap and water are irritants to already dried, cracked, and scaling skir
   The patient should bathe only to keep reasonably clean, and use of soa

should be restricted to such areas as the axillae, groin, and feet. Bland, superfatted, or oil-containing soaps (Basis, Oilatum, Aveeno Oilated) may be useful.

4. **Antihistamines** (see Sec. **XIV.B**) are useful because of their sedative effects. The dosage should thus be raised until the patient is less active than usual and somewhat drowsy. Double doses are recommended at bedtime, when most pruritus occurs.

5. **Secondary bacterial infection** is a common complication of scratching. Obtain cultures from lesions suspected of being suprainfected and institute therapy using systemic antibiotics effective against gram-positive pyogens (see Table 15-2).

II. CONTACT DERMATITIS

A. **Etiology** Sensitization to contact allergens. To cause contact sensitization, an antigen must penetrate the epidermis and contain reactive groups that conjugate with tissue proteins. Many substances satisfy these criteria.

B. **Evaluation** The location, distribution, and shape of the lesions are the most useful features in determining the cause of a contact dermatitis.

C. **Diagnosis**

1. **Subjective findings** A history of contact allergy to several different substances is often obtainable. Pruritus is an early distressing symptom of the eruption.

2. **Objective findings** The earliest change is erythema. Edema, vesiculation, and bullous formation follow in rapid succession. **Linearly distributed vesicles** are pathognomonic of contact dermatitis.

D. **Therapy**

1. **Acute vesicular contact dermatitis**

   a. **Aluminum acetate** (Burow's) solution, 1:20, used as a cool, wet compress for 15 min q1–2h relieves pruritus and loosens crusts.

   b. When oozing and crusting begin to resolve, compresses are decreased to qid, and a **topical fluorinated corticosteroid cream** (see Sec. **XIV.A**) is applied after each compress is removed.

   c. In mild cases without oozing and crusting, calamine lotion with 1% phenol relieves pruritus.

   d. In severe, widespread dermatitis, **prednisone** PO quickly relieves symptoms and prevents progression of the eruption.

      (1) To prevent generalized eczematous dermatitis, a 10-day course of corticosteroid therapy, as described in Table 22-1, should be given. A similar schedule should be given to the patient with a warning that prematurely stopping the medication may cause exacerbation.

      (2) Prednisone may be avoided if the usual contraindications are present. After the dermatitis has resolved, patch testing may be done to define the sensitizing allergen clearly. (Patch testing during the active phase of the process can exacerbate the dermatitis.)

2. **Chronic, lichenified contact dermatitis**

   a. A **fluorinated corticosteroid cream** is applied to the lesions at bedtime and occluded with a plastic wrap overnight (see Sec. **XIV.A.1**).

Table 22-1.   Ten-Day Oral Prednisone Regimen in Contact Dermatitis*

Day of Therapy	Number of 5-Milligram Tablets To Be Taken QID				Total Dos (mg)
	Breakfast	Lunch	Dinner	Bedtime	
1	2	2	2	2	40
2	2	2	2	2	40
3	2	2	2	2	40
4	2	1	2	2	35
5	2	1	2	1	30
6	2	1	1	1	25
7	1	1	1	1	20
8	1	1	0	1	15
9	1	0	0	1	10
10	1	0	0	0	5

* Should be modified proportionately for younger children.

    b. A **lubricating, hydrophilic ointment** (hydrated petrolatum, Eucerin) applied during the day as needed for dryness and scaling.

    c. After the dermatitis has resolved, **patch testing** is done to define th etiology clearly.

IV. DIAPER DERMATITIS

    A. Etiology   Diaper dermatitis is the result of dampness, maceration, an chemical irritation.

    B. Evaluation   Question parents regarding the use of plastic occlusive pant and detergents or disinfectants. Examine the scalp, retroauricular area face, and axillae for evidence of seborrhea or atopic dermatitis. Scrape th moist, erythematous lesion in the diaper area and examine the material fo *Candida albicans.*

    C. Diagnosis   Erythema, scaling, and often erosion and ulceration affec primarily convex surfaces, i.e., the buttocks, genitalia, lower abdomen, an upper thighs. The flexural folds may be spared.

    D. Therapy   Instructions are as follows:

        1. Stop the use of bulky diapers and occlusive plastic pants.

        2. Use disposable paper diapers, or rinse cloth diapers well to remove de tergent, enzymes, and chemical irritants.

        3. Change diapers more often.

        4. With each diaper change, cleanse the diaper area with tepid water.

        5. Apply **nonfluorinated hydrocortisone cream** (see Sec. **XIV.A**).

        6. If *C. albicans* is present, add **nystatin cream** tid.

V. ERYTHEMA MULTIFORME

    A. Etiology   Erythema multiforme is a hypersensitivity reaction to multipl agents. Among the common precipitants are infections with herpe simplex, *Mycoplasma pneumoniae*, vaccinia, adenovirus, *Histoplasma*, and exposures to penicillin, sulfonamides, barbiturates, and butazones. However, in 50 percent of cases an etiologic factor cannot be elicited. Severe erythema multiforme with oral and conjunctival involvement is referred to as the Stevens-Johnson syndrome.

B. Evaluation Review the events of the previous 3 weeks for evidence of the recognized precipitants. Determine if a similar eruption has occurred in the past.

C. Diagnosis

1. Subjective findings Successive crops of lesions may appear for from 10 to 14 days. Mucous membrane erosions are extremely painful and debilitating.

2. Objective findings

a. Painful erosions with hemorrhagic crusts involve the mucous membranes of the mouth, lip, nose, eyes, urethra, vagina, and anus. On the dorsa of the hands, palms, wrists, forearms, feet, and legs are erythematous plaques 1–2 cm in diameter, with violaceous or purpuric centers (so-called target lesions) that may become bullous. Hyperpigmented spots are left as the lesions resolve.

b. Corneal ulcerations with subsequent opacities occur in severe disease.

D. Therapy

1. Mild and moderately severe disease

a. Simple topical care with **hexachlorophene (pHisoHex)** and water prevents secondary bacterial invasion of denuded skin lesions.

b. Topical anesthetics such as dyclonine (Dyclone) mouthwash or lidocaine (Xylocaine) ointments are applied to painful, denuded mucous membranes.

2. Severe disease

a. Prednisone, 1–2 mg/kg/day in divided doses, or IV hydrocortisone in severe cases, will shorten the duration of the disease process.

b. If skin lesions are extensive, 1:20 aluminum acetate (Burow's) solution as wet compresses should be applied for 30 min q3–4h while the patient is awake.

c. If oral lesions preclude fluid intake, maintain fluid and electrolyte balance with IV replacement.

d. If an infectious disease is the underlying cause, treat the infection appropriately.

VI. FUNGAL INFECTIONS See also pp. 363 and 389.

A. Etiology

1. Tinea capitis, tinea corporis (ringworm), tinea versicolor, tinea cruris, tinea pedis (athlete's foot), and tinea unguium (onychomycosis) are superficial infections of the skin, hair, and nails due to keratinophilic fungi.

2. A nonpyogenic, localized hypersensitivity response to inflammatory tinea capitis results in a pustular, follicular eruption termed a *kerion*. A

dry, follicular hyperkeratotic eruption on the trunk and proximal ex‑
tremity may accompany kerion formation.

3. Associated with inflammatory tinea pedis is a vesicular "id" eruption o‑
the fingers and palms.

B. Evaluation

1. Demonstration of fungi   Scrape the active border of skin lesions and col‑
lect fine scales on a glass microscope slide. Apply 1 drop of 15% potassium
hydroxide (KOH), cover with a glass coverslip, and heat without boiling
over an open flame or boiling water. Invert the slide and press onto a
paper towel or gauze to express KOH. Examine under "high-dry" powe‑
(× 40). The proximal ends of plucked hairs and scrapings from beneath
nails are similarly prepared for examination.

2. Culture of fungi   Scrapings or hairs are planted on Sabouraud agar o‑
Dermatophyte Test Media (Pfizer, Difco) and incubated for 2–4 weeks a‑
room temperature.

3. Wood's light examination   In a darkened room, shine a Wood's light o‑
the scalp. Involved hairs show **brilliant green** fluorescence at their base‑
when *Microsporum* is the agent responsible.

C. Specific infections

1. Tinea capitis

a. Diagnosis

(1) Subjective findings   The incubation time to clinically apparen‑
disease is 2–3 weeks. Except in the case of painful kerion forma‑
tion, the infection is slightly pruritic or asymptomatic.

(2) Objective findings   Tinea capitis causes a patchy, scaling alopecia
with dull, lusterless hairs broken off 1–2 mm above the skin ("gray
patch"). Inflammation and erythema are mild or moderate. In ac‑
tively enlarging lesions, vesicles may be seen in the advancing
border. Kerion formation is characterized by the appearance o‑
one or more boggy, edematous, raised plaques with nonpyogenic
purulent material crusting on the surface of the lesion. Infecte‑
hairs pull out easily without pain.

b. Treatment   Microcrystalline griseofulvin (Fulvicin-U/F, Grifulvin V
Grisactin), 10 mg/kg 24 hr PO in single doses or in divided doses.

(1) For children weighing 30–50 lb, 125–250 mg/24 hr.

(2) For children weighing over 50 lb, 250–500 mg/24 hr.

2. Tinea corporis

a. Diagnosis

(1) Subjective findings   Incubation time is 1–3 weeks.

(2) Objective findings   Lesions begin as erythematous papules and
expand centrifugally with a raised, papular scaling and sometimes
vesicular border. They clear from the center outward and resolve
spontaneously after several weeks. Occasionally a deep, inflam‑
matory, nodular reaction occurs (Majocchi's granuloma).

b. Treatment

(1) For mild to moderate involvement, apply an **antifungal agent** (Table
22-2) tid. To prevent recurrence, continue this treatment for 1‑
days after the lesions have resolved.

Table 22-2 Commonly Used Topical Antifungal Agents

Chemical Name	Trade Name	Preparations Available	Sizes
Clotrimazole	Lotrimin	Cream 1% Solution 1%	Tube, 15 gm, 30 gm Bottle 10 ml, 30 ml
Haloprogin	Halotex	Cream 1% Solution 1%	Tube, 30 gm Bottle, 10 ml
Miconazole	MicaTin	Cream 2%	Tube, 1 oz, 15 gm
Tolnaftate	Tinactin	Cream 1% Solution 1% Powder 1%	Tube, 15 gm Bottle, 10 ml Container, 45 gm

      (2) For extensive or deep involvement, give **microcrystalline griseofulvin** (see **1.b**) for 2–3 weeks.

3. Tinea versicolor

  a. Diagnosis

    (1) Subjective findings Disease activity is exacerbated by warm, humid weather. The eruption is slightly pruritic or asymptomatic. Hypopigmentation of affected areas has been attributed to sun screening for overlying scales. After treatment, 3–6 months may be required for complete repigmentation.

    (2) Objective findings A capelike area over the neck, shoulders, and proximal upper extremities is involved by round, finely scaling, hypopigmented or tan macules. The lesions coalesce into extensive, confluent areas over the posterior shoulders. Scraping with a tongue blade or surgical blade raises an abundance of fine white scales.

  b. Treatment Instructions are as follows: Apply **selenium sulfide** (Selsun) directly to affected areas, let dry, and leave on several hours to overnight. Repeat this process daily for 4 days. An overnight application once a month will prevent recurrence.

4. Tinea cruris

  a. Diagnosis

    (1) Subjective findings Inflammation and pruritis may be intense.

    (2) Objective findings Sharply marginated, erythematous, and scaling areas with elevated borders and little central clearing extend down the medial thighs from the inguinal folds. The scrotum, penis, and labia are commonly spared. Candidiasis, on the other hand, is characterized by a brightly erythematous eruption above and below the inguinal fold, by involvement of the scrotum and labia, and by satellite pustules scattered beyond the poorly marginated central lesions.

  b. Treatment

    (1) For mild to moderate involvement An **antifungal solution or cream** (see Table 22-2) is applied tid until the eruption clears, and then is continued bid for 10 days more to prevent recurrence.

    (2) For severe involvement, give **microcrystalline griseofulvin** (see **1.b**) for 3–4 weeks. Initially, if inflammation is severe, cool Burow solution (Domeboro powder) compresses are applied tid–qid.

5. Tinea pedis

a. Diagnosis   Tinea pedis is uncommon before puberty, but should be suspected in any chronic scaling eruption of the feet. Scaling, erythematous changes on the feet of children are most likely to be *noninfectious* eruptions due to sweating and maceration ("sneaker dermatitis"), especially in children with an atopic diathesis, i.e., hay fever, asthma, eczema, urticaria by history.

b. Treatment

(1) For mild involvement, apply an **antifungal agent** (see Table 22-2).

(2) For moderate involvement with scaling and hyperkeratosis, an **antifungal solution or cream** is applied tid on even days. On alternate days, 6% sulfur and 6% salicylic acid in petrolatum are applied bid.

(3) For severe or recurrent involvement, give **microcrystalline griseofulvin** (see **1.b**) for 4–6 weeks.

6. Tinea unguium

a. Diagnosis

(1) Subjective findings   Acquisition of nail infection is probably from antecedent skin dermatophytosis. Thus tinea pedis or tinea manum usually coexists. The dystrophic nails are asymptomatic.

(2) Objective findings   Usually, only one or two nails on one hand are involved. Early white-to-yellow discoloration of the lateral nail tip is seen. With progression of the infection, the nail becomes yellow or brown, thick, and friable. Keratinous debris collects beneath the distal nail plate.

b. Treatment is difficult and relapse is common. Surgical removal of involved nails at the onset of therapy improves the cure rate. Microcrystalline griseofulvin (see **1.b**) is required for 6–12 months.

VII. IMPETIGO

A. Etiology   Impetigo is clinically and bacteriologically classified into two distinct types. The **nonbullous** type is characterized by crusted lesions caused primarily by **streptococci** and sometimes secondarily infected by staphylococci. **Bullous impetigo** is associated with a bulla or a relatively clean, eroded lesion caused by **staphylococci**, usually bacteriophage group II. Glomerulonephritis may result from nonbullous impetigo caused by **streptococci M-type 49 or 55.** Rheumatic fever is not a sequela of cutaneous infection. A primary cutaneous disease may underlie the impetiginous process.

B. Evaluation

1. Gram stain is helpful in bullous but not in nonbullous impetigo, since secondary infection of the latter is frequent.

2. Laboratory evaluation   A CBC and antistreptolysin titer are not helpful. Since nephritogenic strains are propagated by direct contact, throat and skin cultures should be done on family members and close contacts of a patient with impetigo.

C. Diagnosis

1. **Subjective findings** There is often a history of antecedent minor trauma, or insect bites, or exposure to other infected children. The lesions are usually relatively asymptomatic, but occasionally pruritus may be a prominent feature.

2. **Objective findings**

   a. **Nonbullous impetigo** Multiple lesions, more numerous on the face and extremities than elsewhere, are characterized by a thick, adherent, yellowish-brown (honey-colored) crust. Involved areas spread centrifugally and coalesce into large, irregularly shaped lesions with no tendency for central clearing. Regional lymphadenopathy is common.

   b. **Bullous impetigo** Flaccid bullae, 1–2 cm in diameter and containing turbid fluid, occur anywhere on the body. After 2–3 days they rupture, leaving discrete, round lesions and coalescent, polycyclic areas that tend to clear centrally. On Gram stain, fluid contains gram-positive cocci in clusters.

D. Treatment

1. **Nonbullous impetigo**

   a. **Minimal disease** may be treated by **local cool water soaks** to remove crusts. This is followed by hexachlorophene scrubs and the application of a topical antibiotic 2–3 times daily. However, if the lesions do not resolve quickly with topical care, systemic antibiotic therapy is indicated.

   b. **Moderate or extensive disease Benzathine penicillin G (Bicillin),** 600,000 U IM in a single dose, usually is effective therapy. Even if a penicillin-resistant staphylococcus is present in the lesion, treatment of the streptococci with penicillin induces cure. In rare cases, specific antistaphylococcal therapy may be indicated.

2. **Bullous impetigo** Since the causative organism, bacteriophage group II staphylococcus, is generally penicillin resistant, a semisynthetic, **penicillinase-resistant penicillin** must be employed (see Tables 15-1, p. 338, and 15-2, p. 342).

3. **Penicillin allergy Erythromycin** is the alternative drug of choice for bullous or nonbullous impetigo in patients allergic to penicillin.

III. INFESTATIONS

A. Scabies

1. **Etiology** Scabies is caused by infestation with the mite *Sarcoptes scabiei*. Transmission is usually by direct personal contact; however, fomes (bedclothes, towels) transmission is possible.

2. **Evaluation** With a needle point or the tip of a No. 11 surgical blade, attempt to extract a mite from the advancing end of a burrow. Scrape the top from a burrow tract and examine under low power for mites, larvae, or ova. Organisms or ova are often difficult to demonstrate. Thus the clinical pattern (symptoms, distribution of eruption, and morphology of individual lesions) must be the basis for diagnosis.

3. Diagnosis

a. **Subjective findings**   Crowded and unhygienic living conditions ar frequently, but not necessarily, associated with infestation. Chara teristically, pruritus intensifies soon after retiring to bed, and remi 1–2 hr thereafter.

b. **Objective findings**   The most frequent areas of involvement are th interdigital webs of the fingers, hypothenar eminences, volar surfa of the wrists, extensor elbows, periareolar skin, anterior axillar folds, intergluteal fold, penis, scrotum, and, in infants, the soles. Th lesions are

(1) Seen most often on the sides of the fingers are 1–2 cm, curving S-shaped or subcutaneous burrows, which may terminate in a sma vesicle.

(2) Firm, indurated, erythematous, 0.5-cm, excoriated nodules occu most frequently on the interdigital webs, volar surface of th wrists, and penis and scrotum.

(3) On the lower abdomen, buttocks, and thighs are numerous urt carial papules 0.2–0.5 cm in diameter, many of which are cappe by a pinpoint crusted excoriation.

(4) Secondary bacterial infection (impetigo) often dominates the clini cal picture and obscures the individual lesions.

4. Treatment is as follows:

a. Bathe and scrub thoroughly with soap and water.

b. Apply a **scabicide cream or lotion** to all skin from the neck down; 12 h later, without rebathing, repeat the application. Effective scabicide include 1% gamma benzene hexachloride (Kwell) and 10% crotamito (Eurax).

c. Wash bedclothes, towels, and underwear in a detergent and ho water.

d. It is wise to treat contacts prophylactically.

e. An oral antipruritic agent such as **hydroxyzine (Atarax)** or **chlo pheniramine (Chlor-Trimeton)** will help reduce symptoms (Table 22-3

B. Pediculosis

1. Etiology   *Pediculus humanus*, the body louse, and *Phthirus pubis*, th pubic "crab" louse. *P. humanus* occurs in two distinct populations. *P humanus capitis* is transmitted via hats, combs, hairbrushes, and th backs of theater seats. *P. humanus corporus* transmission is via share clothing and bedding. Although *P. pubis* transmission is most commonl through sexual contact, infestation is possible via clothing, bedding, an towels.

2. Diagnosis

a. **Subjective findings**

(1) Infestation with *P. humanus* is associated with intractabl **pruritus** on the scalp or trunk. Secondary infection, especially o the scalp, frequently follows the onset of pruritus. Persons a fected by *P. humanus* often live in a crowded, unhygienic env ronment, but members of all social groups may be infected.

(2) *P. pubis* in particular is common in adolescents and young adult

Chemical Name	Trade Name	Preparations Available	Dosage
Brompheniramine	Dimetane	Tablet, 4 mg Extentab, 8 mg, 12 mg Elixir, 2 mg/5 ml Parenteral, 10 mg/ml, 100 mg/ml	2–4 mg q4–6h 0.5 mg/kg daily maximum
Chlorpheniramine maleate	Chlor-Trimeton	Tablet, 4 mg Repetab, 8 mg, 12 mg Syrup, 2 mg/5 ml Parenteral, 10 mg/ml	2–4 mg q4–6h 0.5 mg/kg daily maximum
Cyproheptadine	Periactin	Tablet, 4 mg Syrup 2 mg/5 ml	2–4 mg q4–6h 0.5 mg/kg daily maximum
Diphenhydramine		Capsule, 25 mg, 50 mg Elixir, 12.5 mg/5 ml Parenteral, 10 mg/ml	25–50 mg q4–6h 5 mg/kg daily maximum
Tripelennamine	Pyribenzamine	Tablet, 25 mg, 50 mg Lontab, 50 mg, 100 mg Elixir, 30 mg/4 ml	25–50 mg q4–6h 5 mg/kg daily maximum
Hydroxyzine hydrochloride pamoate	Atarax Vistaril	Tablet, 10 mg, 25 mg, 50 mg, 100 mg Syrup, 10 mg/5 ml Capsule, 25 mg, 50 mg, 100 mg Suspension, 25 mg/5 ml	25–50 mg q4–6h 5 mg/kg daily maximum

and is associated with the more commonly recognized venere[al] diseases. Every patient with *P. pubis* should be questioned abo[ut] sexual contacts, urethritis, vaginitis, and genital ulcers.

b. Objective findings

(1) Pediculosis capitis   Oval egg capsules ("nits") appear along th[e] hair shafts as highlights that are fixed in position and do n[ot] brush away easily. Adult lice are seen on the scalp. Purulence an[d] matting of the hair often occurs over the occiput and nape of th[e] neck. Occipital and posterior cervical adenitis may be present.

(2) Pediculosis corporis   Excoriated papules, parallel linear excoria[-]tions, and, in chronic cases, scaling, lichenification, and hyperpig[-]mentation are seen across the shoulders, in the interscapula[r] area, and around the waist. The initial lesion is a pinpoint re[d] macule. After 7–10 days, the time required for sensitization to th[e] louse salivary antigens, the bites become urticarial and papula[r.] Lice and ova are found in the seams of clothing.

(3) Pediculosis pubis   Pruritus dominates the clinical picture. Th[e] yellow, translucent 1–3 mm adult louse is seen on close examina[-]tion of the skin. Oval egg capsules (nits) are firmly attached to ha[ir] shafts 1–2 cm above the skin surface. Reddish-brown, particula[te] accumulations of excreted heme pigment deposited on the ski[n] about hair shafts are the most apparent clinical sign. Discret[e] round, bluish-gray macules (maculae caerulae), measuring 0.5–1 cm in diameter, are occasionally seen on the lower abdomen an[d] inguinal areas.

3. Therapy

a. Pediculosis capitis

(1) If secondary bacterial infection is prominent, prescribe an appr[o]priate **antibiotic** directed against gram-positive organisms (se[e] Table 15-2).

(2) Instruct the patient to shampoo the hair and scrub the scal[p] thoroughly with 1% gamma benzene hexachloride (Kwell) sham[-]poo. Repeat in 24 hr.

(3) Towels, bedclothes, caps, and head scarfs should be washed in d[e]tergent and hot water.

(4) Prophylactic treatment of family members and close contacts i[s] indicated.

(5) Although benzene hexachloride kills adult lice and nits, the dea[d] organisms do not fall off the hairs spontaneously. Application of [a] 1:1 solution of white vinegar and water followed by a shower wi[ll] help dissolve the nits cemented to the hairs and wash off the[ir] remains.

b. Pediculosis corporis

(1) The patient should bathe and scrub thoroughly with soap an[d] water.

(2) Clothing and bedding should be decontaminated by boiling or b[y] pressing with a hot iron, especially along seams.

c. Pediculosis pubis

(1) The patient should bathe and scrub thoroughly with soap an[d] water.

(2) A **pediculicidal cream or lotion** should be applied to all skin from the neck down; 12 hr later, without rebathing, the application is repeated. Effective pediculicides include 1% gamma benzene hexachloride (Kwell).

(3) If eyebrows and eyelashes are involved, 0.25% **physostigmine** (eserine) or $1/16$% **phospholine iodide** should be applied until the infestation is eliminated.

(4) Bedclothes, towels, and underwear should be washed in detergent and hot water.

(5) Treat contacts prophylactically.

IX. PITYRIASIS ROSEA

A. Etiology Pityriasis rosea is a superficial, scaling, self-limited eruption of unknown etiology.

B. Evaluation Pityriasis rosea may be virtually indistinguishable from the generalized eruption of secondary syphilis. Thus a serologic test for syphilis is sometimes indicated.

C. Diagnosis

1. Subjective findings Pruritus is generally absent or mild. However, a small percentage of patients complain of significant itching.

2. Objective findings

a. In about 50 percent of cases, a single, primary lesion, the "herald patch," precedes the generalized eruption by 7–10 days. The herald patch is round, 2–4 cm in diameter, slightly raised, scaly, and yellowish brown in color. It occurs on the trunk or proximal extremities.

b. The generalized eruption involves the neck, trunk, and proximal extremities and spares the face and distal extremities. The lesions form a "Christmas-tree" pattern on the back, where they are oriented along skin cleavage lines.

c. The individual lesions are round or oval, 0.5–1.0 cm in diameter, yellowish tan in color, and characterized by a central "cigarette-paper" crinkling of the skin, and by a fine, peripheral collarette of scale. In darkly pigmented skin, the lesions may be papular and more inflammatory than in lighter skin.

D. Therapy Generally, no therapy is indicated. If bothersome, the pruritus is treated with oral antihistamines and with intermittent, cool water compresses. Corticosteroid creams are of no use. Exposure to artificial UVL or sun tanning often speeds resolution of the eruption.

X. PSORIASIS is a disease of the skin characterized by thick, scaling, erythematous plaques associated with a marked increase in the rate of epidermal turnover.

A. Etiology Polygenic inheritance is the causative factor, but is subject to environmental influences. Onset or exacerbation of the disease in children may follow pharyngeal streptococcal infection. Local lesions may be provoked by simple abrasions and thermal burns (Koebner's phenomenon).

B. Diagnosis

1. Subjective findings The family history is positive for psoriasis in 50 per cent of childhood cases. Emotional stress may be associated with exacerbation of disease activity. Pruritus may be present.

2. Objective findings

a. The lesions are elevated, moderately erythematous papules and plaques that are covered with thick, silvery, loosely adherent, micaceous scale. Punctate bleeding points occur when the scale is removed (Auspitz's sign). Extensor surfaces (elbows, knees, buttocks) and the scalp are the areas most often involved. Scalp lesions stop abruptly at the hairline.

b. An erosive, polyarticular arthritis of the distal interphalangeal joint is associated with psoriasis in 10–30 percent of patients.

C. Therapy

1. Limited disease with isolated plaques Instructions are as follows:

a. Paint full-strength **Zetar emulsion** on lesions 1 hr before bathing in water containing 2–4 capfuls of the same emulsion.

b. Apply a **fluorinated corticosteroid cream** under plastic occlusion at bedtime overnight (see **A.1**, p. 518).

c. Arrange to have careful, graded **sunlight** or **artificial UVL** exposure.

2. Scalp

a. Shampoos containing salicylic acid, sulfur, and tar (Zetar, Sebutone, Ionil T) are used daily until scaling is controlled.

b. If the scale is thick and adherent, **warm mineral oil** should be applied to the scalp and the head wrapped turban fashion with a warm, wet towel for 3 hr before shampooing.

c. Fluorinated corticosteroid solutions (see Sec. **XIV.A**) may be applied to the scalp after shampooing.

3. Acute, generalized disease The following instructions should be given:

a. Mix a fluorinated corticosteroid cream half and half with Eucerin cream, apply to the affected skin at bedtime, and occlude with plastic wrap overnight (see Sec. **XIV.A.1**).

b. As the disease activity decreases (in 2–3 days), add a daily tar bath (Zetar, Balnetar) to the treatment regimen.

XI. SEBORRHEIC DERMATITIS

A. Etiology Disease activity is chronologically coincident with androgenic stimulation of sebaceous glands. Hence seborrheic dermatitis is seen in infancy while transplacentally acquired maternal androgens are still present and is also seen after the onset of puberty.

B. Infantile seborrhea This begins in the second or third month of life and resolves spontaneously by the fifth or sixth month. Ordinarily, the disease is limited to the scalp (cradle cap), axillae, and diaper area. Occasionally, it extends to the forehead, ears, trunk, and proximal extremities. Rarely, it erupts into a generalized exfoliative erythroderma (Leiner's disease).

1. Subjective findings There is little discomfort or pruritus. Even with widespread dermatitis, an infant will continue to eat and sleep well. Diarrhea may be associated with generalized, erythrodermic disease.

2. **Objective findings**   A thick, yellow, greasy scale (cradle cap) is present on the scalp. Confluent, scaling erythema involves the intertriginous areas (axillae, inguinal and intergluteal folds, umbilicus). Individual lesions on the extremities and trunk are erythematous papules 0.5–1.0 cm in diameter, capped by an easily removed, yellowish-tan, greasy scale.

C. **Adult-type postpubertal seborrhea** is limited to areas of high sebaceous gland concentration.

D. **Therapy**

1. **Scalp**

   a. Shampoos containing sulfur, salicylic acid, and hexachlorophene (Sebulex, Ionil T, Meted, Sebaveen) are used every 2–3 days until scaling is controlled. Subsequently, shampooing once or twice weekly is sufficient.

   b. If the cradle cap is thick and adherent, **warm mineral oil** should be applied and the head wrapped with a cloth wet with water for 3–4 hr before shampooing.

   c. In resistant cases, a **corticosteroid lotion** (see **XIV.A**, p. 518) applied bid is useful.

2. **Intertriginous areas** should be left open and dry. Plastic pants should not be used, and wet diapers should be changed promptly. A fluorinated corticosteroid cream should be applied qid (see **XIV.A**, p. 518). If *Staphylococcus* or *Candida* is present, an appropriate topical antibiotic cream (neomycin, gramicidin, polymyxin) or nystatin cream is added.

3. **Generalized disease**   The patient should bathe twice daily in a colloidal oatmeal bath (Aveeno). Topical corticosteroid and antibiotic nystatin are indicated as in **2**.

XII. SUNBURN, PHOTOSENSITIVITY, AND SUNSCREENS

A. **Etiology**   Overexposure to UVL of wavelengths 290–320 nm.

B. **Evaluation**

1. Inquire about the ingestion of photosensitizing drugs such as the sulfonamides, sulfonylureas (Orinase, Diabinese), thiazide diuretics, phenothiazines, griseofulvin, tetracyclines, and psoralens.

2. Other causes of photosensitivity are nutritional deficiency (kwashiorkor, pellagra), vitiligo, albinism, porphyria, phenylketonuria, systemic lupus erythematosus, dermatomyositis, xeroderma pigmentosum, and Rothmund, Cockayne, and Bloom syndromes.

C. **Diagnosis**

1. **Subjective findings**   The initial transient erythema is relatively asymptomatic; 6–12 hr later, burning and stinging accompany the appearance of the delayed, prolonged erythema. Malaise, chills, and headache are frequent if sunburn is severe.

2. **Objective findings**   The initial erythema limited to sun-exposed areas fades in 1–2 hr. Prolonged erythema and edema appear at 6–12 hr and reach maximum intensity (bulla formation) at 24 hr. Low-grade fever is not unusual. Hypophidrosis, hyperpyrexia, and hypotension may ensue in severe cases.

D. Therapy

1. Treatment of sunburn

    a. Cool baths with colloidal oatmeal (Aveeno) are soothing.

    b. Damp compresses with cool water relieve burning and stinging.

    c. Aspirin in the usual doses provides symptomatic relief.

    d. Severely affected patients, if treated early, respond rapidly to **predni sone**, 1–2 mg/kg PO per day in divided doses for no more than 2 days

2. Prevention of sunburn

    a. Para-aminobenzoic acid (5%) in alcohol (Pabanol, PreSun) provide maximum screening for the sunburn wavelengths of the spectrum (290–320 nm). However, the preparation photo-oxidizes to a water washable, brown pigment, which colors skin and clothing.

    b. Para-aminobenzoic acid esters (Block-Out, PABA-film) do not stain clothing or skin, but are somewhat less effective as a sunscreen. How ever, PABA esters provide adequate protection for the usual lightl pigmented, sun-sensitive skin.

    c. Benzophenone (10%) (Uval, Solbar) provides screening over a broade spectrum (250–360 nm), but does not protect so adequately in th sunburn part of the spectrum.

    d. Markedly sun-sensitive skin (vitiligo, albinism, porphyria) may re quire an opaque screen such as titanium dioxide or zinc oxide in hydrophilic ointment (Reflecta, Covermark).

XIII. WARTS

A. Etiology
Warts are caused by a DNA-containing virus of the papovaviru group. The localized viral infection can be spread to other sites by au toinoculation and to other people by direct contact.

B. Evaluation
The amount of pain and degree of disability experienced from plantar lesion are important in deciding what treatment, if any, should b employed. Genital and perianal lesions may be spread during sexual con tact. Thus sex partners should be treated simultaneously to preven "Ping-Pong" reinfection.

C. Diagnosis

1. Subjective findings
Plantar warts on weight-bearing surfaces may b painful. Perianal and genital condyloma acuminatum (venereal warts may be friable and tender.

2. Objective findings

    a. Common warts are firm, hyperkeratotic papules containing blac specks of hemosiderin pigment in thrombosed capillary loops.

    b. Periungual warts involve the lateral and proximal nail folds but usu ally do not cause nail plate abnormalities. Punctate, black, throm bosed capillary loops are usually apparent.

    c. Plantar warts are hyperkeratotic, dome shaped, or flat lesions, whic may be distinguished from calluses by paring down the lesions an looking for thrombosed capillaries.

    d. A mosaic wart is a superficial, nontender, confluent plaque, whic may involve a large area of the plantar surface.

e. Filiform warts are small fingerlike growths seen primarily on the face and neck.

f. Condylomata acuminata are soft, friable, pink, elongated, and filiform lesions, which may be seen in any intertriginous area, but are most often found under the prepuce, on the vaginal and labial mucosa, in the urethral meatus, and around the anal mucocutaneous junction. They are often hemorrhagic and the site of secondary infection.

D. Therapy

1. Common warts

a. Apply **liquid nitrogen** with a cotton-tipped applicator. Keep the lesion frozen for 20 seconds. After the lesion has completely thawed, reapply liquid nitrogen for another 20 second freeze. In 6–10 hr a hemorrhagic bulla will form, with the wart in the blister roof.

b. Paint the lesion with **cantharidin (Cantharone),** apply a patch of 40% salicylic acid plaster, and occlude with Blenderm plastic tape for 1–2 days. Although no initial pain results, significant distress may occur within 4 hr, *or*

c. Electrocautery followed by curettage of the lesion may be used. This method may leave more noticeable hypopigmentation and scarring than other techniques, *or*

d. In young children who will not tolerate pain induced by the foregoing techniques, the lesions may be painted with 10% lactic acid in flexible collodion or 12.5% salicylic acid plus 12.5% lactic acid in flexible collodion (duofilm).

2. Periungual warts
Cantharidin used as previously described is helpful for periungual lesions. Trichloroacetic or monochloroacetic acid may be substituted for cantharidin. Two or three treatments at 2-week intervals may be required. Liquid nitrogen should be used with caution about the nails, since freezing the nail matrix that lies beneath the proximal fold may result in permanent nail plate dystrophy.

3. Plantar warts

a. Plantar lesions are extraordinarily difficult to eradicate. Recurrence after repeated and painful treatments is frequent. Therefore, unless the patient is suffering significant pain or disability, it is best to use only repeated daily applications of **40% salicylic acid plaster** under ordinary adhesive tape. This treatment reduces the hyperkeratotic mass of the wart and thus relieves weight-bearing tenderness, but it will not permanently destroy the lesion. If more definitive treatment is desired, trichloroacetic acid or the method in **1.b** is recommended. Repeated treatments will probably be required.

b. Liquid nitrogen freezing of the plantar surface often results in a painful, tense, hemorrhagic bulla. Electrodesiccation or surgical excision may leave a tender hyperplastic scar.

4. Mosaic warts
Mosaic lesions are best treated with repeated applications of 40% salicylic acid plaster (see **3.a**). They are too extensive to use the more destructive methods.

5. Filiform warts
Small filiform warts may be treated as in **D.1.**

6. Condyloma acuminatum
The patient should apply 25% **podophyllin** in compound tincture of benzoin to lesions in moist, intertriginous areas. The areas should be powdered with talc to prevent smearing of podophyllin onto surrounding normal skin. **The medication should be**

thoroughly washed off in 4–6 hr; otherwise, a painful primary irrita[nt] dermatitis will follow. The recurrence rate is high, and repeated week[ly] applications may be required. Podophyllin will not induce resolution [of] verrucae on dry, nonintertriginous skin such as the penile shaft.

XIV. TOPICAL CORTICOSTEROIDS, ANTIHISTAMINES, AND DRESSINGS

A. Topical corticosteroids   These are the most effective topical antiinflam[-] matory preparations available for a broad array of dermatologic condition[s.] Commonly used corticosteroids are listed in Table 22-4.

1. Application

a. Topical corticosteroids are applied sparingly but often throughout th[e] day. Their effectiveness is enormously increased by occluding th[e] treated area with polyethylene plastic wrap (Saran Wrap, Hand[i] Wrap). On the extremities, the plastic is wrapped entirely around th[e] limb in sleevelike fashion and fixed in place at either end with tap[e.] Plastic bags (Baggies) are useful on the feet, and disposable, ligh[t] weight plastic gloves (Dispos-A-Glov) are available for use on th[e] hands. The occlusive wrappings are applied at bedtime and remove[d] in the morning.

b. Occlusion is useful in subacute, dry, nonexudative lesions, as seen [in] psoriasis, lichen planus, and neurodermatitis. **Do not occlude** acut[e,] weeping, exudative processes (e.g., poison ivy contact dermatitis).

c. Ointments that are partially occlusive by their greasy nature a[re] used on dry, nonexudative lesions when plastic occlusion is undesir[a-] ble or impractical.

2. Complications   The use of fluorinated topical corticosteroids under o[c-] clusion or in intertriginous areas effectively occluded by skin folds ca[n] result in the development of atrophic striae or vascular dilatation an[d] telangiectasia. For this reason, **1% hydrocortisone** will suffice for mos[t] cases of mild-to-moderate inflammation, and fluorinated agents shoul[d] be reserved for more severe cases and used for short periods, if possibl[e.] **Percutaneous absorption of corticosteroids in sufficient concentration t[o] suppress elaboration of corticotropin can occur.** However, clinicall[y] significant pituitary suppression with deleterious effects on the patien[t] is virtually unheard of, even after long-term, extensive therapy wit[h] occlusion.

Table 22-4   Commonly Used Topical Corticosteroids

Chemical Name	Trade Name
Betamethasone	
valerate	Valisone
dipropionate	Diprosone
Fluocinolone	Synalar, Fluonid
Fluocinonide	Lidex
	Topsyn
Flurandrenolide	Cordran
Halcinonide	Halog
Hydrocortisone	Hytone, Cort-Dome
Triamcinolone	Kenalog, Aristocort
acetonide	

B. Antihistamines Antihistamines should never be used topically, because they are potent contact sensitizers. Commonly used antihistamines are listed in Table 22-3.

1. Administration

a. The oral route is the usual means of administration. IM injection is useful for rapid relief of generalized urticaria.

b. Since sedation is an important facet of the effectiveness of these drugs in pruritic skin disease, the usually suggested dose may have to be increased toward the recommended maximum daily dose in order to achieve the desired therapeutic result.

2. Side effects include dizziness, tinnitus, blurred vision, nervousness, insomnia, tremors, dry mouth, nausea, tingling of the hands, and hypotension.

C. Wet dressings are useful in suppressing pruritus, in drying moist, oozing lesions, and in removing crusts. Towels, washcloths, strips of bed sheets, or gauze rolls (Kerlix) are satisfactory materials for open, nonoccluded wet dressings, which allow evaporation of water and hence cool and soothe inflamed surfaces.

1. Application Strips of cotton material are soaked in the dressing solutions and wrung out to a point just short of dripping wet. The dressing is wrapped about an extremity or laid on the area to be treated. Dressings are removed and remoistened, q10–15 min to prevent drying. This process is continued for 1–2 hr periods 3 or 4 times per day, depending on the degree of pruritus, oozing, or crusting.

2. Precautions Dressings should not be left in place and remoistened simply by pouring additional solution over them. The process of removal and redressing is instrumental in cooling and debriding. Wet dressings should not be wrapped with plastic or rubber sheets to prevent wetting the bedclothes. If wet dressings are occluded, they *raise* the surface temperature rather than lower it. Also, occlusion prevents evaporation and leads to maceration of tissues.

3. Commonly used solutions

a. Saline One level teaspoon of table salt in 1 pint of tap water approximates normal saline in concentration. It is a physiologic preparation for use on mild to moderate inflammation.

b. Aluminum acetate (Burow's solution) Burow's solution 1:20 is prepared by adding 1 Domeboro packet or tablet to 1 pint of tap water. The only advantage over saline is a mild antibacterial effect. Hence the solution is useful in secondarily infected dermatoses.

c. Silver nitrate A 0.5% solution is very effective as a topical bactericidal agent. It is useful on widely denuded areas such as burns, or on chronic, infected ulcers. A significant disadvantage is that it stains cloth, floors, cabinet tops, skin, and fingernails.

23

Ear, Nose, and Throat Disorders

I. GENERAL PRINCIPLES

A. Airway evaluation   See Tables 23-1 to 23-3.

B. Intubation and tracheotomy   See also Chaps. 2, 5, and 20.

   1. Indications   An airway should be established or preserved as soon as the condition endangering it is recognized.

   2. Methods

      a. Oral or nasotracheal intubation is a rapid method of establishing an airway (see **B.2**, p. 106).

      b. Cricothyrotomy is the fastest way to establish an airway in *total obstruction* at the level of the glottis or above. **This procedure is not possible in neonates and young infants.**

      c. Tracheotomy is the preferred method for managing chronic upper airway obstruction, i.e., subglottic stenosis, an infrequent complication of intubation. If tracheotomy is done in a controlled way, preferably over an endotracheal tube or bronchoscope, the hazards and complications are minimized. Tracheotomy should not be avoided because of fears of surgical trauma.

      d. Problems and complications

         (1) A foreign body partially blocking an airway may shift to a position of total obstruction by intubation.

         (2) A foreign body in the esophagus may occlude the trachea below the endotracheal tube.

         (3) Intubation and cricothyrotomy may be hazardous or impossible with laryngeal and tracheal trauma.

         (4) In epiglottitis, intubation may be difficult to accomplish, especially for the inexperienced. Hypoxia and acidosis predispose the patient to cardiac arrhythmias and laryngospasm. **A bronchoscope and tracheotomy set should be immediately at hand when intubation is attempted.**

         (5) Suctioning of the airway tube as often as necessary (even q10min) and the administration of warm humidified air are essential to preserve a patent airway and minimize complications.

         (6) Cuffed endotracheal tubes are hazardous in children, producing stenosis, and are rarely necessary unless positive end-expiratory pressure (PEEP) is required (see also Chaps. 5 and 20). In all other situations a leak can be compensated for by increasing respiratory volume.

Table 23-1 Causes, Symptoms, and Signs of Obstruction

Site of Obstruction	Nasal or Nasopharyngeal	Oral	Supraglottic	Subglottic	Tracheal
Cause					
Neonate	Choanal atresia	Macroglossia, Pierre Robin syndrome	Laryngomalacia, cyst, hemangioma	Vocal cord paralysis, congenital stenosis, atresia, laryngeal web, hemangioma, fibroma	Stenosis, tracheomalacia, vascular compression, hemangioma, lymphangioma (cystic hygroma)
Child	Adenoid hypertrophy, neoplasm	Tonsillar hypertrophy, tumor, infection (Vincent's and Ludwig's angina), abscess	Foreign body, epiglottitis, recurrent papillomatosis; laryngeal cyst, tumor	Foreign body, trauma; laryngotracheobronchitis (croup), stenosis; hemangioma, tumor, vocal cord paralysis	Foreign body, trauma, vascular compression, thyroid or mediastinal tumor, other tumors, cystic fibrosis, recurrent papillomatosis, tracheoesophageal fistulas and malformations
Symptom or sign					
Alteration in voice	Nasal quality, normal pitch and strength	Unaffected, throaty, or full	Muffled, throaty	Hoarse or husky	Normal
Stridor	Sonorous (snoring) and inspiratory	Inspiratory and coarse; increases with sleep	Snoring, inspiratory fluttering	Inspiratory: early; expiratory: later; to and fro: when	Expiratory with wheezing; to and fro with increased

522

	when asleep	costal, increases to affect the entire chest with severe obstruction and while asleep	then severe	tercostal: later; suprasternal and supraclavicular: severe	xiphoid and sternal: severe obstruction
Alteration in jaw position	Open, jaw forward (except in neonates)	Open, jaw forward	Open, jaw forward	Closed (often); nares flare	May be closed; nares flare
Feeding problem	Poor in neonates and infants; increases with degree of obstruction, with choking and aspiration	Difficult, with pooling of saliva, drooling	Difficult to impossible	Normal except in severe obstruction	Normal unless obstruction is severe or extrinsic pressure involving esophagus (foreign body or tumor) is present
Cardiopulmonary problems	Cor pulmonale follows alveolar hypoventilation		Hyperventilation and sudden bradycardia grave signs	As with supraglottic	
Restlessness	During sleep; improves when awake	During sleep; may avoid sleep			
Cough			None	Barking (croupy)—pathognomonic of subglottic problem	Brassy, dry—pathognomonic of tracheal problem

Table 23-2 Bronchoscope Sizes for Various Ages

Age	Internal Diameter (mm)
Premature	3.0
0–6 months	3.5
6 months–3 years	4.0
3 years–12 years	5.0
12 years and over	6.0

Table 23-3 Tracheotomy Tube Sizes for Various Ages

Age	Tracheotomy Tube Size
Premature	000 or 00
0–6 months	0
6–18 months	1
18 months–4 to 5 years	1 or 2
4 to 5–10 years	2 or 3
10 years and over	3 to 5

C. Tonsillectomy and adenoidectomy

  1. Indications

   a. In cor pulmonale secondary to severe chronic upper airway obstruction, tonsillectomy, adenoidectomy, or both may be required, depending on relative anatomic size and relationships of the tonsils and adenoids.

   b. Tonsillectomy alone is indicated for confirmed **peritonsillar abscess** or **tonsillar hypertrophy** sufficient to cause *severe* dysphagia.

   c. Adenoidectomy alone is indicated in **adenoid hypertrophy,** in which the posterior choana is completely obliterated, resulting in dyspnea and *severe* hyponasality.

  2. Possible indications

   a. Tonsillectomy is of **possible** benefit in recurrent tonsillitis (seven episodes in 1 year, five episodes in each of 2 years). Recurrent streptococcal tonsillitis **must be confirmed** by clinical observation **and** positive culture for group A β-hemolytic streptococcus.

   b. Adenoidectomy is of possible benefit in **recurrent rhinitis** and **rhinosinusitis secondary to obstructive adenoids,** with stagnation of secretions within the nasal cavity.

D. Foreign body aspiration See Table 23-1.

  1. Diagnosis Radiopaque foreign bodies are readily seen. **No statement regarding foreign body aspiration should be ignored.** If the history suggests foreign body aspiration even if x-rays are negative, bronchoscopy must be performed to confirm or rule out the diagnosis.

2. Treatment

a. If obstruction is complete, the **Heimlich emergency maneuver** should be attempted, followed by tracheotomy (see Table 23-3) or cricothyrotomy if unsuccessful, since the object is usually at the glottis.

b. If obstruction is not total, O_2 and respiratory support should be provided.

c. The most experienced endoscopist and anesthesiologist available should be consulted for removal of the foreign body.

d. Cautions

(1) Do not turn the patient upside down or slap or shake the patient, since these maneuvers may cause the foreign body to fall into a position of total occlusion or lacerate the esophagus or trachea.

(2) Do not grope blindly in the throat, since this may push the object into the larynx.

(3) Do not use a Foley or Fogarty catheter to remove a foreign body from the throat, esophagus, or trachea, since the object may flip into the larynx or be wedged there, completely obstructing it.

(4) Do not use bronchodilators, chest percussion, or postural drainage, since the foreign body may be dislodged and become wedged at the glottis, causing asphyxiation. Pneumothorax may also result.

II. DISORDERS OF THE EAR

A. Removal of cerumen

1. Dry techniques

a. A No. 00 blunt ear curet is tiny and can be used to clean out cerumen in children of any age. (**Do not** use the sharp curet, which looks similar. Test it first on your own skin.)

b. The ear canal should be cleaned only under direct vision.

c. If the wax is very hard, it may be softened with hydrogen peroxide or mineral oil for 15 min to allow the wax mass to be moved more easily. The dry technique is successful in 95 percent of children.

2. Wet techniques

a. The water should be body temperature (lukewarm to the touch).

b. A metal ear syringe or a Water Pik may be used. If neither is available, a 10-ml syringe with scalp vein needle tubing cut 1–1½ inches from the hub can be effective.

c. The wet technique should not be used if a tympanic membrane (TM) perforation is suspected, since wax may inadvertently be blown into the middle ear.

B. Tympanometry induces pressure changes in the external canal to assess immobility of the tympanic membrane. It is a quantitative adjunct to inspection and pneumotoscopy.

C. Hearing loss is a common problem in children. It is important to detect it early, so that early treatment can be instituted to alleviate speech defects, learning disabilities, and behavioral changes. Hearing tests can be performed by audiologists in children at any age, including the first day of life. Electrocochleography and brainstem-evoked responses to acoustic stimuli are objective methods of evaluating hearing loss in the neonate and the mentally retarded child.

D. Specific entities

1. External otitis (acute, diffuse) (swimmer's ear)

a. Etiology *Pseudomonas aeruginosa* is usually cultured in this infection.

b. Evaluation Examination of the external canal and TM requires removal of all exudate and discharge. If the TM cannot be seen or otitis media ruled out, treatment for both should be instituted.

c. Diagnosis External otitis is characteristically a diffuse inflammation of the ear canal with or without involvement of the TM. There is frequently moist otorrhea.

d. Treatment

(1) Eardrops 3 drops tid for 1–2 weeks containing cortisone and antibiotics effective against *Pseudomonas* and *Staphylococcus* (see Table 15-2). Half-strength vinegar or Burow's solution drops may be used. A proprietary preparation (VōSol) has been used with success.

(2) Swimming is not permitted.

(3) Cleaning of the ear canal as needed, e.g., 1–2 times a week.

(4) Cotton in the ear canal when there is drainage, to prevent dermatitis of the pinna.

(5) Analgesics (aspirin, codeine) (see Chap. 1).

(6) Systemic antibiotics should be given if facial cellulitis, pinna chondritis, or fever occurs (see Chap. 15).

(7) If treatment is unsuccessful in 2 weeks or symptoms increase, neomycin sensitivity (if the drug is used) should be suspected and other medication substituted. Resistant flora or fungi should be ruled out.

2. Foreign bodies

a. Evaluation The nature of the foreign body should be determined. The TM may be perforated.

b. Treatment

(1) Most foreign bodies may be removed by syringing (see **A.2.b**).

(2) Hygroscopic objects such as nuts and vegetable products swell with moisture. They should be removed with a Ring curet.

(3) Smooth, round objects occluding the external canal may be pushed against the TM by instrumentation, causing injury. They should be removed with the aid of an operating microscope.

(4) Living foreign bodies should be killed with 95% alcohol prior to removal with instruments.

(5) If a foreign body is not easily removed in a few moments, or if the patient fails to cooperate, he or she should be referred to an otolaryngologist. Brief general anesthesia may be required for removal.

(6) Treatment of minor trauma to the external canal should be the same as for external otitis (see **D.1,** p. 526).

3. Bullous myringitis

a. Etiology   *Mycoplasma pneumoniae* is the common agent, but influenza viruses are sometimes suspected.

b. Diagnosis   A blister can be seen on the TM, with the adjacent part of the TM usually normal. A middle ear effusion may be present.

c. Treatment

(1) Analgesics   Aspirin, codeine, and Auralgan eardrops may be used.

(2) A heating pad should be applied to the ear.

(3) Resolution or rupture of the bulla should be awaited.

(4) Erythromycin 30–50 mg/kg/day in qid doses may be helpful.

(5) No myringotomy is needed.

4. Otitis media
Eustachian tube dysfunction causes inadequate ventilation of the middle ear, resulting in a negative middle ear pressure. Persistent negative pressure produces a sterile transudate within the middle ear. Concurrent or subsequent contamination of the middle ear with infected nasopharyngeal contents occurs by aspiration and insufflation during crying and nose blowing.

a. Acute suppurative otitis media (ASOM)

(1) Etiology

(a) *Streptococcus* (diplococcus) *pneumoniae, Haemophilus influenzae,* group A *Streptococcus pyogenes; S. aureus, M. pneumoniae, C. diphtheriae,* and enteric gram-negative bacilli (in neonates) are less frequent causes.

(b) Parainfluenza viruses, respiratory syncytial virus, adenovirus, and coxsackievirus.

(c) *H. influenzae* type B is usually isolated from children less than 6 years of age and is frequently associated with invasive disease. Nontypable *H. influenzae* (nonencapsulated) comprise the majority of middle ear isolates, are not associated with invasive infection, and are responsible for a small but significant proportion of infections in older children and adults.

(2) Evaluation

(a) Pneumotoscopy.

(b) Tympanometry.

(c) Tympanocentesis   Middle ear aspiration should be performed on children who are seriously ill, have a poor response to antibiotics, or have a complication of ASOM. It should also be done in newborns.

Diagnostic tympanocentesis should be performed under semisterile conditions with the aid of an operating microscope; an 18-gauge spinal needle is inserted through the anterior inferior segment of the tympanic membrane.

(3) Diagnosis   There is decreased mobility of the TM. Perforation and a pulsatile discharge may be seen in the anterior inferior segment of the membrane.

(4) Treatment

(a) Antibiotics are prescribed for all symptomatic patients.

   i. Amoxicillin, 20–40 mg/kg/day PO for 10 days, *or*

   ii. Penicillin or erythromycin, 30–50 mg/kg/day, plus sulfisoazole, 100–200 mg/kg/day q6h PO, or phenoxymethyl pecillin, 250 mg qid for 10 days in children over 8 years
   age.

(b) Analgesics (aspirin, Tylenol, codeine) may be indicated in old
children.

(c) Antihistamines and decongestants are not indicated in ASO
except to relieve coryza symptoms.

(d) The patient should be reevaluated 2 weeks after starting the
apy to determine whether effusion persists. If complete reso
tion has occurred, the patient is discharged. Periodic monit
ing is required for patients with repeated episodes of ASOM.
effusion persists after 4 weeks, treatment is the same as th
for chronic serious otitis media.

(e) Repeated episodes of ASOM with **clearing** of middle ear eff
sion between attacks may be managed by the use of proph
lactic antibiotics, trimethoprim-sulfamethoxazole or sulfiso
azole, 100 mg/kg/day. If ASOM develops in a patient who is c
antibiotic prophylactic therapy, myringotomy and inserti
of a ventilation tube are indicated to restore normal midd
ear function.

(f) If the TM is perforated and drainage is occurring, the drainag
should be suctioned and aspirate for culture procured throug
the hole in the TM. Treatment is guided by the results of th
culture. If perforation persists over 3 months, the patie
should be referred to an otologist.

b. Acute and chronic serous otitis media

(1) Etiology

(a) Persistent negative intratympanic pressure results in a steri
transudate within the middle ear. A low-grade inflammato
reaction leads to an exudative "glue" secretion. Bacteria a
present in 50 percent of "glue" effusions; their exact role
unclear.

(2) Evaluation

(a) Pneumotoscopy is essential.

   i. The TM is classically thickened with a gray or amber flu
   in the middle ear. Sometimes, a fluid meniscus, air bubble
   or bluish fluid may appear in the middle ear.

   ii. The mobility of the TM is always impaired.

   iii. Protracted eustachian tube dysfunction leads to the d
   velopment of a cholesteatoma if it is not reversed by r
   storing normal middle ear ventilation.

(b) Tympanometry can be performed when the findings are equi
ocal.

(c) Audiometry may be performed on children over 2 years of ag

(d) Anatomic defects may be present.

(3) Diagnosis   An immobile TM with fluid can be seen on pneumotoscopy.

(4) Treatment

   (a) Attempts can be made to improve ventilation of the middle ear by the Valsalva maneuver, blowing up a balloon, etc.

   (b) The efficacy of decongestants, antihistamines, and adenoidectomy has not been proved.

   (c) An effusion present for 8 weeks should be removed by myringotomy, especially if it is associated with hearing deficit greater than 20 decibels.

   (d) Myringotomy and insertion of ventilation tubes is required if the middle ear is atelectatic, shows retraction pockets, or if effusion is thick with hypertrophic middle ear mucosa.

c. Chronic suppurative otitis media with perforation or cholesteatoma is a sequela of acute suppurative infection and should be referred to an otolaryngologist for evaluation and management.

5. Acute mastoiditis

a. Etiology   Primary, β-hemolytic streptococci, pneumococci, and *H. influenzae*. Less frequently, *S. aureus*.

b. Evaluation and diagnosis

   (1) Medical mastoiditis is an infection of the mastoid bone that accompanies almost all cases of acute otitis media and can be treated medically. Roentgenograms are not needed.

   (2) Surgical mastoiditis   Severe and persistent otalgia is present, associated with swelling and tenderness over the mastoid region. The auricle is displaced anteriorly; inferiorly, there is swelling of the posterosuperior canal wall. This condition may present as an abscess in the neck (Bezold's abscess). Roentgenograms show destruction of the bony walls of the mastoid air cells.

   (3) Masked mastoiditis is an acute mastoiditis that has been rendered "quiet" by antibiotics. However, the infection continues unsuspected and destroys the air-cell bony walls. A mild chronic headache may occur. Progression to intracranial complications may occur without warning.

c. Therapy

   (1) Medical mastoiditis   Treatment is similar to that for acute otitis media [see **4.a.(4).(a)**].

   (2) Surgical mastoiditis

      (a) Antibiotics   Ampicillin, 200 mg/kg/day. If *S. aureus* is suspected, an antistaphylococcal antibiotic should be added until culture results are available.

      (b) Therapy is continued for 3 weeks.

      (c) Consult an otolaryngologist regarding myringotomy, incision and drainage of the abscess, and simple mastoidectomy.

   (3) Masked mastoiditis

      (a) IV antibiotics.

      (b) Myringotomy if effusion is present.

(c) If there is no improvement after 24 hr, a cortical mastoide
tomy should be performed.

6. Acute labyrinthitis

a. Etiology

(1) Viral labyrinthitis, in most instances, follows upper respiratory tra
infection.

(2) Suppurative labyrinthitis is caused by bacterial invasion of tl
inner ear and may complicate acute or chronic otitis media.

b. Evaluation Vertigo is the predominant complaint and is associate
with nausea and vomiting. Horizontal nystagmus is present with tl
fast component to the affected side. Hearing loss may complicate su
purative labyrinthitis. Caloric testing should **never** be performed
the acute phase.

c. Diagnosis Labyrinthine symptoms are associated with upper resp
ratory tract infection, otitis media, or meningitis.

d. Treatment

(1) Viral labyrinthitis Meclizine, 1 tablet qid.

(2) Suppurative labyrinthitis The patient should be admitted to tl
hospital. IV antibiotics (see Chap. 15).

(3) The diazepam (titrated slowly) dosage should **never** exceed 0.!
mg/kg and should be infused at a rate not to exceed 5 mg/min.

(4) An otologist should be consulted.

III. DISORDERS OF THE NOSE

A. Allergic rhinitis See **II.D,** p. 467.

B. Foreign body

1. Evaluation Look for chronic, unilateral purulent nasal discharge that
unresponsive to antibiotics. X-ray studies may be helpful.

2. Therapy The foreign body should be removed on the first try.
struggling begins, the foreign body may be pushed in more posterior
and nasal bleeding may occur.

a. First, assemble all equipment (bright light, nasal speculum, sucti
apparatus and suction tip, a small forceps [avoid large Kelly clamp
a cotton-tipped applicator, ½% phenylephrine, and 4% lidocaine).
blunt darning hook may be helpful.

b. Avoid traumatizing the mucosa; once it bleeds, removal of the forei
body is difficult.

c. Place 4% lidocaine drops in the nose for topical anesthesia. A spr
atomizer is helpful.

d. Constrict the vessels of the mucosa with phenylephrine drops
spray. Wait 5 min.

e. Suction nasal discharge if present.

f. Remove the foreign body with forceps. A blunt darning hook can
used to pass behind the foreign body and pull it forward.

g. Refer the patient to an otolaryngologist if he or she is very resista
if bleeding is a problem, or if the foreign body is difficult to remov

C. Epistaxis

1. Etiology

a. Epistaxis is usually the result of trauma, especially nose picking, or rhinitis, either viral or allergic.

b. Excessive drying or nasal mucous secondary to winter indoor heating, may produce bleeding, as may aberrant nasal air flow with nasal septal deformity.

c. Epistaxis may be due to bleeding diatheses or to hypertension.

2. Evaluation

a. The most common site for bleeding is on the anterior nasal septum. **Look there first.**

b. Bleeding from points not seen is likely of posterior origin.

c. If bleeding is prolonged, signs of hypovolemic shock should be sought and the hematocrit obtained.

3. Therapy

a. Anterior bleeding

(1) Most anterior bleeding can be stopped by pinching the nose gently but firmly with the thumb and finger placed firmly against the cheek bones on either side. Pressure is held securely without release for 10 min. If bleeding has not stopped, other measures are necessary.

(2) Constriction of the nasal vessels and topical anesthesia is achieved with spray or drops of

   (a) 4% cocaine (maximum dose in 1 hr 2.5 mg/kg or 1 ml of spray/15 kg). No epinephrine is necessary with cocaine and may be hazardous.

   (b) 4% lidocaine and ½% phenylephrine (drops or spray).

(3) Suction away blood.

(4) Wait 2–5 min.

(5) Touch a silver nitrate stick to the bleeding vessel and hold 15 sec. Repeat if necessary.

(6) If bleeding is easily controlled, no pack is necessary. If bleeding is not easily controlled, a pack of cotton or ¼ in. packing gauze covered liberally with bacitracin or neomycin ointment may be placed inside the nose against the vessel. The pack should be large, with both ends placed anteriorly to prevent the pack from falling backward and being aspirated. The pack is removed within 48 hr.

(7) Epistaxis in leukemic or renal failure patients may be controlled with oxidized cellulose or gelatin foam packs or with microfibrillar collagen (Avitene) that need not be removed. Regular packs should be avoided unless absolutely necessary, since removal reinitiates the epistaxis.

b. Posterior bleeding, if untreated, can be fatal.

(1) The patient must be hospitalized and observed closely. Transfusion may be necessary.

(2) Hematocrit, prothrombin time, and partial thromboplastin time should be obtained. Vital signs should be checked frequently.

(3) The child must be completely restrained, including the arms.

(4) Hemostasis by gauze pack method   A posterior pack created fr[o]m a rolled-up, tied, $3'' \times 3''$ gauze sponge or half a vaginal tampon c[an] be used. Three tails are made using 0 silk suture sewn through t[he] pack, two tails "up," one "down," each 50 cm in length.

(a) Procedure   Two No. 14F catheters are passed, one per nostr[il] until they are seen in the oral pharynx, where they are grasp[ed] with a clamp, pulled out through the mouth, and each is ti[ed] securely to one of the up tails. Both catheters are withdra[wn] again, pulling the tails out of each nostril and the pack into t[he] nasopharynx. This is verified by palpation through the s[oft] palate. The up tails are tied around a gauze pad placed agai[nst] the columella (the ties should not touch the skin). The down t[ail] exits through the mouth and is taped to the cheek. Both nas[al] passages are packed in layers with bacitracin-covered packi[ng] gauze.

(b) The hematocrit is followed serially until the pack is remove[d.]

(c) Low-flow humidified O_2 is given by mask. The head of the bed [is] elevated.

(d) Mild sedation and analgesia may be necessary for the patien[t's] comfort and to decrease movement and bleeding. **Do not gi[ve] aspirin.**

(e) If epistaxis continues or recurs, an otolaryngologist should [be] consulted on an urgent basis. Surgery may be necessary [to] prevent exsanguination.

(f) The posterior pack is gently removed in 5 days: The balloon [is] deflated and withdrawn or the up tails cut and the posteri[or] pack withdrawn through the mouth with the down tail. If [no] bleeding is seen, the anterior packs are gently removed. A fe[w] drops of blood may be seen, but bleeding should cease in [a] moment.

IV. DISORDERS OF THE PARANASAL SINUSES

A. Acute sinusitis

1. Etiology   Acute sinusitis is usually secondary to pneumococcal, stre[p]tococcal, or staphylococcal infection, or in children under 5 years of a[ge] to *H. influenzae.*

2. Evaluation   A CBC and a culture and smear of the nasal discharge, [as] well as blood cultures, may be helpful. In experienced hands, transill[u]mination may be useful. X-rays will identify the site and severity of t[he] infection.

a. Maxillary sinusitis presents with cheek pain, upper teeth pain, fev[er] and swelling of the lower eyelid.

b. Ethmoid sinusitis presents with central facial and orbital pain, te[n]derness at the medial canthi, and upper-lid or periorbital edema wi[th] fever.

c. Sphenoid sinusitis presents with central vertex or retro-orbital hea[d]ache with fever. Purulent material may drain into the throat.

d. Frontal sinusitis presents with frontal headache, fever, nasal d[is] charge, and increased pain on bending the head forward. Upper-lid edema may be seen.

3. Diagnosis A purulent nasal discharge with pain and fever usually indicates sinusitis. X-ray findings confirm the diagnosis. Multiple-sinus involvement is common.

4. Treatment

   a. Antibiotics are given for 10 days according to culture results (see Table 15-2). Begin with ampicillin, 100 mg/kg/day in 4 divided doses, until the culture results are available. If *S. aureus* is suspected, either clinically or by Gram stain, add dicloxacillin, 50 mg/kg/day in 4 divided doses.

   b. Nasal decongestion is achieved with phenylephrine drops or spray q4h, or 0.05% oxymetazoline (Afrin) spray q8h. Pseudoephedrine elixir may be added. This is continued until the sinusitis is resolved.

   c. Local heat is applied.

   d. Analgesics are given as needed.

5. Complications include osteomyelitis; intraorbital, retro-orbital, and intracranial problems; sepsis; and endocarditis.

   a. Frontal sinusitis complications include **intracranial spread** (meningitis, extradural and subdural abscess, or frontal lobe abscess), periostitis, and osteomyelitis.

   b. Ethmoid and sphenoid sinusitis complications include orbital cellulitis, orbital abscess **(a medical emergency),** cavernous sinus thrombosis and intracranial spread including meningitis, extra and subdural abscess, and frontal lobe abscess.

   c. Maxillary sinusitis complications include facial cellulitis (including the periorbital region), osteomyelitis, oral-antral fistula, cavernous sinus thrombosis, intracranial spread, and loss of teeth.

B. Chronic sinusitis

1. Etiology Anaerobic bacteria are the major pathogens. Allergic rhinosinusitis may be an etiologic factor, as may immunodeficiency syndromes, cystic fibrosis, and diabetes.

2. Evaluation Aspiration is not a routine procedure. Transillumination can be misleading because of the different types of fluid present.

3. Diagnosis Sinus x-ray series show opacification, mucosal thickening, or air fluid levels. The sinuses are not tender.

4. Treatment

   a. Antibiotics Penicillin VK, 50 mg/kg/24 hr in 4 divided doses for 10 days. Almost all bacteria involved in chronic sinusitis are sensitive to penicillin.

   b. Decongestants Pseudoephedrine and/or phenylephrine or 0.05% oxymetazoline hydrochloride (Afrin) nasal spray or drops (see **A.4.b**).

   c. Repeat sinus x-rays in 3 weeks.

   d. Refer the patient to an otolaryngologist for sinus irrigation or surgery if sinusitis persists.

5. Complications See **A.5.**

V. DISORDERS OF THE ORAL CAVITY

A. Herpetic stomatitis (herpetic gingivostomatitis)

1. **Etiology**   Herpes simplex virus is the causative organism.

2. **Evaluation and diagnosis**   Frequently, an upper respiratory infecti◌
   precedes the onset. The painful vesicular lesions of the mucous me◌
   brane are initially yellow and irregular, developing a red base and ri◌
   around each lesion. A smear and Tzanck preparation from the base ◌
   the lesion will reveal characteristic giant cells. Similar lesions (fev◌
   blisters) may recur at the vermilion border of the lips after a late◌
   period, especially after exposure to ultraviolet radiation or sunlight.

3. **Therapy**

   a. Adequate hydration can be a problem. Occasionally, IV fluids may ◌
      necessary.

   b. Cēpacol or 5% phenol Chloraseptic mouthwashes q2h prn are reco◌
      mended.

   c. Glycerine or Gly-Oxide applications to the lips are helpful.

   d. **To relieve pain** (particularly before meals), the following may be use◌

      (1) Viscous lidocaine mouthwash, bid–tid

      (2) Diclonine HCl (Diclone) bid–tid

      (3) Diphenhydramine (Benadryl) elixir and kaolin and pectin (Ka◌
          pectate) in a 50:50 mixture

B. Aphthous stomatitis (canker sores)

1. **Etiology** is unknown. Reiter's and Behçet's diseases must be excluded◌

2. **Evaluation**   A history of recurrent episodes of multiple, painful oral ◌
   sions only over many months, frequently coinciding with physical a◌
   emotional stress.

3. **Diagnosis**   The recurrent painful oral lesions are small, oval, and lig◌
   yellow, with a red margin covered by a fibrinous exudate.

4. **Therapy**

   a. 5% phenol solution (Chloraseptic) or Cēpacol mouthwash q2h prn ◌
      helpful.

   b. Pain relief   See **A.3.c** above.

   c. Each lesion should be cauterized with a silver nitrate stick applied f◌
      15 sec. Topical anesthesia with 4% cocaine, 4% lidocaine, or 4% te◌
      racaine (Pontocaine) solutions on cotton-tipped applicators or cott◌
      is mandatory before cauterization. The relief is dramatic, but lesio◌
      must be recauterized every 2–4 weeks.

C. Acute necrotizing gingivitis (Vincent's infection, trench mouth)

1. **Etiology**   Symbiotic infection with fusiform bacilli and *Borrelia vince◌
   tii*, an oral spirochete, causes the disorder.

2. **Evaluation and diagnosis**   Gingival mucosa and interdental papillae a◌
   painful, tender, hyperemic, ulcerated and friable. A fetid odor is prese◌
   Cultures may confirm the diagnosis.

3. **Treatment**

   a. **Antibiotics**   Penicillin V PO, 50 mg/kg/24 hr in 4 divided doses, is giv◌
      for 10 days.

    b. Local oxygenating agents   3% hydrogen peroxide should be used as a mouthwash q2h.

    c. Local dental care   The teeth should be thoroughly brushed and dental floss used. Dental consultation should be sought for specific problems.

D. Oral candidiasis (thrush)

    1. Etiology   *Candida albicans* is the infecting organism.

    2. Evaluation and diagnosis   Oral candidiasis in a child over 1 year of age, particularly if recurrent, raises the possibility of immunodeficiency. Whitish, curdlike patches and plaques are scattered over all the mucosal surfaces. When these are removed, the underlying mucosa is hyperemic but does not bleed. Culture or microscopic examination confirms the diagnosis.

    3. Treatment

        a. Nystatin (Mycostatin) mouthwash, 100,000 U/ml for 5 days; 1–5 ml is held in the mouth for 5 min if possible, then swallowed. Older children can suck on nystatin tablets or vaginal inserts, which are swallowed when dissolved.

        b. Normal saline or half-strength vinegar mouthwashes q2h are recommended.

E. Tonsillar infections   See Chap. 15.

F. Ludwig's angina is an emergency.

    1. Etiology   Anaerobic bacteria, *Fusobacterium* and *Borrelia vincentii; S. aureus* and gram-negative rods are rarely causative.

    2. Evaluation and diagnosis   A history of recent dental infection, dental work, or oral trauma is usual. There is intense pain, edema, and tenderness in the base of the tongue, floor of the mouth, and in the submental space; these areas feel woody hard to palpation. The tongue is pushed posteriorly, endangering the airway. Drooling and dysphagia are marked. Edema will spread to the larynx, and death can result within 6–10 hr.

    3. Treatment

        a. Establish an airway (oral or nasotracheal intubation or tracheotomy) immediately (see Sec. **I.B**).

        b. Antibiotics   Penicillin, given IV in high doses, is begun immediately.

        c. Consult an otolaryngologist promptly concerning surgical drainage.

        d. Analgesics are given only after an airway is established.

G. Suppurative sialadenitis

    1. Etiology   Bacterial infection, predominantly staphylococcal, causes the disorder.

    2. Evaluation and diagnosis

        a. Marked swelling, tenderness, and eventually fluctuance of a major salivary gland is noted, especially in a debilitated, dehydrated patient. Purulent discharge may be noted at the salivary duct.

        b. The parotid gland is more frequently affected.

        c. Fever is present, and the WBC count is elevated.

        d. Sialography may be helpful but is hazardous.

3. Treatment

a. IV antibiotics Give oxacillin, 100–200 mg/kg/24 hr in 4 divided dose

b. Surgical drainage is mandatory. Consult an otolaryngologist imme ately.

c. Aspiration is contraindicated, since it may endanger the facial nerv

d. Maintain adequate hydration by IV fluid administration.

e. Warm moist heat should be applied for 10 min q2h.

f. Sialagogues Hard candies (diabetic) and lemon wedges should given hourly. Expectorants, saturated solution of potassium chlori (SSKI), or glycerol guaiacolate may be helpful.

g. Elevate the head of the bed 40 degrees.

VI. DISORDERS OF THE PHARYNX   See also Chap. 15.

A. Peritonsillar abscess is a medical emergency.

1. Etiology Gram-positive bacteria, especially staphylococci, are the i fecting organisms.

2. Evaluation and diagnosis

a. These abscesses usually occur in children over age 2. If spontaneo rupture occurs, aspiration pneumonia or death may follow.

b. A soft-palate bulge is usually seen, with deviation of the uvula to t opposite side.

c. The tonsil is inflamed and pushed medially.

d. Drooling of saliva occurs due to severe sore throat. There is mark trismus.

e. A "hot-potato" voice is characteristic (sounds as though the patie has a hot potato in his or her mouth).

f. There are signs and symptoms of infection (increased WBC cou pain, fever).

3. Therapy

a. Hospitalization is required in all cases.

b. IV antibiotics Give oxacillin, 100–200 mg/kg/day in 4 divided doses, select an antibiotic on the basis of the culture results (Table 15-2).

c. Give nothing by mouth.

d. Give IV fluids.

e. Administer a cool mist via face mask or croupette.

f. Give meperidine IM, 1 mg/kg q3–4h prn.

g. Elevate the head of the bed 30 degrees.

h. Incision and drainage or large-bore needle aspiration Incision a drainage through the soft palate **above** the tonsil (not lateral to t tonsil, since the internal carotid artery may be punctured) is prefer ble to aspiration.

i. Surgery Because of the frequency of recurrence, tonsillectomy m be indicated. An otolaryngologist should be consulted.

B. Diphtheria pharyngitis

   1. Etiology   *C. diphtheriae* is the causative agent.

   2. Evaluation and diagnosis

      a. Intense inflammation of the tonsils and pharynx is seen. The structures may be covered by a thick, dirty-gray pseudomembrane that is densely and tenaciously adherent to underlying structures. Its removal yields brisk bleeding.

      b. The membrane can occlude the airway.

      c. Involvement of the larynx must be ruled out.

      d. Microscopic examination of smears and cultures is necessary for diagnosis.

   3. Treatment

      a. Assure an airway. If the larynx is involved, tracheotomy is necessary to minimize laryngeal stenosis.

      b. IV antibiotics   Give penicillin G (see Table 15-2).

      c. Antitoxin must be given early to prevent tissue fixation by the toxin (see Table 15-4).

C. Retropharyngeal abscess is a suppurative adenitis of the nodes of Henle in the buccopharyngeal and prevertebral fascia. These nodes atrophy after age 5.

   1. Etiology   Gram-positive cocci and anaerobes are the causative organisms. Retropharyngeal abscess often follows otitis media.

   2. Evaluation and diagnosis

      a. The abscess is almost always unilateral and does not spread across the midline. It occurs in children under the age of 5.

      b. A bulge of the posterior lateral pharyngeal wall may be seen.

      c. The head and neck may be extended or the neck flexed with prevertebral muscle spasm; the head is extended for a better airway.

      d. Drooling and swallowing difficulties are present.

      e. Gentle palpation may confirm the diagnosis, but is so hazardous (posing the risk of rupture, aspiration, and death) that doing it is contraindicated.

      f. Anteroposterior and lateral soft tissue neck x-rays will support the diagnosis, especially if gas is seen in the retropharyngeal area. Fluoroscopy can be helpful.

   3. Therapy

      a. IV antibiotics   Oxacillin, 100–200 mg/kg/24 hr in 6 divided doses and ampicillin, 200 gm/24 hr in divided doses pending culture results.

      b. Surgical drainage under general anesthesia

         (1) The anesthesiologist must be careful not to rupture the abscess during intubation.

         (2) The neck is hyperextended and the neck and head are held below the level of the chest to prevent drainage of pus into the larynx and the trachea.

24

Eye Disorders

I. STRABISMUS AND AMBLYOPIA The term *strabismus* refers to any abnormal deviation of the eyes from the parallel position. The eyes may be turned in (esotropia) or out (exotropia), or one eye may be higher than the other (hypertropia). *Amblyopia*, a loss of vision without evident organic defect in the visual system, will develop in over one-third of patients with strabismus. In strabismus, amblyopia occurs in the deviating eye when one eye is preferred. Amblyopia may also occur in an eye that has a worse refractive error than its fellow, as well as in visual deprivation early in infancy, as in congenital cataracts or corneal opacities.

A. Evaluation

1. Strabismus can be detected in infancy by observing the corneal light reflex when the patient fixes on a pocket flashlight. The reflexes should be approximately centered in each pupil.

2. Depending on cooperation, the **cover-uncover test** can be used in children as young as 1 year. If, when one eye is covered, the other must move to fix on a light, the patient has strabismus. This and the corneal light reflex test will reveal many cases of strabismus not obvious to gross inspection.

3. The most important single test in patients with strabismus is *visual acuity*. Amblyopia is *not* related to the amplitude of the deviation, so that a very small, inapparent strabismus may lead to profound loss of vision.

B. Therapy

1. Strabismus

a. A hyperopic (farsighted) person must accommodate to achieve clear vision, even at a distance. The patient's eyes may cross (esotropia) because of this accommodative effort, and they may be straightened with glasses that correct the hyperopia.

b. Surgery may be required to straighten the patient's eyes in nonaccommodative esotropia or in exotropia.

c. In the vast majority of patients with strabismus, straightening the eyes will be primarily of cosmetic significance, although many will achieve some partial binocularity. In a few patients, usually those whose eyes began to deviate later in childhood, normal binocular vision can be restored. In many patients with nonaccommodative congenital esotropia, surgery can restore partial binocular cooperation if the eyes are straightened before the age of 2.

d. The early school years are a difficult psychological period for the child with obvious strabismus. The eyes should be straightened by the time the child starts school.

2. Amblyopia

a. The most effective treatment of amblyopia is total occlusion of t preferred eye with an Elastoplast patch. The earlier this treatment begun, the easier and more effective it is. A young infant may learn use two eyes equally well with only a few days of occlusion of tl preferred eye.

b. The usual period of patching in a 3-year-old is several weeks, a previously untreated amblyopia in a 4- or 5-year-old child typica requires several months of patching.

c. Beyond the age of 6, many patients will not respond to any form treatment for amblyopia. However, some older children may st achieve near-normal vision in the amblyopic eye with prolonged (clusion of the preferred eye.

d. Amblyopic patients should be followed into adolescence to detect a treat any recurrence of amblyopia in the successfully treated eye.

e. Parents should never be reassured that strabismus will resolve spo taneously. Although the angle of the deviation may become less ov the years, so that the patient's eyes appear straight, he or she m still be left with a profoundly amblyopic eye.

II. INFLAMMATION   Inflammation may be infectious (bacterial, viral, or fung or secondary to systemic inflammatory disease.

A. Eyelids

1. Hordeolum (stye)

a. Etiology *Staphylococcus aureus.*

b. Evaluation and diagnosis A painful swelling that points at the eyel margin and involves the sebaceous glands of the eyelash follicle.

c. Therapy Frequent hot soaks. Antibiotics are generally not indicate and incision and drainage are rarely required.

2. Chalazion

a. Etiology Foreign body granulomatous reaction to retained meib mian gland secretion.

b. Evaluation and diagnosis A mass anywhere in the tarsus of tl eyelid.

c. Therapy If the lesion is small, it may involute with hot soaks; if it large, it will usually require incision and curettage. In an older chi this can be performed under local anesthesia, but general anesthes is required in younger children.

3. Marginal blepharitis

a. Etiology Seborrhea, *S. aureus.*

b. Evaluation and diagnosis Accumulation of yellowish scales on tl eyelashes associated with erythema and thickening of the lid ma gins. Seborrhea is sometimes present elsewhere.

c. Therapy This condition can be temporarily relieved by application hot soaks to the eyelids to soften the crusts, so that they can l removed with a soft cotton swab, and application of sodium su facetamide eye ointment bid–tid. Treatment of seborrhea should be carried out at the same time (see Chap. 22).

It is important to reassure the patient that although this is an annoying, chronic, recurrent condition, it will not damage the eyes.

4. Herpes simplex blepharitis

  a. Evaluation and diagnosis Finding of either a primary or secondary infection, or a viral culture, or both.

  b. Therapy Idoxuridine (IUdR) eye ointment should be applied to the conjunctival sac prophylactically to prevent the occurrence of herpes simplex keratitis (see **E.4**). **Corticosteroids are contraindicated.**

B. Lacrimal drainage system

 1. Congenital dacryostenosis

  a. Etiology Congenital.

  b. Diagnosis The presence of dacryostenosis is confirmed by chronic tearing from the eye, with or without discharge, in the absence of conjunctivitis. A gush of tears, or mucus (white), or both, may be observed through the lacrimal canaliculi on digital pressure over the lacrimal sac, along the side of the nose just medial to the medial canthus of the eye.

  c. Treatment

   (1) If infection is present (see **2**) it should be treated. In any case, the mother should be taught to perform massage several times a day, with firm pressure over the lacrimal sac to empty it of accumulated tears and mucus, which form an ideal culture medium for bacteria. Massage may also help break down the membrane at the lower end of the nasolacrimal duct.

   (2) Congenital dacryostenosis will resolve spontaneously or with massage in the first few weeks or months of life in most infants. If it has not resolved by a few months of age, or certainly by 8 months of age, probing of the involved nasolacrimal duct should be performed by an ophthalmologist. In younger infants this can be done under topical anesthesia. Older infants will require brief general anesthesia.

 2. Dacryocystitis

  a. Etiology Stasis of tears and mucus in the lacrimal sac due to dacryostenosis; pneumococci; staphylococci.

  b. Evaluation and diagnosis Purulent (yellow or green) matter regurgitates from the tear sac. If edema of the canaliculi prevents regurgitation, the sac is enlarged and may point to the skin surface inferomedial to the medial canthus of the eye. Pressure over the inflamed sac will often cause a gush of purulent material through the canaliculi and temporary relief of the swelling and discomfort. The infection is almost always localized to the area of the lacrimal sac.

  c. Therapy

   (1) Every attempt should be made to drain the sac through the normal orifices. Incision and drainage directly over the pointing area should be avoided, since this may result in a permanent lacrimal fistula to the skin. Local heat and systemic antibiotics may be indicated if the infection is severe (see Table 15-2).

    (2) In nasolacrimal obstruction that has not responded to probing resulting in recurrent dacryocystitis and chronic epiphora, dacryocystorhinostomy (surgical anastomosis of the lacrimal sac directly to the nasal mucosa) is indicated.

C. Orbital cellulitis is a serious and potentially life-threatening infection, usually occurring as a direct spread from infection of the paranasal sinuses most commonly the ethmoids. See also Chaps. 15 and 23.

D. Conjunctivitis

  1. Ophthalmia neonatorum

    a. Etiology *Neisseria gonorrhoeae.* Any conjunctivitis beginning within the first three days of life should be considered gonococcal, although staphylococci, streptococci, pneumococci, and fecal organisms may occasionally cause conjunctivitis during this period.

    b. Evaluation The chemical conjunctivitis from the silver nitrate prophylactic drops may occasionally be confused with gonococcal conjunctivitis, but the inflammation is rarely so severe, and the characteristic copious yellow pus of gonococcal conjunctivitis is absent. Serologic test for syphilis should be obtained.

    c. The **diagnosis** can be made by smear of the pus and identification of the gram-negative intracellular diplococci. In addition, culture on Thayer-Martin medium should yield positive identification.

    d. Therapy If untreated, corneal ulceration with permanent loss of vision or loss of the eye may occur. Treatment with systemic penicillin and frequent instillations of topical sulfacetamide drops will relieve the infection and prevent corneal ulceration and scarring (see also Chap. 15).

  2. Inclusion blennorrhea

    a. Etiology *Chlamydia* or so-called large virus.

    b. Evaluation

      (1) In newborns, inclusion blennorrhea starts at 5–15 days of age and is characterized by acute inflammation of the conjunctiva with swelling of the eyelids; 3–4 weeks later there is enlargement of the lymphoid follicles in the conjunctiva of the lower eyelid, with mucopurulent discharge.

      (2) It may also occur in older children, in whom the follicles in the lower palpebral conjunctiva enlarge early. The infection may be contracted by swimming in a contaminated pool.

      (3) The length of the course of inclusion blennorrhea is about months. Permanent loss of vision does not occur.

    c. The **diagnosis** is made by staining scrapings of the lower conjunctiva with Wright's or Giemsa stain and observing the typical paranuclear red- or blue-staining (or both red and blue) inclusions in epithelial cells.

    d. Therapy Treatment with oral sulfonamides and topical sulfacetamide or tetracycline eye ointment qid will bring about resolution within a week.

  3. Acute catarrhal conjunctivitis

    a. Etiology Common pathogens, including *S. aureus*, pneumococci streptococci, *H. influenzae, Haemophilus aegyptius,* and, rarely, meningococci.

b. Evaluation and diagnosis reveal conjunctival injection and a mucopurulent discharge, which may accumulate on the lashes during sleep, causing them to stick together, but is never so thick and crusting as in typical staphylococcal conjunctivitis. **A gram-stained smear and culture of the conjunctival sac should be obtained before beginning therapy in any variety of bacterial conjunctivitis.** (The culture swab should be immediately placed in a tube of broth because the amount of material is very small and rapidly desiccates. If eye cultures are handled in the routine way, the organism will not grow in most cases.)

c. Treatment

(1) In general, sulfacetamide eyedrops or ointment will be effective. Since most of the causative organisms are gram positive, erythromycin is also useful.

(2) Treatment should not be delayed until the results of the culture are known.

(3) Drops or ointment containing neomycin should generally be avoided because of the toxicity of neomycin to the cornea after prolonged usage and the tendency for allergies to develop. **Antibiotic-corticosteroid combinations are especially to be avoided because of the side effects of topical steroids.**

(4) Depending on the severity of the infection, the conjunctivitis will usually show some improvement within 2–3 days and will generally be completely cleared in a week. If there is no improvement, the results of the previously obtained culture will then be available, and more specific treatment can be directed at the offending organisms. The topical treatment should be continued for a full week or at least for 72 hr after the signs and symptoms of conjunctivitis have resolved. Otherwise, the infection is likely to recur.

(5) Actual failure of therapy due to bacterial resistance is unusual. The concentrations of antibiotic or chemotherapeutic agent achieved by topical therapy in the conjunctival sac are several orders of magnitude higher than that achieved by systemic treatment, so that apparently resistant staphylococci, for example, will respond to topical erythromycin or sulfonamides. However, systemic antibiotics should be added in conjunctivitis due to pneumococci, β-hemolytic streptococci, and meningococci.

4. Trachoma

a. Etiology *Chlamydia.*

b. Evaluation Trachoma is a follicular conjunctivitis that involves the upper lid and upper portion of the globe more severely than the lower. If untreated, infiltration and vascularization of the cornea occur. There may be scarring of the eyelids, with trichiasis (inversion of the lashes rubbing against the globe), and severe visual loss may occur.

c. The **diagnosis** is made from the clinical picture and from finding typical cytoplasmic inclusion bodies in epithelial cells from conjunctival scrapings stained by Wright's or Giemsa stain.

d. Therapy Oral sulfonamides are given for at least 10 days and topical tetracycline eye ointment is applied qid until 72 hr after the inflam-

mation has subsided. If photophobia is severe, the pupil may be (
lated with a mydriatic-cycloplegic agent.

E. Corneal inflammation

1. Bacterial corneal ulcers

  a. Etiology   Common gram-positive or gram-negative pathogens.

  b. Evaluation   These lesions are usually associated with infections (
  the lids, lacrimal sac, or conjunctiva.

  c. The **diagnosis** may be attempted from a Gram stain and smear
  direct scraping from the corneal ulcer itself. Cultures of the ulcer ar
  of the conjunctival sac should also be taken.

  d. Therapy   Topical and systemic treatment should be directed to th
  suspected organism.

  **(1) In no case should treatment be deferred until the organism has bee
  positively identified on culture.**

  (2) When the organism cannot be reasonably identified immediatel
  "shotgun" therapy with antibiotics is completely justified.

  (3) Pneumococcal corneal ulcers should be treated with system:
  penicillin in addition to frequent applications of topical erythrom;
  cin or sulfonamide.

  (4) *Pseudomonas* corneal ulcers should be treated with frequent i
  stillations of polymyxin B eyedrops and systemic gentamicin unt
  sensitivities can be obtained. Once the organism has been pos
  tively identified, systemic and topical treatment can be altered
  necessary (see Table 15-2).

2. Interstitial keratitis

  a. Etiology   Usually, congenital syphilis or tuberculosis; noninfectiou
  varieties have been described.

  b. Evaluation and diagnosis   It is usually a late manifestation of co
  genital syphilis occurring in preadolescent and adolescent childre
  The cornea assumes a ground-glass appearance from edema an
  infiltration, and corneal vascularization proceeds rapidly.

  c. Therapy   Luetic interstitial keratitis is treated with systemic pen
  cillin, topical corticosteroids, and mydriatic-cycloplegic drops.

3. Fungal keratitis occurs following trauma.

  a. Etiology   The organisms most commonly involved are *Cephalosp
  rium* and *Fusarium* species.

  b. Evaluation   These lesions may be difficult to distinguish from bact(
  rial ulcers, but they tend to have more raised borders with radiatin
  lines of infiltrate in the corneal stroma, and satellite lesions ofte
  develop around the primary infection.

  c. The **diagnosis** can be made by scrapings stained for fungi and fung
  cultures.

  d. Therapy   Topical treatment with **pimaricin** is most effective. Topic;
  amphotericin B is not very effective and is irritating to the eye. To
  ical potassium iodide drops may have some effect in some cases. Ny
  tatin is effective only in *Candida* infections. The patients are ofte

left with severe scarring and may require corneal transplant. This is a serious condition. Consult an ophthalmologist for proper treatment.

4. Herpetic keratitis is the most important corneal inflammation.

   a. Etiology Herpes simplex virus.

   b. Evaluation and diagnosis The disease is confirmed by the characteristic appearance of a dendritic figure, which stains with fluorescein. It is a branching, jagged linear infiltrate on the surface of the epithelium, which may resemble branching coral. The patient may be uncomfortable and photophobic, but without much evidence of inflammation.

   c. Therapy Whenever epithelial herpes simplex keratitis is present, topical corticosteroid treatment is contraindicated. In most cases the infection can be controlled with topical applications of idoxuridine ointment. If drops are used, they must be put in around the clock. Thus, the use of the ointment is much more convenient.

F. Uveitis may be *anterior*, involving primarily the iris and ciliary body; or *posterior*, involving the choroid.

   1. Anterior uveitis (iritis, iridocyclitis)

   a. Etiology Juvenile rheumatoid arthritis (JRA). Other causes are the Reiter syndrome, Behçet's disease, and sarcoid. The disease may also be idiopathic. Herpes zoster ophthalmicus may also cause a severe iritis. Many patients will have a much more acute and symptomatic onset of iritis than those with JRA. The eye will generally be injected, more immediately around the cornea than elsewhere, and the patient often complains of severe pain and photophobia.

   b. Evaluation and diagnosis

   (1) In **JRA** the inflammation is insidious and the first symptom is usually visual loss. Because of the insidious course and ultimately severe complications of the iritis in JRA, every child with this illness should be examined carefully with the slit lamp every 4 months in the absence of symptoms.

   (2) Sarcoid may cause a granulomatous iritis. The diagnosis depends on determining the systemic illness.

   (3) Secondary glaucoma is frequently seen in iritis. (Patients with iritis should be examined carefully for inflammation elsewhere in the body and have serologic tests for syphilis,, a tuberculin test, and a chest x-ray.)

   c. Therapy consists of dilation of the pupils with cycloplegic-mydriatic eyedrops (atropine, 1%, or homatropine, 5%) to prevent the formation of posterior synechiae (adhesions of the iris to the lens) and topical corticosteroid drops to control the inflammation. If band keratopathy becomes severe, the calcium can be removed with disodium edetate (EDTA) drops. Do not use Versenate, which is the calcium salt of EDTA. Cataracts may eventually require operation.

   2. Posterior uveitis (choroiditis and chorioretinitis) The most common causes are *Toxoplasma*, congenital syphilis, rubella, cytomegalic inclusion disease, visceral larva migrans, sarcoid, tuberculosis, and sympathetic ophthalmia. The cause can be determined in about 50 percent of cases.

a. **Toxoplasmosis**

(1) **Evaluation and diagnosis**

(a) *Toxoplasma* uveitis is usually a prenatal infection, and the sions are discrete, atrophic areas with pigmented borders a pigmented lines running through them. They may be a where in the retina, but are often found in the macular area congenital toxoplasmosis.

(b) Most commonly, the chorioretinitis is healed when the patie is first seen in the newborn period. These healed lesions cc tain viable parasites, and reactivation of the chorioretini may occur any time during life.

(c) When active inflammation is present, the vitreous becom cloudy, and fluffy white lesions appear, usually at the border an old healed scar.

(d) Presumptive diagnosis of *Toxoplasma* chorioretinitis may made from the clinical appearance and from the Sabi Feldman dye test or the *Toxoplasma* complement fixation tes

(2) **Therapy** Treatment of active *Toxoplasma* chorioretinitis consis of systemic and topical corticosteroids and topical mydriat cycloplegic drops. Treatment with combined pyrimethami (Daraprim) and sulfonamide, although lethal to the organisms, of questionable benefit clinically. If it is undertaken, the patie must be given folinic acid concurrently.

b. **Congenital syphilis**

(1) **Evaluation** consists in systemic examination and serologic tes Syphilis typically causes a diffuse fine pigmentary disturban throughout the fundus.

(2) **Therapy** Systemic penicillin.

3. **Endophthalmitis**

a. **Etiology** Bacterial or fungal contamination of a perforating injury the eye, corneal ulcer, intraocular surgery, or, rarely, generaliz sepsis.

b. **Evaluation** Vision is lost, and the eye becomes painful and intense inflamed, with chemosis of the conjunctiva, corneal haze, hypopyo and vitreous opacity.

c. **Therapy** If untreated, the infection may spread to the orbit. Occ sionally, the globe, and even some vision, may be preserved by prom antibiotic therapy early in the course of the disease.

III. GLAUCOMA

A. **Etiology** Glaucoma (increased intraocular pressure) may be inherited, d to trauma, secondary to inflammation, or due to topical corticosteroid a plication.

B. **Evaluation**

1. Congenital glaucoma should be suspected in any infant with excessi tearing and photophobia, without evidence of ocular inflammation. general pediatric examination should be performed to rule out ass ciated primary disease.

2. A complete ophthalmic examination should also include measurement of the corneal diameters to rule out abnormal enlargement, inspection of the corneas for cloudiness, inspection of the optic nerve heads for cupping produced by an elevated intraocular pressure, and measurement of the intraocular pressures.

C. The **diagnosis** is confirmed by increased intraocular pressure.

D. **Therapy**

1. **Medical** Acetazolamide (Diamox) 15 mg/kg PO daily; pilocarpine HCl, 2–4%, applied topically q6h.

2. **Surgical** Goniotomy for infantile glaucoma, filtration surgery, and cyclocryotherapy.

Index

Maalox, 254
Magnesium
in dialysis solution, 214
hypermagnesemia, 181, 195
hypomagnesemia, 181, 195
in newborn, 136
from parenteral nutrition, 249
and seizures in neonates, 489
plasma levels of, 181
poisoning from, dimercaprol in, 74
recommended daily allowances in
diet, 19
Magnesium hydroxide antacids, 254
Magnesium sulfate
dosage in neonatal disorders, 148
during EEG in neonatal seizures, 491
Majocchi's granuloma, in tinea corporis, 506
Malabsorption, intestinal, 251
Malaria, 415–417
diagnostic features of, 400
differentiation of parasites in, 416
parasite detection in, 401
relapsing, 417
treatment of, 405, 416–417
Malformed infants, 146
Malt soup extract, as stool softener, 21
Manganese poisoning, EDTA in, 74
Mannitol
in cerebral edema, 44
in renal failure, acute, 205
in shock, 38, 39
Marihuana, slang terms for, 60
Mastoiditis, acute, 529
masked, 529
medical, 529
surgical, 529
Maxillary sinusitis, 532–533
Measles
gamma globulin prophylaxis in, 350
and immunization schedule, 24
Mebendazole
adverse effects of, 406
in hookworm, 408
in pinworm, 409
Meclizine, in labyrinthitis, 530
Meconium aspiration, 115–116
prevention of, 115
treatment of, 116
Meconium ileus, 258
Medic Alert identification tag
in adrenal disorders, 275, 294
in anaphylaxis, 466
in diabetes, 275, 328
Medical orders, for hospitalized
patient, 2
Medications. *See* Drugs

Megacolon, aganglionic, 267–268
Melena, 251
Meningitis, 374–376
bacterial causes of, 335
in candidal infections, 387
cryptococcal, 391
gonococcal, treatment of, 389
intravenous therapy in, 203
in newborn, 139–141
seizures in, 42–43
in neonates, 489
treatment of, 375–376
tuberculous, treatment of, 385
Meningococcal disease, antimicrobial
agents in, 339, 353
Meningococcal polysaccharide vaccine
26
Menstruation
and amenorrhea, 307–308
and dysfunctional uterine bleeding
309
and dysmenorrhea, 309–310
Meperidine, 8
dosage for pediatric use, 7
in neonatal disorders, 148
in lytic cocktail, 8, 11, 12
in peritonsillar abscess, 536
Mephobarbital, as anticonvulsant drug
485, 486
Mercury poisoning, treatment of, 74
Mesenteric artery syndrome, superior
vomiting in, 274
Mestinon, in myasthenia gravis, 497
Mestranol, in oral contraceptives, 311
Metabolic disorders, in newborn, 133
Metaproterenol, in respiratory diseases, 472–473
Methadone, 9
dosage for pediatric use, 7
for drug withdrawal in newborn, 14
Methanol poisoning, ethanol in, 75
Methemoglobinemia, drug-induced,
methylene blue in, 75
Methenamine, metabolism and excretion of, 346
Methicillin
in cervical adenitis, 369
dosage of, 342
renal function affecting, 348
penetration into CSF, 344
Methimazole, in hyperthyroidism,
289–290
Methsuximide, as anticonvulsant drug
486, 487
Methyldopa
in hypertension, 218
in hypertensive crisis, 217